Aspects of synaptic transmission: LTP, galanin, opioids, autonomic and 5-HT

Aspects of synaptic transmission: LTP, galanin, opioids, autonomic and 5-HT

Edited by

T.W. Stone
Department of Pharmacology, University of Glasgow, Scotland

Taylor & Francis
London • New York • Philadelphia
1991

UK Taylor & Francis Ltd, 4 John St., London WC1N 2ET

USA Taylor & Francis Inc., 1900 Frost Road, Suite 101, Bristol, PA 19007

British Library Cataloguing in Publication Data

Aspects of synaptic transmission.
1. Mammals. Neurotransmitters
I. Stone, T.W. II. Series
591.188

ISBN 0-85066-828-X

Library of Congress Cataloging in Publication Data

is available

Printed in Great Britain by Burgess Science Press, Basingstoke on paper which has a specified pH value on final paper manufacture of not less than 7·5 and is therefore 'acid free'.

Contents

Preface

This volume is a collection of general reviews on selected areas of synaptic transmission. It is emphatically not a volume of symposium proceedings. Scientific conferences increasingly fall into two categories: first, those huge, international meetings which are so diverse, superficial and fatiguing that it is difficult to learn anything new either in one's own special area or in other unrelated topics, and secondly, the smaller specialist or satellite symposia which tend to be rather exclusive due to space limitations and so specialized and established that new, younger recruits may find difficulty in breaking in. With this background the Kelvin Conferences on Synaptic Transmission were initiated in July 1990 with the several objectives of:

(a) providing an opportunity for younger scientists to meet with established figures in an informal setting,
(b) providing those younger scientists with a forum at which they could present an extended review lecture,
(c) providing the opportunity for scientists from several unrelated areas of neurotransmitter research to meet and exchange ideas with each other.

The first of the Kelvin Conferences proved enormously successful. The present volume is being produced in association with that meeting and contains review chapters written by the participants. All are up-to-date but broadly based reviews grouped into the five themes of the meeting, and should provide useful background research and teaching material for new research workers, postgraduate and senior undergraduate students and those neuroscientists who simply wish to broaden their knowledge base.

The subjects included were deliberately selected to encompass both mainstream reviews (e.g. LTP, opioid receptors, 5-HT_3 receptors), topics which frequently receive less detailed consideration than they deserve (e.g. opioids and memory, opioids and respiratory depression), the slightly esoteric (β-casomorphins) or the very new (e.g. nitric oxide as a transmitter). I challenge anyone to read a Kelvin volume and not learn something new or have a new idea.

I am deeply grateful to staff and students of the University of Glasgow who helped make the Kelvin Conference a success, and to my wife for adopting the joint roles of conference organizer, administrative assistant and secretary.

I would also like to thank the following organizations for their financial support: Astra Laboratories Sweden, Glaxo, The International Society for Neurochemistry, The Royal Society and SmithKline Beecham.

T.W. Stone
Glasgow
September 1990

Contributors*

Peter J. Barnes	National Heart and Lung Institute, Dovehouse Street, London SW3 6LY, UK
John A. Bevan	Department of Pharmacology, University of Vermont, Burlington VT 05405, USA
Lynn Bindman	Department of Physiology, University College, Gower Street, London WC1E 6BT, UK
A.H. Bom	Department of Pharmacology, Erasmus University Rotterdam, 3000 DR Rotterdam Box 1738, The Netherlands
P.A. Colley	Department of Psychology, Northwestern University College of Arts and Sciences, Evanston, IL 60208, USA
J.R. Docherty	Department of Clinical Pharmacology, 123 St Stephens Green, Dublin 2 Ireland
A. Dresse	Laboratoire de Pharmacologie, University of Liege, Liege 1 Belgium
P. Dutar	INSERM U161, 2 rue d'Alesia, Paris 75014, France
M. Göthert	Institut für Pharmakologie und Toxicologie, Universitat Bonn, Reuterstrasse 26, 5300 Bonn 1, Germany
William D. Hutchison	Division of Neurosciences, John Curtin School of Medical Research, Australian National University, Canberra, Australia

* First named author of each chapter.

I. Izquierdo — Departmento de Bioquimica, Centro de Memoria, Instituto de Biociencias, UFRGS (centro), 90049 Porto Alegre, RS, Brazil

Ole Kiehn — The Panum Institute, DK-2200 Copenhagen, Denmark

Christer Köhler — Astra Research Centre AB, CNS 2 R & D, S-151 85 Sodertalje, Sweden

W. Martin — Department of Pharmacology, University of Glasgow, Glasgow G12 8QQ, Scotland, UK

S.J. Paterson — Department of Pharmacology, United Medical School of Guy's and St Thomas', Lambeth Palace Road, London SE1 7EH, UK

J.A. Peters — Neuroscience Research Group, Department of Pharmacology and Clinical Pharmacology, Ninewells Hospital and Medical School, Dundee, DD1 9SY, Scotland

K. Ramabadran — Department no. 426 AP9A-1, Abbott Laboratories, 1 Abbott Park Road, IL 60064, USA

R. Samanin — Instituto di Richerche Farmacologiche 'Mario Negri', via Eritrea 62, 20157 Milan, Italy

Alan N. Sandler — Department of Anaesthesia, Toronto General Hospital, Toronto, Ontario, Canada M5G 2C4

R. Simantov — Department of Molecular Genetics and Virology, Weizmann Institute of Science, Rehovot 76100, Israel

T.W. Stone — Department of Pharmacology, University of Glasgow, Glasgow G12 8QQ, Scotland UK

Part I

Long-term potentiation

Chapter 1

Long-term potentiation (LTP) and depression (LTD) in the neocortex and hippocampus: an overview

Lynn Bindman, Geri Christofi, Kerry Murphy and Alex Nowicky

1.1. *Introduction: LTP and LTD in hippocampus and neocortex*

1.1.1. **Definitions**

Long-term potentiation (LTP) is an activity-dependent, long-lasting increase in the efficacy of synaptic transmission; long-term depression (LTD) is, conversely, a long-lasting decrease in the efficacy of synaptic transmission. LTP can be produced by brief tetanic stimulation of an excitatory monosynaptic pathway (Bliss and Lomo, 1973) and the enhancement of synaptic transmission is manifest by an increased depolarizing slope and an increased amplitude of the excitatory postsynaptic potentials evoked by test stimuli in that pathway. LTP lasts for tens of minutes or hours, as observed in acute experiments in neocortex and hippocampus, and apparently for days or weeks, as recorded with chronically implanted electrodes in the hippocampus of freely moving animals.

LTD in neocortex and hippocampus can be produced by seemingly identical afferent tetani to those inducing LTP; LTD can be homosynaptic (affecting synapses in the stimulated pathway) or heterosynaptic (affecting synapses on the postsynaptic cells that are inactive during the afferent stimulation) (Lynch *et al.*, 1977; Dunwiddie and Lynch, 1978). Its duration has been measured in tens of minutes and hours.

The introductory section (1.1) of this review includes a review of the possible sites for long-term modulation of synaptic transmission. Sections 1.2 and 1.3 focus on the mechanisms involved in the induction and maintenance of neocortical LTP, in particular on recent intracellular studies of LTP in neocortex. Section 1.4 examines LTD, particularly new work on the induction of LTD in neocortex.

Although this review is primarily concerned with neocortex, much of the work on LTP and LTD has been carried out in the hippocampus, with its simpler and more highly organized anatomical and histological structure. Therefore studies of hippocampal as well as neocortical LTP and LTD, and particularly recent investigations, are described where relevant. The reader is also referred to reviews of hippocampal LTP by Swanson *et al.* (1982), Bliss and Lynch (1988), Lynch *et al.* (1988), Voronin (1989) and Brown *et al.* (1990); reviews of LTP in neocortex are given by Teyler and DiScenna (1987) and Teyler *et al.* (1990). The latter review is limited to experiments in which neocortical LTP and LTD are induced by tetanic stimulation of afferents.

1.1.2. **Possible behavioural correlates of LTP and LTD**

There is currently great interest in the mechanisms underlying the induction and the maintenance of LTP and LTD in various areas of the brain especially the hippocampus and the neocortex. What is the basis for this interest? The neocortex and the hippocampus are areas known to be involved in learning and memory; activity-dependent, long-lasting changes in the efficacy of synaptic transmission could provide a neural substrate for learning and the memory trace. This suggestion has become more compelling since it has been shown that associative LTP could be induced in both neocortex and hippocampus: the experimental paradigm mimicked at cellular level that of classical, associative or Pavlovian conditioning. Pavlov's dogs, which naturally salivated at the taste or smell of food, were conditioned to salivate (when hungry) in response to previously insignificant sensory stimuli, such as the sight of a food bowl or the sound of the footsteps of the man bringing their food, or, in experiments, to musical sounds. The conditioned salivation only occurred after the conditioning stimulus had been repeatedly presented in temporal association with the arrival of food. The conditioning was dependent on the cerebral cortex for the analysis of the sensory inputs (Pavlov, 1928).

In neocortex or in hippocampus, a weak test input (analogous to the conditioning sound) in one afferent pathway to a single neurone was repetitively associated with a strong input (analogous to the smell or taste of the food) in another pathway to the cell; after tens of pairings, the weak input elicited a persistently potentiated synaptic response — LTP.

Further experiments revealed that the process of induction of LTP conformed to a Hebbian model of learning (Hebb, 1949): only those synaptic inputs that were associated in time with depolarization and firing of the postsynaptic cell were potentiated, while those inputs that occurred hundreds of milliseconds or seconds apart from cell depolarization were not potentiated. The induction of LTP was thereby demonstrated to be postsynaptic, input-specific and associative (Wigstrom and Gustafsson, 1986; Kelso *et al.*, 1986, in hippocampus; Baranyi and Feher, 1981a,b; Baranyi and Szente, 1987; Bindman *et al.*, 1988b, in neocortex).

Other experiments have revealed parallels between aspects of LTP and of memory (see Bliss and Lynch, 1988). To take one example, the drug D-L-2-amino-phosphonopentanoic acid (AP5) that selectively blocks a glutamate-receptor subtype, the *N*-methyl-D-aspartate (NMDA) receptor, could prevent spatial learning (Morris, 1989). AP5 also interferes with the induction of LTP (see Sections 1.2.2 and 1.2.2(g)). It should be noted that NMDA receptors are widespread in the central nervous system (CNS), and AP5 was shown to cause disturbance of sensorimotor function. However, in these experiments it did not, at least, interfere with visual discrimination learning. It selectively impaired spatial learning which is an important function of the rat hippocampus (O'Keefe and Nadel, 1978).

When the strength of transmission at some synapses is increased by the conjunction of postsynaptic depolarization with the synaptic activity, there is often concomitant depression at other inactive synapses — heterosynaptic LTD. The physiological rules for homosynaptic and heterosynaptic LTD are not entirely clear at present, but like the induction of LTP, the induction of LTD is postsynaptic (see Kano and Kato, 1987; Stanton and Sejnowski, 1989; Pockett *et al.*, 1990, for different experimental conditions under which LTD can be produced in the cerebellum and hippocampus, and Bindman *et al.*, 1988b; Berry *et al.*, 1989; and particularly Artola *et al.*, 1990, for neocortex). Neural network modelling of learning predicts such down-regulation, and behaviourally habituation and extinction are possible correlates of decreased responsiveness of synapses in LTD (Morris and Willshaw, 1989).

1.1.3. **Sites for long-lasting modulation of synaptic transmission**

Figure 1.1 illustrates sites at which synaptic transmission can be modulated. Each site is further described in this section, and in Section 1.1.4 we look at what evidence exists for such modulation in LTP.

When a nerve impulse reaches the terminal, Ca^{2+} enters via voltage-sensitive channels and transmitter is liberated from site a into the synaptic cleft. Alterations in the action potential amplitude and duration can affect the amount of calcium ions entering the terminal, and hence the amount of transmitter liberated following the nerve impulse. Transmitter diffuses across the synaptic cleft (approximately 20 nm) and some of it binds to postsynaptic receptors. The amount of transmitter available for binding may be limited because it may diffuse away or be taken up from the extracellular space by nerve terminals in the vicinity (site b_1) or by glial cells (b_2). The number of receptors (site c) available for binding, and/or the affinity of the receptors for the transmitter, affects the number of ionic channels opened by excitatory or inhibitory transmitter postsynaptically. Receptors mediating either excitatory or inhibitory postsynaptic actions could be affected. Other substances present in the neurones or extracellular space, i.e. modulators

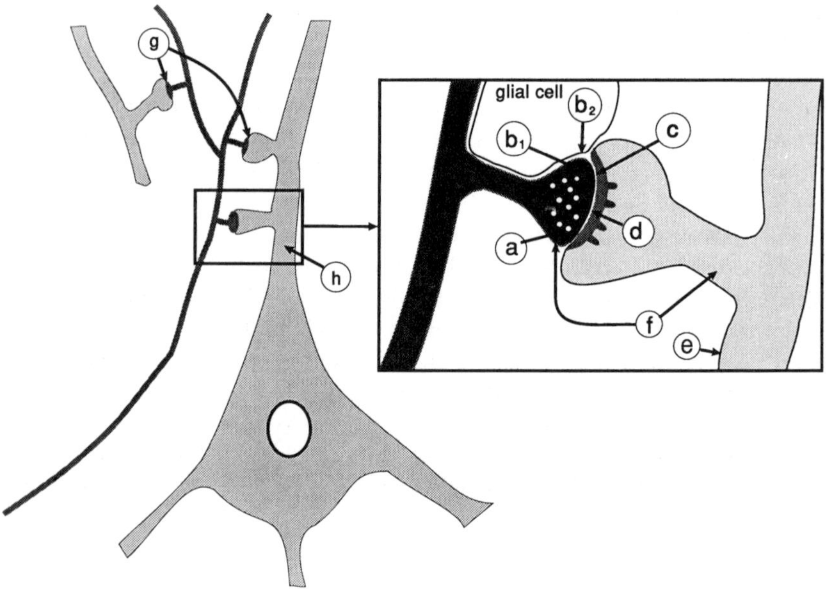

Figure 1.1. Diagram identifying sites at which neuronal transmission could be modified. Illustrated are synaptic contacts between an afferent axon and spines of postsynaptic apical dendrites. Rectangle shows enlarged synapse. (a) Presynaptic terminal with vesicles containing transmitter; (b) sites for reuptake of transmitter 1, into presynaptic terminal, 2, into adjacent glial cell; (c) site of receptors at postsynaptic membrane; (d) site of ionic channels in postsynaptic membrane; (e) neuronal membrane in which conductance changes can occur; (f) sites of possible structural change, e.g. presynaptic knob and postsynaptic dendritic spine; (g) additional synapses; (h) cytoplasm where biochemical changes could occur.

and coagonists, can alter the transmitter–receptor reaction. The channels themselves could be blocked internally (site d) thus modifying the synaptic currents. The biophysical properties of the postsynaptic membrane such as the membrane resistance (site e) affect the spread of synaptic current (excitatory or inhibitory postsynaptic currents) to the initial segment where integration of currents occurs, thereby determining whether the cell fires an impulse or not. This coupling between the excitatory postsynaptic potential (EPSP) and spike generation is referred to as E–S coupling. The structure of the synaptic region (f) could change, e.g. the size of the presynaptic knob and hence the amount of transmitter released, or the shape of the dendritic spine could alter, affecting the distribution of postsynaptic currents. The total number of active synapses (g) could change hence allowing more cells to fire. Finally, the biochemistry of the postsynaptic neurone (h) or the presynaptic terminals (a) might alter in an enduring fashion. The effect of the biochemical alteration could be expressed as a further structural or chemical change at any one of the sites described in a–g, thus producing a long-term alteration in transmission at modifiable synapses.

1.1.4. Experimental evidence for sites at which transmission is affected in LTP

Let us now look at some of the key areas of the experimental evidence for modulation of synaptic transmission during LTP at each of the sites mentioned in Section 1.1.3. The sites at which changes occur in LTD have not been explicitly investigated.

(a) The amount of transmitter released can be increased for tens of minutes by brief high-frequency tetani applied to the axon. The increased synaptic transmission which immediately follows the tetanic stimulation and which decays over about 10 min in the hippocampus and neocortex is called post-tetanic potentiation (PTP); it has been shown from studies at the neuromuscular junction to be due to the entry of either Ca^{2+} or Na^{+} into the nerve (Lev-Tov and Rahamimoff, 1980). However, there can also be a post-tetanic depression (PTD; e.g. in Figure 1.3) when the tetani are at high frequency or are of long duration. Following PTP or PTD is the long-lasting increase in synaptic transmission of LTP (e.g. Figures 1.2–1.4) or the long-lasting decrease in transmission of homosynaptic LTD. Bliss and his colleagues have obtained evidence from three areas of the hippocampus that increased transmitter release could be a factor not only in PTP, but also in the maintenance of LTP (Dolphin *et al.*, 1982; Bliss *et al.*, 1986, for the dentate gyrus; see Bliss and Lynch, 1988, for data obtained from CA1 and CA3).

Malinow and Tsien (1990) using whole-cell, voltage-clamp recordings in CA1, analysed the synaptic variability of EPSCs before and after postsynaptic induction of synapse-specific LTP. On their analytic model, the changes in the distribution of EPSC amplitudes and the decreased proportion of synaptic failures they observed during LTP were consistent with an increased probability of transmitter release. The changes in variability paralleled those produced by increasing extracellular Ca^{2+}, which enhances transmitter release. The changes in variability would not be explained by an increase in postsynaptic responsiveness. The elegant demonstration of presynaptic changes in transmitter release does not rule out some postsynaptic modifications in LTP under other experimental conditions. Malinow and Tsien (1990) used Cs^{+} in the recording electrodes to block postsynaptic potassium channels; this would also be likely to block the postsynaptic modifications in potassium current (I_K) seen in LTP by Baranyi *et al.* (1990) (see Section 1.3). However, Edwards (1991) and Larkman *et al.* (1991) have criticized Malinow and Tsien's deductions, which were based on a simple binomial distribution of EPSC amplitudes. More recent models of synaptic transmission in the brain make the interpretation of binomial parameters unclear. Whether enhanced synaptic transmission is pre- or postsynaptic is still an open question!

Increased amounts of transmitter collected from the tissue during LTP may not be entirely due to increased release from each axon terminal, because an increased quantity of transmitter may be due to decreased uptake into neighbouring axon terminals and glial cells, as discussed below.

(b) If LTP is induced postsynaptically (see Section 1.1), but maintained by increased release of transmitter following each presynaptic action potential, there has to be a retrograde messenger released from the postsynaptic cell. Arachidonic acid, which is an unsaturated fatty acid released during LTP is one candidate for a retrograde messenger.

An interesting recent observation is that arachidonic acid inhibited the uptake of the amino acid transmitter glutamate into glial cells in the salamander retina (Barbour *et al.*, 1989) for tens of minutes. However, inhibition of glial glutamate uptake is not likely to play an important role in the results of Malinow and Tsien (1990), i.e. a decreased probability of failures of synaptic transmission in LTP, etc. [see Section 1.1.4(a)]. Inhibition of uptake would be seen as increased quantal size, not increased probability of transmitter release.

When arachidonic acid was applied to the hippocampus to assess its effectiveness as a retrograde messenger, it did induce an activity-dependent enhancement of transmission and an increase in glutamate release (Williams *et al.*, 1989) but it took tens of minutes for it to take effect. Important questions that remain are: (1) what concentration of arachidonic acid is released at synapses and (2) how fast and at what concentration applied arachidonic acid reached synapses within the slice?

(c) An increase in the number of glutamate receptors in LTP was proposed to occur by Baudry *et al.* (1980), but their method of measurement of glutamate receptor density was inappropriate (Sastry and Goh, 1984; Lynch *et al.*, 1985). Indeed, the latter authors reported a reduced dendritic responsiveness to iontophoresis of glutamate in the dentate gyrus of the hippocampus during LTP, and in similar experiments in the CA1 region of hippocampus no effect was found during the first 30 min of LTP (Schwartzkroin and Taube, 1986; Taube and Schwartzkroin, 1988;. However, more recently Davies *et al.* (1989) have found an increased responsiveness of hippocampal neurones during LTP to iontophoresis of a glutamate agonist, which acts on a non-NMDA subtype of glutamate receptor (excited by quisqualate and by a drug called AMPA, or α-amino-3-hydroxy-5-methyl-4-isoxazolpropionic acid). This increased sensitivity of non-NMDA glutamate receptors did not arise until about 45 min or longer after the induction of LTP.

A decrease in inhibition, e.g. in the number of affinity of γ-amino butyric acid (GABA) receptors, may play a part in enhancement of transmission, but cannot account for the increase in slope at the onset of monosynaptic EPSPs during the LTP in hippocampus and neocortex.

Little is known about changes in the release or effectiveness of modulators or coagonists in LTP and LTD. Candidates are noradrenaline and acetylcholine, which are known to modify postsynaptic potassium currents in neocortex and hippocampus [see Section 1.2.2(h)], vasopressin, which modulates the action of noradrenaline on β-receptors in hippocampus (Brinton and McEwen, 1989) and glycine which acts on the NMDA receptors (see Thomson, 1990).

(d) Mg^{2+} ions are known to block NMDA receptor-activated membrane channels in a voltage-dependent manner so that a depolarization is required to allow Na^+ and Ca^{2+} to enter. There is no evidence for change in channel block in LTP or LTD, but the persistent membrane depolarization seen in some cells *in vivo* in LTP (Baranyi and Szente, 1987) would enhance the effectiveness of glutamate in opening NMDA receptor-activated channels.

(e) There is evidence that biophysical properties of the postsynaptic membrane may be modified in LTP. If membrane conductances are reduced, then an increased membrane resistance, and a measured increase in input resistance of the neurone, would result. Depending on which conductances are altered, the membrane potential, V_m, could change. It has been reported that the input resistance of neurones did not change in LTP (Andersen *et al.*, 1980, in hippocampus; Bindman *et al.*, 1988b, in neocortex). However these measurements were made in the hyperpolarizing direction from resting potential in isolated slices of brain. *In vivo*, V_m is depolarized relative to neurones in slice preparations. Following associative LTP in the neocortex of anaesthetized cats, a proportion of neurones showed an increased input resistance together with a depolarized V_m (see Baranyi and Szente, 1987). The significance of the increased membrane resistance is that the length or space constant would thereby be increased, synaptic potentials at the soma would be larger and E–S coupling enhanced. Evidence for enhanced E–S coupling was observed in the earliest extracellular studies of hippocampal LTP (Bliss and Lomo, 1973) and these observations have been extended by Taube and Schwartzkroin (1988). A decreased membrane conductance in neocortex has been observed following acetylcholine application together with spike discharges (Woody *et al.*, 1978); following Pavlovian eyeblink conditioning in awake cats (Woody, 1984); following a few minutes of high-frequency firing induced by intracellular current stimulation (Bindman *et al.*, 1988a) and in LTP (Baranyi *et al.*, 1990; 1991) but in the LTP experiments in undrugged cortex, the change was moderate and not statistically significant.

(f) The structure of the synaptic region has been compared in control tissue with that in which LTP has been induced, and correlated changes in synaptic structure have been noted (Lee *et al.*, 1980). Desmond and Levy (1988) critically review the structural changes observed in the hippocampus during LTP, and report their work on the dentate gyrus demonstrating six noteworthy structural changes in LTP: an increased incidence of concave spine heads, fewer synapses, an increased spine head area, increased area of the postsynaptic density, shorter and wider spine stems, and an increase in the number of front-line synaptic vesicles. They caution that when LTP is recorded, it is probably not the only modification of synaptic transmission that occurs. They propose that the decreased number of synapses (reflecting a change in the small non-concave spine synapses) may be correlated with inactive, heterosynaptically depressed synapses, while the other changes could support LTP of active synapses.

(g) A suggestion that there may be latent synapses which become active during LTP in CA1 has been made by Voronin *et al.* (1990) and is based on measurements of minimal EPSPs that incremented in step-like fashion with increased stimulus strength, and were also incremented following the postsynaptic induction of LTP.

(h) Many long-term changes in the biochemistry of both the postsynaptic neurone and presynaptic terminals, triggered by an essential entry of Ca^{2+}, have been proposed to underlie the production and maintenance of activity-induced LTP. One example is an early activation of calcium-dependent calmodulin kinase (Nelson *et al.*, 1988; Reymann *et al.*, 1988; Malenka *et al.*, 1989). Another important example is the activation of protein kinase C (PKC) which modifies membrane currents when phosphorylated; experimentally this activation can be brought about by a phorbol ester (see Baranyi *et al.*, 1987, 1988, for a postsynaptic effect in neocortex). Increases in both membrane PKC activity, and phosphorylation of the PKC-substrate protein B50 (also called protein F1 or GAP 43), as well as other presynaptic proteins, have been observed in LTP (for references see Lovinger and Routtenberg, 1988; Melchers *et al.*, 1988; Nelson *et al.*, 1988; Routtenberg, 1989). Lovinger and Routtenberg (1988) reported that PKC stimulating drugs prolonged LTP in the dentate gyrus by acting specifically at synapses given high-frequency stimulation, while not affecting synapses given low-frequency stimulation, or affecting postsynaptic membrane excitability, as assessed by extracellular recordings.

A later stage in the maintenance of LTP (>5 h) is vulnerable to protein synthesis inhibitors such as anisomycin (Frey *et al.*, 1988; see Matthies, 1989).

1.2. *Activity-dependent LTP in the neocortex*

1.2.1. **Historical background**

Long-lasting, activity-dependent changes in the efficacy of synaptic transmission in the neocortex *in vivo* were reported in the 1960s: potentiation of the somatosensory cortical response to test stimuli applied to the skin was found to persist, undiminished, for tens of minutes in the anaesthetized rat following a few minutes of local cortical stimulation by weak steady current (Bindman *et al.*, 1964). Activity-dependent persisting increases and decreases in synaptic transmission were produced in undercut slabs of neocortex in the anaesthetized cat (Bliss *et al.*, 1968). In the 1970s Pavlovian conditioning of eyeblink responses was found to be associated with increased excitability of neurones in the motor cortex of awake cats, selectively within the region projecting to muscles involved in the conditioned response (see

Woody, 1984). Progress on LTP as such in the neocortex was delayed until the 1980s when isolated slice preparations were developed, and intracellular recording and induction of LTP were used.

1.2.2. Experimental conditions for the production of neocortical activity-dependent LTP

Essentially the induction of LTP in the hippocampus occurs when the afferent input excites a threshold number of excitatory synapses (Friedlander *et al.*, 1990; Malinow, 1991) and when the postsynaptic dendrite in the region of the active synapses is sufficiently depolarized to permit Ca^{2+} entry (Malenka *et al.*, 1988). There is no reason to suppose that the situation is different in the neocortex, but the means by which Ca^{2+} entry is achieved varies in different regions of the hippocampus. For example NMDA receptor-mediated activity is essential in dentate and CA1, but not at the mossy fibre input to CA3. There are other examples of regional variation (see Bliss and Lynch, 1988) so it is important to investigate each region of neocortex separately to uncover the appropriate experimental conditions for the induction and maintenance of LTP.

Tetanic stimulation of an afferent pathway has been used to elicit LTP in a variety of experimental situations in the neocortex and olfactory cortex (Teyler *et al.*, 1990). We shall consider a number of questions about these experimental conditions.

a. *Does the age of the animal or developmental stage of the neocortex matter?*

The ease with which LTP can be induced was thought to be age-dependent. For example in visual cortex (areas 17 and 18) of kittens, using field potential studies, Komatsu *et al.* (1988) obtained LTP only in the critical period. The highest probability of induction (0·8 in field potential experiments) occurred between 21 and 34 days. However, LTP has been induced in adult rat visual cortex *in vitro* when a $GABA_A$ receptor blocker such as bicuculline was used (Artola and Singer, 1987, 1990). LTP has been produced in adult cat motor cortex under anaesthesia in about 30% of EPSPs (Baranyi and Szente, 1987; see also for references to Baranyi's earlier work) and in adult rat sensorimotor cortex *in vitro* (Bindman *et al.*, 1988b). In the latter preparation the probability of inducing LTP of field potentials by afferent tetani was >50%, but for EPSPs in layer V cells it was about 20%. A recent study in motor cortex of adult, awake cats (Baranyi *et al.*, 1991) found that LTP could be induced associatively in >50% of EPSPs.

b. *Anaesthetic*

Neocortical LTP has been induced in animals under anaesthesia (Baranyi and Feher, 1981a,b) but it has also been elicited in awake rabbits (see

Voronin, 1988) and cats (Baranyi *et al.*, 1991) and in isolated slices of cortex *in vitro* without additional drugs.

c. *Where in the neocortex can LTP be produced?*

As previously mentioned, LTP has been produced in visual, somatosensory and motor cortex. More recently non-primary areas have been investigated; Sutor and Hablitz (1989a,b) produced LTP in frontal cortex, Hirsch and Crepel (1990) in prefrontal cortex and Sah and Nicoll (1991) in limbic cortex (anterior cingulate) of the rat.

d. *What connections onto neocortical neurones can be potentiated?*

Intracellular recordings suggest that transmission at many excitatory synapses onto cells in various layers of cortex can be modified over tens of minutes and hours. In the cat motor cortex, EPSPs in layer V neurons (many of which projected into the pyramidal tract) could be potentiated when elicited by either stimulation of thalamic nucleus VL, or the pyramidal tract, or the contralateral radial nerve, or the contralateral homotypic area, activating callosal fibres. The associative LTP occurred in some monosynaptic responses (Baranyi and Szente, 1987; Baranyi *et al.*, 1991). Normal afferent pathways would be excited when stimulating the radial nerve, and in the other situations normal afferents but also corticofugal axons running past the stimulus site and having recurrent collaterals into neocortex would be excited.

In slice preparations *in vitro*, high frequency stimulation of subcortical white matter has been used to elicit EPSPs that were subsequently potentiated in layers II and III of visual cortex (Artola and Singer, 1987, 1990) and layers III, V and VI of sensorimotor cortex (Bindman *et al.*, 1988b). Stimulation of the white matter can excite normal afferents, corticofugal axons with recurrent collaterals into the grey matter, cortico-cortical fibres and callosal axons. It is not surprising that the postsynaptic potentials are often complex mixtures of EPSPs and inhibitory postsynaptic potentials (IPSPs).

In frontal cortex, Sutor and Hablitz (1989a) stimulated layer IV electrically and recorded from layers II and III; the LTP they produced by high frequency stimulation was most often (in 11/14 neurones) in polysynaptic components of the EPSP (a late EPSP of latency between 20 and 60 ms). Hirsch and Crepel (1990) recorded monosynaptic EPSPs in layer V of prefrontal cortex resulting from stimulation of intracortical circuitry: they stimulated axons in layer II above the recording electrode in layer V. Interestingly they obtained LTP following afferent tetani in 10/28 of monosynaptic EPSPs, expressed as an increased slope of depolarization, but also obtained LTD in another 14/28 monosynaptic EPSPs.

Bindman and Murphy (1990) suggested that the terminals onto neurones in sensorimotor cortex may be heterogeneous: those responsible for the shortest latency depolarizing slope of the EPSPs in layer V cells evoked by stimulation of subcortical white matter may not be capable of sustaining LTP (see 1.3.1).

e. *How long does neocortical LTP last?*

A number of experimenters have observed LTP that continued, undiminished, for several hours. For example, Sutor and Hablitz (1989a) in their intracellular study of LTP in frontal layer II and III neurones reported LTP lasting up to 5 h, undiminished at the end of the observation period.

f. *Is it necessary to block inhibition?*

Most experimenters inducing LTP in slices of hippocampus used a $GABA_A$ blocking drug to facilitate the induction of LTP. In neocortex, as mentioned above, it is necessary for the induction of LTP in visual cortex after the critical period (Teyler *et al.*, 1990; Artola and Singer, 1987, 1990), but in sensorimotor cortex it does not improve the probability of inducing LTP in layer V neurones, speculatively because there is also potassium-mediated ($GABA_B$) inhibition (Bindman *et al.*, 1988b; Bindman and Murphy, 1990). In frontal cortex also, Sutor and Hablitz (1989a,b) found that block of $GABA_A$ inhibition was not required for the induction of LTP. Importantly, associated LTP can be produced with an incidence of 50 to 60% in awake cats, using no drugs (Baranyi *et al.*, 1991).

g. *The role of NMDA receptor-mediated activity in neocortical EPSPs, and in the induction and maintenance of neocortical LTP*

The major difference found between the NMDA receptor-mediated component of the EPSPs in the hippocampal CA1 region and the neocortex (visual, sensorimotor, frontal and prefrontal) was that in the neocortex it was not necessary to resort to Mg^{2+}-free bathing medium, high frequency stimulation or depolarization of neurones in order to reveal NMDA receptor-mediated activity. It could be seen in normal [Mg^{2+}] (1 mM as in cerebrospinal fluid) at low frequency stimulation and at a V_m only a few millivolts depolarized above the resting potential of about 80 mV. Moreover, it was not always necessary to use a $GABA_A$ blocker to uncover the NMDA receptor-mediated component (Artola and Singer, 1987, 1990; Aram *et al.*, 1987; Sutor and Hablitz, 1989b; Hirsch and Crepel, 1990). In some experimental preparations the NMDA receptor-mediated component of the EPSP had the same latency of onset as a non-NMDA receptor-mediated component (Artola and Singer, 1990; Hirsch and Crepel, 1990) while in others it started from milliseconds to tens of milliseconds after the onset of the non-NMDA receptor-mediated EPSP (Aram *et al.*, 1987; Sutor and Hablitz, 1989b). The non-NMDA receptor-mediated component of neocortical EPSPs may be mediated largely by glutamate as transmitter since it was blocked by kynurenate (a non-selective glutamate antagonist; Aram *et al.*, 1987; Jones and Baughman, 1988) or by 6,cyano-7-nitroquinoxaline-3,3-dione (CNQX) (Artola and Singer, 1990; Hirsch and Crepel, 1990).

However, as in the hippocampus (Collingridge *et al.*, 1983) antagonists of NMDA receptor-mediated activity block the induction of LTP (Artola and Singer, 1987, 1990; Bindman and Murphy, 1988b; Sutor and Hablitz, 1989b). The importance of the NMDA receptor-mediated activity lies in the fact that it allows Ca^{2+} to enter the cell (Mayer and Westbrook, 1987).

In view of the presence of an NMDA receptor-mediated component in neocortical EPSPs prior to potentiation, it is not surprising that, unlike in the hippocampus (Gustafsson *et al.*, 1987), NMDA receptor-mediated activity participated in the expression of LTP (Bindman and Murphy, 1988a; Artola and Singer, 1990). Following application of AP5 it was seen that in some cells the LTP was manifest as both an enhanced non-NMDA receptor-mediated component and a later, enhanced NMDA receptor-mediated component (Bindman and Murphy, 1990 and Figures 1.2–1.4; also Artola and Singer, 1990) while in other cells the LTP was expressed only as an NMDA receptor-mediated enhancement (Artola and Singer, 1990).

h. *Are neuromodulators able to induce long-lasting changes in neocortical synaptic transmission?*

Noradrenaline

Noradrenaline (NA) produced a long-lasting enhancement of transmission in the dentate region of hippocampus both *in vivo* and *in vitro* (Lacaille and Harley, 1985), but not in the CA1 region (Sarvey, 1988). What of its action in neocortex? It is clear from field potential studies and intracellular recordings that NA acting on β-receptors, enhances synaptic transmission at some, but not all, synapses in both the visual cortex (Nowicky *et al.*, 1990a,b) and sensorimotor cortex (Bindman *et al.*, 1990). However the enhancement declines to control levels when the NA is washed out. Foehring *et al.* (1989) have studied its action on layer V pyramidal cells in slices *in vitro* taken from the motor cortex of cats. NA and the β-agonist isoprenaline reduced some potassium currents thereby increasing firing rate and cell excitability. We have found that NA and isoprenaline had no effect on the depolarizing slope of EPSPs evoked in layer V neurones in somatosensory cortex, or layer III cells in visual cortex by white matter stimulation. In some EPSPs there was an enhancement of late portions of the EPSP which may have been due to an enhanced di- or polysynaptic transmission consequent on membrane conductance changes (Nowicky *et al.*, 1990a,b).

Acetylcholine

Woody *et al.* (1987) showed that extracellular iontophoresis of acetylcholine (ACh), or of cGMP intracellularly, caused an increased input resistance,

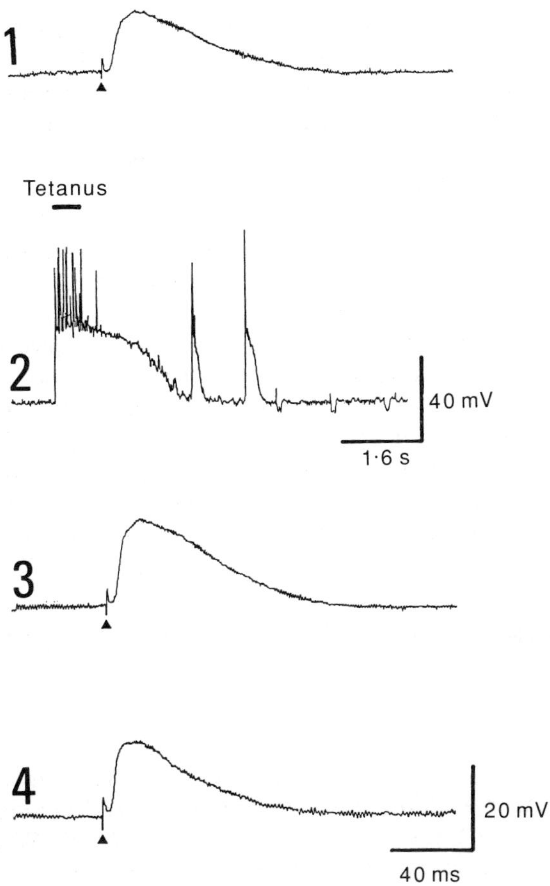

Figure 1.2. Intracellular records from layer V neurone in slice of rat sensorimotor neocortex. 1,3,4: averages of four successive EPSPs evoked by stimulation of sub-cortical white matter (at time shown at arrow) at 0·1 Hz. (1) In control period; (3) 18 min after the induction of LTP. Note enhanced slope of depolarizing phase, increased amplitude and duration of averaged EPSPs. EPSPs with action potentials were excluded from the average. (4) 38 min after the induction of LTP showing effect of bath-applied 20 μM D-AP5 on the potentiated response. 40 ms and 20 mV calibration bars apply to 1, 3 and 4. (2) Single trace at slower time base showing effect of first of four conditioning tetani applied at time shown by horizontal black bar (100 Hz for 0·5 s). Action potentials attenuated by digitizing procedure. No $GABA_A$ antagonist used in this experiment.

R_m, in half the neurones tested in the motor cortex of the awake cat, but only when associated with spike discharges elicited by intracellular current. The increased R_m lasted for tens of minutes. With single-electrode, voltage-clamp techniques, they showed that ACh, and cGMP together with cGMP-dependent protein kinase, reduced net outward currents induced by depolarizing voltage steps (Woody and Gruen, 1987). These changes enhance the excitability of the neurone.

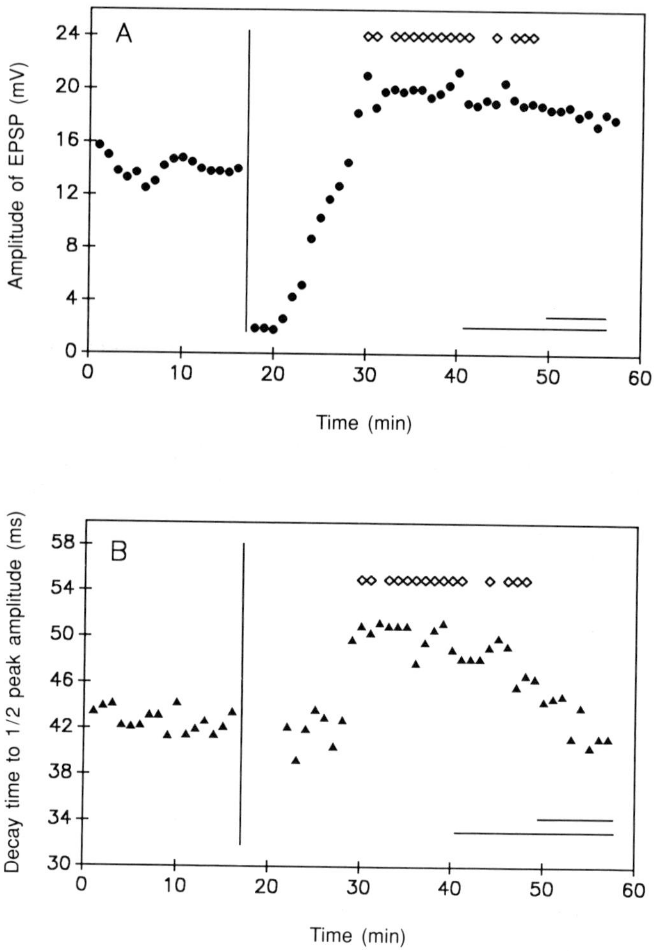

Figure 1.3. Time course of experiment shown in Figure **1.2**. (A) Average peak amplitude of EPSPs (n=6, ●) plotted against time. After 16 min of control, four conditioning tetani were applied at 10-s intervals starting at vertical line. Immediately after conditioning there was a post-tetanic depression, followed by LTP. ◇, Occurrence of action potentials on one or more constituent EPSPs of each average. D-AP5 bath applied at 10 μM (lower horizontal line and) 20 μM (upper line). (B) Same experiment as (A) plotting time taken (measured from onset of averaged EPSP) to decay to half the peak amplitude. This measure shows the effect of AP5 is greater on the duration of EPSPs than on amplitude.

1.3. *Associative LTP in the neocortex*

1.3.1. **Associative, postsynaptic induction of LTP**

This was demonstrated in motor cortex of anaesthetized cats by Baranyi and Szente (1987). They paired repetitively mono- and oligosynaptic EPSPs with postsynaptic action potentials induced in the same cell. Weak test stimuli

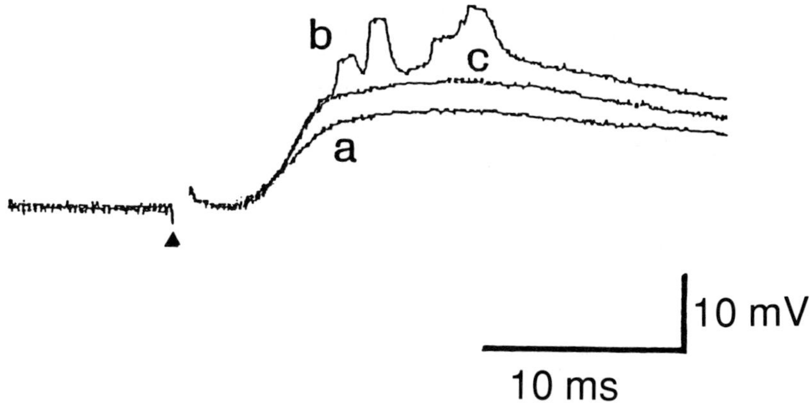

Figure 1.4. Same experiment as in Figures 1.2 and 1.3. Three superimposed averages of eight successive EPSPs. (a) During control, latency of onset of EPSP 3·7 ms; (b) during LTP, showing enhanced depolarizing slope of EPSP starting at 5 ms (action potentials on EPSPs distorted in average); (c) effect of bath-applied 20 μM D-AP5, apparent in the averaged response at 8 ms. The drug reveals the enhanced EPSP in LTP consisted of a non-NMDA-receptor mediated component followed by an NMDA-receptor mediated component.

were at one of the following sites: thalamic, callosal, somatosensory or pyramidal tract pathways, while stronger conditioning stimuli were either applied to one of these pathways or were postsynaptically injected depolarizing currents. LTP was elicited in 28% of 533 cells. The average duration of the enhancement was 49 min and extinction of the enhancement was often seen. However, in 43 cells the EPSP did not decrement until the end of the recording (mean duration of LTP 116 min). In a recent paper, Baranyi Szente and Woody (1991) analysed in detail the production of input-specific, associative LTP in motor cortex of conscious cats. The postsynaptic induction of LTP occurred with a high probability (0.5 to 0.6) greatly strengthening the proposal that associative LTP could be the neural basis of learning.

Postsynaptic induction of LTP in slices of sensorimotor *in vitro* has been observed (Bindman *et al.*, 1988b; Bindman and Murphy, 1990). Two EPSPs were elicited in each cell by stimulation of separate pathways in the subcortical white matter, and LTP was only induced in the EPSP paired with intracellular current stimulation. However, a lower percentage of EPSPs, about 15–20%, were potentiated in the slice *in vitro* (loc. cit.) than in the *in vivo* studies cited above presumably due to the loss of modulatory inputs in the slices.

Bindman and Murphy (1990) found that the potentiated EPSPs had a non-NMDA (AP5 insensitive) component followed by an NMDA receptor-mediated component. The onset of the (non-NMDA receptor-mediated) potentiated depolarizing slope, however, was delayed by a few milliseconds from the start of the EPSP (see Figure 1.4). We think the shortest latency inputs onto the cells may not form modifiable synapses. The delay in onset of the potentiation is not likely to be a reflection of a polysynaptic LTP (i.e.

LTP happening at an earlier synapse in the test pathway) because it was also manifest in EPSPs in which LTP was induced postsynaptically. For example, in nine short latency EPSPs (mean onset latency 2·8 ms) the mean onset latency of the potentiated component during postsynaptically induced LTP was 7·8 ms. The delay between EPSP onset and onset of potentiated component (5 ms; range: 1·7–16·4 ms) was significant at $P < 0{\cdot}01$ (unpublished observations). We wondered whether there was a voltage-sensitive component to the expression of potentiation in the EPSPs but were unable to find changes in the onset of the potentiated component with changed V_m. Heterogeneous synaptic inputs onto the postsynaptic neurone, with the fastest conducting inputs forming non-modifiable synapses, seems the most likely explanation.

1.3.2. **Postsynaptic calcium ions**

An important observation by Baranyi and Szente (1987) concerning the induction of LTP was that when the Ca^{2+} chelator EGTA was injected intracellularly in 53 cells, no LTP was observed following pairing. EGTA was no longer effective after 30 min, and then LTP was successfully induced in 10 out of 24 of these cells. A rise in postsynaptic $[Ca^{2+}]$ was presumably needed for the induction of LTP, as previously shown by Lynch *et al.* (1983) in hippocampus.

1.3.3. **Neuronal transport**

Effects of the neuronal transport blocker colchicine were also examined in cortical cells *in vivo* by Baranyi and Szente (1987). Colchicine was injected intracellularly; it caused a gradual increase in neuronal excitability after about 15 min. Its effect on induction of LTP was studied therefore in the first 10 min. In 44 cells colchicine was injected before pairing and in only three EPSPs was LTP induced (the expected number would be 12). The drug effects were not reversible in 2–3 h. This interesting observation suggests that postsynaptic tubular transport may play a part in the induction of LTP.

1.3.4. **Postsynaptic conductance changes**

These may be involved in the maintenance of LTP in neocortical cells. In awake cats Baranyi *et al.* (1990) have found that postsynaptic induction of synapse-specific LTP is associated with a reduction in outward currents in the potentiated but not the unpaired EPSCs. The current was identified as the potassium-mediated A current; LTP induction was blocked with intracellular Cs^+ or aminopyridine, but not by apamin or TEA (see also Woody *et al.*, 1989).

1.4. *Activity-dependent LTD in the neocortex*

Homosynaptic, activity-dependent LTD has been seen in neocortex, in neuronally-isolated slabs *in vivo* (Bliss *et al.*, 1968), in slices of sensorimotor cortex *in vitro* (Bindman *et al.*, 1988b), in prefrontal cortex (Hirsch and Crepel, 1990) and in visual cortex (Berry *et al.*, 1989; Artola *et al.*, 1990). No difference was detected in the stimulus parameters inducing LTP from those eliciting LTD.

However Artola *et al.* (1990) analysed the postsynaptic action of the afferent tetani and proposed that LTP was elicited when the postsynaptic depolarization was strong enough to activate NMDA channels, but LTD was evoked when the postsynaptic depolarization was not as great, and did not reach the threshold for opening the NMDA receptor-activated channels. They tested their hypothesis in two ways: (1) they modified the postsynaptic depolarizing response by reducing inhibition pharmacologically (using bicuculline) or by applying postsynaptic depolarizing current, or by altering the tetanic stimulus intensity; (2) they blocked NMDA receptor-mediated activity with AP5.

As predicted for adult visual cortex, tetanic stimulation in normal medium produced no change ($n = 12$) while in 0·1–0·2 μM bicuculline, tetanic stimulation gave rise to pathway-specific LTD ($n = 7$) and in 0·3μM bicuculline, post-tetanic LTP resulted ($n = 20$). In contrast, tetanic stimulation produced LTD in 13 of 14 cells treated with 0·3 μM bicuculline and AP5. After the AP5 was washed out, a second tetanic stimulus, >1 h after the first, induced LTP. Teyler *et al.* (1990) also reported that tetanic stimulation in the presence of AP5 gave rise to LTD.

The results of the postsynaptic current application during the tetanus showed that the induction of the homosynaptic LTD depended on the level of depolarization and was postsynaptic (Artola *et al.*, 1990). They concluded that LTD had a different (lower) depolarization threshold from that required for induction of LTP. The results of the experiments with bicuculline and AP5 suggested that postsynaptic depolarization together with reduction of Ca^{2+} entry leads to LTD. A similar inference was drawn by Kimura *et al.* (1990) who injected EGTA (a Ca^{2+} chelator) into visual cortical neurones. Tetanic stimulation of afferent axons gave rise to LTD in the injected cells but to LTP in field potentials derived from cells with no EGTA. They suggested the LTD resulted from the reduction in intracellular Ca^{2+}. Note this was the same experimental paradigm used previously in hippocampus and neocortex to deduce that Ca^{2+} was needed for LTP, but no LTD was observed! Presumably the precise $[Ca^{2+}]$ is the critical factor in determining whether LTP, LTD or no change ensues.

Interestingly, LTD was also reliably induced in CA1 neurones by high frequency postsynaptic firing in the presence of sufficient extracellular Mg^{2+} (25 mM) to block synaptic transmission during the tetani (Pockett *et al.*, 1990). Increased postsynaptic activity was brought about by antidromic tetani. The LTD lasted for as long as the recording period (up to 2 h) in eight out of eleven cells, but decayed to control levels within 20, 30 or 60 min in the remaining three cells. In normal medium LTD was induced by antidromic stimulation in six out of nine cells. Recently Christofi *et al.* (1991) showed that extracellular Ca^{2+} was needed for the postsynaptic induction of LTD.

In these experiments, the LTD was induced postsynaptically, and was heterosynaptic by definition since was no increase in activity in an afferent pathway. The postsynaptic depression of synaptic responses seen once the raised [Mg^{2+}] was washed out would presumably be generalized to all regions of the postsynaptic neurone that were sufficiently depolarized. It may be that heterosynaptic depression and a component of homosynaptic depression are the same activity-dependent postsynaptic phenomenon, which is overcome or converted to LTP when synaptic activity is sufficiently intense.

Acknowledgement

We thank the Wellcome Trust for financial support of research.

References

Andersen, P., Sundberg, S.H., Sveen, O., Swann, J.W. and Wigstrom, H. (1980). Possible mechanisms for long-lasting potentiation of synaptic transmission in hippocampal slices from guinea-pigs. *Journal of Physiology (London)*, **302**, 463–482.

Aram. J., Bindman, L.J., Lodge, D. and Murphy, K.P.S.J. (1987). Glutamate-receptor-mediated e.p.s.p.s. in layer V neurones in rat neocortical slices. *Journal of Physiology (London)*, **394**, 117P.

Artola, A. and Singer, W. (1987). Long-term potentiation and NMDA receptors in rat visual cortex. *Nature*, **330**, 649–652.

Artola, A. and Singer, W. (1990). The involvement of *N*-methyl-D-aspartate receptors in induction and maintenance of long-term potentiation in rat visual cortex. *European Journal of Neuroscience*, **2**, 254–269.

Artola, A., Brocher, S. and Singer, W. (1990). Different voltage-dependent thresholds for the induction of long-term depression and long-term potentiation in slices of the rat visual cortex. *Nature*, **347**, 69–72.

Baranyi, A. and Feher, O. (1981a). Intracellular studies on cortical synaptic plasticity. *Experimental Brain Research*, **41**, 124–134.

Baranyi, A. and Feher, O. (1981b). Selective facilitation of synapses in the neocortex by heterosynaptic activation. *Brain Research*, **212**, 164–168.

Baranyi, A. and Szente, M.B. (1987). Long-lasting potentiation of synaptic transmission requires postsynaptic modifications in the neocortex. *Brain Research*, **423**, 378–384.

Baranyi, A., Szente, M.B. and Woody, C.D. (1987). Intracellular injection of phorbol ester increases the excitability of neurons of the motor cortex of awake cats. *Brain Research*, **424**, 396–401.

Baranyi, A., Szente, M.B. and Woody, C.D. (1988). Activation of protein kinase C induced long-term changes of postsynaptic currents in neocortical neurons. *Brain Research*, **440**, 341–347.

Baranyi, A., Szente, M.B. and Woody, C.D. (1990). Dependence on A current of input-specific, associative synaptic potentiation in neocortex. (Abstract 5B.) European Science Foundation (ESF) *Open Network Conference on Neural Mechanisms of Learning and Memory*, University College, London, 4–6 April.

Baranyi, A., Szente, M.B. and Woody, C.D. (1991). Properties of associative long-lasting potentiation induced by cellular conditioning in the motor cortex of conscious cats. *Neuroscience*, **42**, 321–334.

Barbour, B., Szatkowski, M., Ingledew, N. and Attwell, D. (1989). Arachidonic acid induces a prolonged inhibition of glutamate uptake into glial cells. *Nature*, **342**, 918–920.

Baudry, M., Oliver, M., Creager, R., Wierasko, A. and Lynch, G. (1980) Increase in glutamate receptors following repetitive electrical stimulation in hippocampal slices. *Life Sciences*, **27**, 325–330.

Berry, R., Teyler, T.J. and Taizhen, H. (1989). Induction of LTP in primary visual cortex: tetanus parameters. *Brain Research*, **481**, 221–227.

Bindman, L.J. and Murphy, K.P.S.J. (1988a). NMDA-receptors participate in the maintenance of long-term potentiation of synaptic transmission in slices of rat neocortex *in vitro*. *Journal of Physiology* (*London*), **406**, 176P.

Bindman, L.J. and Murphy, K.P.S.J. (1988b). NMDA-receptor-mediated and long-term potentiation (LTP) in rat neocortex. *Society for Neuroscience, Abstracts*, **14**, 567.

Bindman, L.J. and Murphy, K.P.S.J. (1990). Delayed onset of potentiation in neocortical EPSPS during long-term potentiation (LTP) — a postsynaptic mechanism or heterogeneous synaptic inputs? In: *Excitatory Amino Acids and Neural Plasticity*, edited by Y. Ben Ari. *Advances in Experimental Medicine and Biology*, **268**, 307–312.

Bindman, L.J., Lippold, O.C.J. and Redfearn, J.W.T. (1964). The action of brief polarizing currents on the cerebral cortex of the rat (1) during current flow and (2) in the production of long-lasting after-effects. *Journal of Physiology* (*London*), **172**, 369–382.

Bindman, L.J., Meyer, T. and Prince, C.A. (1988a). Postsynaptic events associated with long-lasting activity-induced changes in excitability of cortical neurons. In: *Cellular Mechanisms of Conditioning and Behavioral Plasticity*, edited by C.D. Woody, D.L. Alkon and J.L. McGaugh. London: Plenum Press. pp. 379–390.

Bindman, L.J., Murphy, K.P.S.J. and Pockett, S. (1988b). Postsynaptic control of the induction of long-term changes in efficacy of transmission at neocortical synapses in slices of rat brain. *Journal of Neurophysiology*, **60**, 1053–1065.

Bindman, L.J., Dedicoat, M., Hamiduddin, R., Harnett, P.R. and Pegna, A. (1990). The effect of noradrenaline on synaptic transmission in slices of rat neocortex *in vitro*. *Journal of Physiology* (*London*), **423**, 97P.

Bliss, T.V.P. and Lomo, T. (1973). Long-lasting potentiation of synaptic transmission in the dentate area of the anaesthetized rabbit following stimulation of the perforant path. *Journal of Physiology* (*London*), **232**, 331–356.

Bliss, T.V.P. and Lynch, M. (1988). Long-term potentiation of synaptic transmission in the hippocampus: properties and mechanisms. In: *Long-term Potentiation: From Biophysics to Behavior*. New York: Alan R. Liss, Inc. pp. 3–72.

Bliss, T.V.P., Burns, B.D. and Uttley, A.M. (1968). Factors affecting the conductivity of pathways in the cerebral cortex. *Journal of Physiology (London*), **232**, 331–356.

Bliss, T.V.P., Douglas, R.M., Errington, M.L. and Lynch, M. (1986). Correlation between long-term potentiation and release of endogenous amino-acids from dentate gyrus of anaesthetized rats. *Journal of Physiology* (*London*), **377**, 391–408.

Brinton, R.E. and McEwen, B. (1989). Vasopressin neuromodulation in the hippocampus. *Journal of Neuroscience*, **9**, 752–759.

Brown, T.H., Kairiss, E.W. and Keenan, C.L. (1990). Hebbian Synapses: biophysical mechanisms and algorithms. *Annual Review of Neuroscience*, **13**, 475–511.

Christofi, G., Nowicky, A.V. and Bindman, L.J. (1991). The postsynaptic induction of long-term depression (LTD) of synaptic transmission in isolated rat hippocampal slices requires extracellular calcium. *Journal of Physiology*, in press.

Collingridge, G.L., Kehl, S.J. and McLennan, H. (1983). Excitatory amino acids in synaptic transmission in the Scaffer collateral-commissural pathway of the rat hippocampus. *Journal of Physiology* (*London*), **334**, 33–46.

Davies, S.N., Lester, R.A.J., Reymann, K.G. and Collingridge, G.L. (1989). Temporally distinct pre- and postsynaptic mechanisms maintain long-term potentiation. *Nature*, **338**, 500–503.

Desmond, N.L. and Levy, W.B. (1988). Anatomy of associative long-term synaptic modification. In: *Long-term Potentiation: From Biophysics to Behavior*. New York: Alan R. Liss Inc. pp. 265–305.

Dolphin. A.C., Errington, M.L. and Bliss, T.V.P. (1982). Long-term potentiation of the perforant path *in vivo* is associated with increased glutamate release. *Nature*, **297**, 496–498.

Dunwiddie, T. and Lynch, G. (1978). Long-term potentiation and depression of synaptic responses in the rat hippocampus: localization and frequency dependency. *Journal of Physiology* (*London*), **276**, 353–367.

Edwards, F. (1991). LTP is a long-term problem, *Nature*, **350**, 271–272.

Foehing, R.C., Schwindt, P.C. and Crill, W.E. (1989). Norepinephrine selectively reduces slow Ca^{2+}- and Na^{+}-mediated K^{+} currents in cat neocortical neurons. *Journal of Neurophysiology*, **61**, 245–256.

Friedlander, M.J., Sayer, R.J. and Redman, S.J. (1990). Evaluation of long-term potentiation of small compound and unitary EPSPs at the hippocampal CA3–CA1 synapse. *Journal of Neuroscience*, **10**, 814–825.

Frey, U., Krug, M., Reymann, K. and Matthies, H. (1988). Anisomycin, an inhibitor of protein synthesis, blocks late phases of LTP-phenomena in the hippocampal CA1 region *in vitro*. *Brain Research*, **452**, 57–65.

Gustafsson, B., Wigstrom, H., Abraham, W.C. and Huang, Y.-Y. (1987). Long-term potentiation in the hippocampus using depolarizing current pulses as the conditioning stimulus to single volley synaptic potentials. *Journal of Neuroscience*, **7**, 774–780.

Hebb, D.O. (1949). *The Organization of Behaviour*. New York: Wiley.

Hirsch, J.C. and Crepel, F. (1990). Use-dependent changes in synaptic efficacy in rat prefrontal neurones *in vitro*. *Journal of Physiology* (*London*), **427**, 31–49.

Jones, K.A. and Baughman, R.W. (1988). NMDA- and non-NMDA-receptor components of excitatory synaptic potentials recorded from cells in layer V of rat visual cortex. *Journal of Neuroscience*, **8**, 3522–3534.

Kano, M. and Kato, M. (1987). Quisqualate receptors are specifically involved in cerebellar synaptic plasticity. *Nature*, **325**, 276–279.

Kelso, S.R., Ganong, A.H. and Brown, T.H. (1986). Hebbian synapses in the hippocampus. *Proceedings of the National Academy of Sciences USA*, **83**, 5326–5330.

Kimura, F., Tsumoto, T., Nishigori, A. and Yoshimura, Y. (1990). Long-term depression but not potentiation is induced in Ca^{2+}-chelated visual cortex neurons. *NeuroReport*, **1**, 65–68.

Komatsu, Y., Fujii, K., Maeda, J., Sakaguchi, H. and Toyama, K. (1988). Long-term potentiation of synaptic transmission in kitten visual cortex. *Journal of Neurophysiology*, **59**, 124–141.

Lacaille, J.-C. and Harley, C. (1985). The action of norepinephrine in the dentate gyrus: beta-mediated facilitation of evoked potentials *in vitro*. *Brain Research*, **358**, 210–220.

Larkman, A., Stratford, K. and Jack, J. (1991). Quantal analysis of excitatory synaptic action and depression in hippocampal slices. *Nature*, **350**, 344–347.

Lee, K.S., Schottler, F., Oliver, M. and Lynch, G.S. (1980). Brief bursts of high frequency stimulation produce two types of structural change in the hippocampus. *Journal of Neurophysiology*, **44**, 247–258.

Lev-Tov, A. and Rahamimoff, R. (1980). A study of tetanic and post-tetanic potentiation of miniature end-plate potentials at the frog neuromuscular junction. *Journal of Physiology* (*London*), **309**, 247–273.

Lovinger, D.M. and Routtenberg, A. (1988). Synapse-specific protein kinase C activation enhances maintenance of long-term potentiation in rat hippocampus. *Journal of Physiology* (*London*), **400**, 321–333.

Lynch, G.S., Dunwiddie, T. and Grybkoff, V. (1977). Heterosynaptic depression: a postsynaptic correlate of long-term potentiation. *Nature*, **266**, 737–739.

Lynch, G., Muller, D., Seubert, P. and J. Larson (1988). Long-term potentiation: persisting problems and recent results. *Brain Research Bulletin*, **21**, 363–372.

Lynch, G., Larson, J., Kelso, S., Barrionuevo, G. and Schottler, F. (1983). Intracellular injection of EGTA blocks induction of hippocampal long-term potentiation. *Nature*, **305**, 719–721.

Lynch, M.A., Errington, M.L. and Bliss, T.V.P. (1985). Long-term potentiation of synaptic transmission in the dentate gyrus: increased release of [^{14}C]-glutamate without increase in receptor binding. *Neuroscience Letters*, **62**, 123–129.

Malenka, R.C., Kauer, J.A., Zucker, R.S. and Nicoll, R.A. (1988). Postsynaptic calcium is sufficient for potentiation of hippocampal synaptic transmission. *Science*, **242**, 81–87.

Malenka, R.C., Kauer, J.A., Perkel, D.J., Mauk, M.D., Kelly, P.T., Nicoll, R.A. and Waxham, M.N. (1989). A essential role for postsynaptic calmodulin and protein kinase activity in long-term potentiation. *Nature*, **340**, 554–557.

Malinow, R. (1991). Transmission between pairs of hippocampal slice neurons: quantal levels, oscillations, and LTP. *Science*, **252**, 722–724.

Malinow, R. and Tsien, R.W. (1990). Presynaptic enhancement shown by whole-cell recordings of long-term potentiation in hippocampal slices. *Nature*, **346**, 177–180.

Matthies, H. (1989). Neurobiological aspects of learning and memory. *Annual Review of Psychology*, **40**, 381–404.

Mayer, M.L. and Westbrook, G.L. (1987). Permeation and block of *N*-methyl-D-aspartatic acid receptor channels by divalent cations in mouse cultured central neurones. *Journal of Physiology* (*London*), **394**, 501–527.

Melchers, B.P.C., DeGraan, P.N.E., Schrama, L.H., Wadman, W.J., Lopes da Silva, F.H. and Gispen, W.-H. (1988). Synaptic potentiation and membrane phosphoproteins. In: *Long-term Potentiation: From Biophysics to Behavior*. New York: Alan R. Liss, Inc. pp. 307–327.

Morris, R.G.M. (1989). Synaptic plasticity and learning: selective impairment of learning in rats and blockade of long-term potentiation *in vivo* by the *N*-methyl-D-aspartate receptor antagonist AP5. *Journal of Neuroscience*, **9**, 3040–3057.

Morris, R.G.M. and Willshaw, D.J. (1989). Must what goes up come down? *Nature*, **339**, 175–176.

Nelson, R.B., Linden, D.J., Hyman, C., Pfenniger, K.H., Reymann, K.G., Brodemann, R., Kase, H. and Matthies, H. (1988). Inhibitors of calmodulin and protein kinase C block different phases of hippocampal long-term potentiation. *Brain Research*, **461**, 388–392.

Nowicky, A.V., Berry, R. and Teyler, T.J. (1990a). Noradrenaline and isoprenaline produce reversible enhancement of synaptic responses in rat visual cortex *in vitro*. *Journal of Physiology (London)*, **424**, 62P.

Nowicky, A.V., Christofi, G. and Bindman, L.J. (1990b). The neuromodulatory actions of noradrenaline on synaptic transmission in the rat sensorimotor cortical slice. *E.S.F. Open Network Conference on Neural Mechanisms of Learning and Memory*, University College London, 4–6 April.

O'Keefe, J. and Nadel, L. (1978). *The Hippocampus as a Cognitive Map*. Oxford: Oxford University Press.

Pavlov, I.P. (1928). *Lectures on Conditioned Reflexes*, Vol. I, translated and edited by W. Horsley Gantt. New York: International.

Pockett, S. Brookes, N.H. and Bindman, L.J. (1990). Long-term depression at synapses in slices of rat hippocampus can be induced by bursts of postsynaptic activity. *Experimental Brain Research*, **80**, 196–200.

Reymann, K.G., Brodemann, R., Kase, H. and Matthies, H. (1988). Inhibitors of calmodulin and protein kinase C block different phases of hippocampal long-term potentiation. *Brain Research*, **461**, 388–392.

Routtenberg, A. (1989). The two major phosphoproteins in growth cones are probably identical to two protein kinase C substrates correlated with persistence of long-term potentiation. *Journal of Neuroscience*, **9**, 381–389.

Sah, P. and Nicoll, R. (1991). Mechanisms underlying potentiation of synaptic transmission in rat anterior cingulate cortex *in vitro*. *Journal of Physiology (London)*, **370**, 531–549.

Sarvey, J.M. (1988). Protein synthesis in long-term potentiation and norepinephrine-induced long-lasting potentiation in hippocampus. In: *Long-term Potentiation: From Biophysics to Behavior*. New York: Alan R. Liss, Inc. pp. 329–353.

Sastry, B.R. and Goh, J.W. (1984). Long-lasting potentiation in the hippocampus is not due to an increase in glutamate receptors. *Life Sciences*, **34**, 1497–1501.

Schwartzkroin P.A. and Taube, J.S. (1986). Mechanisms underlying long-term potentiation. In: *Neural Mechanisms of Conditioning*, edited by D.L. Alkon and C.D. Woody, London: Plenum Press, pp. 319–329.

Stanton, P.K. and Sejnowski, T.J. (1989). Associative long-term depression in the hippocampus induced by hebbian covariance. *Nature*, **339**, 215–218.

Swanson, L.W., Teyler, T.J. and Thompson, R.F. (1982). Hippocampal long-term potentiation: mechanisms and implications for memory. *Neuroscience Research Progress Bulletin*, **20**, 611–769.

Sutor, B. and Hablitz, J.J. (1989a). EPSPs in rat neocortical neurons *in vitro*. I. Electrophysiological evidence for two distinct EPSPs. *Journal of Neurophysiology*, **61**, 607–620.

Sutor, B. and Hablitz, J.J. (1989b.) EPSPs in rat neocortical neurons *in vitro*. II. Involvement of *N*-methyl-D-aspartate receptors in the generation of EPSPs. *Journal of Neurophysiology*, **61**, 621–634.

Taube, J.S. and Schwartzkroin, P.A. (1988). Mechanisms of long-term potentiation: EPSP/spike dissociation, intradendritic recordings, and glutamate sensitivity. *Journal of Neuroscience*, **8**, 1632–1644.

Teyler, T.J. and DiScenna, P. (1987). Long-term potentiation. *Annual Review of Neuroscience*, **10**, 131–161.

Teyler, T.J., Aroniadou, V., Berry, R.L., Borroni, A., DiScenna, P., Grover, L. and Lambert, N. (1990). LTP in neocortex. In: *Seminars in the Neurosciences*, Vol. 2, edited by B. Gustafsson and H. Wigstrom, in press.

Thomson, A.R. (1986). A magnesium-sensitive post-synaptic potential in rat cerebral cortex resembles neuronal responses to N-methylaspartate *Journal of Physiology* (*London*), **370**, 531–549.

Thomson, A.M. (1990). Glycine is a coagonist at the NMDA receptor/channel complex. *Progress in Neurobiology*, **35**, 53–74.

Voronin, L.L. (1988). Investigations of neurophysiological mechanisms of plasticity and Learning. *Soviet Science Reviews, Section F, Physiology and General Biology*, **2**, 529–596.

Voronin, L.L. (1989). Principles of long-term potentiation in mammalian brain. *Progress in Zoology*, **37**, 175–188.

Voronin, L.L., Kuhnt, U., Davletshin, R.N. and Hess, G. (1990). Latent synapses in hippocampal slices. *Proceedings of the E.S.F. Open Network Conference on Neural Mechanisms of Learning and Memory*, University College London, 4–6 April.

Wigstrom, H. and Gustaffson, B. (1986). Postsynaptic control of hippocampal long-term potentiation. *Journal of Physiology* (*Paris*), **81**, 228–236.

Williams, J.H., Errington, M.L., Lynch, M. and Bliss, T.V.P. (1989). Arachidonic acid induces a long-term activity-dependent enhancement of synaptic transmission in the hippocampus. *Nature*, **341**, 739–742.

Woody, C.D. (1984). The electrical excitability of nerve cells as an index of learned behavior. In: *Primary Neural Substrates of Learning and Behavioral Change*, edited by D.L. Alkon and J. Farley. Cambridge: Cambridge University Press, pp. 101–127.

Woody, C.D. and Gruen, E. (1987). Acetylcholine reduces net outward currents measured *in vivo* with single electrode voltage clamp techniques in neurons of the motor cortex of cats. *Brain Research*, **424**, 193–198.

Woody, C.D., Swartz, B.E. and Gruen, E. (1978). Effects of acetylcholine and cyclic GMP on input resistance of cortical neurons in awake cats. *Brain Research*, **158**, 373–395.

Woody, C.D., Baranyi, A., Szente, M.B., Gruen, E., Holmes, W., Nenov, V. and Strecker, G.J. (1989). An aminopyridine-sensitive, early outward current — recorded *in vivo* in neurons of the pericruciate cortex of cats using single-electrode voltage-clamp techniques. *Brain Research*, **480**, 72–81.

Chapter 2

Persistence of hippocampal long-term potentiation: regulation by protein kinase C

Patricia A. Colley

2.1. *Introduction*

2.1.1. **Hippocampal long-term potentiation: a model of information storage and processing**

Brief tetanic stimulation of any one of the excitatory pathways in the hippocampus produces a rapid and persistent enhancement of either the population (or intracellular) excitatory postsynaptic potential (EPSP) or the population spike to subsequent afferent stimulation of the same pathway (Bliss and Gardner-Medwin, 1973; Bliss and Lomo, 1973). This example of synaptic plasticity has been labelled hippocampal long-term potentiation (LTP). The physiology and biochemical correlates of hippocampal LTP have been studied as a means to identify the neural and molecular events underlying information storage and memory. Although it is unlikely that the processes regulating LTP are identical to those which occur with the acquisition of a learning task, or that the study of an individual pathway in the hippocampus, or even a single brain region, will identify the mechanisms regulating all forms of neural plasticity, LTP may provide a general model of neural plasticity which can be applied to different systems with only slight modification of the sequence of events and/or substitution of appropriate enzymes and substrates.

2.1.2. **Electrophysiological components of LTP**

The electrophysiological features of LTP can be divided into at least two components which are defined by their different time courses of onset and decay, and by their differential sensitivity to electrophysiological and pharmacological manipulations. The first component is the initial potentiation of LTP which is typically measured within the first 5–15 min after tetanic stimulation. Initial potentiation should not be confused with the rapid and transient increase in synaptic efficacy which is referred to as post-tetanic potentiation (PTP) and thought to be mediated by mobilization of neurotransmitter within the presynaptic terminal (McNaughton, 1982).

The second component, the persistence of LTP, consists of the maintenance of the initial potentiation over a time course of hours to days. It is the persistence of LTP which appears to be regulated, at least in part, by activation of protein kinase C (PKC) (Routtenberg *et al.*, 1986). The persistence component itself may be divided into two phases: an earlier phase which is correlated with post-translational alterations in synaptic proteins (Browning *et al.*, 1979; Bar *et al.*, 1982; Tielen *et al.*, 1983; Routtenberg *et al.*, 1985) and a later phase which appears to be mediated by protein synthesis (Krug *et al.*, 1984; Stanton and Sarvey, 1984; Frey *et al.*, 1988). Both these processes may be PKC-regulated mechanisms (Reymann *et al.*, 1988b; Colley *et al.*, 1990).

2.2. *Proposed Physiological and Biochemical Mechanisms of LTP*

2.2.1. **Activation of postsynaptic NMDA receptors**

The induction of LTP requires activation of postsynaptic *N*-methyl-D-aspartate (NMDA) receptors (Harris *et al.*, 1984; Collingridge, 1985) allowing for an influx of Ca^{2+} (Mayer and Westbrook, 1981; Jahr and Stevens, 1987). The importance of Ca^{2+} for the induction of LTP has been demonstrated by postsynaptic ejection of Ca^{2+} chelators which block LTP (Lynch *et al.*, 1983; Malenka *et al.*, 1988), and by the induction of a synaptic enhancement which is indistinguishable from LTP in time course with high extracellular Ca^{2+} concentrations (Turner *et al.*, 1982; Reymann *et al.*, 1986) or by selectively increasing postsynaptic free Ca^{2+} levels (Malenka *et al.*, 1988). In addition, synaptic enhancement produced by either high Ca^{2+} or tetanic stimulation will occlude further enhancement by the other (Reymann *et al.*, 1986).

Although NMDA receptor activation may be necessary, it is not sufficient for persistent potentiation. D-2-Amino-5-phosphonovalerate (APV), an NMDA receptor blocker, blocks LTP when delivered before tetanic stimulation, but has no effect on LTP if delivered after tetanic stimulation (Collingridge *et al.*, 1983; Harris *et al.*, 1984). Thus, LTP requires mechanisms in addition to NMDA receptor activation. This was demonstrated further by the application of an NMDA dose sufficient for postsynaptic depolarization which produced only a transient enhancement of transmission with a decay rate of about 30 min at Schaffer collateral–CA1 synapses (Kauer *et al.*, 1988).

The evidence suggests that a Ca^{2+}-stimulated event is required for persistent potentiation. In addition to a Ca^{2+} influx through NMDA receptor-associated channels, potentiating tetanic stimulation also results in an increase in intracellular Ca^{2+} concentrations at the presynaptic terminal for the regulation of neurotransmitter release (McNaughton, 1982). Thus, a Ca^{2+} signal, pre- or postsynaptically, may activate a CaM-dependent kinase(s), Ca^{2+}-dependent lipase(s); e.g. phospholipase A2 (PLA2) or the Ca^{2+}/phospholipid-stimulated PKC, all of which may play a role in the regulation of LTP.

2.2.2. **CaM-dependent processes regulate early components of LTP**

Membrane bound CaM is increased from 5 to 30 min and then decreased 0·5–5 h after LTP induction with either tetanic or high Ca^{2+} stimulation (Popov *et al.*, 1988). Thus, translocation of CaM to the membrane is proposed to regulate enzyme activity important for early components of LTP (Popov *et al.*, 1988). This hypothesis is supported by observations that a CaM inhibitor (50 μM calmidazolium) selectively blocked the initial potentiation of LTP in CA1 pyramidal cells (Reymann *et al.*, 1988a). However, calmidazolium may have direct effects on voltage-dependent Ca^{2+} channels (Greenberg *et al.*, 1987). Possible CaM-dependent mechanisms which may underly early components of LTP are enhanced neurotransmitter release (DeLorenzo, 1982; Lynch and Bliss, 1986) and enhanced receptor sensitivity (Gnegy, 1982).

2.2.3. **Activation of protein kinase C**

The translocation and activation of the Ca^{2+}/phospholipid-stimulated PKC, and subsequent substrate phosphorylation, have been proposed to regulate the persistence of LTP (Routtenberg *et al.*, 1986). PKC has been identified as a class of several closely related enzymes (Coussens *et al.*, 1986; Nishizuka, 1988) which can be differentiated on the basis of sensitivity to activators (Nishizuka, 1988; Sekiguchi *et al.*, 1987), as well as regional (Brandt *et al.*, 1987; Huang *et al.*, 1987, 1988) and subcellular localization in the brain (Wolf *et al.*, 1986; Wood *et al.*, 1986; Worley *et al.*, 1986). PKC has been detected in a wide range of mammalian tissues and organs as well as in other organisms, and shown to catalyse the phosphorylation of a range of substrates, which include receptors, ion channels, cytoskeletal proteins and metabolic enzymes (for review see Nishizuka, 1986).

PKC has been linked to signal transduction by the observation that the enzyme is activated with receptor-mediated breakdown of inositol phospholipids (PI) (Takai *et al.*, 1979; Kishimoto *et al.*, 1980). Full activation of PKC requires the enzyme to be translocated from the cytosol to the plasma membrane in a Ca^{2+}-dependent fashion (Kraft and Anderson, 1983). Phospholipase C catalysed breakdown of phosphatidylinositol 4,5-biphosphate results in the transient production of diacylglycerol (DAG) which increases the affinity of PKC for Ca^{2+} (Takai *et al.*, 1979; Kishimoto *et al.*, 1980), and inositol 1,4,5-triphosphate (IP3). IP3 also acts as second messenger releasing Ca^{2+} from non-mitochondrial intracellular stores (Berridge and Irvine, 1984). Thus, PKC can be activated by exogenous compounds which can mimic the effects of DAG, e.g. synthetic diacylglycerols or tumour-promoting phorbol esters.

An alternative pathway for PKC activation has been revealed (Murakami and Routtenberg, 1985; Murakami *et al.*, 1986). The *cis*-fatty acids, oleate and arachidonate, can activate PKC in the absence of Ca^{2+} and phospholipids. Free *cis*-fatty acids are released from the 2-acyl position of membrane phospholipids *in vivo* by PLA2. Thus, the translocation of PKC to membrane has been proposed to activate the enzyme via its association with membrane-bound phospholipids, or unsaturated fatty acids (Murakami and Routtenberg, 1985).

2.2.4. **Protein kinase C regulates the persistence of LTP**

Activation of PKC following LTP has been measured as either an increase in *in vitro* substrate phosphorylation or an increase in membrane PKC activity. In rats, which received eight trains of 400-Hz stimulation to induce LTP, an increase in the *in vitro* phosphorylation of a 47kDa protein, designated as protein F1, was detected 5 min, but not 1 min after tetanic stimulation (Routtenberg *et al.*, 1985). Increases in the *in vitro* phosphorylation of protein F1 was also measured 1 h and 3 days after LTP induction (Lovinger *et al.*, 1985, 1986). In each study, the level of phosphorylation was related to a persistence measure and not to the magnitude of initial potentiation. In addition, there was no difference in the level of protein F1 phosphorylation in animals whose potentiation decayed to baseline and low frequency controls.

As would be predicted if LTP requires PKC activation, an increase in membrane PKC activity was detected 60 min, but not 1 min, after high frequency stimulation (Akers *et al.*, 1986). With the increase in membrane activity there was a concomitant decrease in cytosol activity, and thus no change in total PKC activity. The increase in membrane PKC activity following tetanic stimulation was associated with the persistence of LTP, and was not seen in animals which did not show persistent potentiation.

Post-translational modification of proteins is an attractive mechanism for the regulation of synaptic plasticity in that changes can be restricted to potentiated synapses, and it does not require targeting of newly synthesized proteins to specific sites. Thus, in accordance with these data, a translocation of PKC activity to the plasma membrane and the subsequent phosphorylation of protein F1 was proposed to be a biochemical mechanism regulating a persistence phase of LTP (Routtenberg *et al.*, 1986).

If PKC does play a role in LTP, then direct manipulation of the kinase with PKC activators should alter the LTP response. Phorbol esters which mimic the role of DAG in the translocation of PKC to the membrane (Castagna *et al.*, 1982) have been used in an attempt to modify or induce LTP. It should be noted, however, that unlike DAG which is a transient membrane signal, phorbol esters are not easily degraded. An initial study in which 12-tetradecanoyl phorbol-13-acetate (TPA) was iontophoretically applied to the intact hilar dentate gyrus prior to abbreviated tetanic stimulation (stimulation parameters were sufficient to elicit an initial potentiation of typical magnitude, but which decays to baseline within 2 h) reported enhanced potentiation persistence with no effect on initial potentiation (Routtenberg *et al.*, 1986; see also Figure 2.1A). There was no effect of TPA on baseline synaptic activation. This enhancement of LTP was shown to be synapse specific, and thus not due merely to overall increases in postsynaptic excitability (Lovinger and Routtenberg, 1988). These data led to the hypothesis that phorbol esters were working synergistically with a Ca^{2+}-mediated event induced with tetanic stimulation to produce LTP. This conclusion was supported by the observations that the unsaturated fatty acid, oleate, also enhanced the persistence of potentiation without having an effect on initial potentiation, and under no conditions was oleate alone sufficient to induce LTP (Linden *et al.*, 1986, 1987). In addition, protein F1 phosphorylation levels following the application of TPA in combination with abbreviated tetanic stimulation were increased as compared to controls receiving abbreviated tetanic stimulation alone (Routtenberg *et al.*, 1986).

Other reports demonstrated that relatively high concentrations of phorbol 12,13-dibutyrate (PDBu) or phorbol 12,13-diacetate (PDA) applied to the intact hippocampus or hippocampal slice was sufficient for synaptic enhancement (Malenka *et al.*, 1986; Colley *et al.*, 1989; see also Figure 2.1B). Phorbol ester enhancement occluded subsequent potentiation by tetanic stimulation (Malenka *et al.*, 1986; Colley *et al.*, 1989) and was blocked by the PKC inhibitor polymyxin B (Reymann *et al.*, 1988c) suggesting that the two forms of synaptic enhancement require similar mechanisms. Although high doses of phorbol ester alone will produce a slowly developing synaptic enhancement and it too appears to be regulated by PKC activation, current evidence suggests that phorbol ester enhancement differs from LTP produced with tetanic stimulation (Gustafsson *et al.*, 1988; Muller *et al.*, 1988; Colley *et al.*, 1989).

Protein kinase inhibitors have also been tested to determine the role of PKC activation in the regulation of LTP (Lovinger *et al.*, 1987; Malinow *et al.*, 1988; Muller *et al.*, 1988; Reymann *et al.*, 1988a,b; Colley *et al.*, 1990; see Table 2.1). In evaluating the effects of inhibitors, however, one must take into consideration that these inhibitors are not specific. Although all of them inhibit protein kinases other than PKC, each inhibits a different subset of protein kinases. For example, the inhibitors polymyxin B, mellitin (Mazzei *et al.*, 1982) and sphingosine (Hannun *et al.*, 1986) which compete with phosphatidylserine at the regulatory subunit also inhibit Ca^{2+}/CaM-dependent kinases. H-7, on the other hand, competes with ATP at the catalytic phosphotransferase site and inhibits cyclic nucleotide-dependent kinases as well as PKC (Hidaka *et al.*, 1984).

In the first inhibitor study (Lovinger *et al.*, 1987), application of 50 pmol of polymyxin B, H-7 or mellitin to the intact dentate gyrus prior to tetanic

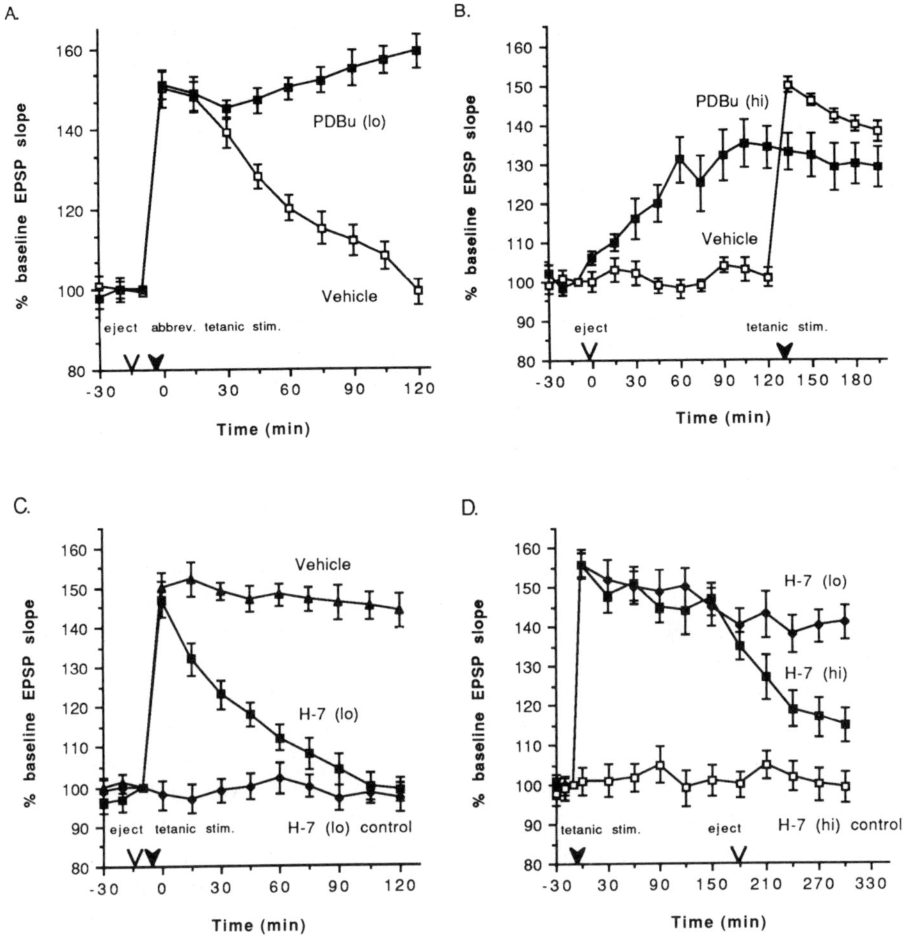

Figure 2.1. The effects of PKC activators and inhibitors on LTP. (A) Abbreviated tetanic stimulation (abbrev. tetanic stim.) of perforant path fibres produced potentiation of intact dentate granule cells which decayed within 2 h. As was previously observed with TPA (Routtenberg, *et al.*, 1986), a low (lo) dose of phorbol 12,13-dibutyrate (PDBu) iontophoretically ejected 15 min before abbreviated tetanic stimulation enhanced the persistence of potentiation, but had no effect on the initial potentiation. (B) A high (hi) dose of PDBu ejected alone into the intact dentate gyrus was sufficient for synaptic enhancement. Initial PDBu enhancement occluded subsequent potentiation produced with tetanic stimulation. (C) H-7 micropressure ejected 15 min before tetanic stimulation into the intact dentate gyrus inhibited the persistence of LTP while leaving the initial potentiation intact. H-7 had no effect on low frequency synaptic activation. (D) Unlike a low dose of H-7, a high dose of H-7 inhibited the persistence of LTP when delivered as late as 3 h after tetanic stimulation. A high dose of H-7 also had no effect on baseline synaptic activation.

Table 2.1. Summary of PKC inhibitor studies.

Study	Preparation	Inhibitor	Application[a]	Effect[b] on LTP persistence
Extracellular				
Colley *et al.*, 1990	Dentate *in vivo*	Polymyxin B, H-7	25–250 pmol ejections	Inhibit up to 240 min
Lovinger *et al.*, 1987	Dentate *in vivo*	Polymyxin B, mellitin, H-7	50 pmol ejections	Inhibit but not at 240 min
Malinow *et al.*, 1988	CA1 slice	H-7	300 μM 3–8 h perfusion	Inhibit up to 3 h
Muller *et al.*, 1988	CA1 slice	H-7	100 μM 20 min static bath	No inhibition
Reymann *et al.*, 1988a,b	CA1 slice	Polymyxin B	20 μM 60 min perfusion	Inhibit
Intracellular				
Malenka *et al.*, 1989	CA1 slice	H-7	20 μM leaking	Inhibit
Malinow *et al.*, 1989	CA1 slice	H-7	300 μM leaking	Inhibit but not at 240 min
			300 μM 3 h perfusion	Inhibit

[a] The parameters of inhibitors application include the dose of inhibitors used, the duration of application and the method of application.
[b] References to time indicate the time after LTP induction at which inhibitors are still effective in producing decay of LTP.

stimulation produced decay of LTP to baseline within 60 min. None of the inhibitors had an effect on the initial potentiation. These observations were repeated by Reymann *et al.* (1988a,b) with application of K-252b or polymyxin B delivered during tetanic stimulation of the Schaffer collateral–CA1 synapses in the slice preparation. Pretreatment with sphingosine (10 μM) or H-7 (300 μM) also caused total decay of LTP at Schaffer collateral–CA1 synapses in the slice preparation 30–45 min after LTP induction (Malinow *et al.*, 1988). A 100 μM concentration of H-7, however, failed to inhibit LTP in the same preparation (Muller *et al.*, 1988).

A second issue which can be explored with the use of PKC inhibitors is the time at which PKC activation is no longer necessary for persistent potentiation. Initial reports demonstrated an inability of mellitin to affect LTP persistence if delivered *in vivo* 4 h after LTP induction (Lovinger *et al.*,

1987). An *in vitro* study, however, reported a reversible inhibition of persistence with 300 μM H-7 3 h after LTP induction (Malinow *et al.*, 1988).

In a study which compared different doses and time points of inhibitor application in the same preparation, the effects of polymyxin B and H-7 on the initial potentiation and persistence of LTP were shown to be both dose- and time-dependent (Colley *et al.*, 1990). Polymyxin B (25 pmol) or H-7 (50 pmol) micropressure ejected into the intact dentate gyrus caused decay of LTP if delivered before or up to 30 min after tetanic stimulation (Figure 2.1C). H-7 had no effect on initial potentiation even at a higher does (250 pmol). Interestingly, unlike 25 pmol of H-7, this high dose did cause decay of LTP persistence if delivered 3–4 h after tetanic stimulation (Figure 2.1D). The dose-dependent effects of H-7 on LTP suggest that the persistence of LTP is made up of at least two phases, both of which are regulated by PKC, but which show differential susceptibility to PKC inhibitors. The effectiveness of inhibitors in blocking the two persistence phases may be determined by the subtype of PKC involved, the site of PKC regulation (plasma membrane vs. nuclear membrane), or the state of the PKC molecule (translocated, cleaved or autophosphorylated) at the different time points.

Recent studies which injected PKC and CaM-dependent kinase inhibitors intracellularly into CA1 pyramidal cells showed blockade of LTP suggesting a postsynaptic locus for PKC and CaM-dependent processes underlying LTP (Malinow *et al.*, 1989; Malenka *et al.*, 1989). However, H-7 inhibition of the late persistence phase of LTP (3 h after LTP induction) was not seen with intracellular injection in the postsynaptic cell, but was seen with bath application of H-7 suggesting a presynaptic locus of this effect (Malinow *et al.*, 1989).

2.2.5. Presynaptic PKC regulation of the persistence component of LTP: proposed functions of protein F1

Protein F1 immunoreactivity in the hippocampus (Oestreicher and Gispen, 1986; Snipes *et al.*, 1987; Benowitz *et al.*, 1988) and *in situ* hybridization of protein F1 mRNA (Rosenthal *et al.*, 1987) suggest that the protein is localized to presynaptic terminals. This conclusion agrees well with a study (Goslin *et al.*, 1988) using immunofluorescence staining which demonstrated the selective localization of protein F1 (GAP 43) in hippocampal axonal growth cones, and not in developing dendrites or dendritic growth cones.

Evidence suggesting a function for protein F1 comes from studies of proteins with which it has been coidentified. These include regeneration and growth-associated proteins (Basi *et al.*, 1987; Benowitz and Routtenberg, 1987; Karns *et al.*, 1987). Protein F1 has also been implicated in CaM sequestration (Alexander *et al.*, 1987) as P57 (Wakim *et al.*, 1987), and regulation of phosphoinositide (PI) metabolism as B50 (Gispen *et al.*, 1985).

Protein F1/GAP-43 is associated with the processes of axonal growth and regeneration (Benowitz and Routtenberg, 1987). Protein F1 may regulate LTP by mediating growth processes such as expansion of pre-existing terminals or sprouting of new terminals (Routtenberg, 1985). Development and regeneration, however, are coupled with increases in protein synthesis; whereas the initial changes in protein F1 phosphorylation following LTP occur too rapidly to be explained by increased synthesis and transport of protein F1. An alternative scenario is based on the theory that the negatively-charged, rod-like carboxy terminal of protein F1 is involved in the interactions between cytoskeletal elements and plasma membrane (Allsopp and Moss, 1989; LeBate and Skene, 1989). Phosphorylation of protein F1 may then mediate reorganization of cytoskeletal elements which have been proposed to occur with LTP (Routtenberg, 1985).

In addition, protein F1 has been proposed to play a sequestering role, maintaining CaM near the membrane where it can rapidly act once it is released by protein F1 phosphorylation (Alexander *et al.*, 1987). Protein F1 in an unphosphorylated state binds to CaM, an association which is hindered by increased Ca^{2+} concentrations (Alexander *et al.*, 1987). Activation of presynaptic PKC and subsequent protein F1 phosphorylation may trigger the release of CaM and activation of CaM-dependent processes at the membrane and/or in the cytosol which underly LTP. Alternatively, an influx of Ca^{2+} may directly, without protein F1 phosphorylation, cause the dissociation of protein F1 and CaM. Either scenario allows for parallel processes, regulated by protein F1 and CaM, which may be required for persistent potentiation.

The regulation of LTP persistence has been proposed to be mediated by increased neurotransmitter release (Skrede and Malthe-Sorenssen, 1981; Dolphin *et al.*, 1982; Bliss *et al.*, 1986). An increase in neurotransmitter release may be regulated by the combined effects of PKC and CaM-dependent activities (Lynch and Bliss, 1986). Both CaM and a synthetic DAG increased the release of [^{3}H]-glutamate from synaptosomes prepared from the CA3 region (Lynch and Bliss, 1986). The increase in release was occluded by prior LTP treatment of hippocampal tissue. More specifically, presynaptic application of phorbol esters was observed to produce an enhancement of synaptic transmission which decayed with a time course similar to that of increased neurotransmitter release (Malenka *et al.*, 1987).

Dual regulation of neurotransmitter release by PKC and CaM-dependent kinase(s) can be explained if protein F1 is indeed involved in the sequestration of CaM (Alexander *et al.*, 1987). A presynaptic Ca^{2+} influx may result in the phosphorylation of protein F1 and release of CaM (Alexander *et al.*, 1987). CaM may trigger neurotransmitter release by phosphorylation of vesicle proteins by CaM-dependent protein kinases (DeLorenzo, 1982). In addition, phosphorylated protein F1, by affecting cytoskeletal organization (Allsopp and Moss, 1989; LeBate and Skene, 1989), may increase the accessibility of the vesicle to the synaptic membrane. A role of protein F1 in neurotransmitter release is suggested by the observation that noradrenaline release from synaptosomes was blocked with antibodies to protein F1 (Dekker *et al.*, 1989).

2.2.6. Postsynaptic PKC in the regulation of the persistence of LTP: PKC regulation of protein synthesis

A role of postsynaptic PKC activity in the regulation of LTP has also been suggested. Injection of PKC into pyramidal cells produced a LTP-like enhancement of synaptic activation at Schaffer collateral–CA1 synapses which persisted for at least 30 min (Hu *et al.*, 1987). PKC inhibitors injected postsynaptically blocked LTP in CA1 pyramidal cells (Malenka *et al.*, 1989; Malinow *et al.*, 1989). Although these data do not substantiate that endogenous PKC is present postsynaptically, PKC has been detected in the apical dendrites of pyramidal cells (Saito *et al.*, 1988), and found to be a major component in postsynaptic densities from rat brain (Wolf *et al.*, 1986). A proposed role of postsynaptic PKC is to mediate enhanced quisqualate sensitivity following LTP induction (Davies *et al.*, 1989).

Protein synthesis has been proposed to underly the persistence of LTP over several hours to days (for review see Matthies, 1989). Anisomycin, a blocker of protein synthesis, has been shown to block a later phase (>3 h) of LTP both in CA1 slice preparation (Frey *et al.*, 1988) and in the dentate gyrus in freely moving animals (Krug *et al.*, 1984).

Presynaptically, protein synthesis may underly a morphological alteration and/or sprouting of presynaptic terminals (Routtenberg, 1985). However, postsynaptic protein synthesis has been implied by both electrophysiological and morphological studies. Frey *et al.* (1989) observed that LTP induced in dendrites separated from CA1 pyramidal cell bodies decayed to baseline within 3 h compared to intact cells in which LTP persisted for 8–10 h. The authors concluded that a later phase of LTP which appears to be mediated by protein synthesis requires postsynaptic cell bodies. However, there is a selective distribution of polyribosomes, the machinery for protein synthesis, beneath postsynaptic sites (Steward and Levy, 1982) suggesting that LTP-induced changes in postsynaptic protein synthesis may not require nuclear synthetic processes. This hypothesis is supported by the observation that anisomycin, a protein synthesis inhibitor, but not actinomycin D, an mRNA synthesis inhibitor, blocked the persistence of LTP (Otani *et al.*, 1989). In addition, anisomycin blocked LTP when injected into the dentate gyrus, but not the entorhinal cortex (Otani and Abraham, 1989). These studies imply that LTP persistence is dependent upon postsynaptic protein synthesis from already existing mRNA. Thus, postsynaptic protein synthesis may mediate morphological changes which are observed following LTP, such as increases in the number of shaft and sessile spine synapses at Schaffer collateral-commissural projections to CA1 following potentiating tetanic stimulation (Lee *et al.*, 1980; Chang and Greenough, 1984).

Recent data suggest that if protein synthesis underlies the persistence of LTP, whether it occurs presynaptically, postsynaptically or both, it may be regulated by PKC. PKC has been implicated in the regulation of protein synthesis by studies which show phorbol ester-induced increases in mRNA (Bjorge *et al.*, 1989) or transcription of mRNA activated by the transcription factor AP2 (Imagawa *et al.*, 1987). With regard to LTP, high doses of the PKC inhibitor, H-7, produce decay of LTP when applied 3–4 h after LTP induction, a time period in which protein synthesis appears to be important for LTP persistence (Malinow *et al.*, 1988; Colley *et al.*, 1990).

2.3. *Conclusion*

Activation of PKC regulates the persistence of LTP, but not its initial potentiation. In addition, LTP persistence can be divided into at least two phases. Translocation of PKC activity to the synaptic membrane and subsequent substrate phosphorylation has been proposed to mediate an early phase of LTP persistence. A later phase of LTP persistence appears to be mediated by protein synthesis; a process which may also be regulated by PKC activation.

Acknowledgement

This work was supported by MH25281-12 and AFOSR 87-0046 to Dr Aryeh Routtenberg.

References

Akers, R.F., Livinger, D.M., Colley, P.A., Linden, D.J. and Routtenberg, A. (1986). Translocation of protein kinase C activity may mediate hippocampal long-term potentiation. *Science*, **231**, 374–378.

Alexander, K.A., Cimler, B.M., Meier, K.E. and Storm, D.R. (1987). Regulation of calmodulin binding to P-57, a neurospecific calmodulin-binding protein. *Journal of Biological Chemistry*, **262**, 6108–6113.

Allsopp, T.E. and Moss, D.J. (1989). A developmentally regulated chicken neuronal protein associated with the cortical cytoskeleton. *Journal of Neuroscience*, **9**, 13–24.

Bar, P.R., Tielen, A.M., Lopes da Silva, F.H., Zwiers, H. and Gispen, W.H. (1982). Membrane phosphoproteins of rat hippocampus: sensitivity to tetanic stimulation and enkephalin. *Brain Research*, **245**, 69–79.

Basi, G.S., Jacobson, R.G., Virag, I., Schilling, J. and Skene, J.H.P. (1987). Primary structure and transcriptional regulation of GAP-43: a protein associated with nerve growth. *Cell*, **49**, 785–793.

Benowitz, L.I. and Routtenberg, A. (1987). A membrane phosphoprotein associated with neural development, axonal regeneration, phospholipid metabolism and synaptic plasticity. *Trends in Neuroscience*, **10**, 527–532.

Benowitz, L.I., Apostolides, P.J., Perrone-Bizzozero, N., Finklestein, S.P. and

Zwiers, H. (1988). Anatomical distribution of the growth-associated protein GAP-43/B50 in the adult rat brain. *Journal of Neuroscience*, **8**, 339–352.
Berridge, M.J. and Irvine, R.F. (1984). Inositol triphosphate, a novel second messenger in cellular signal transduction. *Nature*, **312**, 315–321.
Bjorge, J.D., Paterson, A.J. and Kudlow, J.E. (1989). Phorbol ester or epidermal growth factor (EGF) stimulates the concurrent accumulation of mRNA for the EGF receptor and its ligand transforming growth factor-alpha in a breast cancer cell line. *Journal of Biological Chemistry*, **264**, 4021–4027.
Bliss, T.V.P. and Gardner-Medwin, A.R. (1973). Long-lasting potentiation of synaptic transmission in the dentate area of the unanesthetized rabbit following stimulation of the perforant path. *Journal of Physiology* (*London*), **232**, 357–374.
Bliss, T.V.P. and Lomo, T. (1973). Long-lasting potentiation of synaptic transmission in the dentate area of the anesthetized rabbit following stimulation of the perforant path. *Journal of Physiology* (*London*), **233**, 334–356.
Bliss T.V.P., Douglas, R.M., Errington, M.L. and Lynch, M.A. (1986). Correlation between long-term potentiation and release of endogenous amino acids from dentate gyrus of anesthetized rats. *Journal of Physiology* (*London*), **377**, 391–408.
Brandt, S.J., Niedel, J.E., Bell, R.M. and Young III, W.S. (1987). Distinct patterns of expression of different protein kinase C mRNAs in rat tissue. *Cell*, **49**, 57–63.
Browning, M., Dunwiddie, T., Bennett, W., Gispen, W. and Lynch, G. (1979). Synaptic phosphoproteins: specific changes after repetitive stimulation of the hippocampal slice. *Science*, **203**, 60–62.
Castagna, M., Takai, Y., Kaibuchi, K., Sano, K., Kikkawa, U. and Nishizuka, Y. (1982). Direct activation of calcium-activated, phospholipid-dependent protein kinase by tumor-promoting phorbol esters. *Journal of Biological Chemistry*, **257**, 7847–7851.
Chang, E.-L. and Greenough, W.T. (1984). Transient and enduring morphological correlates of synaptic activity and efficacy change in the rat hippocampal slice. *Brain Research*, **309**, 35–46.
Colley, P.A., Sheu, F.-S. and Routtenberg, A. (1989). Dose-dependent phorbol ester facilitation or blockade of hippocampal long-term potentiation: relation to membrane/cytosol distribution of protein kinase C activity. *Brain Research*, **495**, 205–216.
Colley, P.A., Sheu, F.-S. and Routtenberg, A. (1990). Protein kinase C inhibitors block the persistence of hippocampal long-term potentiation: an interaction of dose- and time-dependent effects. *Journal of Neuroscience*, **10**, 3353–3360.
Collingridge, G.L. (1985). Long-term potentiation in the hippocampus: mechanisms of initiation and modulation by neurotransmitters. *Trends in Pharmacological Science*, **6**, 407–411.
Collingridge, G.L., Kehl, S.L. and McLennan, H. (1983). Excitatory amino acids in synaptic transmission in the Schaffer collateral–commissural pathway of the rat hippocampus. *Journal of Physiology* (*London*), **334**, 33–46.
Coussens, L., Parker, P.J., Rhee, L., Yang-Feng, T.L., Chen, E., Waterfield, M.D., Francke, U. and Ullrich, A. (1986). Multiple distinct forms of bovine and human protein kinase C suggest diversity in cellular signalling pathways. *Science*, **233**, 859–866.
Davies, S.N., Lester, R.A.J., Reymann, K.G. and Collingridge, G.L. (1989). Temporally distinct pre- and post-synaptic mechanisms maintain long-term potentiation. *Nature*, **338**, 500–503.
Dekker, L.V., DeGraan, P.N.E., Oestreicher, A.B. Versteeg, D.H.G. and Gispen W.H. (1989). Inhibition of noradrenaline release by antibodies to B-50 (GAP-43). *Nature*, **342**, 74–76.

DeLorenzo, R. (1982). Calmodulin in neurotransmitter release and synaptic function. *Federation Proceedings*, **41**, 2265–2272.
Dolphin, A.C., Errington, M.L. and Bliss, T.V.P. (1982). Long-term potentiation of the perforant path *in vivo* is associated with increased glutamate release. *Nature*, **297**, 496–498.
Frey, U., Krug, M., Reymann, K.G. and Matthies, H. (1988). Anisomycin, an inhibitor of protein synthesis blocks late phases of LTP phenomena in the hippocampal CA1 region *in vitro*. *Brain Research*, **452**, 57–65.
Frey, U., Krug, M., Brodemann, R., Reymann, K. and Matthies, H. (1989). Long-term potentiation induced in dendrites separated from rat's CA1 pyramidal somata does not establish a late phase. *Neuroscience Letters*, **97**, 135–139.
Gispen, W.H., Leunissen, J.L.M., Oestricher, A.B., Verkleij, A.J. and Zwiers, H. (1985). Presynaptic localization of B-50 phosphoprotein: the (ACTH)-sensitive protein kinase substrate involved in rat brain polyphosphoinositide metabolism. *Brain Research*, **328**, 381–385.
Gnegy, N.E. (1982). The relationship of calmodulin and dopaminergic activity in the striatum. *Federation Proceedings*, **41**, 2273–2277.
Goslin, K., Schreyer, D.J., Skene, J.H.P. and Banker, G. (1988). Development of neuronal polarity: GAP-43 distinguishes axonal from dendritic growth cones. *Nature*, **336**, 672–674.
Greenberg, D.A., Carpenter, C.L. and Messing, R.O. (1987). Interaction of calmodulin inhibitors and protein kinase C inhibitors with voltage-dependent calcium channels. *Brain Research*, **404**, 401–404.
Gustafsson, B., Huang, Y.-Y. and Wigstrom, H. (1988). Phorbol ester-induced synaptic potentiation differs from long-term potentiation in the guinea pig hippocampus *in vitro*. *Neuroscience Letters*, **85**, 77–81.
Hannun, Y.A., Loomis, C.R., Merrill, A.H. and Bell, R.M. (1986). Sphingosine inhibition of protein kinase C activity and of phorbol dibutyrate binding *in vitro* and in human platelets. *Journal of Biological Chemistry*, **261**, 1264–1269.
Harris, E.W., Ganong, A.H. and Cotman, C.W. (1984). Long-term potentiation in the hippocampus involves activation of *N*-methyl-D-aspartate receptors. *Brain Research*, **323**, 132–137.
Hidaka, H., Inagaki, M., Kawamoto, S. and Sasaki, Y. (1984). Isoquinolinesulfonamides, novel and potent inhibitors of cyclic nucleotide-dependent protein kinase and protein kinase C. *Biochemistry*, **23**, 5036–5041.
Hu, G.-Y., Hvalby, O., Walaas, S.I., Albert, K.A., Skjeflo, P., Andersen, P. and Greengard, P. (1987). Protein kinase C injection into hippocampal pyramidal cells elicits features of long-term potentiation. *Nature*, **328**, 426–429.
Huang, F.L., Yoshida, Y., Nakabayashi, H. & Huang, K.-P. (1987). Differential distribution of protein kinase C isozymes in the various regions of brain. *Journal of Biological Chemistry*, **262**, 15714–15720.
Huang, F.L., Yoshida, Y., Nakabayashi, H., Young, W.S. and Huang, K.-P. (1988). Immunocytochemical localization of protein kinase C isozymes in rat brain. *Journal of Neuroscience*, **8**, 4734–4744.
Imagawa, M., Chiu, R. and Karin, M. (1987). Transcription factor AP-2 mediates induction by two different signal–transduction pathways: protein kinase C and cAMP. *Cell*, **51**, 251–260.
Jahr, C.E. and Stevens, C.F. (1987). Glutamate activates multiple single-channel conductances in hippocampal neurones. *Nature*, **325**, 522–525.
Karns, L.R., Ng, S.-C., Freeman, J.A. and Fishman, M.C. (1987). Cloning of complementary DNA for GAP-43: a neuronal growth-related protein. *Science*, **236**, 597–600.
Kauer, J.A. Malenka, R.C. and Nicoll, R.A. (1988). NMDA application potentiates synaptic transmission in the hippocampus. *Neuron*, **324**, 250–252.

Kishimoto, A., Takai, Y., Mori, T., Kikkawa, U. and Nishizuka, Y. (1980). Activation of calcium and phospholipid-dependent protein kinase by diacylglycerol, its possible relation to phosphatidylinositol turnover. *Journal of Biological Chemistry*, **255**, 2273–2276.

Kraft, A.S. and Anderson, W.B. (1983). Phorbol esters increase the amount of CA^{2+}/phospholipid dependent protein kinase associated with plasma membrane. *Nature*, **301**, 621–623.

Krug, M., Lossner, B. and Ott, T. (1984). Anisomycin blocks the late phase of long-term potentiation in the dentate gyrus of freely moving rats. *Brain Research*, **13**, 39–42.

LeBate, M.E. and Skene, J.H.P. (1989). Selective conservation of GAP-43 structure in vertebrate evolution. *Neuron*, **3**, 299–310.

Lee, K.S., Schottler, F., Oliver, M. and Lynch, G. (1980). Brief bursts of high-frequency stimulation produce two types of structural change in rat hippocampus. *Journal of Neurophysiology*, **44**, 247–258.

Linden, D.J., Murakami, K. and Routtenberg, A. (1986). A newly discovered protein kinase C activator (oleic acid) enhances long-term potentiation in the intact hippocampus. *Brain Research*, **379**, 358–363.

Linden, D.J., Wong, K.L., Sheu, F.-S. and Routtenberg, A. (1987). Enhancement of long-term potentiation by *cis*-unsaturated fatty acid: relation to protein kinase C and phospholipase A_2. *Journal of Neuroscience*, **7**, 3783–3792.

Lovinger, D.M. and Routtenberg, A. (1988). Synapse specific protein kinase C activation enhances maintenance of long-term potentiation in rat hippocampus. *Journal of Physiology*, **400**, 321–333.

Lovinger, D.M., Wong, K.L. and Routtenberg, A. (1987). Protein kinase C inhibitors eliminate hippocampal long-term potentiation. *Brain Research*, **436**, 177–183.

Lovinger, D.M., Colley, P.A., Akers, R.F., Nelson, R.B. and Routtenberg, A. (1986). Direct relation of long-term synaptic potentiation of phosphorylation of membrane protein F1, a substrate for membrane protein kinase C. *Brain Research*, **399**, 205–211.

Lovinger, D., Akers, F., Nelson, R., Barnes, C., McNaughton, B. and Routtenberg, A. (1985). Selective increase in hippocampal protein F1 phosphorylation directly related to three day growth of long-term enhancement. *Brain Research*, **343**, 137–143.

Lynch, M.A. and Bliss, T.V.P. (1986). Long-term potentiation of synaptic transmission in the hippocampus of the rat: effect of calmodulin and oleoyl-acetylglycerol on release of [^{3}H]-glutamate. *Neuroscience Letters*, **65**, 171–176.

Lynch, G., Larson, J., Kelso, S., Barrioneuvo, G. and Schottler, F. (1983). Intracellular injections of EGTA block induction of hippocampal long-term potentiation. *Nature*, **305**, 719–721.

McNaughton, B.L. (1982). Long-term synaptic enhancement and short-term potentiation in rat fascia dentata act through different mechanisms. *Journal of Physiology*, **324**, 249–262.

Malenka, R.C., Madison, D.V. and Nicoll, R.A. (1986). Potentiation of synaptic transmission in the hippocampus by phorbol esters. *Nature*, **321**, 175–177.

Malenka, R.C., Ayoub, G.S. and Nicoll, R.A. (1987). Phorbol esters enhance transmitter release in rat hippocampal slices. *Brain Research*, **403**, 198–203.

Malenka, R.C., Kauer, J.A., Zucker, R.S. and Nicoll, R.A. (1988). Postsynaptic calcium is sufficient for potentiation of hippocampal synaptic transmission. *Science*, **242**, 81–84.

Malenka, R.C., Kauer, J.A., Parkel, D.J., Mauk, M.D., Kelly, P.T., Nicoll, R.A. and Waxham, M.N. (1989). An essential role for postsynaptic calmodulin and protein kinase activity in long-term potentiation. *Nature*, **340**, 554–557.

Malinow, R., Madison, D.V. and Tsien, R.W. (1988). Persistent protein kinase activity underlying long-term potentiation. *Nature*, **335**, 820–824.

Malinow, R., Schulman, H. and Tsien, R.W. (1989). Inhibition of postsynaptic PKC or CaMKII blocks induction but not expression of LTP. *Science*, **245**, 862–866.

Matthies, H. (1989). In search of cellular mechanisms of memory. *Progress in Neurobiology*, **32**, 277–349.

Mayer, M.L. and Westbrook, G.L. (1987). Permeation and block of *N*-methyl-D-aspartic acid receptor channels by divalent cations in mouse central neurones. *Journal of Physiology*, **394**, 501–528.

Mazzei, G.J., Katoh, N. and Kuo, J.F. (1982). Polymyxin B is a more selective inhibitor for phospholipid-sensitive, calcium-dependent protein kinase than for calmodulin-sensitive, calcium-dependent protein kinase. *Biochemical and Biophysical Research Communications*, **109**, 1129–1133.

Muller, D., Turnbull, J., Baudry, M. and Lynch, G. (1988). Phorbol ester-induced synaptic facilitation is different than long-term potentiation. *Proceedings of the National Academy of Sciences USA*, **85**, 6997–7000.

Murakami, K. and Routtenberg, A. (1985). Direct activation of purified protein kinase C by the unsaturated fatty acids (oleate and arachidonate) in the absence of phospholipids and Ca^{2+}. *FEBS Letters*, **192**, 189–193.

Murakami, K., Chan, S.Y. and Routtenberg, A. (1986). Protein kinase C activation by *cis*-fatty acid in the absence of Ca^{2+} and phospholipids. *Journal of Biological Chemistry*, **261**, 15424–15429.

Nishizuka, Y. (1986). Studies and perspectives of protein kinase C. *Science*, **233**, 305–312.

Nishizuka, Y. (1988). The molecular heterogeneity of protein kinase C and its implication for cellular regulation. *Nature*, **334**, 661–665.

Oestreicher, A.B. and Gispen, W.H. (1986). Comparison of the immunocytochemical distribution of the phosphoprotein B-50 in the cerebellum and hippocampus of immature and adult rat brain. *Brain Research*, **375**, 267–279.

Otani, S. and Abraham, W.C. (1989). Inhibition of protein synthesis in the dentate gyrus, but not the entorhinal cortex, blocks maintenance of long-term potentiation in rats. *Neuroscience Letters*, **106**, 175–180.

Otani, S., Marshall, C.J., Tate, W.P., Goddard, G.V. and Abraham, W.C. (1989). Maintenance of long-term potentiation in rat dentate gyrus requires protein synthesis but not messenger RNA synthesis immediately post-tetanization. *Neuroscience*, **28**, 519–526.

Popov, N.S., Reymann, K.G., Schulzeck, K., Schulzeck, S. and Matthies, H. (1988). Alterations in calmodulin content in fractions of rat hippocampal slices during tetanic- and calcium-induced long-term potentiation. *Brain Research Bulletin*, **21**, 201–206.

Reymann, K.G., Brodemann, R., Kase, H. and Matthies, H. (1988a). Inhibitors of calmodulin and protein kinase C block different phases of hippocampal long-term potentiation. *Brain Research*, **461**, 388–392.

Reymann, K.G., Frey, U., Jork. R. and Matthies, H. (1988b). Polymyxin B, an inhibitor of protein kinase C, prevents the maintenance of synaptic long-term potentiation in hippocampal CA1 neurons. *Brain Research*, **440**, 305–314.

Reymann, K.G., Schulzeck, K., Kuse, H. and Matthies, H. (1988c). Phorbol ester-induced hippocampal long-term potentiation is counteracted by inhibitors of protein kinase C. *Experimental Brain Research*, **71**, 227–230.

Reymann, K.G. Matthies, H.K., Frey, U., Vorobyev, V.S. and Matthies, H. (1986). Calcium-induced long-term potentiation in the hippocampal slice: characterization of the time course and conditions. *Brain Research Bulletin*, **17**, 291–296.

Rosenthal, A., Chan, S.Y., Henzel, W., Haskell, C., Kuang, W.-J., Chen, E., Wilcox, J.N., Ullrich, A., Goeddel, D.V. and Routtenberg, A. (1987). Primary structure and mRNA localization of protein F1, a growth-related protein kinase

C substrate associated with synaptic plasticity. *European Molecular Biology Organization*, **6**, 3641–3646.
Routtenberg, A. (1985). Protein kinase C activation leading to protein F1 phosphorylation may regulate synaptic plasticity by presynaptic terminal growth. *Behavioral and Neural Biology*, **44**, 186–200.
Routtenberg, A., Lovinger, D. and Steward, O. (1985). Selective increase in the phosphorylation of a 47kD protein (F1) directly related to long-term potentiation. *Behavioral Neural Biology*, **43**, 3–11.
Routtenberg, A., Colley, P., Linden, D., Lovinger, D., Murakami, K. and Sheu, F.-S. (1986). Phorbol ester promotes growth of synaptic plasticity. *Brain Research*, **378**, 374–378.
Saito, N., Kikkawa, U., Nishizuka, Y. and Tanaka, C. (1988). Distribution of protein kinase C-like immunoreactive neurons in rat brain. *Journal of Neuroscience*, **8**, 369–382.
Sekiguchi, K., Tsukuda, M., Ogita, K., Kikkawa, U. and Nishizuka, Y. (1987). Three distinct forms of rat brain protein kinase C: differential response to unsaturated fatty acids. *Biochemical and Biophysical Research Communications*, **145**, 797–802.
Skrede, K.K. and Malthe-Sorenssen, D. (1981). Increased resting and evoked release of transmitter following repetitive electrical tetanization in hippocampus: a biochemical correlate to long-lasting synaptic potentiation. *Brain Research*, **208**, 436–441.
Snipes, G.J., Chan, S.Y., McQuire, C.B., Costello, B.R. Norden, J.J., Freeman, J.A. and Routtenberg, A. (1987). Evidence for the coidentification of GAP-43, a growth-associated protein, and F1, a plasticity-associated protein. *Journal of Neuroscience*, **7**, 4066–4075.
Stanton, P.K. and Sarvey, J.M. (1984). Blockade of long-term potentiation in rat hippocampal CA1 region by inhibitors of protein synthesis. *Journal of Neuroscience*, **4**, 3080–3088.
Steward, O. and Levy, W.B. (1982). Preferential localization of polyribosomes under the base of dendritic spines in granule cells of the dentate gyrus. *Journal of Neuroscience*, **2**, 284–291.
Takai, Y., Kishimoto, A. Kikkawa, Y., Mori, T. and Nishizuka, Y. (1979). Unsaturated diacylglycerol as a possible second messenger for the activation of calcium-activated, phospholipid-dependent protein kinase system. *Biochemical Biophysical Research Communications*, **90**, 1218–1224.
Tielen, A.M., DeGraan, P.N.E., Mollevanger, W.J., Lopes da Silva, F.H. and Gispen, W.H. (1983). Quantitative relationship between post-tetanic biochemical and electrophysiological changes in rat hippocampal slices. *Brain Research*, **277**, 189–912.
Turner, R.W., Baimbridge, K.G. and Miller, J.J. (1982). Calcium-induced long-term potentiation in the hippocampus. *Neuroscience*, **7**, 1411–1416.
Wakim, B.T., Alexander, K.A., Masure, H.R., Cimler, B.M., Storm, D.R. and Walsh, K.A. (1987). Amino acid sequence of P-57, a neurospecific calmodulin-binding protein. *Biochemistry*, **26**, 7466–7470.
Wolf, M., Burgess, S., Misra, U.K. and Sahyoun, N. (1986). Postsynaptic densities contain a subtype of protein kinase C. *Biochemical and Biophysical Research Communications*, **140**, 691–698.
Wood, J.G., Girard, P.R., Mazzei, G.J. and Kuo, J.F. (1986). Immunocytochemical localization of protein kinase C in identified neuronal compartments of the rat brain. *Journal of Neuroscience*, **6**, 2571–2577.
Worley, P.F., Baraban, J.M., De Souza, E.B. and Snyder, S.H. (1986). Mapping second messenger systems in the brain: differential localizations of adenylate cyclase and protein kinase C. *Proceedings of the National Academy of Sciences USA*, **83**, 4053–4057.

Part II

Galanin

Chapter 3

Galanin: localization, release and putative functions

*W.D. Hutchison and C.R. Morton**

3.1. *Introduction*

Galanin is a peptide of 29 amino acid residues, the sequence of which bears little resemblance to other known peptide families (Figure 3.1). Galanin was originally isolated from porcine intestine (Tatemoto *et al.*, 1983), and subsequently immunoreactive (ir)-galanin has been found to be widely distributed in the central and peripheral nervous systems of several species including humans (Bauer *et al.*, 1986c; Tainio *et al.*, 1987; Gibson *et al.*, 1988; Johansson *et al.*, 1988; Gentleman *et al.*, 1989), other primates (Melander and Staines, 1986; Beal *et al.*, 1988), dog (Dunning *et al.*, 1986), cat (Bauer *et al.*, 1986b; Kummer, 1987; Garry *et al.*, 1989; Lindh *et al.*, 1989), pig (Cheung *et al.*, 1984; Ch'ng *et al.*, 1985; Gibson *et al.*, 1985; Bauer *et al.*, 1986b), and rat (Rökaeus *et al.*, 1984; Ch'ng *et al.*, 1985; Skofitsch and Jacobowitz, 1985a,b, 1986; Melander *et al.*, 1985b, 1986b,c,d; Ju *et al.*, 1987a,b; Holets *et al.*, 1988; Tuchscherer and Seybold, 1989; Stenfors *et al.*, 1989; Suzuki *et al.*, 1989). The use of chromatographic procedures and antibodies directed against specific portions of the galanin molecule suggested some interspecies differences in the amino acid sequence in the C-terminal region, and also the existence of more than one molecular form (Bauer *et al.*, 1986a,b). Molecular biological studies have established that galanin is derived from preproGal, a large precursor peptide of 123 (pig) or 124 (rat) amino acids, containing a signal peptide, a single galanin sequence, and a galanin mRNA-associated peptide of 59 (pig) or 60 (rat) amino acids (Rökaeus and Brownstein, 1986; Kaplan *et al.*, 1988). The amino acid sequences of pig galanin and rat galanin are shown in Figure 3.1.

* Author for correspondence.

3.2. *Localization of galanin*

3.2.1. **Brain**

The use of immunoreactive techniques has revealed a widespread and uneven distribution of ir-galanin in the central nervous system (CNS). The regional concentrations and the distribution of neural elements containing this peptide have been most extensively investigated in the rat (Rökaeus *et al.*, 1984; Ch'ng *et al.*, 1985; Skofitsch and Jacobowitz, 1985a, 1986; Melander *et al.*, 1986b; Stenfors *et al.*, 1989). In this species, high levels of ir-galanin have been found in the amygdaloid nuclei, septum, bed nuclei of the stria terminalis, hypothalamus, locus coeruleus and the posterior pituitary (Rökaeus *et al.*, 1984; Ch'ng *et al.*, 1985; Skofitsch and Jacobowitz, 1986; Stenfors *et al.*, 1989). Dense accumulations of perikarya, fibres and terminals containing ir-galanin have been observed mainly in the hypothalamus, medulla oblongata and spinal cord, with fewer stained structures in the telencephalon, thalamus, mesencephalon and pons (Melander *et al.*, 1986b). Regions particularly rich in cell bodies containing ir-galanin include the septal and diagonal band nuclei, bed nucleus of stria terminalis, the preoptic, arcuate, periventricular and dorsomedial nuclei, medial forebrain bundle area, the tubular, caudal, accessory, supraoptic and paraventricular magnocellular nuclei, the locus coeruleus and dorsal raphe nucleus, various cranial motor nuclei, and the medullary ventral raphe nuclei, caudal spinal trigeminal nucleus and the nucleus of the solitary tract (Ch'ng *et al.*, 1985; Skofitsch and Jacobowitz, 1985a; Melander *et al.*, 1985b, 1986b; Köhler *et al.*, 1986; Holets *et al.*, 1988; Moore, 1989). Ir-galanin-positive fibres generally have a similar distribution, with extensive networks in the septal region, in the bed nucleus of stria terminalis, throughout the hypothalamus (especially the median eminence), the dorsal parabrachial area and locus coeruleus, the nucleus of the solitary tract and the posterior pituitary (Ch'ng *et al.*, 1985; Skofitsch and Jacobowitz, 1985a; Melander *et al.*, 1986b,d; Sawchenko and Pfeiffer, 1988).

A substantially similar pattern of distribution of ir-galanin has been reported in other species studied, e.g. in pig (Ch'ng *et al.*, 1985), owl monkey (Melander and Staines, 1986) and baboon (Beal *et al.*, 1988). In humans, ir-galanin-containing cells were found restricted to the basal nucleus of Meynert and hypothalamic areas, but with fibre staining in the additional regions of the diagonal band, septum, amygdala, hippocampus, stria terminalis, and fornix (Gentleman *et al.*, 1989). In some studies, ir-galanin has been found co-localized with other neurochemicals or their synthesizing enzymes: with vasopressin in neurones of the parvocellular and magnocellular paraventricular nuclei, with tyrosine hydroxylase in arcuate nucleus and locus coeruleus neurones, with glutamic acid decarboxylase in fibres in the median eminence external layer and in cell bodies in the tuberal and caudal magnocellular nuclei, with histidine decarboxylase in tuberomammillary

p Galanin

Gly-Trp-Thr-Leu-Asn-Ser-Ala-Gly-Tyr-Leu-Leu-Gly-Pro-His-Ala-

Ile-Asp-Asn-His-Arg-Ser-Phe-His*-Asp-Lys-Tyr*-Gly-Leu-Ala*-NH_2

r Galanin

Gly-Trp-Thr-Leu-Asn-Ser-Ala-Gly-Tyr-Leu-Leu-Gly-Pro-His-Ala-

Ile-Asp-Asn-His-Arg-Ser-Phe-Ser*-Asp-Lys-His*-Gly-Leu-Thr*-NH_2

Figure 3.1. Amino acid sequences of porcine galanin (p Galanin) and rat galanin (r Galanin). The residues which differ in the two species are marked with asterisks.

nucleus neurones, and with serotonin in mesencephalic and medullary raphe neurones (Brownstein and Mezey, 1986; Köhler *et al.*, 1986; Melander *et al.*, 1986c). In addition, ir-galanin is present in cholinergic neurones of basal forebrain regions which project to the hippocampus (Melander *et al.*, 1985b, 1986d; Melander and Staines, 1986).

3.2.2. **Spinal cord and sensory neurones**

Immunohistochemical studies demonstrated the presence of ir-galanin in the spinal cord. In the rat, cell bodies and fibres containing ir-galanin are concentrated in the superficial laminae of the dorsal horn at all spinal levels (Rökaeus *et al.*, 1984; Ch'ng *et al.*, 1985; Skofitsch and Jacobowitz, 1985a,b; Melander *et al.*, 1986b). In addition, ir-galanin has been detected in some motoneurones and in fibres in the intermediolateral cell column region (Ch'ng *et al.*, 1985). The concentration of ir-galanin in the sacral cord of the rat is increased following thoracic cord transection, suggesting accumulation of the peptide in an ascending pathway (Ch'ng *et al.*, 1985). In fact, immunostained cells and fibres have been identified in the areas around the central canal (Rökaeus *et al.*, 1984; Ch'ng *et al.*, 1985; Melander *et al.*, 1986b), regions where spinothalamic neurones containing both ir-cholecystokinin and ir-galanin have been detected (Ju *et al.*, 1987b). A similar distribution pattern of ir-galanin has been observed in human spinal cord (Gibson *et al.*, 1988).

Dorsal rhizotomy or neonatal capsaicin administration produces a marked loss of ir-galanin-containing fibres and axonal varicosities from the superficial dorsal horn, indicating a primary afferent origin for a significant proportion of these fibres (Ch'ng *et al.*, 1985; Skofitsch and Jacobowitz, 1985b; Tuchscherer and Seybold, 1989). Accordingly, ir-galanin has been detected in a subpopulation of sensory ganglion neurones in the rat (Ch'ng *et al.*, 1985; Skofitsch and Jacobowitz, 1985b; Ju *et al.*, 1987a; Hökfelt *et al.*, 1987;

Suzuki *et al.*, 1989), pig (Ch'ng *et al.*, 1985; Gibson *et al.*, 1985) and cat (Garry *et al.*, 1989). Coexistence of neuropeptides within dorsal root ganglion (DRG) cells is well documented: ir-galanin has been found coexisting in DRG neurones with ir-substance P (ir-SP), ir-calcitonin gene-related peptide (ir-CGRP) and ir-neurokinin A in the rat (Grunditz *et al.*, 1987; Ju *et al.*, 1987a), with ir-SP and ir-CGRP in the pig (Gibson *et al.*, 1985), and — to a limited extent — with ir-somatostatin in the cat (Garry *et al.*, 1989). There is evidence that such coexistence patterns are preserved at the central terminals of these cells, since in the superficial dorsal horn of the rat, axonal varicosities of primary afferent neurones have been found to contain both ir-galanin and ir-SP (Tuchscherer and Seybold, 1989). In several species, the DRG neurones containing ir-galanin are of the small type, with cell diameters of 20–50 μm (300–2000 μm^2 cross-sectional area), suggesting that the majority give rise to unmyelinated axons (Ch'ng *et al.*, 1985; Ju *et al.*, 1987a; Garry *et al.*, 1989). This is consistent with the severe depletion in the number and intensity of these immunoreactive neurones observed in rats treated neonatally with capsaicin, a selective neurotoxin for a subpopulation of C-type DRG cells (Skofitsch and Jacobowitz, 1985b). Moreover, ir-galanin-positive sensory nerves identified in human skin were noted to be of small diameter (Johansson *et al.*, 1988).

3.2.3. **Binding sites**

Biochemical and autoradiographic techniques have been used to study the distribution of binding sites for galanin in the CNS of the rat (Skofitsch *et al.*, 1986; Servin *et al.*, 1987; Melander *et al.*, 1986a, 1988), monkey and humans (Köhler *et al.*, 1989a,b). Such binding sites were found throughout the CNS, concentrated in the prefrontal cortex, basal forebrain regions, the amygdala and hippocampus, the hypothalamus including the median eminence, and certain thalamic and brain-stem cell groups such as the dorsal raphe nucleus, periaqueductal grey, substantia nigra zona compacta, locus coeruleus, parabrachial nuclei, the dorsal vagal complex and the sensory and motor trigeminal nuclei (Skofitsch *et al.*, 1986; Melander *et al.*, 1986a, 1988; Servin *et al.*, 1987; Köhler *et al.*, 1989a,b). In the spinal cord, ^{125}I-galanin binding sites were observed in the superficial laminae of the dorsal horn and also lamina X (Skofitsch *et al.*, 1986; Melander *et al.*, 1988). In the neocortex, binding sites were detected in the monkey and humans but not in the rat; in other brain regions, however, the distribution of binding sites was similar in the two species (Skofitsch *et al.*, 1986; Melander *et al.*, 1986a, 1988; Köhler *et al.*, 1989a,b). In general, a good correlation has been found between the regions exhibiting a high density of binding sites and the location of ir-galanin-containing fibres in the CNS (see above), e.g. neurones of the septum–basal forebrain complex containing ir-galanin and ir-choline acetyltransferase project to the hippocampus (Melander *et al.*, 1985b, 1986d; Melander and Staines, 1986), where ^{125} I-galanin binding sites are concentrated (Skofitsch *et al.*, 1986; Melander *et al.*, 1988; Köhler *et al.*, 1898a,b).

3.2.4. **Periphery**

In addition to sensory neurones, ir-galanin has been detected in neural structures in a number of peripheral systems and organs (Rökaeus, 1987). In the cat, ir-galanin has been found in cell bodies of the parasympathetic submandibular and sphenopalatine ganglia, and also in paravertebral sympathetic ganglia coexisting with ir-tyrosine hydroxylase and ir-neuropeptide Y in the majority of neurones (Kummer, 1987; Lindh *et al.*, 1989). The autonomic innervation of human sweat glands also exhibits galanin immunoreactivity (Tainio *et al.*, 1987). In several species, ir-galanin is present in intrinsic neurones innervating all layers of the gut (Rökaeus *et al.*, 1984; Ekblad *et al.*, 1985b; Melander *et al.*, 1985a; Bishop *et al.*, 1986; Furness *et al.*, 1987; Hoyle and Burnstock, 1989), and in nerve fibres in the respiratory tract, especially the trachea and bronchi (Cheung *et al.*, 1985; Ghatei *et al.*, 1987; Luts *et al.*, 1989). Immunostained fibres have also been demonstrated in the smooth muscle layers of various organs of the male and female urogenital systems of rats and humans (Bauer *et al.*, 1986c; Stjernquist *et al.*, 1988; Papka and Traurig, 1989). In the canine pancreas, a dense network of ir-galanin-containing fibres has been observed in association with the islets of Langerhans (Dunning *et al.*, 1986), while the thyroid gland of the rat has been shown to possess fibres derived from various ganglia and co-containing ir-galanin with ir-neurokinin A, ir-SP and ir-CGRP, or, instead, ir-galanin with ir-vasoactive intestinal peptide (VIP) (Grunditz *et al.*, 1987). Galanin has also been localized in the feline and porcine adrenal medulla, by immunoreactive and *in situ* hybridization histochemical techniques (Bauer *et al.*, 1986b; Rökaeus and Brownstein, 1986).

3.3. *Release of galanin*

With most neuropeptides (including galanin), the literature is dominated by immunoreactive localization studies, with relatively few investigations of the release of these substances. Although anatomical knowledge of the structures and pathways containing particular peptides, and their binding sites, is important for drawing inferences about function, a more direct approach is to study the physiological conditions under which neuropeptides are released in the body.

3.3.1. **Pancreas**

In the dog, nerve fibres innervating the islets of Langerhans contain ir-galanin, and infusion of porcine galanin into the pancreatic artery or intravenously decreases the pancreatic output of ir-insulin and ir-somatostatin and increases that of ir-glucagon (Dunning *et al.*, 1986). Intrapancreatic release of galanin might therefore influence pancreatic hormone secretion, a hypothesis which has been tested by measuring ir-galanin in the pancreatic venous circulation of the dog during mixed autonomic pancreatic nerve stimulation (Dunning and Taborsky, 1989). Such stimulation elevated pancreatic venous ir-galanin levels, and produced similar effects on the pancreatic output of ir-insulin, ir-somatostatin and ir-glucagon as administration of galanin into the pancreatic artery (Dunning and Taborsky, 1989). These experiments have provided evidence for galanin release from pancreatic neurones in the dog, possibly as a regulatory control of islet function.

3.3.2. **Pituitary**

Relatively high levels of ir-galanin have been detected in the pituitary (Ch'ng *et al.*, 1985), from which release of ir-galanin has been examined using a perfused *in vitro* preparation of rat anterior pituitaries (Calvo *et al.*, 1990). The addition of adrenocorticotropin (ACTH) to the perfusion medium produced alterations in the levels of ir-galanin (and ir-VIP) detected in the perfusate: low concentrations of ACTH (0·02–0·4 μM) elevated ir-galanin release (and ir-VIP release) while higher ACTH concentrations (1–2 μM) suppressed release of these peptides (Calvo *et al.*, 1990). Although the functional significance of this biphasic effect of ACTH on pituitary peptides such as galanin is not clear, it could represent a paracrine control system whereby ACTH could influence the release of other pituitary hormones such as growth hormone and prolactin, the secretions of which are stimulated by galanin (Bauer *et al.*, 1986d; Ottlecz *et al.*, 1986; Murakami *et al.*, 1987; Koshiyama *et al.*, 1987).

3.3.3. **Cortex**

Decreased levels of neuropeptides in particular CNS regions have been used as an indirect index of release. Although levels of ir-galanin in the rat cerebral cortex are relatively low (Skofitsch and Jacobowitz, 1986), ir-galanin concentrations in the frontal cortex were noted to be reduced following a repeated handling procedure (Stenfors *et al.*, 1989). One interpretation of this observation is that stress produces release of galanin in the frontal cortex, a hypothesis which will require confirmation with more direct methods of release measurement.

3.3.4. **Spinal cord**

The localization of ir-galanin in a subpopulation of small capsaicin-sensitive DRG neurones and in the superficial dorsal horn where many unmyelinated primary afferent fibres terminate (Ch'ng *et al.*, 1985; Skofitsch and Jacobowitz, 1985b; Melander *et al.*, 1986b; Ju *et al.*, 1987a; Garry *et al.*, 1989) has suggested that this peptide might be released during the spinal transmission of sensory, possibly nociceptive, information. Release of ir-galanin in the spinal cord under *in vivo* conditions has been investigated with the antibody microprobe technique (Morton and Hutchison, 1989). Antibody microprobes are glass micropipettes coated on their outer surfaces with antibodies to a particular peptide (Duggan *et al.*, 1988a). After microprobe placement in the CNS, released peptide binds to that part of the microprobe shaft traversing the region of release. Subsequent incubation of the microprobe tips in a radiolabelled form of the peptide, and exposure of the tips to X-ray film highlights regions of endogenous peptide release as localized deficits of tracer binding. Microdensitometry of the autoradiograms enables quantification of peptide release (Hendry *et al.*, 1988). The sensitivity of microprobes is determined by measuring the degree of suppression of tracer binding produced by prior incubation of microprobes in known concentrations of unlabelled peptide (Figure 3.2A,E).

The use of this technique in the lower lumbar spinal cord of anaesthetized cats has revealed a basal, ongoing release of ir-galanin, in the absence of intentional somatic stimulation. This release has been detected in the region of the substantia gelatinosa, and also in the overlying pia mater at or just beneath the dorsal surface of the cord. Figure 3.2B illustrates computer-compiled mean image density scans of antibody microprobes which show these two zones of ir-galanin release in the cat spinal cord. A basal release of other neuropeptides, including ir-SP (Duggan *et al.*, 1987, 1988b), ir-somatostatin (Morton *et al.*, 1988, 1989), ir-CGRP (Morton and Hutchison, 1989) and ir-dynorphin A (Hutchison *et al.*, 1990), has also been detected in the superficial lumbar dorsal horn under similar experimental conditions.

The intraspinal release of several of these peptides is not influenced by impulses evoked in non-nociceptive primary afferent fibres, but is increased by impulses evoked in somatic nociceptive afferents by various forms of noxious stimulation or peripheral nerve stimulation procedures (Duggan *et al.*, 1988b, 1990; Morton *et al.*, 1988, 1989; Morton and Hutchison, 1989; Hutchison *et al.*, 1990). With ir-galanin, however, release detected in the substantia gelatinosa was of similar magnitude as basal release when measured during innocuous or noxious cutaneous stimulation (thermal or mechanical) or during electrical stimulation of a mixed muscle–cutaneous nerve (Figure 3.2B–D). Figure 3.2 compares this lack of evoked release of ir-galanin with release of ir-CGRP in the same spinal region produced by nociceptive afferent stimulation.

Ir-galanin occurs in a subpopulation of small DRG neurones (Ch'ng *et al.*, 1985; Ju *et al.*, 1987a; Garry *et al.*, 1989), the majority of which terminate in the superficial spinal laminae (Sugiura *et al.*, 1986). The basal release of ir-galanin in the superficial dorsal horn could therefore originate from the central terminals of ir-galanin-containing primary sensory neurones tonically active in this experimental preparation. In addition to afferents conveying non-nociceptive information from skin, muscle and viscera, the lower lumbar segments would have received continuous nociceptive input from areas subjected to surgery. Another possible source is ir-galanin-containing intrinsic spinal neurones which are localized in the upper dorsal horn (Rökaeus

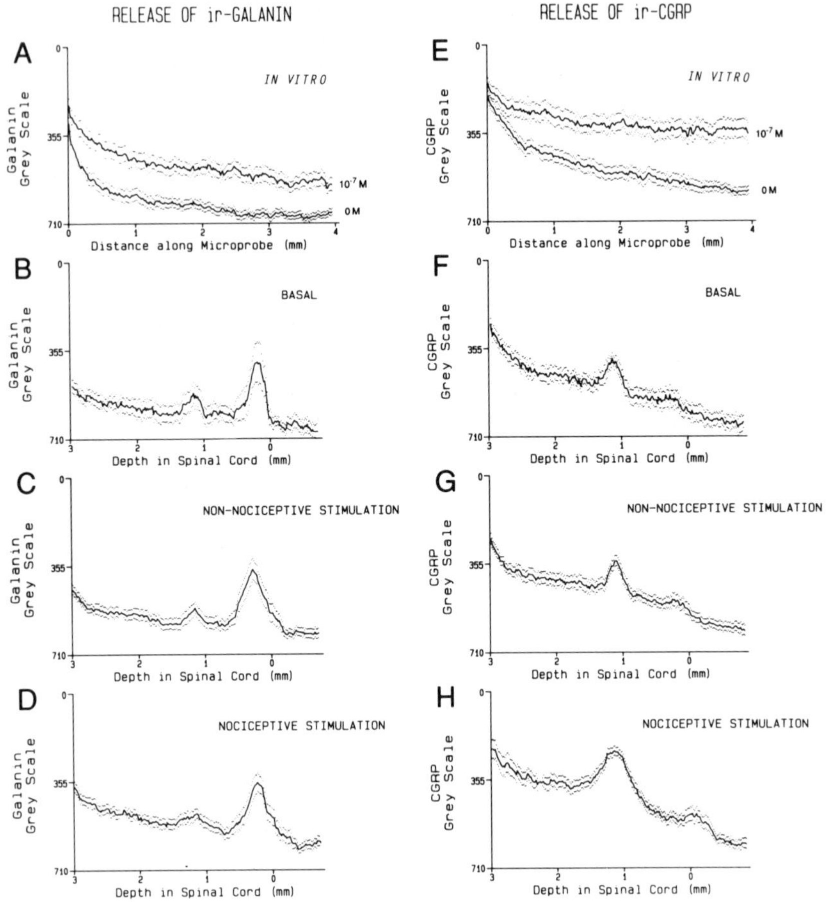

Figure 3.2. Release of ir-galanin and ir-CGRP in the lower lumbar spinal cord of cats. Digitized optical density values have been obtained for each microprobe autoradiogram (image density scans), and mean density scans (unbroken lines) and SEM (broken lines), calculated for groups of microprobes, have been plotted with respect to distance from the tip. (A,E) Mean image density scans of *in vitro* microprobes. Microprobes were exposed to 10^{-7} M galanin for 30 min (A, $n = 20$) or 10^{-7}M CGRP for 10 min (E, $n = 20$) prior to incubation in the appropriate radioiodinated peptide. The 0 M mean scans are of microprobes merely incubated in ^{125}I-galanin (A, $n = 31$) or ^{125}I-CGRP (E, $n = 31$) (*in vitro* zeros). (B,F) The mean scans (and SEM) of microprobes detecting ir-galanin release for 30 min (B, $n = 11$) or ir-CGRP release for 10 min (F, $n = 11$) in the absence of peripheral stimulation procedures. In B–D and F–H, microprobes were inserted 3 mm into the spinal cord; the cord surface is at 0 mm. (C,G) The mean scans (and SEM) of microprobes detecting ir-galanin release for 30 min (C, $n = 28$) or ir-CGRP release for 10 min (G, $n = 28$) during stimulation of non-nociceptive afferent fibres (innocuous cutaneous thermal or mechanical stimulation, or low-intensity tibial nerve stimulation). (D,H) The means scans (and SEM) of microprobes detecting ir-galanin release for 30 min (D, $n = 28$) or ir-CGRP release for 10 min (H, $n = 28$) during nociceptive afferent (noxious cutaneous thermal or mechanical, or high-intensity tibial nerve) stimulation. Non-nociceptive stimulation did not affect the basal release of either peptide in the substantia gelatinosa, whereas nociceptive stimulation significantly increased the release of ir-CGRP, but not that of ir-galanin.

Figure 3.2B reproduced, with permission, from Morton and Hutchison, 1989.

et al., 1984; Ch'ng *et al.*, 1985; Skofitsch and Jacobowitz, 1985a,b; Melander *et al.*, 1986b) and which may be driven from primary afferent or central sources. These experiments did not differentiate between these two possible sources of release. The origin and significance of the ir-galanin release detected at the spinal cord surface are less clear. Release of other neuropeptides in this region has also been noted, prompting the suggestion of release from pial afferent nerve endings in response to a local inflammation at sites of microprobe insertion (Duggan *et al.*, 1988b; Morton *et al.*, 1988, 1989; Morton and Hutchison, 1989; Hutchison *et al.*, 1990). Indeed, ir-galanin has been detected in sensory nerves in association with pial arteries in the rat (Suzuki *et al.*, 1989). However, regions of inflammation could also contain other substances which may interfere with the immunoassay at this site on microprobes, and further investigations are required to confirm the presence of ir-galanin release at the spinal cord surface.

It is clear that the question of galanin release in both the peripheral and central nervous systems deserves much more investigation.

3.4. *Putative functions of galanin*

The majority of investigations aimed at elucidating the possible physiological functions of galanin have concentrated on three main areas, each of which is discussed below.

3.4.1. **Hypothalamus**

Numerous studies have been directed at identifying a possible neuroendocrine role for galanin in hypothalamic-pituitary function, regions where ir-galanin has been localized (Ch'ng *et al.*, 1985; Skofitsch and Jacobowitz, 1985a, 1986; Köhler *et al.*, 1986; Melander *et al.*, 1986b). Intracerebroventricular administration of galanin to rats has produced a dose-dependent elevation of plasma levels of growth hormone and prolactin (Ottlecz *et al.*, 1986, 1988; Koshiyama *et al.*, 1987; Melander *et al.*, 1987; Murakami *et al.*, 1987, 1989) while similar administration of galanin antiserum has altered the normal pulsatile pattern of growth hormone secretion (Maiter *et al.*, 1990). Intravenous administration of galanin to rats and humans has also produced growth hormone release (Bauer *et al.*, 1986d; Ottlecz *et al.*, 1988; Murakami *et al.*, 1989). The inability of galanin to induce growth hormone release from *in vitro* anterior pituitary preparations has suggested that the stimulatory action of this peptide on growth hormone secretion probably operates through the hypothalamus (Ottlecz *et al.*, 1986, 1988; but see Gabriel *et al.*, 1988). There is evidence that the effect of galanin on growth hormone release is mediated by release of growth hormone-releasing factor, since pretreatment with antiserum to growth hormone-releasing factor blocks the galanin effect (Murakami *et al.*, 1987,

1989; Cella *et al.*, 1988), although a galanin-induced inhibition of somatostatin release may also contribute (Davis *et al.*, 1987; Cella *et al.*, 1988). The concensus from these studies is that hypothalamic galanin may regulate the secretion of anterior pituitary hormones under normal physiological conditions.

3.4.2. **Spinal cord**

The question of the function of galanin in the spinal cord has been the subject of numerous studies. Clearly, the inability of peripheral somatic stimulation to evoke intraspinal release of ir-galanin (Morton and Hutchison, 1989) does not preclude a role for this peptide in spinal synaptic transmission. It is possible, for example, that galanin may be present in visceral rather than cutaneous or muscle primary afferent fibres. Visceral afferents, although not yet demonstrated to contain ir-galanin, exhibit immunostaining for both ir-SP and ir-CGRP (Molander *et al.*, 1987), peptides which coexist with ir-galanin in some small DRG neurones (Ju *et al.*, 1987a). If this is the case, then the basal intraspinal release of ir-galanin (Morton and Hutchison, 1989) could well be increased under conditions of visceral nociception.

The possible participation of galanin in spinal sensory transmission has also been investigated using electrophysiological and behavioural models for nociception in rodents. It is well documented that lumbar intrathecal administration of SP to rats and mice evokes a caudally-directed scratching/biting behavioural response suggestive of pain perception, and increases the excitability of nociceptive flexion reflexes (Hylden and Wilcox, 1981; Seybold *et al.*, 1982; Wiesenfeld-Hallin *et al.*, 1984; Gamse and Saria, 1986; Woolf and Wiesenfeld-Hallin, 1986). As ir-SP is localized in small sensory neurones (reviewed in Nicoll *et al.*, 1980) and is released in the superficial spinal laminae during acute nociception (Duggan *et al.*, 1987, 1988b), these data collectively suggest that the exogenous SP may act upon structures normally activated by SP released from unmyelinated primary afferent terminals during nociceptive transmission. With intrathecal somatostatin, a similar behavioural response has been observed, but thermal rather than mechanical nociceptive reflexes were potentiated (Seybold *et al.*, 1982; Wiesenfeld-Hallin, 1985, 1986), a finding consistent with release of this peptide in the upper dorsal horn during noxious thermal, but not mechanical, cutaneous stimulation (Morton *et al.*, 1989).

Although intrathecal administration of galanin to rats also evokes behavioural signs of nociception (Cridland and Henry, 1988), the effects on spinal cord function are more complex (Figure 3.3). In unanaesthetized spinalized rats, low doses (10–100 ng) of intrathecal galanin facilitate a nociceptive flexor reflex (Wiesenfeld-Hallin *et al.*, 1988, 1989a), possibly mimicking sensory transmission. Increased doses (1–10 μg), however, have a biphasic effect (facilitation, then depression) while large doses (100 μg) are purely

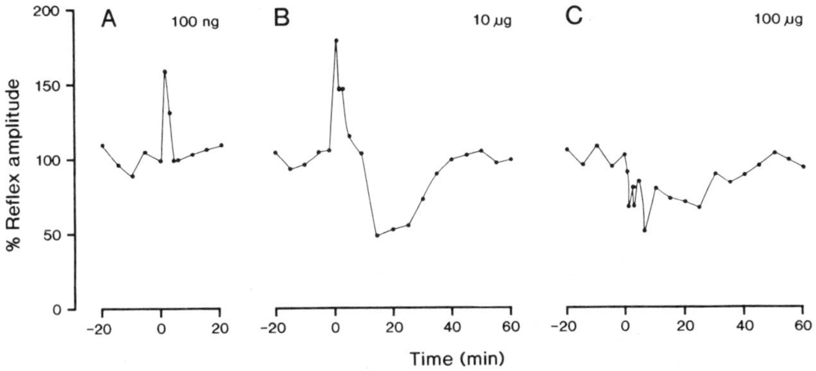

Figure 3.3. Effect of galanin on flexor reflex excitability in decerebrate, spinalized, unanaesthetized rats. The flexor reflex was elicited by electrical stimulation (1/min) of a sural nerve at an intensity suprathreshold for unmyelinated afferent fibres, and recorded as electromyogram activity in the ipsilateral biceps femoris/semitendinosus muscles. Integrated numbers of action potentials have been plotted with respect to time, with baseline reflex amplitude represented as 100%. Galanin 100 ng (A), 10 μg (B), or 100 μg (C), was injected intrathecally at the level of the lumbar enlargement (L_4–L_5) at 0 min.
Reproduced, with permission, from Wiesenfeld-Hallin *et al.*, 1989a.

depressive (Wiesenfeld-Hallin *et al.*, 1989a), and these higher doses have produced hypoalgesic effects in standard analgesic testing procedures (tail flick, hot plate) (Cridland and Henry, 1988; Post *et al.*, 1988). Moreover, intrathecal galanin antagonizes the nociceptive flexor reflex facilitation produced by conditioning stimulation of unmyelinated primary afferents or by intrathecal administration of SP or CGRP (Wiesenfeld-Hallin *et al.*, 1989a; Xu *et al.*, 1989, 1990b). These spinal effects of galanin appear to be mediated by the N-terminal portion of the peptide (Xu *et al.*, 1990a), but the mechanism involved is not known. It is possible that the galanin-induced antagonism of the conditioning stimulation-induced reflex facilitation could involve presynaptic inhibition of transmitter release from primary afferent terminals. There is evidence from other studies that galanin may inhibit release of neuroactive substances in the CNS (Fisone *et al.*, 1987; Nordström *et al.*, 1987; Dutar *et al.*, 1989; Tsuda *et al.*, 1989; Ben-Ari, 1990) and from sensory neurones (Giuliani *et al.*, 1989). Moreover, axotomy of a peripheral nerve enhances both galanin synthesis in DRG neurones and the inhibitory effect of intrathecal galanin, responses which have been suggested to occur to counteract, by inhibition of release from primary afferents, the increased nociceptive afferent input following nerve section (Hökfelt *et al.*, 1987; Villar *et al.*, 1989; Wiesenfeld-Hallin *et al.*, 1989b; Xu *et al.*, 1990b). This may also explain the relatively low level of ir-galanin release detected in the dorsal horn of non-axotomized animals (Morton and Hutchison, 1989). However, the inhibitory interactions of galanin with exogenous SP and CGRP (Xu *et al.*, 1989, 1990b) suggest a postsynaptic action of galanin in the spinal cord. A direct action on motoneurones has been suggested (Cridland and Henry, 1988), and in fact galanin has produced inhibition of a monosynaptic reflex in the neonatal rat spinal cord *in vitro* (Yanagisawa *et al.*, 1986), but this was not observed in adult rats *in vivo* (Wiesenfeld-Hallin *et al.*, 1989a). It is conceivable that galanin could act on interneurones in polysynaptic reflex pathways, but this will require experimental confirmation. With some neuropeptides (e.g. somatostatin, dynorphin A), the interpretation of their effects following direct administration to the spinal cord is made more difficult by the possibility of neurotoxicity secondary to alterations in spinal cord blood flow (Long *et al.*, 1988; Mollenholt *et al.*, 1988), but such circulatory effects were not observed following application of galanin to the lumbar cord surface (Wiesenfeld-Hallin *et al.*, 1989a). The extent to which galanin penetrates into the spinal cord to access intraspinal structures is unknown, and the interpretation of the observed spinal effects of this peptide is also complicated by the possibility of an action of intrathecal galanin in the pia mater where ir-galanin is localized (Suzuki *et al.*, 1989) and released (Morton and Hutchison, 1989). Further studies are required to clarify the relationships between the pharmacological effects of this peptide on spinal cord function, and its role in spinal cord physiology.

3.4.3. **Periphery**

Initial pharmacological experiments in the dog revealed that galanin, infused intravenously, produced hyperglycaemia (Tatemoto *et al.*, 1983), which was found to be associated with inhibition of insulin secretion (McDonald *et al.*, 1985). This finding was subsequently confirmed in rodents (Schnuerer *et al.*, 1987; Lindskog and Ahrén, 1987). Electrical stimulation of the mixed autonomic pancreatic nerves in the dog increased pancreatic venous ir-galanin concentrations and also altered the pancreatic secretion of ir-insulin (decreased), ir-somatostatin (decreased), and ir-glycogen (increased), effects which were mimicked by infusion of an appropriate dose of galanin into the pancreatic artery (Dunning and Taborsky, 1989). These effects may be species specific, however, since similar stimulation of the mixed pancreatic nerves in pigs elevated the pancreatic venous levels of ir-neuropeptide Y, but not ir-galanin (Ahrén *et al.*, 1989). In any event, electrical stimulation of nerves is an unphysiological procedure, and the normal conditions under which these pancreatic nerves might release galanin (and thereby influence pancreatic hormone output) remain to be determined. Nevertheless, it appears that galanin in intrapancreatic nerves may play some role in the regulation of pancreatic hormone secretion.

Evidence for functional roles for galanin in the other tissues in which it is localized is sparse at present. For example, pharmacological experiments have failed to demonstrate any effect of exogenous galanin on isolated guinea-pig respiratory tissues (Ekblad *et al.*, 1985a), where ir-galanin-containing nerve fibres have been localized in this species (Cheung *et al.*,

1985). Fibres containing ir-galanin have been identified in the urinary bladder (Bauer *et al.*, 1986c), and galanin has been reported to evoke dose-dependent contractions of the isolated bladder of the rat (Tatemoto *et al.*, 1983). This effect may be species or receptor specific, since similar concentrations of galanin were subsequently found to inhibit the atropine-sensitive component of contractions induced by field stimulation of human bladder, suggesting a prejunctional action of inhibition of acetylcholine release (Maggi *et al.*, 1987). In the rat vas deferens, there is also evidence for a presynaptic action of galanin to enhance noradrenaline release from sympathetic nerve terminals (Ohhashi and Jacobowitz, 1985). The precise role of this peptide in urogenital function, however, remains to be fully elucidated. The innervation of the gastrointestinal tract by intrinsic neurones which immunostain for ir-galanin (Rökaeus *et al.*, 1984; Ekblad *et al.*, 1985b; Melander *et al.*, 1985a; Bishop *et al.*, 1986; Furness *et al.*, 1987; Hoyle and Burnstock, 1989), and the responses produced by galanin in various gut preparations *in vitro* (Tatemoto *et al.*, 1983; Ekblad *et al.*, 1985a; Fox *et al.*, 1986), suggest that galanin may regulate or modulate gastrointestinal function. The exact nature of this proposed action, however, has yet to be established. Similarly, the physiological roles of galanin in autonomic ganglia and/or autonomic control of various target organs (Tainio *et al.*, 1987; Kummer, 1987; Lindh *et al.*, 1989), and in the adrenal medulla (Bauer *et al.*, 1986b; Rökaeus and Brownstein, 1986) and the thyroid gland (Grunditz *et al.*, 1987), are still conjectural.

From the published literature to date, it is clear that there is widespread interest in the neuropeptide galanin. The majority of this work concerns the localization of galanin in various tissues and species, with much less evidence available for the physiological *raison d'être* of this peptide in particular tissues and systems. Our understanding of the functional significance of many of the biological observations of galanin will be enhanced by increased knowledge of the physiological conditions under which galanin is released in the body and the relevance of pharmacological actions to physiological function.

References

Ahrén, B., Martensson, H. and Ekman, R. (1989). Pancreatic nerve stimulation releases neuropeptide Y- but not galanin- or calcitonin gene-related peptide-like immunoreactivity from the pig pancreas. *Journal of the Autonomic Nervous System*, **27**, 11–16.

Bauer, F.E., Adrian, T.E., Christofides, N.D., Ferri, G.-L., Yanaihara, N., Polak, J.M. and Bloom, S.R. (1986a). Distribution and molecular heterogeneity of galanin in human, pig, guinea pig, and rat gastrointestinal tracts. *Gastroenterology*, **91**, 877–883.

Bauer, F.E., Adrian, T.E., Yanaihara, N., Polak, J.M. and Bloom, S.R. (1986b). Chromatographic evidence for high-molecular-mass galanin immunoreactivity in pig and cat adrenal glands. *FEBS Letters*, **201**, 327–331.

Bauer, F.E., Christofides, N.D., Hacker, G.W., Blank, M.A., Polak, J.M. and Bloom, S.R. (1986c). Distribution of galanin immunoreactivity in the genitourinary tract of man and rat. *Peptides*, **7**, 5–10.

Bauer, F.E., Ginsberg, L., Venetikou, M., MacKay, D.J., Burrin, J.M. and Bloom, S.R. (1986d). Growth hormone release in man induced by galanin, a new hypothalamic peptide. *Lancet*, **2**, 192–195.

Beal, M.F., Gabriel, S.M., Swartz, K.J. and MacGarvey, U.M. (1988). Distribution of galanin-like immunoreactivity in baboon brain. *Peptides*, **9**, 847–851.

Ben-Ari, Y. (1990). Galanin and glibenclamide modulate the anoxic release of glutamate in rat CA3 hippocampal neurons. *European Journal of Neuroscience*, **2**, 62–68.

Bishop, A.E., Polak, J.M., Bauer, F.E., Christofides, N.D., Carlei, F. and Bloom, S.R. (1986). Occurrence and distribution of a newly discovered peptide, galanin, in the mammalian enteric nervous system. *Gut*, **27**, 849–857.

Brownstein, M.J. and Mezey, É. (1986). Multiple chemical messengers in hypothalamic magnocellular neurons. In: *Progress in Brain Research*, Vol. 68, edited by T. Hökfelt, K. Fuxe and B. Pernow. Amsterdam: Elsevier, pp. 161–168.

Calvo, J.J., Freire de Carvalho, L., Gonzalez, R., Burnet, P.W.J., Ghatei, M.A. and Bloom, S.R. (1990). Effect of ACTH on VIP and galanin release from the pituitary. *Endocrinology*, **126**, 1283–1287.

Cella, S.G., Locatelli, V., De Gennaro, V., Bondiolotti, G.P., Pintor, C., Loche, S., Provezza, M. and Müller, E.E. (1988). Epinephrine mediates the growth hormone-releasing effect of galanin in infant rats. *Endocrinology*, **122**, 855–859.

Ch'ng, J.L., Christofides, N.D., Anand, P., Gibson, S.J., Allen, Y.S., Su, H.C., Tatemoto, K., Morrison, J.F., Polak, J.M. and Bloom, S.R. (1985). Distribution of galanin immunoreactivity in the central nervous system and the responses of galanin-containing neuronal pathways to injury. *Neuroscience*, **16**, 343–354.

Cheung, A., Bauer, E., Christofides, N., Bloom, S.R. and Polak, J.M. (1984). Immunocytochemical localization of galanin in the porcine respiratory tract. *Regulatory Peptides*, **9**, 327.

Cheung, A., Polak, J.M., Bauer, F.E., Cadieux, A., Christofides, N.D., Springall, D.R. and Bloom, S.R. (1985). Distribution of galanin immunoreactivity in the respiratory tract of pig, guinea pig, rat, and dog. *Thorax*, **40**, 889–896.

Cridland, R.A. and Henry, J.L. (1988). Effects of intrathecal administration of neuropeptides on a spinal nociceptive reflex in the rat: VIP, galanin, CGRP, TRH, somatostatin and angiotensin II. *Neuropeptides*, **11**, 23–32.

Davis, T.M., Burrin, J.M. and Bloom, S.R. (1987). Growth hormone (GH) release in response to GH-releasing hormone in man is 3-fold enhanced by galanin. *Journal of Clinical Endocrinology and Metabolism*, **65**, 1248–1252.

Duggan, A.W., Morton, C.R., Zhao, Z.Q. and Hendry, I.A. (1987). Noxious heating of the skin releases immunoreactive substance P in the substantia gelatinosa of the cat: a study with antibody microprobes. *Brain Research*, **403**, 345–349.

Duggan, A.W., Hendry, I.A., Green, J.L., Morton, C.R. and Hutchison, W.D. (1988a). The preparation and use of antibody microprobes. *Journal of Neuroscience Methods*, **23**, 241–247.

Duggan, A.W., Hendry, I.A., Morton, C.R., Hutchison, W.D. and Zhao, Z.Q. (1988b). Cutaneous stimuli releasing immunoreactive substance P in the dorsal horn of the cat. *Brain Research*, **451**, 261–273.

Duggan, A.W., Hope, P.J., Jarrott, B., Schaible, H.-G. and Fleetwood-Walker, S.M. (1990). Release, spread and persistence of immunoreactive neurokinin A in the dorsal horn of the cat following noxious cutaneous stimulation. Studies with antibody microprobes. *Neuroscience*, **35**, 195–202.

Dunning, B.E. and Taborsky, G.J. (1989). Galanin release during pancreatic nerve

stimulation is sufficient to influence islet function. *American Journal of Physiology*, **256**, E191–E198.
Dunning, B.E., Ahrén, B., Veith, R.C., Böttcher, G., Sundler, F. and Taborsky, G.J. (1986). Galanin: a novel pancreatic neuropeptide. *American Journal of Physiology*, **251**, E127–E133.
Dutar, P., Lamour, Y. and Nicoll, R.A. (1989). Galanin blocks the slow cholinergic EPSP in CA1 pyramidal neurons from ventral hippocampus. *European Journal of Pharmacology*, **164**, 355–360.
Ekblad, E., Håkanson, R., Sundler, F. and Wahlestedt, C. (1985a). Galanin: neuromodulatory and direct contractile effects on smooth muscle preparations. *British Journal of Pharmacology*, **86**, 241–246.
Ekblad, E., Rökaeus, Å., Håkanson, R. and Sundler, F. (1985b). Galanin nerve fibers in the rat gut: distribution, origin and projections. *Neuroscience*, **16**, 355–363.
Fisone, G., Wu, C.F., Consolo, S., Nordström, Ö., Brynne, N., Bartfai, T., Melander, T. and Hökfelt, T. (1987). Galanin inhibits acetylcholine release in the ventral hippocampus of the rat: Histochemical, autoradiographic, *in vivo*, and *in vitro* studies. *Proceedings of the National Academy of Sciences USA*, **84**, 7339–7343.
Fox, J.E., McDonald, T.J., Kostolanska, F. and Tatemoto, K. (1986). Galanin: an inhibitory neural peptide of the canine small intestine. *Life Sciences*, **39**, 103–110.
Furness, J.B., Costa, M., Rökaeus, A., McDonald, T.J. and Brooks, B. (1987). Galanin-immunoreactive neurons in the guinea-pig small intestine: their projections and relationships to other enteric neurons. *Cell and Tissue Research*, **250**, 607–615.
Gabriel, S.M., Milbury, C.M., Nathanson, J.A. and Martin, J.B. (1988). Galanin stimulates rat pituitary growth hormone secretion *in vitro*. *Life Sciences*, **42**, 1981–1986.
Gamse, R. and Saria, A. (1986). Nociceptive behavior after intrathecal injections of substance P, neurokinin A and calcitonin gene-related peptide in mice. *Neuroscience Letters*, **70**, 143–147.
Garry, M.G., Miller, K.E. and Seybold, V.S. (1989). Lumbar dorsal root ganglia of the cat: a quantitative study of peptide immunoreactivity and cell size. *Journal of Comparative Neurology*, **284**, 36–47.
Gentleman, S.M., Falkai, P., Bogerts, B., Herrero, M.T., Polak, J.M. and Roberts, G.W. (1989). Distribution of galanin-like immunoreactivity in the human brain. *Brain Research*, **505**, 311–315.
Ghatei, M.A., Springall, D.R., Richards, I.M., Oostveen, J.A., Griffin, R.L., Cadieux, A., Polak, J.M. and Bloom, S.R. (1987). Regulatory peptides in the respiratory tract of *Macaca fascicularis*. *Thorax*, **42**, 431–439.
Gibson, S.J., McCrossan, M.V. and Polak, J.M. (1985). A subset of calcitonin gene-related peptide (CGRP)-immunoreactive cells contain substance P (SP), somatostatin (SOM) or galanin (GAL) immunoreactivity in pig dorsal root ganglia. *Regulatory Peptides*, **13**, 68.
Gibson, S.J., Polak, J.M., Katagiri, T., Su, H., Weller, R.O., Brownell, D.B., Holland, S., Hughes, J.T., Kikuyama, S., Ball, J., Bloom, S.R., Steiner, T.J., de Belleroche, J. and Rose, F.C. (1988). A comparison of the distributions of eight peptides in spinal cord from normal controls and cases of motor neurone disease with special reference to Onuf's nucleus. *Brain Research*, **474**, 255–278.
Giuliani, S., Amann, R., Papini, A.M., Maggi, C.A. and Meli, A. (1989). Modulatory action of galanin on responses due to antidromic activation of peripheral terminals of capsaicin-sensitive sensory nerves. *European Journal of Pharmacology*, **163**, 91–96.

Grunditz, T., Håkanson, R., Sundler, F. and Uddman, R. (1987). Neurokinin A and galanin in the thyroid gland: neuronal localization. *Endocrinology*, **121**, 575–585.

Hendry, I.A., Morton, C.R. and Duggan, A.W. (1988). Analysis of antibody microprobe autoradiographs by computerized image processing. *Journal of Neuroscience Methods*, **23**, 249–256.

Hökfelt, T., Wiesenfeld-Hallin, Z., Villar, M. and Melander, T. (1987). Increase of galanin-like immunoreactivity in rat dorsal root ganglion cells after peripheral axotomy. *Neuroscience Letters*, **83**, 217–220.

Holets, V.R., Hökfelt, T., Rökaeus, Å., Terenius, L. and Goldstein, M. (1988). Locus coeruleus neurons in the rat containing neuropeptide Y, tyrosine hydroxylase or galanin and their efferent projections to the spinal cord, cerebral cortex and hypothalamus. *Neuroscience*, **24**, 893–906.

Hoyle, C.H. and Burnstock, G. (1989). Galanin-like immunoreactivity in enteric neurons of the human colon. *Journal of Anatomy*, **166**, 23–33.

Hutchison, W.D., Morton, C.R. and Terenius, L. (1990). Dynorphin A: *in vivo* release in the spinal cord of the cat. *Brain Research*, **532**, 299–306.

Hylden, J.L.K. and Wilcox, G.L. (1981). Intrathecal substance P elicits a caudally-directed biting and scratching behavior in mice. *Brain Research*, **217**, 212–215.

Johansson, O., Vaalasti, A., Tainio, H. and Ljungberg, A. (1988). Immunohistochemical evidence of galanin in sensory nerves of human digital skin. *Acta Physiologica Scandinavica*, **132**, 261–263.

Ju, G., Hökfelt, T., Brodin, E., Fahrenkrug, J., Fischer, J.A., Frey, P., Elde, R.P. and Brown, J.C. (1987a). Primary sensory neurons of the rat showing calcitonin gene-related peptide immunoreactivity and their relation to substance P-, somatostatin-, galanin-, vasoactive intestinal polypeptide- and cholecystokinin-immunoreactive ganglion cells. *Cell and Tissue Research*, **247**, 417–431.

Ju, G., Melander, T., Ceccatelli, S., Hökfelt, T. and Frey, P. (1987b). Immunohistochemical evidence for a spinothalamic pathway co-containing cholecystokinin- and galanin-like immunoreactivities in the rat. *Neuroscience*, **20**, 439–456.

Kaplan, L.M., Spindel, E.R., Isselbacher, K.J. and Chin, W.W. (1988). Tissue-specific expression of the rat galanin gene. *Proceedings of the National Academy of Sciences USA*, **85**, 1065–1069.

Köhler, C., Hallman, H., Melander, T., Hökfelt, T. and Norheim, E. (1989a). Autoradiographic mapping of galanin receptors in the monkey brain. *Journal of Chemical Neuroanatomy*, **2**, 269–284.

Köhler, C., Persson, A., Melander, T., Theodorsson, E., Sedvall, G. and Hökfelt, T. (1989b). Distribution of galanin-binding sites in the monkey and human telencephalon: preliminary observations. *Experimental Brain Research*, **75**, 375–380.

Köhler, C., Ericson, H., Watanabe, T., Polak, J., Palay, S.L., Palay, V. and Chan-Palay, V. (1986). Galanin immunoreactivity in hypothalamic histamine neurons: further evidence for multiple chemical messengers in the tuberomammillary nucleus. *Journal of Comparative Neurology*, **250**, 58–64.

Koshiyama, H., Kato, Y., Inoue, T., Murakami, Y., Ishikawa, Y., Yanaihara, N. and Imura, H. (1987). Central galanin stimulates pituitary prolactin secretion in rats: possible involvement of hypothalamic vasoactive intestinal polypeptide. *Neuroscience Letters*, **75**, 49–54.

Kummer, W. (1987). Galanin- and neuropeptide Y-like immunoreactivities coexist in paravertebral sympathetic neurones of the cat. *Neuroscience Letters*, **78**, 127–131.

Lindh, B., Lundberg, J.M. and Hökfelt, T. (1989). NPY-, galanin-, VIP/PHI-, CGRP- and substance P-immunoreactive neuronal subpopulations in cat autonomic and sensory ganglia and their projections. *Cell and Tissue Research*, **256**, 259–273.

Lindskog, S. and Ahrén, B. (1987). Galanin: effects on basal and stimulated insulin and glucagon secretion in the mouse. *Acta Physiologica Scandinavica*, **129**, 305–309.

Long, J.B., Martinez-Arizala, A., Echevarria, E.E., Tidwell, R.E. and Holaday, J.W. (1988). Hindlimb paralytic effects of prodynorphin-derived peptides following spinal subarachnoid injection in rats. *European Journal of Pharmacology*, **153**, 45–54.

Luts, A., Uddman, R. and Sundler, F. (1989). Neuronal galanin is widely distributed in the chicken respiratory tract and coexists with multiple neuropeptides. *Cell and Tissue Research*, **256**, 95–103.

Maggi, C.A., Santicioli, P., Patacchini, R., Turini, D., Barbanti, G., Beneforti, P., Giuliani, S. and Meli, A. (1987). Galanin: a potent modulator of excitatory neurotransmission in the human urinary bladder. *European Journal of Pharmacology*, **143**, 135–137.

Maiter, D.M., Hooi, S.C., Koenig, J.I. and Martin, J.B. (1990). Galanin is a physiological regulator of spontaneous pulsatile secretion of growth hormone in the male rat. *Endocrinology*, **126**, 1216–1222.

McDonald, T.J., Dupre, J., Tatemoto, K., Greenberg, G.R., Radziuk, J. and Mutt, V. (1985). Galanin inhibits insulin secretion and induces hyperglycemia in dogs. *Diabetes*, **34**, 192–196.

Melander, T. and Staines, W.A. (1986). A galanin-like peptide coexists in putative cholinergic somata of the septum-basal forebrain complex and in acetylcholinesterase-containing fibers and varicosities within the hippocampus in the owl monkey (*Aotus trivirgatus*). *Neuroscience Letters*, **68**, 17–22.

Melander, T., Fuxe, K., Härfstrand, A., Eneroth, P. and Hökfelt, T. (1987). Effects of intraventricular injections of galanin on neuroendocrine functions in the male rat. Possible involvement of hypothalamic catecholamine neuronal systems. *Acta Physiologica Scandinavica*, **131**, 25–32.

Melander, T., Hökfelt, T., Nilsson, S. and Brodin, E. (1986a). Visualization of galanin binding sites in the rat central nervous system. *European Journal of Pharmacology*, **124**, 381–382.

Melander, T., Hökfelt, T. and Rökaeus, Å. (1986b). Distribution of galanin-like immunoreactivity in the rat central nervous system. *Journal of Comparative Neurology*, **248**, 475–517.

Melander, T., Hökfelt, T., Rökaeus, Å., Cuello, A.C., Oertel, W.H., Verhofstad, A. and Goldstein, M. (1986c). Coexistence of galanin-like immunoreactivity with catecholamines, 5-hydroxytryptamine, GABA and neuropeptides in the rat CNS. *Journal of Neuroscience*, **6**, 3640–3654.

Melander, T., Hökfelt, T., Rökaeus, Å., Fahrenkrug, J., Tatemoto, K. and Mutt, V. (1985a). Distribution of galanin-like immunoreactivity in the gastro-intestinal tract of several mammalian species. *Cell and Tissue Research*, **239**, 253–270.

Melander, T., Köhler, C., Nilsson, S., Hökfelt, T., Brodin, E., Theodorsson, E. and Bartfai, T. (1988). Autoradiographic quantitation and anatomical mapping of ^{125}I-galanin binding sites in the rat central nervous system. *Journal of Chemical Neuroanatomy*, **1**, 213–233.

Melander, T., Staines, W.A., Hökfelt, T., Rökaeus, Å., Eckenstein, F., Salvaterra, P.M. and Wainer, B.H. (1985b). Galanin-like immunoreactivity in cholinergic neurons of the septum-basal forebrain complex projecting to the hippocampus of the rat. *Brain Research*, **360**, 130–138.

Melander, T., Staines, W.A. and Rökaeus, Å. (1986d). Galanin-like immunoreactivity in hippocampal afferents in the rat, with special reference to cholinergic and noradrenergic inputs. *Neuroscience*, **19**, 223–240.

Molander, C., Ygge, J. and Dalsgaard, C.-J. (1987). Substance P-, somatostatin- and calcitonin gene-related peptide-like immunoreactivity and fluoride resistant acid phosphatase-activity in relation to retrogradely labeled cutaneous, muscular and visceral primary sensory neurons in the rat. *Neuroscience Letters*, **74**, 37–42.

Mollenholt, P., Post, C., Rawal, N., Freedman, J., Hökfelt, T. and Paulsson, I. (1988). Antinociceptive and 'neurotoxic' actions of somatostatin in rat spinal cord after intrathecal administration. *Pain*, **32**, 95–105.

Moore, R.Y. (1989). Cranial motor neurons contain either galanin- or calcitonin gene-related peptide-like immunoreactivity. *Journal of Comparative Neurology*, **282**, 512–522.

Morton, C.R. and Hutchison, W.D. (1989). Release of sensory neuropeptides in the spinal cord: studies with calcitonin gene-related peptide and galanin. *Neuroscience*, **31**, 807–815.

Morton, C.R., Hutchison, W.D. and Hendry, I.A. (1988). Release of immunoreactive somatostatin in the spinal dorsal horn of the cat. *Neuropeptides*, **12**, 189–197.

Morton, C.R., Hutchison, W.D., Hendry, I.A. and Duggan, A.W. (1989). Somatostatin: evidence for a role in thermal nociception. *Brain Research*, **488**, 89–96.

Murakami, Y., Kato, Y., Koshiyama, H., Inoue, T., Yanaihara, N. and Imura, H. (1987). Galanin stimulates growth hormone (GH) secretion via GH-releasing factor (GRF) in conscious rats. *European Journal of Pharmacology*, **136**, 415–418.

Murakami, Y., Kato, Y., Shimatsu, A., Koshiyama, H., Hattori, N., Yanaihara, N. and Imura, H. (1989). Possible mechanisms involved in growth hormone secretion induced by galanin in the rat. *Endocrinology*, **124**, 1224–1229.

Nicoll, R.A., Schenker, C. and Leeman, S.E. (1980). Substance P as a transmitter candidate. *Annual Review of Neuroscience*, **3**, 227–268.

Nordström, Ö., Melander, T., Hökfelt, T., Bartfai, T. and Goldstein, M. (1987). Evidence for an inhibitory effect of the peptide galanin on dopamine release from the rat median eminence. *Neuroscience Letters*, **73**, 21–26.

Ohhashi, T. and Jacobowitz, D.M. (1985). Galanin potentiates electrical stimulation and exogenous norepinephrine-induced contractions in the rat vas deferens. *Regulatory Peptides*, **12**, 163–171.

Ottlecz, A., Samson, W.K. and McCann, S.M. (1986). Galanin: evidence for a hypothalamic site of action to release growth hormone. *Peptides*, **7**, 51–53.

Ottlecz, A., Snyder, G.D. and McCann, S.M. (1988). Regulatory role of galanin in control of hypothalamic-anterior pituitary function. *Proceedings of the National Academy of Sciences USA*, **85**, 9861–9865.

Papka, R.E. and Traurig, H.H. (1989). Galanin-immunoreactive nerves in the female rat paracervical ganglion and uterine cervix: distribution and reaction to capsaicin. *Cell and Tissue Research*, **257**, 41–51.

Post, C., Alari, L. and Hökfelt, T. (1988). Intrathecal galanin increases the latency in the tail-flick and hot-plate tests in mouse. *Acta Physiologica Scandinavica*, **132**, 583–584.

Rökaeus, Å. (1987). Galanin: a newly isolated biologically active neuropeptide. *Trends in Neuroscience*, **10**, 158–164.

Rökaeus, Å. and Brownstein, M.J. (1986). Construction of a porcine adrenal medullary cDNA library and nucleotide sequence analysis of two clones encoding a galanin precursor. *Proceedings of the National Academy of Sciences USA*, **83**, 6287–6291.

Rökaeus, Å., Melander, T., Hökfelt, T., Lundberg, J.M., Tatemoto, K., Carlquist, M. and Mutt, V. (1984). A galanin-like peptide in the central nervous system and intestine of the rat. *Neuroscience Letters*, **47**, 161–166.

Sawchenko, P.E. and Pfeiffer, S.W. (1988). Ultrastructural localization of neuropeptide Y and galanin immunoreactivity in the paraventricular nucleus of the hypothalamus in the rat. *Brain Research*, **474**, 231–245.

Schnuerer, E.M., McDonald, T.J. and Dupre, J. (1987). Inhibition of insulin release by galanin and gastrin-releasing peptide in the anaesthetized rat. *Regulatory Peptides*, **18**, 307–320.

Servin, A.L., Amiranoff, B., Rouyer-Fessard, C., Tatemoto, K. and Laburthe, M. (1987). Identification and molecular characterization of galanin receptor sites in rat brain. *Biochemical and Biophysical Research Communications*, **144**, 298–306.

Seybold, V.S., Hylden, J.L.K. and Wilcox, G.L. (1982). Intrathecal substance P and somatostatin in rats: behaviors indicative of sensation. *Peptides*, **3**, 49–54.

Skofitsch, G. and Jacobowitz, D.M. (1985a). Immunohistochemical mapping of galanin-like neurons in the rat central nervous system. *Peptides*, **6**, 509–546.

Skofitsch, G. and Jacobowitz, D.M. (1985b). Galanin-like immunoreactivity in capsaicin sensitive sensory neurons and ganglia. *Brain Research Bulletin*, **15**, 191–195.

Skofitsch, G. and Jacobowitz, D.M. (1986). Quantitative distribution of galanin-like immunoreactivity in the rat central nervous system. *Peptides*, **7**, 609–613.

Skofitsch, G., Sills, M.A. and Jacobowitz, D.M. (1986). Autoradiographic distribution of ^{125}I-galanin binding sites in the rat central nervous system. *Peptides*, **7**, 1029–1042.

Stenfors, C., Theodorsson, E. and Mathé, A.A. (1989). Effect of repeated electroconvulsive treatment on regional concentrations of tachykinins, neurotensin, vasoactive intestinal polypeptide, neuropeptide Y, and galanin in rat brain. *Journal of Neuroscience Research*, **24**, 445–450.

Stjernquist, M., Ekblad, E., Owman, C. and Sundler, F. (1988). Immunocytochemical localization of galanin in the rat male and female genital tracts and motor effects *in vitro*. *Regulatory Peptides*, **20**, 335–343.

Sugiura, Y., Lee, C.L. and Perl, E.R. (1986). Central projections of identified, unmyelinated (C) afferent fibers innervating mammalian skin. *Science*, **234**, 358–361.

Suzuki, N., Hardebo, J.E., Kåhrström, J. and Owman, C. (1989). Galanin-positive nerves of trigeminal origin innervate rat cerebral vessels. *Neuroscience Letters*, **100**, 123–129.

Tainio, H., Vaalasti, A. and Rechardt, L. (1987). The distribution of substance P-, CGRP-, galanin- and ANP-like immunoreactive nerves in human sweat glands. *Histochemical Journal*, **19**, 375–380.

Tatemoto, K., Rökaeus, Å., Jörnvall, H., McDonald, T.J. and Mutt, V. (1983). Galanin — a novel biologically active peptide from porcine intestine. *FEBS Letters*, **164**, 124–128.

Tsuda, K., Yokoo, H. and Goldstein, M. (1989). Neuropeptide Y and galanin in norepinephrine release in hypothalamic slices. *Hypertension*, **14**, 81–86.

Tuchscherer, M.M. and Seybold, V.S. (1989). A quantitative study of the coexistence of peptides in varicosities within the superficial laminae of the dorsal horn of the rat spinal cord. *Journal of Neuroscience*, **9**, 195–205.

Villar, M.J., Cortés, R., Theodorsson, E., Wiesenfeld-Hallin, Z., Schalling, M., Fahrenkrug, J., Emson, P.C. and Hökfelt, T. (1989). Neuropeptide expression in rat dorsal root ganglion cells and spinal cord after peripheral nerve injury with special reference to galanin. *Neuroscience*, **33**, 587–604.

Wiesenfeld-Hallin, Z. (1985). Intrathecal somatostatin modulates spinal sensory and reflex mechanisms; behavioral and electrophysiological studies in the rat. *Neuroscience Letters*, **62**, 69–74.

Wiesenfeld-Hallin, Z. (1986). Substance P and somatostatin modulate spinal cord excitability via physiologically different sensory pathways. *Brain Research*, **372**, 172–175.

Wiesenfeld-Hallin, Z., Villar, M.J. and Hökfelt, T. (1988). Intrathecal galanin at low doses increases spinal reflex excitability in rats more to thermal than mechanical stimuli. *Experimental Brain Research*, **71**, 663–666.

Wiesenfeld-Hallin, Z., Villar, M.J. and Hökfelt, T. (1989a). The effects of intrathecal galanin and C-fiber stimulation on the flexor reflex in the rat. *Brain Research*, **486**, 205–213.

Wiesenfeld-Hallin, Z., Xu, X.-J., Villar, M.J. and Hökfelt, T. (1989b). The effect of intrathecal galanin on the flexor reflex in rat: increased depression after sciatic nerve section. *Neuroscience Letters*, **105**, 149–154.

Wiesenfeld-Hallin, Z., Hökfelt, T., Lundberg, J.M., Forssmann, W.G., Reinecke, M., Tschopp, F.A. and Fischer, J.A. (1984). Immunoreactive calcitonin gene-related peptide and substance P coexist in sensory neurons to the spinal cord and interact in spinal behavioral responses of the rat. *Neuroscience Letters*, **52**, 199–204.

Woolf, C. and Wiesenfeld-Hallin, Z. (1986). Substance P and calcitonin gene-related peptide synergistically modulate the gain of the nociceptive flexor withdrawal reflex in the rat. *Neuroscience Letters*, **66**, 226–230.

Xu, X.-J., Wiesenfeld-Hallin, Z., Villar, M.J. and Hökfelt, T. (1989). Intrathecal galanin antagonizes the facilitatory effect of substance P on the nociceptive flexor reflex in the rat. *Acta Physiologica Scandinavica*, **137**, 463–464.

Xu, X.-J., Wiesenfeld-Hallin, Z., Fisone, G., Bartfai, T. and Hökfelt, T. (1990a). The N-terminal 1–16, but not C-terminal 17–29, galanin fragment affects the flexor reflex in rats. *European Journal of Pharmacology*, **182**, 137–141.

Xu, X.-J., Wiesenfeld-Hallin, Z., Villar, M.J., Fahrenkrug, J. and Hökfelt, T. (1990b). On the role of galanin, substance P and other neuropeptides in primary sensory neurons of rat: studies on spinal reflex excitability and peripheral axotomy. *European Journal of Neuroscience*, **2**, 733–743.

Yanagisawa, M., Yagi, N., Otsuka, M., Yanaihara, C. and Yanaihara, N. (1986). Inhibitory effects of galanin on the isolated spinal cord of the newborn rat. *Neuroscience Letters*, **70**, 278–282.

Chapter 4

Brain galanin receptors: anatomical localization and possible functional role

Christer Köhler and Victoria Chan-Palay

4.1. *Introduction*

Galanin is a 29-amino acid peptide first isolated and characterized by Tatemoto *et al.* (1983) from pig intestine and was given its name from the existence of a *glycine* and an *alanine* at positions 1 and 29 of the molecule, respectively. Subsequent work has shown the peptide to be highly conserved among animal species, since only three amino acids differ in the sequence from porcine, rat and bovine galanin between amino acid sequences 1–15. Galanin has a wide range of biological actions, including the inhibition of insulin release from pancreatic β-cells (McDonald *et al.*, 1985; Ahrén *et al.*, 1986), possibly through the activation of ATP-dependent potassium channels (De Weille *et al.*, 1988). Galanin has also been shown to inhibit neurotransmitter and hormone release through an action in the central nervous system (CNS) (Rökaeus, 1987). Galanin most likely participates in the regulation of a wide range of functions since it is present in several organs throughout the body (Rökaeus *et al.*, 1984; Rökaeus, 1987), and findings from recent studies show that many different physiological functions are affected after the administration of this peptide.

Since the discovery of galanin in the CNS (Rökaeus *et al.*, 1984) considerable interest has been focused on its role in brain function. In this chapter we review the current status of understanding of galanin systems in the brain, with special emphasis on the distribution of putative receptors for galanin in various animal species including the human.

4.2. *Galanin pathways*

Galanin immunoreactivity in brain tissue and neurons has been detected in both the rodent and primate, including the human brain (Melander *et al.*, 1986b; Skofitsch and Jacobowitz, 1986; Beal *et al.*, 1988b; Chan-Palay, 1988; Chan-Palay *et al.*, 1990a,b). The distribution of central pathways containing galanin is best known in the rat (Melander *et al.*, 1986b; Skofitsch and

Jacobowitz, 1986). In this species immunoreactive-galanin (ir-galanin) cells and axons are present throughout the neuraxis, but the relative density of galanin-containing cells and terminals show substantial variation among brain areas. The basal forebrain, hypothalamus and the brain-stem are particularly rich in galanin-containing cells and fibres. More specifically, numerous ir-galanin cell bodies are present in the medial septum/diagonal band complex, bed nucleus of stria terminalis, substantia innominata/ventral pallidum. The ir-galanin cells constitute a continous band which extends from the basal forebrain into the hypothalamus. In the hypothalamus, ir-galanin cells are present in large numbers in the preoptic, supraoptic, paraventricular, periventricular, tuberomammillary nuclei, the dorsomedial, ventromedial nuclei as well as in the lateral hypothalamic area (Melander *et al.*, 1986b; Skofitsch and Jacobowitz, 1986). Extensive terminal networks are found in the preoptic and periventricular areas, paraventricular nucleus, dorsomedial nucleus and the lateral hypothalamus. A dense plexus of ir-galanin axons is present in the median eminence. Recent studies have shown a rich galanin innervation of the hypothalamus also in the human brain (Chan-Palay and Jentsch, 1990). In the hypothalamus, galanin is co-localized with oxytocin in the supraoptic nucleus, with vasopressin in the paraventricular nucleus, with tyrosine hydroxylase in presumed dopamine cells of the A12 region, with γ-aminobutyric acid (GABA) in the arcuate nucleus and with histamine in the tuberomammillary nuclei (Köhler *et al.*, 1986; Cecatelli *et al.*, 1989). Galanin-positive cells have been detected in the cingulate cortex, the caudate nucleus, and the bed nucleus of stria terminalis. The deep layers of the cortical mantle as well as the hippocampus also harbour some cells. In colchicine-treated rats, a large number of medium sized cells are present in the hilus of the area dentata (Melander *et al.*, 1986b; C. Köhler, unpublished). The size and position of these cells suggest that they are indentical with somatostatin and neuropeptide Y (NPY) cell found in this area. Since visualization of the cortical ir-galanin cells requires substantial colchicine treatment, the localization of galanin mRNA in these cells is essential in order to establish them as galanin containing.

In contrast to the relatively dense innervation of the basal forebrain and hypothalamus, the basal ganglia and thalamus appear to be poorly endowed with galanin-positive cells and fibres, although scattered cells are present in the striatum and a dense galanin plexus is found in the habenula. In the brain-stem, on the other hand, galanin is present in the central grey substance, the mesencephalic and pontine 5-hydroxytryptamine (5-HT) cell-groups as well as in the noradrenergic nucleus locus coeruleus and in adrenergic cells of the lower medulla. Terminal plexuses are present in the nucleus of solitary tract, the substantia gelatinosa of the trigeminal nucleus, as well as in the dorsal horn of the spinal cord (Melander *et al.*, 1986b; Skofitsch and Jacobowitz, 1986).

Overall, substantial amounts of galanin appear to be present in subcortical cells with long ascending or descending projections.

In both the monkey and the post-mortem human brain, ir-galanin is heterogeneously distributed among regions as shown by radioimmunoassay (Beal *et al.*, 1988a; Gentleman *et al.*, 1989), but detailed understanding of the exact distribution patterns in different brain areas has to await the application of immunohistochemistry. Studies performed on the human brain have shown a prominent galaninergic system of both cells and terminals in the nucleus basalis of Meynert (Chan-Palay, 1988; Chan-Palay *et al.*, 1990a,b) and in the hypothalamus (Vogels *et al.*, 1989; Chan-Palay and Jentsch, 1990), but today little is known about galanin systems in other parts of the human CNS.

In the rat (Melander *et al.*, 1985; Senut *et al.*, 1989a,b), monkey (Melander and Staines, 1986; Walker *et al.*, 1989) and post-mortem human (Chan-Palay, 1988; Kowall and Beal, 1989; Vogels *et al.*, 1989; Chan-Palay *et al.*, 1990a,b) brain galanin is co-localized with acetylcholine (ACh) in a subset of neurones situated in the medial septum/diagonal band of Broca and in the basal nucleus of Meynert. Since these systems have been implied in certain aspects of cognition (Crawley and Wenk, 1989) and since they degenerate in dementing human diseases such as senile dementia of the Alzheimer type (SDAT) (Chan-Palay, 1988), galanin has been hypothesized to play a role in memory and learning.

The widespread distribution of galanin-containing neurones and the localization of this peptide within cholinergic and monoaminergic neuronal systems suggests participation of galanin in different brain functions. Pharmacological studies have shown a wide range of biological effects (for review see Rökaeus, 1987) of galanin suggesting that galanin may act through specific receptors in the periphery as well as in the brain. Indeed, ligand binding experiments have provided evidence that high affinity binding sites for ^{125}I-galanin exist in the brain.

4.3. *Galanin receptors*

4.3.1. **General comments**

By using ^{125}I-galanin, several groups have shown the existence of high affinity binding sites in homogenates from pancreatic β-cells (Lagny-Pourmir *et al.*, 1989) as well as from rat brain (Servin *et al.*, 1987; Fisone *et al.*, 1989). The ventral hippocampus is among the areas best characterized so far with regard to ^{125}I-galanin binding. In homogenates from this area, ^{125}I-galanin was found to bind with high affinity (K_d *c.* 2 nM) to a single population of binding sites (B_{max} *c.* 100 fmol mg protein^{-1}) (Fisone *et al.*, 1989). These values are well within the range of other studies in other tissues (Servin *et al.*, 1987). The hippocampal ^{125}I-galanin binding site was found to be a heat-and trypsin-sensitive membrane protein (Fisone *et al.*, 1989). The sensitivity of the ^{125}I-galanin binding to GTP and to ADP-ribosylation,

Table 4.1. Comparison between the density of ir-galanin terminals and specific ^{125}I-galanin binding sites in some regions in the rat brain.

Brain area	ir-galanin	^{125}I-galanin binding
Frontal cortex	+	+
Piriform cortex	+	++
Septum, lateral	+++	+++
Septum, dorso lateral	+	+++
Bed nucleus of stria terminalis	+++	+++
Preoptic area	+++	+++
Paraventricular nucleus	+++	+
Dorso medial nucleus	+++	++
Median eminence	+++	+++
Thalamus, centro-medial	+	+++
Superior collicullus (stratum opticus)	+	+++
Central grey	++	+++
Nucleus ruber	–	–
Reticular formula	+	++
Parabrachial nucleus	+++	+++
Nucleus of the solitary tract	++	+++
Spinal cord (dorsal horn)	+++	+++
Spinal cord (ventral horn)	+	–
Hippocampus (subiculum)	++	+++
Entorhinal cortex (layer 2)	+	+++
Fornix	++	+++
Stria terminalis	++	+++

–, No fibres/binding detected.
+, Single fibres/low density.
++, Medium density.
+++, High density.
Table based on data from Melander *et al.*, 1986b, 1988.

suggests that the receptor is coupled to an inhibitory G-protein (Gi). In pancreatic tumour cells (Lagny-Pourmir *et al.*, 1989) and in the ventral hippocampus, the N-terminal sequence (galanin 21–29) seems to be of importance for the interaction of galanin with the receptor. Apparently, the *Trp* in position 2 plays a crucial role for the binding, in peripheral tissue as well as in the CNS (Fisone *et al.*, 1989; Lagny-Pourmir *et al.*, 1989).

4.3.2. **Anatomical localization**

a. *Rat*

Application of *in vitro* receptor autoradiography has revealed the anatomical distribution of specific ^{125}I-galanin binding sites (Skofitsch and Jacobowitz, 1986; Melander *et al.*, 1986a, 1988). These studies show a striking concordance between the distribution of ir-galanin processes as revealed by immunohistochemistry and the relative density of putative galanin receptors (Table 4.1), which is in contrast to the relative lack of such concordance noted for several other peptides (Herkenham and McLean, 1986).

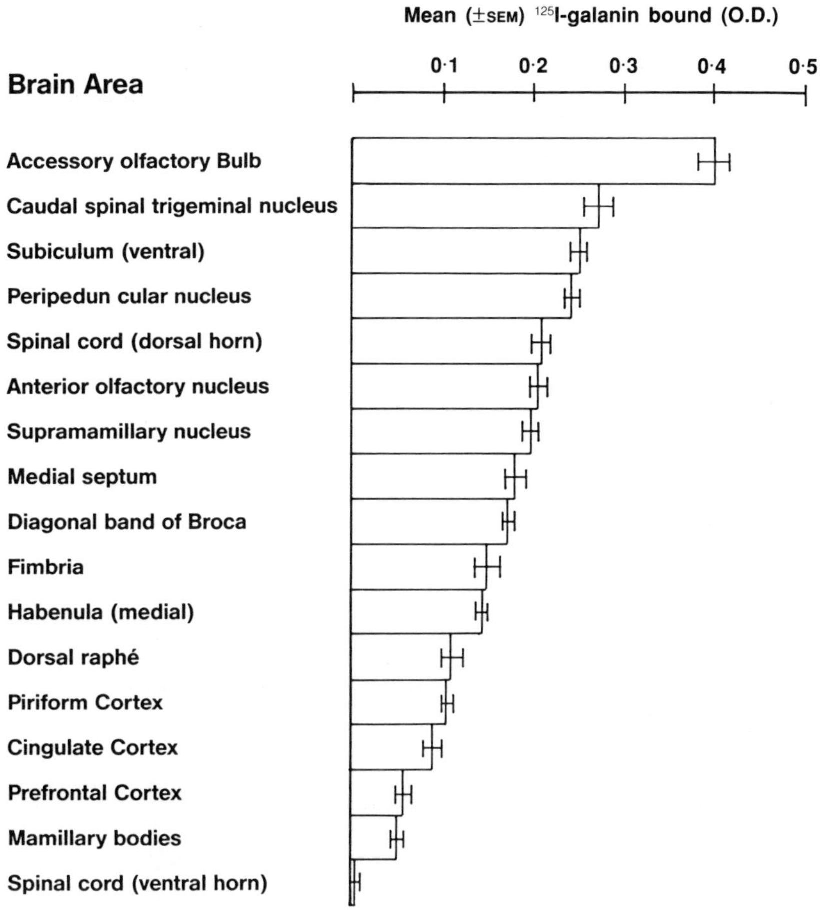

Figure 4.1. Histogram of the distribution of specifically bound ^{125}I-galanin (mean ± SEM; optical density) in various regions of the rat brain. The concentration of ^{125}I-galanin was 0·5 nM. Specific binding was defined by 1 μM unlabelled galanin.

In the rat, high densities of specific ^{125}I-galanin binding is present throughout the basal forebrain, including the septum, ventral pallidum, the bed nucleus of striae terminalis, in most, if not all, parts of the hypothalamus as well as the cortical and central nuclei of amygdala. The basal ganglia, most nuclei of the thalamus (except the centromedial and paraventricular nuclei) and the neocortex (except the infralimbic, piriform and entorhinal cortices) were found to be virtually devoid of specific binding sites. In the temporal hippocampus, there are high densities of ^{125}I-galanin binding sites while far lower densities are present in the septal part (see Figures 4.1–4.3).

Further caudally, the highest binding densities are present in the ventral tegmental area, substantia nigra, central grey substance and parts of the

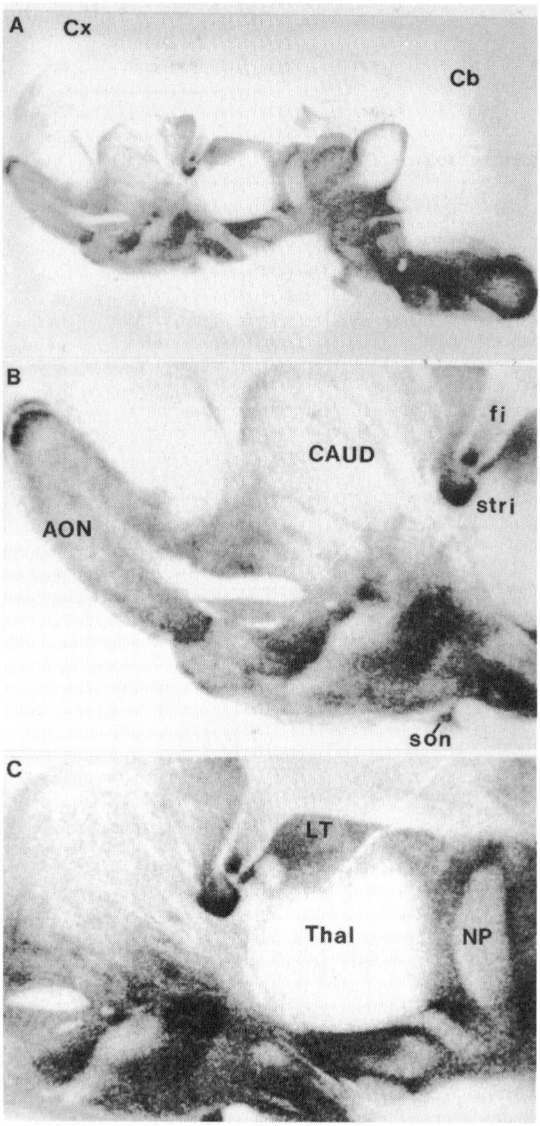

Figure 4.2. (A,C) Photomicrographs of the distribution of ^{125}I-galanin binding sites in the rat brain, saggital sections. Total binding is shown. (B,C) Enlarged details of the binding. Cx, Neocortex; Cb, cerebellum; CAUD, caudate nucleus; fi, fimbria; stri, stria terminalis; AON, anterior olfactory nuclues; son, supraoptic nucleus; Thal, thalamus; NP, nucleus posterior.

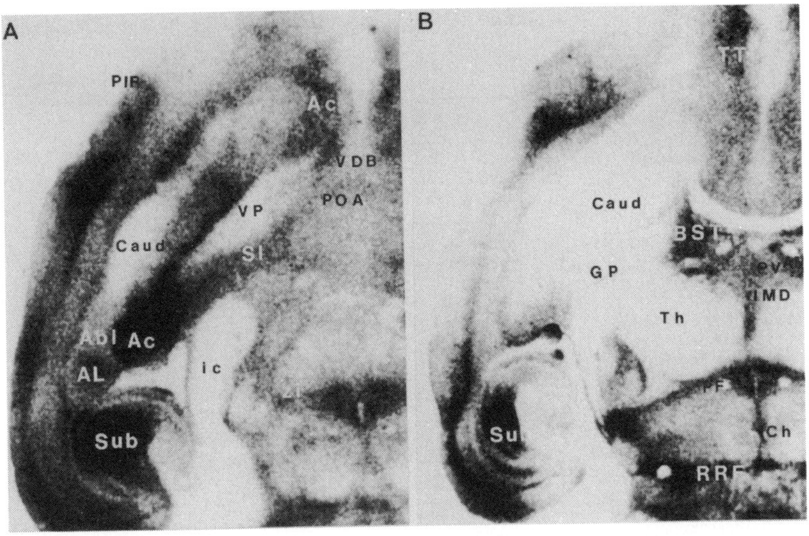

Figure 4.3. (A,B) Photomicrographs of the distribution of ^{125}I-galanin (0·5 nM) binding sites in the rat brain, horizontal sections. Total binding is shown. PIR, piriform cortex; Ac, amygdala central nucleus; VDB, diagonal band of Broca, ventral; Caud, caudate nucleus; SI, substantia innominata; Abl, amygdala basolateral nucleus; AL, amygdala lateral nucleus; ic, internal capsule; Sub, subiculum; BST, bed nucleus stria terminalis; GP, globus pallidum; IMD, intermediodorsal thalamic nuclei; PF, parafascicular nucleus; RRF, retrorubral fields.

reticular formation. In the tectum, the stratum opticus of the superior collicullum harbours most, while the inferior colliculus is poor in binding sites. The parabrachial nuclei, pontine raphe nuclei, locus coeruleus, the nucleus of the solitary tract and the caudal spinal trigeminal nucleus are all rich in ^{125}I-galanin binding. In the spinal cord dense binding is found in the dorsal horn, while no specific binding is found in the ventral horn (Skofitsch *et al.*, 1986; Melander *et al.*, 1988).

The fimbria and stria terminalis contain numerous ^{125}I-galanin binding sites (Figure 4.3) suggesting that galanin receptors are transported in these tracts. It is also possible that some of the binding in the lateral hypothalamus partly represents receptors associated with axons of the medial forebrain bundle. In the medial part of the brain-stem, high densities of binding are present just over the ascending bundles from the median and dorsal raphe nucleus. This observation further indicates an association of galanin receptors with major fibre tracts. A comparison between the density of ^{125}I-galanin binding and galanin nerve terminals, suggests a good concordance between the two measures, although a few exceptions do exist (Table 4.1). This could indicate that galanin receptors are found to a large extent on ir-galanin nerve terminals.

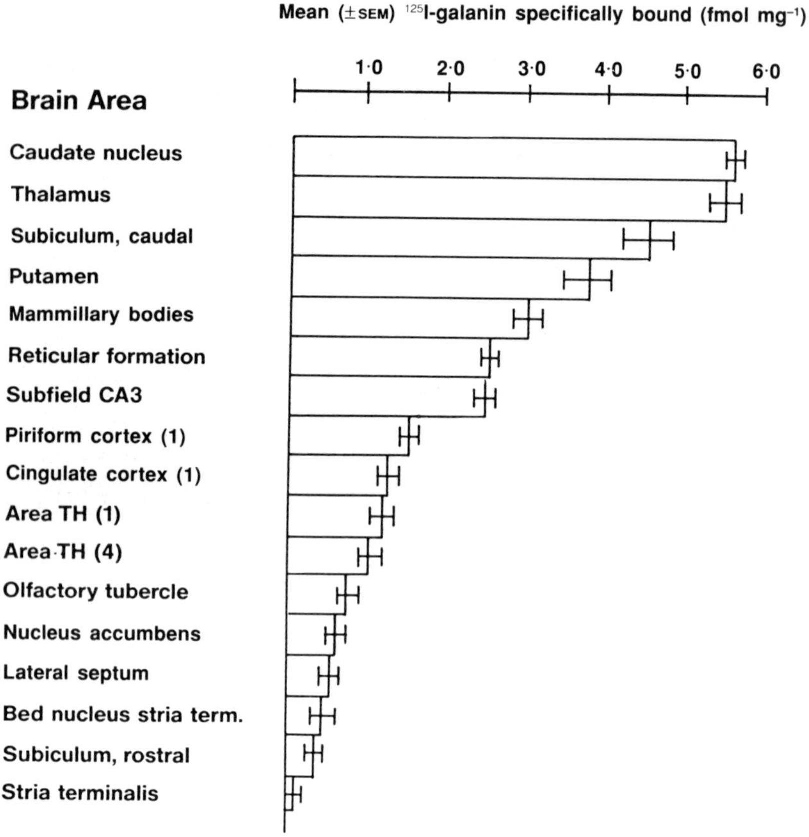

Figure 4.4. Histogram of the distribution of specifically bound ^{125}I-galanin (mean ± SEM; fmol mg^{-1}) in various regions of the monkey brain. Concentration of ^{125}I-galanin, 0·5 nM.

b. *Monkey*

Specific ^{125}I-galanin binding sites are heterogeneously distributed throughout the monkey brain (Figure 4.4). The major difference between the monkey and rat is the high density of ^{125}I-galanin binding sites present in the neocortex of the primate brain. In the monkey, the binding appears as a dense band in layer 4 throughout all cortical areas examined, except in the visual cortex. In the latter cortical area, the binding is highly stratified with the highest densities present in laminae 3, 4c, 5–6 (Figures 4.5 and 4.9). Exactly which neuronal elements in layer 4 may contain the ^{125}I-galanin binding sites is unknown at present. Layer 4 harbours the basal dendrites of cortico-cortical projection cells, local interneurones and dendrites of cells in layers 5 and 6. In addition, thalamo-cortical afferents terminate in layer 4. The galanin receptor may be associated with any of these elements. The high density of ^{125}I-galanin binding sites in layers 2 and 3 of the visual

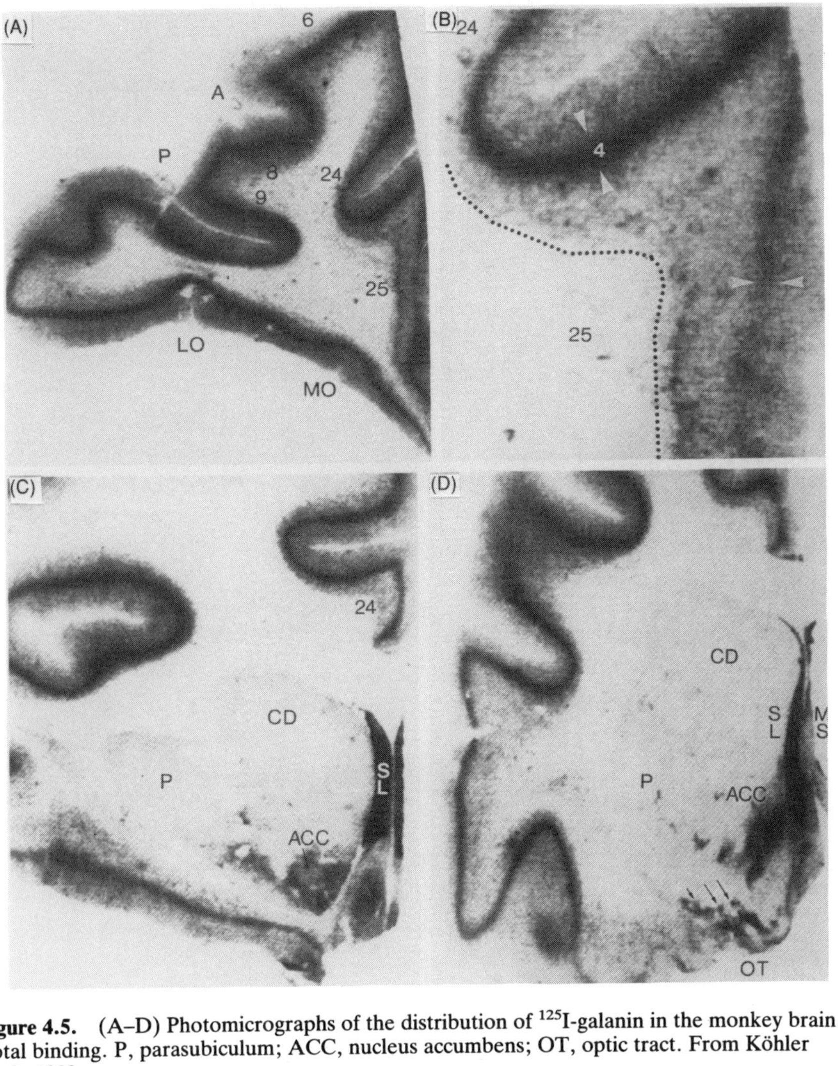

Figure 4.5. (A–D) Photomicrographs of the distribution of ^{125}I-galanin in the monkey brain. Total binding. P, parasubiculum; ACC, nucleus accumbens; OT, optic tract. From Köhler *et al.*, 1989.

cortex indicates an association with cortico-cortical projection systems. In layers 4 to 6 the binding may be associated with any of a wide range of different neural structures: interneurones, subcortical projection neurones or afferents from the lateral geniculate body. Lesion studies will be required to identify the exact location of these binding sites.

Another difference from binding patterns observed in the rat is the relatively lower densities of binding in the most temporal aspect of the hippocampus (e.g. entorhinal cortex) compared to the very high densities found in the rat ventral hippocampus. In the monkey, as in the rat, high

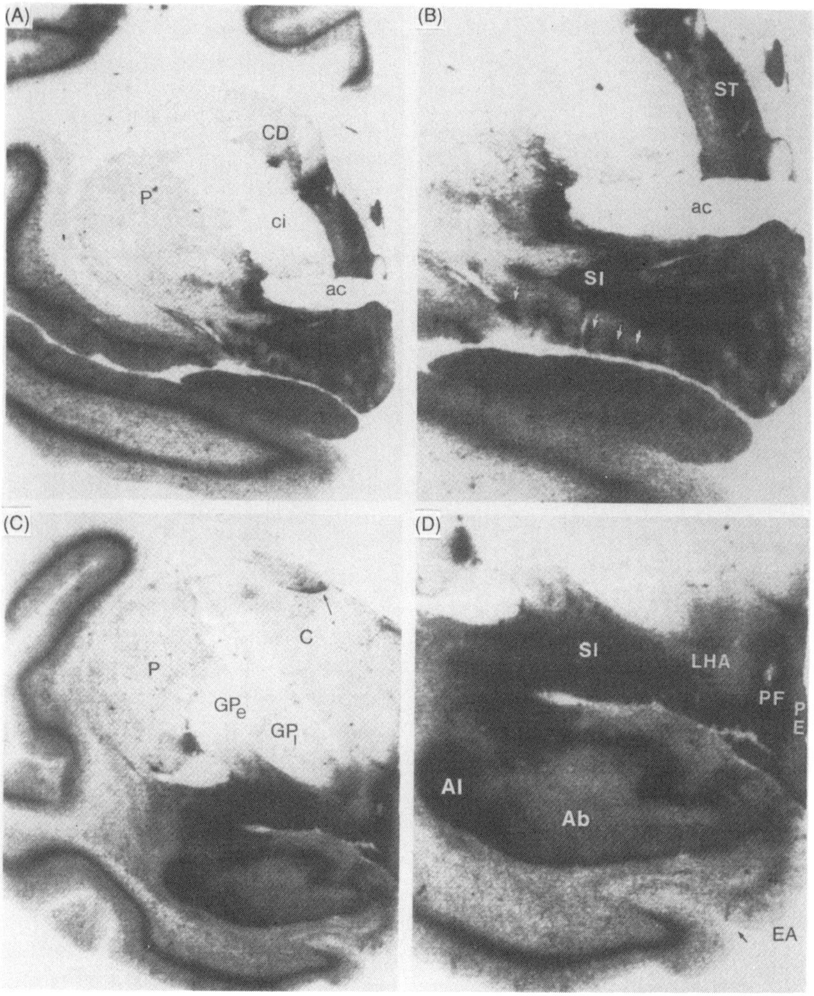

Figure 4.6. (A–D) Photomicrographs of the distribution of ^{125}I-galanin binding in the monkey brain. P, parasubiculum; ac, amygdala central nucleus; ST, stria terminalis; SI, substantia innominata; C, commisura anterior; PF, parafascicular nucleus; Al, amygdala lateral nucleus. From Köhler *et al.*, 1990.

binding densities were recorded in the hippocampal-amygdala area and in the most rostral parts of the subiculum (see below). High binding density is present in the lateral septum, nucleus accumbens and above the islands of Calleja in the olfactory tubercle. The basal nucleus of Meynert also harboured high ^{125}I-galanin binding densities. In the hypothalamus the binding clsoely resembles that reported in the rat (Melander *et al.*, 1988).

^{125}I-Galanin binding sites are enriched in the superior colliculus where the binding appears as dense zones separate from areas with less dense binding. The binding in the inferior colliculus enwraps the structure as a peripheral band. High binding densities are found in the central grey substance, dorsal and median raphe, locus coeruleus, parabrachial nucleus, reticular formation, solitary tract nucleus, the principal nucleus of the trigeminal nerve and the dorsal horn of the spinal cord (Figure 4.4).

c. *Human*

The distribution of specific ^{125}I-galanin binding sites in the human brain shows a pattern similar to that in the monkey, and with some exceptions, to that in the rat. The galanin receptors appear, thus, to be well conserved through phylogeny. In the human brain the basal forebrain, hypothalamus and the entire cortical mantle stand out as particularly rich in ^{125}I-galanin binding sites (Figure 4.7). In the amygdala, medial and central nuclei are rich in binding sites. The basal ganglia and most of the thalamus are, however, poorly endowed with specific ^{125}I-galanin receptors (Figure 4.7). A heterogeneous pattern of binding is present in the brain-stem. Strikingly high densities are present in the central grey substance, the raphe nuclei, the locus coeruleus, parabrachial nuclei, substantia nigra and reticular formation. In the brain-stem, delicate strands of galanin binding can be seen radiating out from the dorsal raphe suggesting the existence of ^{125}I-galanin binding sites in or on axons (Figure 4.8).

The distribution of cortical binding sites resembles that seen in the monkey. Thus, high densities are present in layers 4 to 6. In the visual cortex (area 17) the highest densities are present in layers 2 and 3, 4a and 4cα,β to 6 (Figure 4.9).

The basal nucleus of Meynert is rich in ^{125}I-galanin binding sites. At rostral levels the binding is associated primarily with the peripheral zones of the individual cholinergic subgroups, while in the caudal subgroups the binding sites appears to be associated more with the central core. The binding density is not reduced significantly in cases suffering from SDAT, as shown in single concentration autoradiographic experiments (Köhler and Chan-Palay, 1990b). In one case of multi-infarct dementia a reduction of ^{125}I-galanin binding was noted. These findings suggest that the majority of galanin receptors may not be located on cholinergic somata in the human nucleus basalis Meynert.

d. *The hippocampal region*

In the rat hippocampus, most of the specifically bound ^{125}I-galanin is present in the temporal parts. Indeed, the same is true in the monkey and the post-mortem human brain. In the rat and the primate brain, the most temporal part of subiculum and the amygdala-hippocampal area are very rich in specific ^{125}I-galanin binding. In the post-mortem human brain, high binding densities are found in the uncal region.

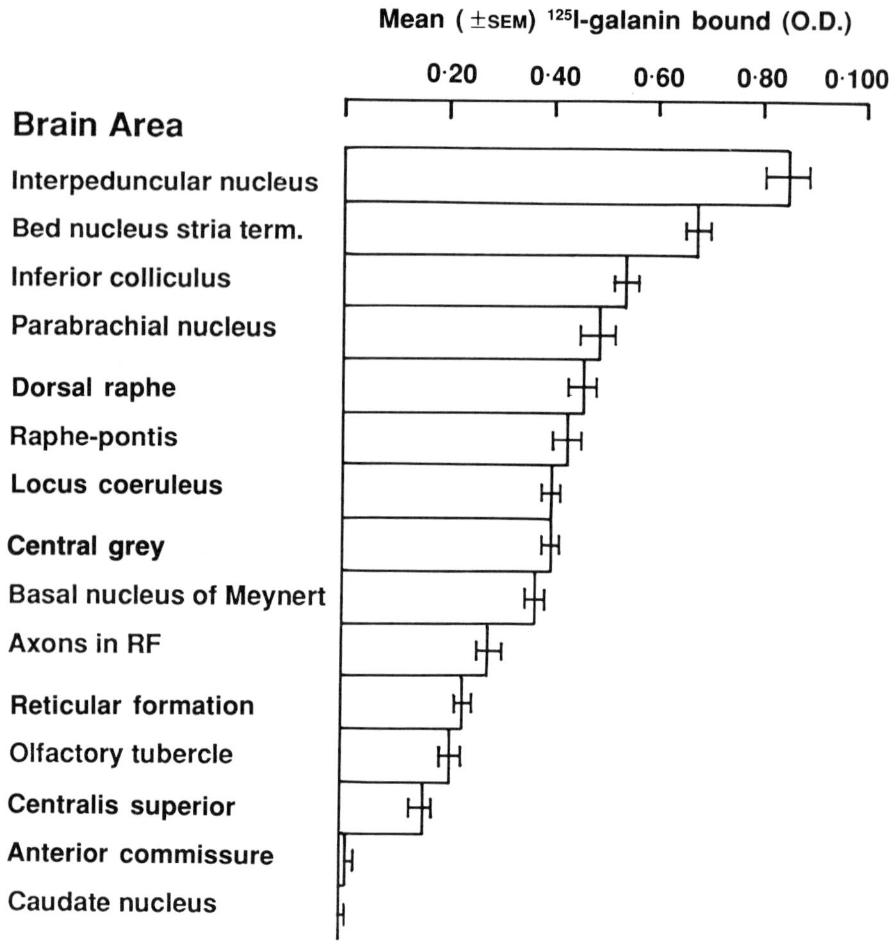

Figure 4.7. Histogram of the distribution of specifically bound ^{125}I-galanin (mean ± SEM; optical density) in the various regions of the human brain. Concentration of galanin 0·5 nM.

In the rat, the highest binding densities are found in the subiculum and entorhinal cortex (EC) (Figures 4.10 and 4.11). In the EC most of the binding occurs in the lateral part (layers 2b, 4 and 6) with moderate to low densities in layers 1, 2a, 3 and 5. In the medial EC, layers 4 and 6 harbour some of binding sites. The binding density increases in all layers of EC at the most ventral layers. Indeed, an increase of specifically bound ^{125}I-galanin is present in all layers of the Ammon's horn and area dentata, (Figures 4.10 and 4.11) at the most ventral levels.

In the monkey and in the human hippocampus the highest binding densities occur in the subiculum and in the most rostral parts of the EC. At these rostral levels, the binding in the lateral EC predominates: layers 2b, 4

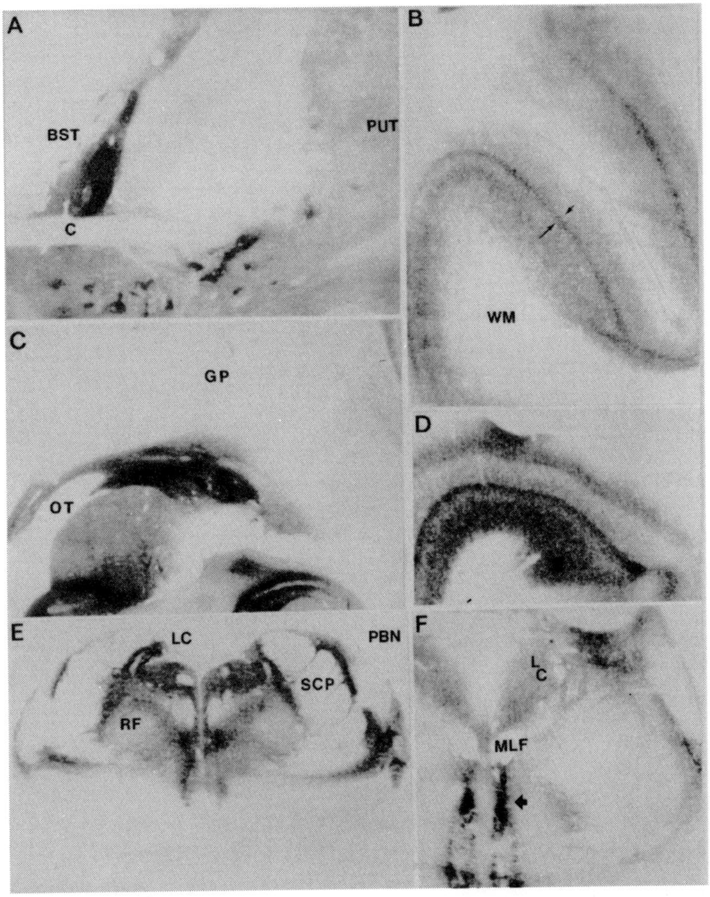

Figure 4.8. Photomicrographs of the distribution of ^{125}I-galanin binding sites in the human brain. Total binding. (A) Binding in the bed nucleus of stria terminalis (BST). (B) Binding in layer 4 of neocortex. (C) High density binding in the basal nucleus of Meynert. (D) Laminar distribution of binding sites in the striate cortex. A band of high density in layer 4c is shown. (E,F) Binding sites in the brain-stem. C, Cerebellum; WM, white matter; GP, globus pallidum; OT, optical tract; LC, locus coeruleus; RF, reticular formation; SCP, superior cerebellar peduncle; PBN, parabrachial nucleus; MLF, medial longitudinal fasciculus; LC, locus coeruleus.

and 6 do show slightly higher binding than the other layers. The medial EC harbours little, if any, specifically bound ^{125}I-galanin.

The exact localization of the hippocampal ^{125}I-galanin binding sites remains to be established. Galanin is present in a subset of cholinergic cells in the diagonal band of Broca (Melander *et al.*, 1985) which project to the ventral hippocampus. The position of these axons in the fimbria corresponds to the localization of ^{125}I-galanin binding sites, suggesting an association of the binding with galanin- and ACh-containing axons. Indeed, transections of

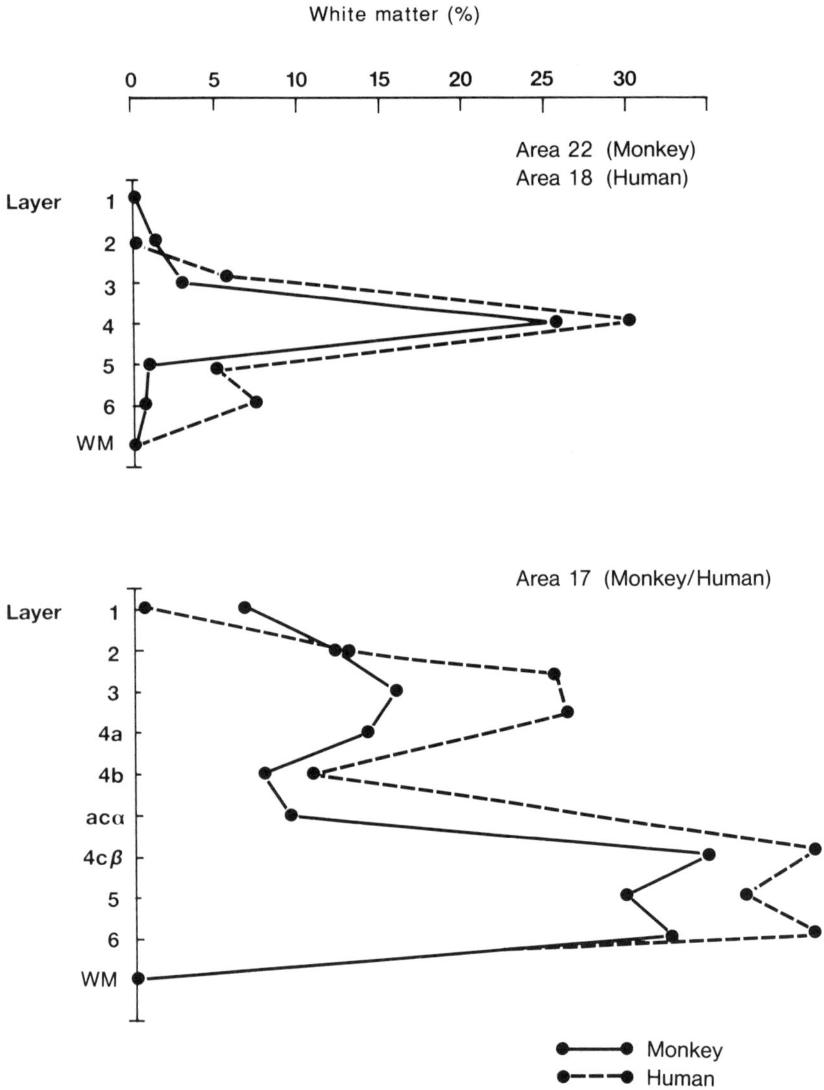

Figure 4.9. The distribution of specific ^{125}I-binding sites in various laminae of the human and the monkey neocortex. Values are expressed as per cent of binding in white matter (WM).

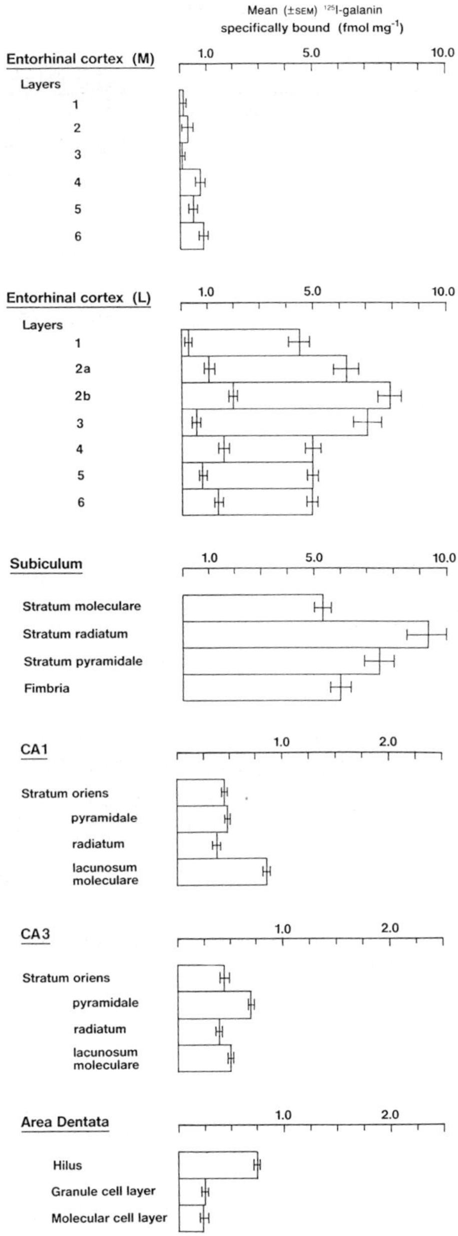

Figure 4.10. Histograms of the regional distribution of specific ^{125}I-galanin (mean ± SEM; fmol mg^{-1}) binding sites in the different laminae of the hippocampal region of the rat brain. The short graphs in the entorhinal cortex (L) represent binding at mid-temporal levels.

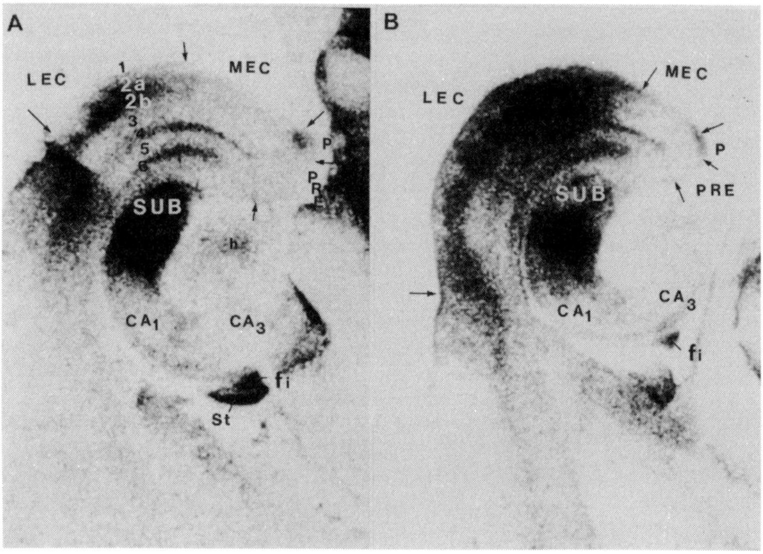

Figure 4.11. Photomicrographs of the distribution of ^{125}I-galanin binding sites in the midtemporal (A) and ventral (B) hippocampal regions of the rat brain. LEC, Lateral entorchinal cortex; MEC, medial entorhinal cortex; SUB, subiculum; P, parasubiculum; PRE, presubiculum; CA_1 and CA_3, subfields of Ammon's horn; St, stria terminalis; fi, fimbria.

the fimbria or massive lesions of the septum reduce the ^{125}I-galanin binding in the ventral hippocampus by approximately 30% (Melander *et al.*, 1989).

Further support for an association of some of the ^{125}I-galanin binding sites with septo-hippocampal axons is the fact that the laminar distribution in the EC corresponds partly to the cholinergic innervation in layers 2 and 4. It is unknown at present with which other hippocampal elements ^{125}I-galanin binding may be associated.

The ^{125}I-galanin binding on the galanin- and/or ACh-containing septo-hippocampal system may represent functional receptors. Thus, galanin is able to inhibit the release of ACh in the ventral, but not in the dorsal, hippocampus *in vitro* (Fisone *et al.*, 1987). Futhermore, electrophysiological studies have shown a presynaptic action of galanin in the ventral hippocampus (Dutar *et al.*, 1989). *In vivo* studies carried out with microdialysis have shown that the galanin fragments found to be most potent in displacing ^{125}I-galanin binding from hippocampal membranes were also the most potent in blocking scopolamine-induced ACh release (Fisone *et al.*, 1990). In a different paradigm, Ben-Ari (1990) has provided evidence that galanin may reduce release of glutamate induced by anoxic condition.Taken together, these findings suggest that galanin may play an important role as a modulator of hippocampal transmitter-release under normal as well as pathological conditions.

4.4. *Summary*

The neuropeptide galanin is widely and heterogenously distributed in the brain of several animal species, including the human. Using *in vitro* receptor autoradiographic technique, presumed receptors for galanin have been localized in the rat, monkey and post-mortem human brains. In all three species, a good concordance exists between the distribution of galanin immunoreactive processes and binding sites. The distribution of binding sites showed small differences between the rodent and the primate brain. The highest density of specific ^{125}I-galanin binding was found in the basal forebrain, substantia innominata, hypothalamus, raphe nuclei, parabrachial nucleus, nucleus of the solitary tract and the dorsal horn of the spinal cord. The primate cortex, in contrast to that of the rat, harboured a large number of binding sites concentrated in layer 4 and in the visual cortex to layers 2, 3 and 4c to 6. In the hippocampus, most of the binding was found in the ventral subiculum and lateral entorhinal cortex, possibly on galanin-/ACh-containing afferents from the septum.

References

Ahrén, B., Arkhammar, P., Berggren, P.O. and Nilsson, T. (1986). Galanin inhibits glucose-stimulated insulin release by a mechanism involving hyperpolarization and lowering of cytoplasmic free Ca^{2+} concentration. *Biochemical and Biophysical Research Communication,* **140**, 1059–1063.

Baner, F.E., Ginsberg, L., Venetikoum, M., Mackay, D.J., Burrnin, J.M. & Bloom, S.R. (1986). Preliminary communication. Growth hormone release in the man induced by galanin, a new hypothalamic peptide. *Lancet* II, 198.

Beal, M.F., Gabriel, S.M., Swartz, K.J. and MacGarvey, U.M. (1988a). Distribution of galanin-like immunoreactivity in baboon brain. *Peptides*, **9**, 847–851.

Beal, M.F., Clevens, R.A., Chattha, G.K., MacGarvey, U.M., Mazurek, M.F. and Gabriel, S.M. (1988b). Galanin-like immunoreactivity is unchanged in Alzheimer's disease and Parkinson's disease dementia cerebral cortex. *Journal of Neurochemistry*, **51**, 1935–1941.

Ben-Ari, Y. (1990). Galanin and glibenclamide modulate the anoxic release of glutamate in rat CA3 hippocampal neurons. *European Journal of Neuroscience*, **2**, 62–68.

Cecatelli, S., Eriksson, M. and Hökfelt, T. (1989). Distribution and coexistence of corticotropin-releasing factor and vasoactive intestinal polypeptide-histidine isoleucine-like peptides in the parvocellular part of the paraventricular nucleus. *Neuroendocrinology*, **49**, 309–323.

Chan-Palay, V. (1988). Galanin hyperinnervates surviving neurons of the human basal nucleus of Meynert in dementias of Alzheimer's and Parkinson's disease: A hypothesis for the role of galanin in accentuating cholinergic dysfunction in dementia. *Journal of Comparative Neurology*, **273**, 543–551.

Chan-Palay, V. and Jentsch, B. (1990). Galanin neurons in the tuberomammillary hypothalamic nucleus in Alzheimer's and Parkinson's disease. *Dementia*, in press.

Chan-Palay, V., Ernfors, P. and Persson, H. (1990a). Galanin gene expression in the nucleus basalis Meynert in senile demenitia of the Alzheimer type. *Dementia*, **1**, 3.

Chan-Palay, V., Köhler C., Ernfors, P. and Persson, H. (1990b). Senile dementia of the Alzheimer type is accompanied by hypertrophy of galanin axons, preservation of receptors and tissue specific expression of the galanin gene in the nucleus basalis Meynert. In press.

Ch'ng, J.L.C., Christofides, N.D., Anand, P., Gibson, S.J., Allen, Y.S., Su, H.C., Tatemoto, K., Morrison, J.F.B., Polak, J.M. & Bloom, S.R. (1985) Distribution of galanin immunoreactivity in the central nervous system and the response of galanin-containing neuronal pathways to injury. *Neuroscience* 16, 343–354.

Crawley, J.N. and Wenk, G.L. (1989). Co-existence of galanin and acetylcholine: is galanin involved in memory precesses and dementia? *Trends in Neuroscience*, **12**, 278–281.

De Weille, J., Schmid-Antomarchi, H., Fosset, M. and Lazdunski, M. (1988). ATP-sensitive K^+ channels that are blocked by hypoglycemia-inducing sulfonylureas in insulin secreting cells are activated by galanin, a hyperglucemia-inducing hormone. *Proceedings of the National Academy of Sciences USA*, **85**, 1312–1316.

Dutar, P., Lamour, Y. and Nicoll, R.A. (1989). Galanin blocks the slow cholinergic EPSP in CA1 pyramidal neurons from ventral hippocampus. *European Journal of Pharmacology*, **164**, 355–360.

Fisone, G., Wu, C.F., Consolo, S., Nordström, Ö., Brynne, N., Bartfai, F., Melander, T. and Hökfelt, T. (1987). Galanin inhibits acetylcholine release in the ventral hippocampus of the rat: histochemical, autoradiographic *in vivo* and *in vitro* studies. *Proceedings of the National Academy of Sciences USA*, **84**, 7339–7343.

Fisone, G., Langel, U., Carlquist, M., Bergman, T., Consolo, S., Hökfelt, T., Undèn, A., Andell, S. and Bartfai, T. (1989). Galanin receptor and its ligands in the rat hippocampus. *European Journal of Biochemistry*, **181**, 269–276.

Fisone, G., Berthold, M., Bedecs, K., Undèn, A., Bartfai, T., Bertorelli, R., Consolo, S., Crawley, J., Martin, B., Nilsson, S. and Hökfelt, T. (1990). N-terminal galanin-(1–16) fragment is an agonist at the hippocampal galanin receptor. *Proceedings of the National Academy of Sciences USA*, **86**, 9588–9591.

Fuxe, K., Euler, G., Agnati, L.F. and Ögren, S.O. (1988). Galanin selectively modulates 5-hydroxytryptamine 1A receptors in the rat ventral limbic cortex. *Neuroscience Letters*, **85**, 163–167.

Fuxe, K., Ögren, S.O., Jansson, A., Cintra, A., Härfstrand, A. and Agnati, L.F. (1988). Intraventricular injections of galanin reduces 5-HT metabolism in the ventral limbic cortex, the hippocampal formation and the fronto-parietal cortex of the male rat. *Acta Physiologica Scandinavica*, **133**, 579–581.

Gabriel, S.M., Kaplan, L.M., Martin, J.B. and Koenig, J.I. (1989). Tissue-specific sex differences in galanin-like immunoreactivity and galanin mRNA during development in the rat. *Peptides*, **10**, 369–374.

Gardiner, S.M., Compton, A.M. and Bennett, T. (1988). Renal vasodilatation after central administration of galanin. *Brain Research*, **458**, 176–179.

Gentleman, S.M., Falkai, P., Bogerts, B., Herrero, M.T., Polak, J.M. and Roberts, G.W. (1989). Distribution of galanin-like immunoreactivity in the human brain. *Brain Research*, **505**, 311–315.

Herkenham, M. and McLean, S. (1986). Mismatches between receptor and transmitter localizations in the brain. In: *Quantitative Receptor Autoradiography*, edited by C.A. Boast, E.W. Gnowhill and A.C. Altar. New York: Alan Liss, pp. 137–171.

Inoue, T., Kato, Y., Koshiyama, H., Yanaihara, N. & Imura, H. (1988) Galanin stimulates the release of vasoactive intestinal polypeptide from perifused hypothalamic fragments *in vitro* and from periventricular structures into the cerebrospinal fluid *in vivo* in the rat. *Neuroscience Letters*, **85**, 95–100.

Kaplan, L.M., Gabriel, S., Koenig, J.I., Sunday, M.E., Spinder, E.R., Martin, J.B. and Chin, W.W. (1988). Galanin is an estrogen-inducible, secretory product of the rat anterior pituitary. *Proceedings of the National Academy of Sciences USA*, **85**, 7408–7412.

Koshiyama, H., Kato, Y., Inoue, T., Murakami, Y., Ishikawa, Y., Yanaihara, N. and Imura, H. (1987). Central galanin stimulates pituitary prolactin secretion in rats: possible involvement of hypothalamic vasoactive intestinal polypeptide. *Neuroscience Letters*, **75**, 49–574.

Koshiyama, H., Shimatsu, A., Kato, Y., Assadian, H., Hattori, N., Ishikawa, Y., Tanoh, T., Yanaihara, N. and Imura, H. (1990). Galanin-induced prolactin release in rats: pharmacological evidence for the involvement of α-adrenergic and opiodergic mechanisms. *Brain Research*, **507**, 321–324.

Köhler, C. and Chan-Palay, V. (1988). Cholecystokinin octapeptide (CCK-8) receptors in the hippocampal region: a comparative *in vitro* autoradiographic study in the monkey and the postmortem human brain. *Neuroscience Letters*, **90**, 51–56.

Köhler, C. and Chan-Palay, V. (1989). Neuropeptide receptors in the hippocampal region. In: *Hippocampus: New Vistas*. Edited by V. Chan-Palay and C. Köhler. New York: Alan R. Liss, pp. 171–189.

Köhler, C. and Chan-Palay, V. (1990a). Galanin receptors in the post-mortem human brain. Regional distribution of ^{125}I-galanin binding sites using the method of *in vitro* receptor autoradiography. *Neuroscience Letters*, in press.

Köhler, C. and Chan-Palay V. (1990b). Preservation of galanin receptors in the human basal nucleus of Meynert in senile dementia of the Alzheimer type. *Dementia*, in press.

Köhler, C., Persson, A., Melander, T., Theodorsson-Norheim, E., Sedvall, G. and Hökfelt, T. (1988). Distribution of galanin binding sites in the monkey and human telencephalon. Preliminary observations. *Exp. Brain Res.*, in press.

Köhler, C. Eriscon, H., Watanabe, T., Polak, J., Palay, S.L., Palay, V. and Chan-Palay, V. (1986). Galanin immunoreactivity in hypothalamic histamine neurons; further evidence for multiple chemical messengers in the tuberomammillary nucleus. *Journal of Comparative Neurology*, **250**, 58–64.

Kowall, N.W. and Beal, M.F. (1989). Galanin-like immunoreactivity is present in human substantia innominata and in senile plaques in Alzheimer's disease. *Neuroscience Letters*, **98**, 118–123.

Kyrkhouli, S.E., Stanley, B.G. and Leibowitz, S.F. (1986). Galanin: stimulation of feeding induced by medial hypothalamic injections of this novel peptide. *European Journal of Pharmacology*, **122**, 159–160.

Lagny-Pourmir, I., Lorinet, A.M., Yanaihara, N. and Laburhte, M. (1989). Structural requirements for galanin interaction with receptors from pancreatic beta cells and from brain tissue of the rat. *Peptides*, **10**, 757–761.

Lamour, Y., Senut, M.C., Dutar, P. & Bassant, M.H. (1989) Neuropeptides and septo-hippocampal neurones: electrophysiological effects and distributions of immunoreactivity. *Peptides*, **9**, 1351–1359.

Levin, M.C., Sawchenko, P.E., Howe, P.R.C., Bloom, S.R. and Polak, J.M. (1987). Organization of galanin-immunoreactive inputs to the paraventricular nucleus with special reference to catecholaminergic afferents. *Journal of Comparative Neurology*, **261**, 562–582.

Lindskog, S. and Ahrèn, B. (1987). Galanin: effects on basal and stimulated insulin and clucagon secretion in the mouse. *Acta Physiologica Scandinavica*, **129**, 305–309.

Mastropaolo, J., Nadi, N.S., Ostrowski, N.L. and Crawley, J.N. (1988). Galanin antagonizes acetylcholine on a memory task in basal forebrain-lesioned rats. *Proceedings of the National Academy of Sciences USA*, **85**, 9841–9485.

McDonald, T.J., Dupre, J. Tatemoto, K., Greenberg, G.R., Radziuk, J. and Mutt, V. (1985). Galanin inhibits insulin secretion and induced hyperglycemia in dogs. *Diabetes*, **34**, 192–196.

Melander, T. and Staines, W.A. (1986). A galanin-like peptide coexists in putative cholinergic somata of the septum-basal forebrain complex and in acetylcholinesterase-containing fibers and varicosities within the hippocampus in the owl monkey. *Neuroscience Letters*, **68**, 17–22.

Melander, T., Hökfelt, T., Nilsson, S. and Brodin, E. (1986a). Visualization of galanin binding sites in the rat central nervous system. *European Journal of Pharmacology*, **124**, 381–382.

Melander, T., Hökfelt, T. and Rökaeus, Å. (1986b). Distribution of galanin-like immunoreactivity in the rat central nervous system. *Journal of Comparative Neurology*, **248**, 475–577.

Melander, T., Fuxe, K., Härfstrand, A., Eneroth, P. and Hökfelt, T. (1987). Effects of intraventricular injections of galanin on neuroendocrine functions in the male rat. Possible involvement of hypothalamic catecholamine terminal systems. *Acta Physiologica Scandinavica*, **131**, 25–32.

Melander, T., Bartfai, T., Brynne, N., Consolo, S., Fisone G., Hökfelt, T., Köhler C., Nordström, Ö., Norheim-Theodorsson, E., Persson, A., Sedvall, G., Stains, W.A. and Wu, C.F. (1989). Galanin in the cholinergic basal forebrain: histochemical autoradiographic and *in vivo* studies. In: *Progress in Brain Research*, Vol. 79, edited by A. Nordberg, B. Holmstedt, and A. Sundwall, Amsterdam: Elsevier, pp. 85–91.

Melander, T., Köhler, C., Nilsson, S., Hökfelt, T., Brodin, E. and Norheim-Theodorson, E. (1988). Autoradiographic quantitation and anatomical mapping of ^{125}I-galanin binding sites in the rat central nervous system. *Journal of Chemical Neuroanatomy*, **1**, 213–233.

Melander, T., Staines, W.A., Hökfelt, T., Rökaeus, Å., Eckenstein, F., Salvaterra, P.M. and Wainer, B.H. (1985). Galanin-like immunoreactivity in cholinergic neurons of the septum–basal forebrain complex projecting to the hippocampus of the rat. *Brain Research*, **360**, 130–138.

Nishibori, M., Oishi, R., Itoh, Y. and Saeki, K. (1988). Galanin inhibits noradrenaline-induced accumulation of cyclic AMP in the rat cerebral cortex. *Journal Neurochemistry*, **51**, 1953–1955.

Nordström, Ö., Melander, T., Hökfelt, T., Bartfai, T. and Goldstein, M. (1987). Evidence for an inhibitory effect of the peptide galanin on dopamine release from the rat median eminence. *Neuroscience Letters*, **73**, 21–26.

Ohashi, T. and Jacobowitz, D.M. (1985). Galanin potentiates electrical stimulation and exogenous norepinephrine-induced contractions in the rat vas deferens. *Regul. Peptides* **12**, 1633–171.

Ottlecz, A., Samson, W.K. and McCann, S.M. (1986). Galanin: evidence for a hypothalamic site of action to release growth hormone. *Peptides*, **7**, 51–53.

Palazzi, E., Fisone, G., Hökfelt, T., Bartfai, T. & Consolo, S. (1988) Galanin inhibits the muscarinic stimulation of phosphoinositide turnover in rat ventral hippocampus. *European Journal of Pharmacology*, **148**, 479–480.

Rökaeus, A. (1987). Galanin: a newly isolated biologically active neuropeptide. *Trends in Neuroscience*, **10**, 158–163.

Rökaeus, A., Melander, T., Hökfelt, T., Lundberg, J., Tatemoto, K., Carlquist, M. and Mutt, V. (1984). A galanin-like peptide in the central nervous system and intestine of the rat. *Neuroscience Letters*, **47**, 161–166.

Senut, M.C., de Bilbao, F. and Labour, Y. (1989a). Age-related loss of galanin-immunoreactive cells in the rat septal area. *Neuroscience Letters*, **105**, 257–262.

Senut, M.C., Menetrey, D. and Labour, Y. (1989b). Cholinergic and peptidergic projections from the medial septum and the nucleus of the diagonal band of Broca to dorsal hippocampus, cingulate cortex and olfactory bulb: a combined wheat-germ agglutinin–horseradish peroxidase–gold immunohistochemical study. *Neuroscience*, **30**, 385–403.

Servin, A.L., Amiranoff, B., Rouyer-Fessard, C., Tatemoto, K. and Laburthe, M. (1987). Identification and molecular characterization of galanin receptor sites in rat brain. *Biochemical and Biophysical Research Communications*, **144**, 298–306.

Skofitsch, G. and Jacobowitz, D.M. (1985). Immunohistochemical mapping of galanin-like neurons in the rat central nervous system. *Peptides*, **6**, 509–516.

Skofitsch, G. and Jacobowitz, D.M. (1986). Quantitative distribution of galanin-like immunoreactivity in the rat central nervous system. *Peptides*, **7**, 609–613.

Skofitsch, G., Sills, M.A. and Jacobowitz, DM. (1986). Autoradiographic distribution of ^{125}I-galanin binding sites in the rat central nervous system. *Peptides*, **7**, 1029–1042.

Skofitsch, G., Jacobowitz, D.M., Amann, R. and Lembeck, F. (1989). Galanin and vasopressin coexist in the rat hypothalamo-neurohypophyseal system. *Neuroendocrinology*, **49**, 419–227.

Sundström, E. and Melander, T. (1988). Effects of galanin on 5-HT neurons in the rat CNS. *European Journal of Pharmacology*, **146**, 327–329.

Tatemoto, K., Rökaeus, Å., Jörnvall, H., McDonald, T.J. and Mutt, V. (1983). Galanin — a novel biologically active peptide from porcine intestine. *FEBS Letters*, **164**, 124–128.

Vogels, O.J.M., Renkawek, K., Broere, C.A.J., ter Laak, H.J. and van Workum, F. (1989). Galanin-like immunoreactivity within Ch2 neurons in the vertical limb of the diagonal band of Broca in aging and Alzheimer's disease. *Acta Neuropathalogica*, **78**, 90–95.

Walker, L.C., Koliatsos, V.E., Kitt, C.A., Richardson, R.T., Rökaeus, Å. and Price, D.L. (1989). Peptidergic neurons in the basal forebrain magnocellular complex of the rhesus monkey. *Journal of Comparative Neurology*, **280**, 272–282.

Chapter 5

Electrophysiological studies of the actions of galanin in the central nervous system

Patrick Dutar, Marie-Claude Senut, Brigitte Potier, Fabienne De Bilbao, Yvon Lamour and Roger A. Nicoll*

5.1. *Introduction*

Galanin is a 29-amino acid peptide initially isolated from the small intestine of the pig (Tatemoto *et al.*, 1983). Galanin has been visualized in the autonomic innervation of the gut, in the enteric nervous system and also in the central nervous system (CNS) of several mammalian species using immunohistochemical techniques. Putative 'galaninergic' pathways have been described in the CNS particularly the septo-hippocampal pathway (for references see Rökaeus, 1987). The biochemistry and anatomy of galanin are detailed in other chapters of this book.

The physiological actions of galanin include the contraction of smooth muscle and the stimulation or inhibition of the release of several hormones. For example, the best known role of galanin is its inhibition of insulin secretion in the endocrine pancreas causing hyperglycaemia. The physiological role of galanin in the CNS is less precisely defined, but its widespread distribution in the brain, the presence of specific galanin-binding sites, the distribution of the peptide at the pre- and postsynaptic level and the co-localization of galanin with classical neurotransmitters, strongly suggest a role for this peptide in the regulation of central synaptic transmission. In this chapter, we describe the physiological effects of galanin in the CNS; and discuss the possible role this peptide plays in the brain and its possible implication in age-related processes.

5.2. *Physiological Effects of Galanin*

5.2.1. **Action of galanin in peripheral tissues**

Physiological actions of galanin have been demonstrated in myenteric neurones of the small intestine (Yau *et al.*, 1986; Tamura *et al.*, 1988), in

* Author for correspondence.

PC12 chromaffin cells (De Weille *et al.*, 1989) and in insulinoma cells (De Weille *et al.*, 1988; Dunne *et al.*, 1989). Electrophysiological experiments in these various systems provide important information concerning the mechanism of galanin action. In the myenteric neurones of the guinea-pig small intestine, galanin induces a hyperpolarization associated with a decrease in membrane input resistance (Tamura *et al.*, 1988). Galanin also abolishes the calcium spike. The authors conclude that the peptide has two major mechanisms of action in those cells: galanin opens potassium channels (inducing hyperpolarization and decreases in membrane input resistance) and blocks voltage-gated calcium channels. These effects lead to a suppression of excitability. Galanin's mechanism of action in insulinoma cells is probably the best understood. Galanin hyperpolarizes the cells and reduces excitability. Using membrane patches and patch-clamp recordings, it has been demonstrated that galanin added to the outside of the membrane activates ATP-sensitive potassium channels (gK_{ATP}) (DeWeille *et al.*, 1988; Dunne *et al.*, 1989). In pancreatic cells, glucose induces the closure of gK_{ATP} by elevating intracellular ATP leading to the depolarization of the cell, to calcium entry through voltage-dependent calcium channels and finally to insulin release (see Ashcroft, 1988; Figure 5.1). Galanin, by activating gK_{ATP} could hyperpolarize the cell, decrease calcium entry and thus insulin release (Figure 5.1). The mechanism of activation of gK_{ATP} by galanin is unknown. Some experiments indicate that the effect of the peptide on the channels is indirect, possibly involving an intracellular coupling factor (Ahrén *et al.*, 1989). It has recently been demonstrated that a pertussis toxin-sensitive G-protein is involved in these effects of galanin (Dunne *et al.*, 1989; Sharp *et al.*, 1989). In addition, it appears that there is no direct effect of galanin on calcium channels (Ahrén *et al.*, 1989). In PC12 chromaffin cells, galanin inhibits dopamine release by activating an inwardly rectifying potassium channel (De Weille *et al.*, 1989). Galanin does not act directly on calcium channels in these cells.

5.2.2. **Action of galanin in the central nervous system**

Galanin is widely distributed in the CNS where most of its effects are related to neurotransmitter release. Indeed, galanin is able to stimulate or inhibit the release of various transmitters or peptides.

a. *Stimulation of release*

Galanin stimulates the secretion of growth hormone in cultures of rat anterior pituitary cells (Gabriel *et al.*, 1988). A comparable result has been observed *in vivo*: intracerebroventricular (i.c.v.) injection of galanin increases prolactin and growth hormone secretion (Melander *et al.*, 1987; Koshiyama *et al.*, 1990). However, the mechanism of this effect is unknown. This effect on release may be indirect as suggested by Inoue and collabor-

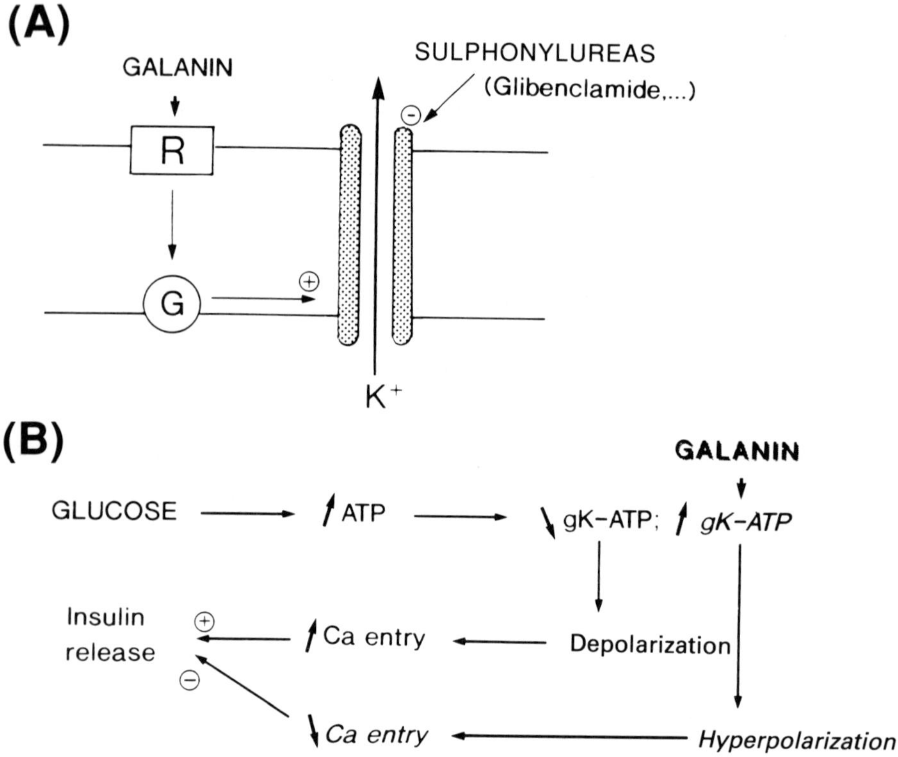

Figure 5.1. Schematic representation of the putative action of galanin on the release of insulin in pancreatic β-cells. (A) Galanin, acting on its receptor (R), activates the gK_{ATP} through a pertussi toxin-sensitive G-protein (G). The channel is inactivated by sulphonylureas such as glibenclamide. (B) In pancreatic β-cells, glucose increases intracellular ATP which inhibits gK_{ATP}: this induces a membrane depolarization, an increase in calcium entry and an increase in insulin release. Galanin activates gK_{ATP} (as described in A), induces hyperpolarization of the membrane and inhibition of calcium entry, and inhibits insulin secretion.

ators (1988) who showed that pituitary prolactin secretion could result from a previous galanin-induced release of hypothalamic vasoactive intestinal polypeptide (VIP). The implication of α-adrenergic and opioid mechanisms has also been suggested in the release of prolactin induced by galanin (Koshiyama *et al.*, 1990). The nature of the mechanism, direct or indirect, on release and the possible implication of intracellular factors remain to be determined.

b. *Inhibition of the release of neurotransmitters*

Several laboratories, using double immunohistochemical techniques, have demonstrated that in some areas of the CNS galanin is co-localized with either classical neurotransmitters or with other peptides. One of the best examples is, without doubt, the co-localization of galanin with the neurones expressing cholinergic enzymes such as the degradative enzyme of acetylcholine (ACh), acetylcholinesterase (AChE), or the synthesizing enzyme of ACh, choline acetyltransferase (ChAT). The first evidence came from the study of Melander *et al.* (1985) who demonstrated the simultaneous presence of ChAT and galanin in septo-hippocampal neurones. The coexistence of galanin and ChAT is not specific to the rodent, since their co-localization has also been described in the septum–basal forebrain complex and in the hippocampus of the monkey (Melander and Staines, 1986; Walker *et al.*, 1989) and of humans (Chan-Palay, 1988b). It is noteworthy that some interspecies differences exist: galanin and ChAT coexist in the cells of the nucleus basalis of Meynert in owls and rhesus monkeys (Melander and Staines, 1986; Walker *et al.*, 1989), but not in the nucleus basalis magnocellularis in the rat (Melander *et al.*, 1985).

Galanin is also co-localized with noradrenaline in the locus coeruleus, with serotonin in the mesencephalic and medullary raphe nuclei, with the synthesizing enzyme of γ-aminobutyric acid (GABA); the glutamic acid decarboxylase (GAD), in the posterior aspects of the arcuate nucleus, the median eminence and the tuberal and caudal magnocellular nuclei, with tyrosine hydroxylase in the arcuate nucleus, with dopamine in the median eminence, and with GABA in the hypothalamus (Melander *et al.*, 1986). Galanin also coexists with other neuropeptides: vasopressin in the rat hypothalamo-hypophyseal system (Melander *et al.*, 1986; Skofitsch *et al.*, 1989) and with pituitary hormones in the rat anterior pituitary gland (Steel *et al.*, 1989). One of the primary effects of galanin in these neurones could be a presynaptic inhibitory effect on neurotransmitter release.

i. Aminergic systems

Galanin inhibits the potassium-induced release of dopamine from the rat median eminence *in vitro* (Nordström *et al.*, 1987). Galanin may act on presynaptic receptors located on dopamine nerve endings and act as a brake to prevent any excess of release of dopamine. The mechanism of action of galanin at the presynaptic level, however, is unknown.

Interactions between galanin and 5-hydroxytryptamine (5-HT) have been reported. *In vitro*, galanin decreases the K_d value of 5-HT_{1A} binding sites in the rat ventral limbic cortex (Fuxe *et al.*, 1988a). *In vivo*, i.c.v. injections of galanin lead to a reduction of 5-HT metabolism in some cortical and hippocampal regions (Fuxe *et al.*, 1988b). Other authors report a presynaptic inhibitory effect of galanin on central 5-HT neurones (Sundström and Melander, 1988).

Finally, galanin decreases the spontaneous activity of noradrenergic locus coeruleus neurones *in vitro* (Seutin *et al.*, 1989).

ii. Cholinergic systems

The effect of galanin on cholinergic mechanisms in the CNS has been studied more extensively. One of the main reasons is that galanin is co-localized with ACh in cholinergic pathways known to be altered during degenerative diseases such as Alzheimer's disease. The localization of galanin in cholinergic neurones of the septo-hippocampal pathway raises the question of the role of galanin in the hippocampus and of the possible interactions between galanin and ACh. To answer these questions, we studied the effect of galanin on CA1 pyramidal neurones from the ventral hippocampus where the galanin binding sites are located. We used intracellular recordings in the *in vitro* slice preparation.

c. *Studies of the actions of galanin in hippocampus*

i. The postsynaptic action of galanin

Galanin had no direct postsynaptic action on pyramidal neurones. It had no obvious effect on membrane polarization (except for a small hyperpolarization in 50% of the cases) and no effect on the after-hyperpolarization (AHP) which follows a train of spikes. This AHP is due to the activation of a calcium-dependent potassium conductance (see Figure 5.2A).

Galanin did not behave as an antagonist of ACh or carbachol in the hippocampus. ACh or carbachol induced a depolarization of the membrane potential, a blockade of the AHP and of the accommodation of the spike discharge and a depression of the excitatory postsynaptic potential (EPSP) elicited by electrical stimulation of afferents located in the stratum radiatum. In the presence of galanin, all these effects of ACh or carbachol were unchanged suggesting that galanin did not interact with muscarinic receptors at the postsynaptic site (Dutar *et al.*, 1989).

Galanin has been shown to inhibit the muscarinic stimulation of phosphoinositide (PI) turnover in the ventral hippocampus (Palazzi *et al.*, 1988). This result suggests that galanin and ACh might interact at the level of intracellular or intramembrane mechanisms. Previously, we implicated PI turnover activation in the muscarinic suppression of a voltage-dependent potassium current, called the M-current (Dutar and Nicoll, 1988). If galanin blocks the muscarinic stimulation of PI turnover, then it could also inhibit the muscarinic suppression of the M-current. We tested the effect of galanin on the carbachol-induced suppression of the M-current in slices from ventral hippocampus using the voltage-clamp technique. We observed that galanin was unable to block or to reverse the cholinergic blockade of the M-current (Dutar *et al.*, unpublished results; see Figure 5.2B). One possible explanation could be that the inhibition of the muscarinic stimulation of PI turnover is only partial. Indeed, galanin decreases the ability of carbachol to stimulate the accumulation of inositol phosphate by only 20–36% (Palazzi *et al.*, 1988).

ii. Action of galanin on synaptic potentials

We tested the effect of galanin on synaptic events in the ventral hippocampus (Dutar *et al.*, 1989). By stimulating the stratum radiatum, it was possible

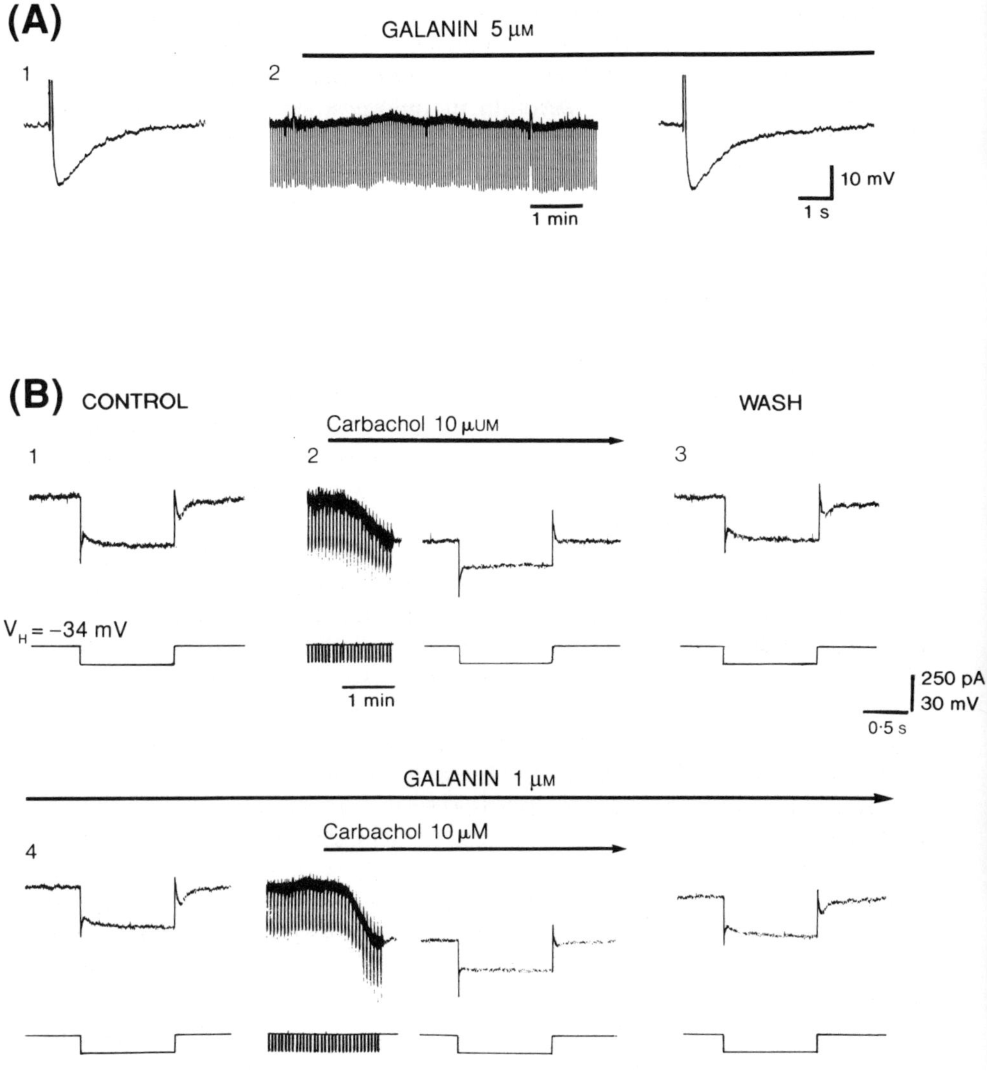

Figure 5.2. (A) Intracellular recording from a CA1 pyramidal neurone from ventral hippocampus. (1) The after-hyperpolarization (AHP) is elicited in response to a brief (60 ms) depolarizing pulse. (2) Constant current hyperpolarizing pulses are applied at 0·3 Hz to measure the membrane input resistance; galanin (5 μM) applied in the superfusion bath induces no change in the membrane potential, in the membrane resistance or in the size of the AHP. (B) Lack of effect of galanin on the muscarinic suppression of the M-current. (1) A cell is held in voltage clamp at a potential of −34 mV and stepped to −50 mV for 1 s. This step results in a time-dependent inward relaxation of membrane current due to the closure of M-current channels. (2) The chart speed is then reduced and the M-current is elicited every 4 s. Carbachol (10 μM) is applied by superfusion through the bath and induces a large inward current, a decrease in instantaneous conductance and reversibly blocks the M-current. (3) These effects recover after washing carbachol from the bath. (4) Galanin (1 μM) is applied for 20 min and the M-current is elicited. Carbachol is then applied and induces comparable effects as in control.

to record synaptic events in CA1 pyramidal cells which included a fast EPSP due to the release of excitatory amino acids and a biphasic inhibitory postsynaptic potential (IPSP) due to the action of GABA released from nerve terminals. It was also possible to induce a slow cholinergic EPSP (cholEPSP) by electrical stimulation of the cholinergic fibres located in stratum oriens. This cholEPSP was induced in the pyramidal neurones by the action of endogenous acetylcholine released from electrically stimulated cholinergic afferents.

Galanin had a weak effect on EPSPs and IPSPs triggered by stimulation of the stratum radiatum, depressing them by only 20–25%, on average. In contrast, galanin was able to antagonize the cholEPSP by 60%, on average (Figure 5.3). This effect was unlikely to result from a postsynaptic action of the peptide, as the resting membrane potential and the input resistance of the neurones were only slightly affected by the peptide. This result suggests that galanin could have a presynaptic inhibitory effect in the hippocampus. This is consistent with the data obtained by Fisone *et al.* (1987) who showed, using a microdialysis technique, that galanin administered i.c.v. inhibited the scopolamine-induced release of ACh in the ventral hippocampus and also inhibited the *in vitro* release of ACh evoked in the hippocampus by high potassium. The presynaptic effect of galanin preferentially affected the cholinergic terminals since the depression of the EPSP triggered by stimulation of Schaffer collaterals/commissural fibres was less consistent and less potent (Figure 5.3A).

Under which physiological conditions could galanin regulate the release of ACh? Although the conditions under which galanin can be released from the septo-hippocampal terminals are unknown, one can hypothesize that it would be released when the septo-hippocampal pathway is stimulated at high frequency. As a consequence, the release of ACh would be controlled by ACh itself acting on muscarinic presynaptic receptors at low rates of firing, whereas both ACh and galanin would act together to inhibit ACh release at high rates of firing (Figure 5.4).

5.2.3. **What are the cellular mechanisms underlying the galanin effects?**

The precise mechanism by which galanin inhibits central neurotransmitter release is still unknown. Earlier in this chapter we emphasized the role of ATP-sensitive potassium channels (potassium channels inhibited by intracellular ATP, gK_{ATP}) in the control of insulin release by pancreatic β-cells. Galanin acting on these conductances produces hypoglycaemia. In the CNS, galanin may act on the same kind of potassium conductance, inhibiting the release of neurotransmitters. Interestingly, the presence of gK_{ATP}, initially described in cardiac ventricular cells, in pancreatic β-cells and in skeletal muscle (for references see Ashcroft, 1988), has also been demonstrated in the CNS, although with different properties (Ashford *et al.*, 1988). Moreover, substances known to interact with this class of potassium channels,

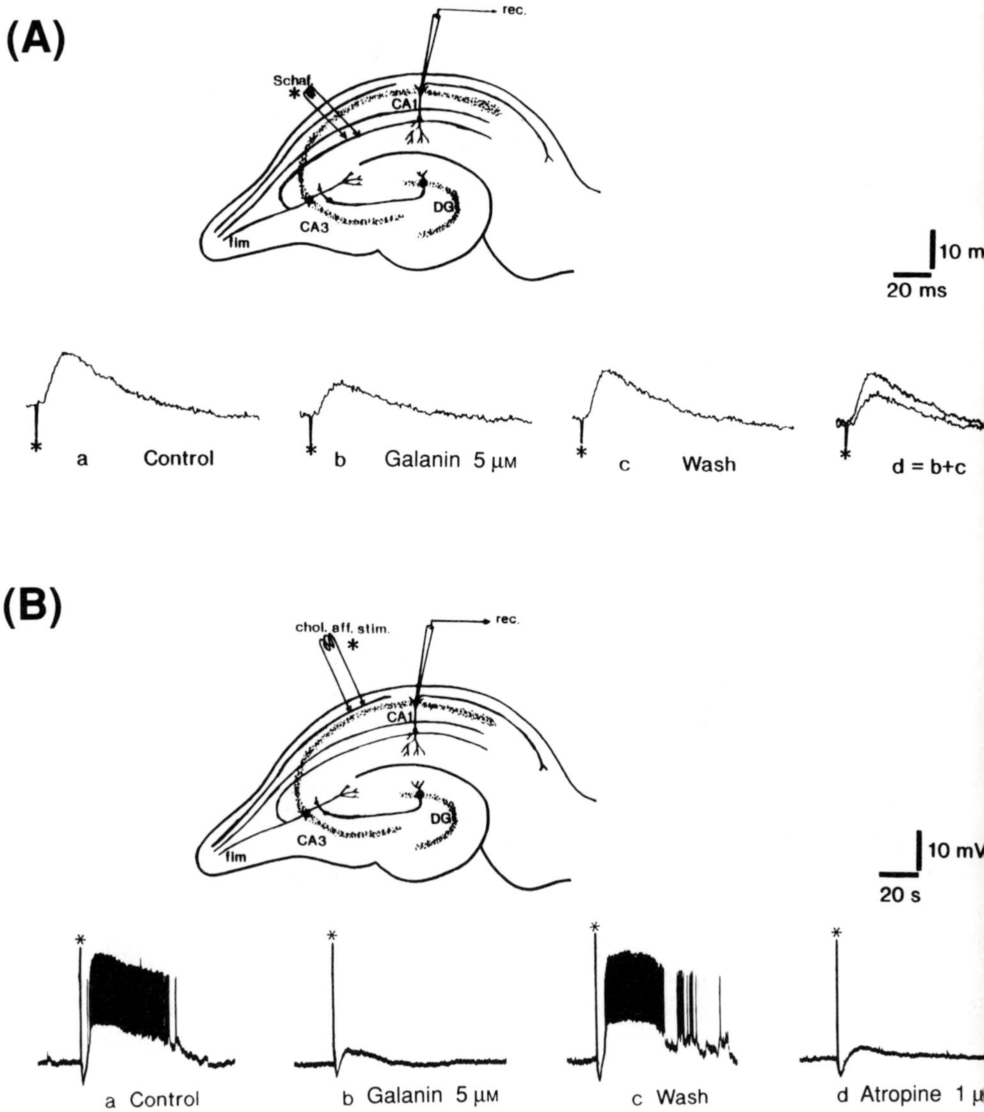

Figure 5.3. Effect of galanin on synaptic events in the ventral hippocampal slices. (A) Effect of galanin on EPSP induced by electrical stimulation of Schaffer collaterals and commissural fibres. Top: schematic location of the stimulating and recording electrodes in hippocampus. Bottom: (a) an EPSP is induced by stimulation of stratum radiatum; (b) 20 min after superfusion with galanin, the EPSP is reduced; (c) the control size of the EPSP recovers after washing galanin from the bath; (d) the trace recorded in (c) is superimposed on the trace recorded in (b). (B) Effect of galanin on the cholinergic EPSP induced by electrical stimulation of cholinergic afferents located in stratum oriens. Top: schematic location of the electrodes. Bottom: (a) the slow cholinergic EPSP is elicited by stimulating the cholinergic fibres in the presence of eserine (2 μM) in the medium; (b) the cholinergic EPSP is depressed after superfusion of galanin for 20 min; (c) it recovers 30 min after washing galanin from the bath and (d) is blocked by application of atropine.
Asterisks indicate stimulation artifacts; fim: fimbria; DG: Dentate Gyrus; rec: recording; chol. aff. stim.: cholinergic afferents stimulation.

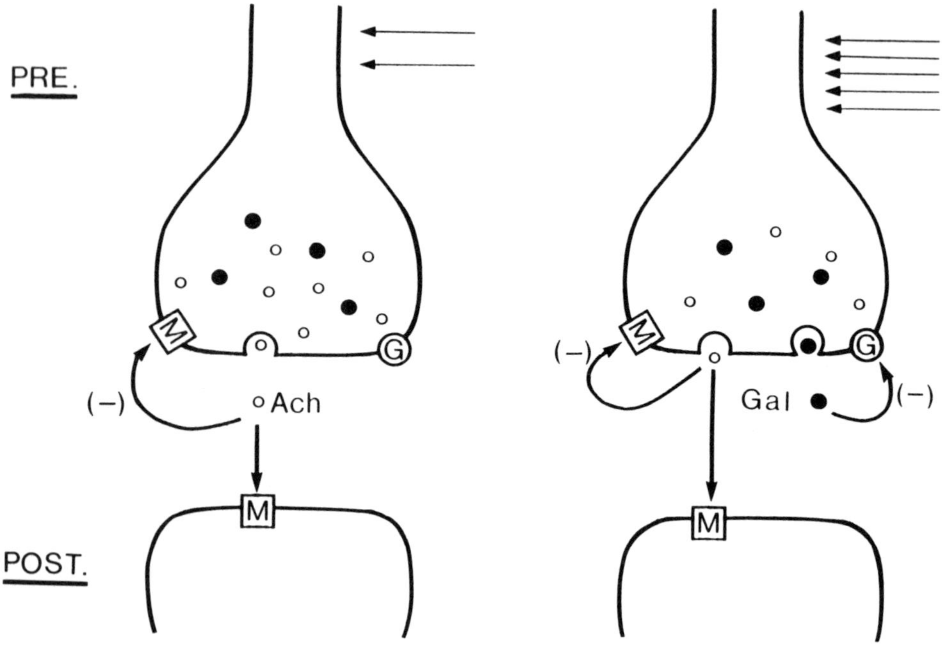

Figure 5.4. Schematic representation of the possible role for galanin-mediated presynaptic inhibition. Left: acetylcholine (○, ACh) is released at low rates of stimulation. ACh induces a postsynaptic (POST.) effect as well as presynaptic (PRE.) inhibitory effect on muscarinic receptors (M). Right, at high discharge frequencies, galanin (•, Gal) is released from large dense core vesicles and acts in synergy with ACh to further reduce the release of ACh by acting on galanin receptors (G).

such as sulphonylureas, have numerous binding sites in the CNS (Mourre *et al.*, 1989). Sulphonylureas stimulate insulin release in pancreatic β-cells. As in insulin-secreting cells and cardiac cells, the binding sites of sulphonylureas may be coupled to ATP-regulated potassium channels in brain cells (Bernardi *et al.*, 1988). These substances have been shown to have potent actions in brain cells (particularly on neurotransmitter release) strongly suggesting a physiological role of gK_{ATP} in nerve terminals (Amoroso *et al.*, 1990; Ben Ari, 1990).

Therefore, the action of galanin on neurotransmitter release in the CNS may involve ATP-dependent potassium channels. Recently it has been demonstrated in CA3 hippocampal pyramidal neurones that galanin reduces the depolarization induced by anoxia, probably through a decrease in the release of glutamate (Ben Ari, 1990). In contrast, the potent sulphonylurea glibenclamide, which blocks gK_{ATP}, augmented the anoxic depolarization. These results are compatible with an effect of galanin in central neurones comparable to the one described in insulinoma cells where galanin blocks the release of transmitters through activation of gK_{ATP}.

5.2.4. **Galanin, behaviour and ageing**

a. *Behaviour*

The septo-hippocampal pathway plays an important role in learning and memory. The presence of galanin in cholinergic medial septal neurones projecting to the hippocampal formation and of receptors for galanin in the hippocampal formation, led to the hypothesis that this peptide might have a functional role in the septo-hippocampal pathway. Therefore, much attention has been given to the possible effects of galanin on learning and memory processes (for a review see Crawley and Wenk, 1989). It has been shown that the i.c.v. administration of galanin in normal rats induces a significant deficit in the acquisition of a modified Morris swim maze task, with no modification in retrieval (Sundström *et al.*, 1988). In contrast, Mastropaolo *et al.* (1988) using a T-maze delayed alternation task reported that galanin had no effect on performances. Another set of experiments demonstrated that in rats with lesions of the nucleus basalis–medial septal area, the intraventricular or intrahippocampal injection of galanin partially antagonized the ability of acetylcholine to reverse the memory deficit in a T-maze delayed alternation task (Mastropaolo *et al.*, 1988).

In conclusion, it is not yet clear if galanin by itself plays a role in learning and memory processes; available data are rather compatible with an action of galanin as an inhibitory modulator of cholinergic function in the septo-hippocampal pathway.

b. *Ageing*

Alterations in the function of the central cholinergic systems in ageing are likely (see Decker, 1987). Numerous studies in animals and humans have examined possible age-related changes in cholinergic neurones. It has been shown that the morphology of the cholinergic neurones in the basal forebrain is altered in aged rodents (Flood and Coleman, 1988). Since galanin coexists in the cholinergic neurones of the medial septal area, it was of interest to determine if galanin-positive cells are modified with ageing in the rat. We examined the morphology and the number of galanin-positive cells in the medial septum and the nucleus of the diagonal band of Broca, as well as their involvement in the septo-hippocampal pathway in young (3-month-old) and old (27–30-month-old) male Sprague–Dawley rats (Senut *et al.*, 1989). A significant and substantial loss of the galanin-containing cells was observed in the rat medial septal area (Figure 5.5). The optical density of the immunoreactive product was markedly reduced. Some galanin-positive somata were also morphologically altered, with a shrunken appearance. The reduction in the number of cells immunoreactive for galanin in aged rats ranged from 30 to 85%, as compared to young animals (Figure 5.5). In aged rats, the proportion of septo-hippocampal neurones containing galanin was

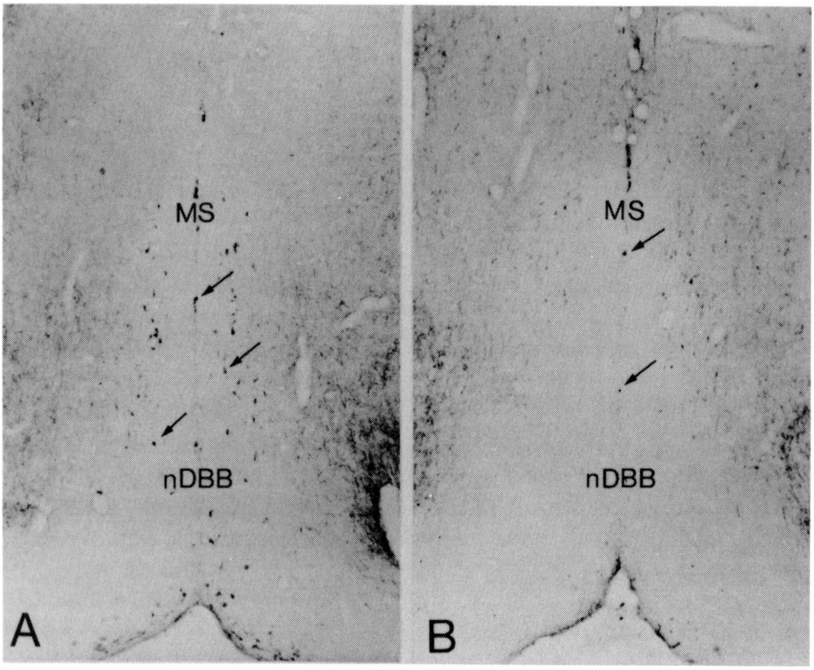

Figure 5.5 Bright-field photomicrographs of transversal sections through the medial septal area illustrating the distribution of cell bodies immunoreactive for galanin in 3-month-old (A) and 26-month-old (B) rats. (A) Numerous galanin-positive cell bodies can be observed in the medial septum (MS) and the nucleus of the diagonal band of Broca (nDBB; arrows). (B) Only a few galanin-positive cells (arrows) are present in the MS–nDBB complex (compare with A). × 33.

reduced (13% versus 22% in young animals). This difference, however, failed to reach statistical significance (Senut *et al.*, 1989). In order to determine the time of onset of this cell loss, we studied the distribution pattern, the morphology and the number of galanin-positive cell bodies in the medial septal region of young (3-month old) and 6–9-, 10–12- and 16–18-month-old rats. There was a significant loss of galanin cell somata in 16–18-month-old rats. In addition, a reduction in the number of galanin-positive cells was already observed in a few 12-month-old rats. In contrast, the density and the distribution pattern of galanin-immunoreactivity was similar at 3, 6–9 and 9–12 months. It remains to be determined if this reduction in the number of galanin-positive cells in the medial septal area in aged rats corresponds to a true cell loss and/or to a decreased expression of the galanin gene. Nevertheless, our results demonstrate that galanin-positive cells in the rat medial septal area undergo alterations with ageing.

Galanin-immunoreactivity has also been demonstrated in the basal forebrain in humans. Changes in the pattern of galanin-immunoreactivity have been described in Alzheimer's disease (Chan-Palay, 1988a; Vogels *et al.*,

1989). Among other things, an increase of galanin innervation of the cholinergic neurones in the nucleus basalis of Meynert has been reported (Chan-Palay, 1988a). This finding, taken together with the demonstration of an inhibitory effect of galanin on ACh release, raised the hypothesis that the galaninergic hyperinnervation observed in this nucleus might reinforce the cholinergic deficit described in Alzheimer's disease. However, the function of endogenous galanin in behaviour has to be more precisely defined before we understand the significance of these observations.

Acknowledgement

This work was supported in part by a grant from Bayer-Pharma, France.

References

Ahrén, B., Berggren, P.O., Bokvist, K. and Rorsman, P. (1989). Does galanin inhibit insulin secretion by opening of the ATP-regulated K^+ channel in the β-cell? *Peptides*, **10**, 453–457.

Amoroso, S., Schmid-Antomarchi, H., Fosset, M. and Lazdunski, M. (1990). Glucose, sulfonylureas, and neurotransmitter release: role of ATP-sensitive K^+ channels. *Science*, **247**, 852–854.

Ashcroft, F.M. (1988). Adenosine-5′-triphosphate-sensitive potassium channels. *Annual Review of Neuroscience*, **11**, 97–118.

Ashford, M.L.J., Sturgess, N.C., Trout, N.J., Gardner, N.J. and Hales, C.N. (1988). Adenosine-5′-triphosphate-sensitive ion channels in neonatal rat cultured central neurones. *Pflügers Archives*, **412**, 297–304.

Ben Ari, Y. (1990). Galanin and glibenclamide modulate the anoxic release of glutamate in rat CA3 hippocampal neurons. *European Journal of Neuroscience*, **2**, 62–68.

Bernardi, H., Fosset, M. and Lazdunski, M. (1988). Characterization, purification, and affinity labeling of the brain [^{3}H]glibenclamide-binding protein, a putative neuronal ATP-regulated K^+ channel. *Proceedings of the National Academy of Sciences USA*, **85**, 9816–9820.

Chan-Palay, V. (1988a). Galanin hyperinnervates surviving neurons of the human basal nucleus of Meynert in dementias of Alzheimer's and Parkinson's disease: a hypothesis for the role of galanin in accentuating cholinergic dysfunction in dementia. *Journal of Comparative Neurology*, **273**, 543–557.

Chan-Palay, V. (1988b). Neurons with galanin innervate cholinergic cells in the human basal forebrain and galanin and acetylcholine coexist. *Brain Research Bulletin*, **21**, 465–472.

Crawley, J.N. and Wenk, G.L. (1989). Co-existence of galanin and acetylcholine: is galanin involved in memory processes and dementia? *Trends in Neuroscience*, **12**, 278–282.

Decker, M.W. (1987). The effect of aging on hippocampal and cortical projections of the forebrain cholinergic system. *Brain Research Review*, **12**, 423–438.

De Weille J.R., Fosset, M., Schmid-Antomarchi, H. and Lazdunski, M. (1989). Galanin inhibits dopamine secretion and activates a potassium channel in pheochromocytoma cells. *Brain Research*, **485**, 199–203.

De Weille J.R., Schmid-Amtomarchi, H., Fosset, M. and Lazdunski, M. (1988).

ATP-sensitive K^+ channels that are blocked by hypoglycemia-inducing sulfonylureas in insulin-secreting cells are activated by galanin, a hyperglycemia-inducing hormone. *Proceedings of the National Academy of Sciences USA*, **85**, 1312–1316.

Dunne, M.J., Bullet, M.J., Li, G., Wollhheim, C.B. and Petersen, O.H. (1989). Galanin activates nucleotide-dependent K^+ channels in insulin-secreting cells via a pertussis toxin-sensitive G-protein. *EMBO Journal*, **8**, 413–420.

Dutar, P. and Nicoll, R.A. (1988). Stimulation of phosphatidylinositol (PI) turnover may mediate the muscarinic suppression of the M-current in hippocampal pyramidal cells. *Neuroscience Letters*, **85**, 89–94.

Dutar, P., Lamour, Y. and Nicoll, R.A. (1989). Galanin blocks the slow cholinergic EPSP in CA1 pyramidal neurons from ventral hippocampus. *European Journal of Pharmacology*, **164**, 355–360.

Fisone, G., Wu, C.F., Consolo, S., Nordström O., Brynne, N., Bartfai, T., Melander, T. and Hökfelt, T. (1987). Galanin inhibits acetylcholine release in the ventral hippocampus of the rat: histochemical, autoradiographic, *in vivo*, and *in vitro* studies. *Proceedings of the National Academy of Sciences USA*, **84**, 7339–7343.

Flood, D.G. and Coleman, P.D. (1988). Neuron numbers and sizes in aging brain: comparisons of human, monkey, and rodent data. *Neurobiology of Aging*, **9**, 453–463.

Fuxe, K., Von Euler, G., Agnati, L.F. and Ogren, S.-O. (1988a). Galanin selectively modulates 5-hydroxytryptamine 1A receptors in the rat ventral limbic cortex. *Neuroscience Letters*, **85**, 163–167.

Fuxe, K., Ogren, S.-O., Jansson, A., Cintra, A., Härfstrand, A. and Agnati, L.F. (1988b). Intraventricular injections of galanin reduces 5-HT metabolism in the ventral limbic cortex, the hippocampal formation and the frontoparietal cortex of the male rat. *Acta Physiologica Scandinavica*, **133**, 579–581.

Gabriel, S.M., Milbury, C.M., Nathanson, J.A. and Martin, J.B. (1988). Galanin stimulates rat pituitary growth hormone secretion *in vitro*. *Life Sciences*, **42** 1981–1986.

Inoue, T., Kato, Y., Koshiyama, H., Yanaihara, N. and Imura, H. (1988). Galanin stimulates the release of vasoactive intestinal polypeptide from perifused hypothalamic fragments *in vitro* and from periventricular structures into the cerebrospinal fluid *in vivo* in the rat. *Neuroscience Letters*, **85**, 95–100.

Koshiyama, H., Shimatsu, A., Kato, Y., Assadian, H., Hattori, N., Ishikawa, Y., Tanoh, T., Yanaihara, N. and Imura, H. (1990). Galanin-induced prolactin release in rats: pharmacological evidence for the involvement of α-adrenergic and opioidergic mechanisms. *Brain Research*, **507**, 321–324.

Mastropaolo, J., Nadi, N.S., Ostrowski, N.L., and Crawley J.N. (1988). Galanin antagonizes acetylcholine on a memory task in basal forebrain-lesioned rats. *Proceedings of the National Academy of Sciences USA*, **85**, 9841–9845.

Melander, T. and Staines, W.A. (1986). A galanin-like peptide coexists in putative cholinergic somata of the septum-basal forebrain complex and in acetylcholinesterase-containing fibers and varicosities within the hippocampus in the owl monkey. *Neuroscience Letters*, **68**, 17–22.

Melander, T., Fuxe, K., Härfstrand, A., Eneroth, P. and Hökfelt, T. (1987). Effects of intraventricular injections of galanin on neuroendocrine functions in the male rat. Possible involvement of hypothalamic catecholamine neuronal systems. *Acta Physiologica Scandinavica*, **131**, 25–32.

Melander, T., Staines, W.A., Hökfelt, T., Rökaeus, A., Eckenstein, F., Salvaterra, P.M. and Wainer, B.H. (1985). Galanin-like immunoreactivity in cholinergic neurons of the septum–basal forebrain complex projecting to the hippocampus of the rat. *Brain Research*, **360**, 130–138.

Melander, T., Hökfelt, T., Rökaeus, Å., Cuello, A.C., Oertel, W.H., Verhofstad, A. and Goldstein, M. (1986). Coexistence of galanin-like immunoreactivity with catecholamines, 5-hydroxytryptamine, GABA and neuropeptides in the rat CNS. *Journal of Neuroscience*, **6**, 3640–3654.

Mourre, C., Ben Ari, Y., Fosset, M. and Lazdunski, M. (1989). Antidiabetic sulfonylureas: localization of binding sites in the brain and effects on the hyperpolarization induced by anoxia in hippocampal slices. *Brain Research*, **486**, 159–164.

Nordström, O., Melander, T., Hökfelt, T., Bartfai, T. and Goldstein, M. (1987). Evidence for an inhibitory effect of the peptide galanin on dopamine release from the rat median eminence. *Neuroscience Letters*, **73**, 21–26.

Palazzi, E., Fisone, G., Hökfelt, T., Bartfai, T. and Consolo, S. (1988). Galanin inhibits the muscarinic stimulation of phosphoinositide turnover in rat ventral hippocampus. *European Journal of Pharmacology*, **148**, 479–480.

Rökaeus, Å. (1987). Galanin: a newly isolated biologically active neuropeptide. *Trends in Neuroscience*, **10**, 158–164.

Senut, M.C., de Bilbao, F. and Lamour, Y. (1989). Age-related loss of galanin-immunoreactive cells in the rat septal area. *Neuroscience Letters*, **105**, 257–262.

Seutin, V., Verbanck, P., Massote, L. and Dresse, A. (1989). Galanin decreases the activity of locus coeruleus neurons *in vitro*. *European Journal of Pharmacology*, **164**, 373–376.

Sharp, G.W.G., Le Marchand-Brustel, Y., Yada, T., Russo, L.L., Bliss, C.R., Cormont, M., Monge, L. and Van Obberghen E. (1989). Galanin can inhibit insulin release by a mechanism other than membrane hyperpolarization or inhibition of adenylate cyclase. *Journal of Biological Chemistry*, **264**, 7302–7309.

Skofitsch, G., Jacobowitz, D.M., Amann, R. and Lembeck, F. (1989). Galanin and vasopressin coexist in the rat hypothalamo-neurohypophyseal system. *Neuroendocrinology*, **49**, 419–427.

Steel, J.H., Gon, G., O'Halloran, D.J., Jones, P.M., Yanaihara, N., Ishikawa, H., Bloom, S.R. and Polack, J.M. (1989). Galanin and vasoactive intestinal polypeptide are colocalized with classical pituitary hormones and show plasticity of expression. *Histochemistry*, **93**, 183–189.

Sundström, E. and Melander, T. (1988). Effects of galanin on 5-HT neurons in the rat CNS. *European Journal of Pharmacology*, **146**, 327–329.

Sundström, E., Archer, T., Melander, T. and Bartfai, T. (1988). Galanin impairs acquisition but not retrieval of spatial memory in rats studied in the Morris swim maze. *Neuroscience Letters*, **88**, 331–335.

Tamura, K., Palmer, J.M., Winkelmann, C.K. and Wood, J.D. (1988). Mechanism of action of galanin on myenteric neurons. *Journal of Neurophysiology*, **60**, 966–979.

Tatemoto, K., Rökaeus, Å., Jörnvall, H., McDonald, T.J. and Mutt, V. (1983). Galanin — a novel biologically active peptide from porcine intestine. *FEBS Letters*, **164**, 124–128.

Vogels, O.J.M., Renkawek, K., Broere, C.A.J., ter Laak, H.J. and van Workum, F. (1989).Galanin-like immunoreactivity within Ch2 neurons in the vertical limb of the diagonal band of Broca in aging and Alzheimer's disease. *Acta Neuropathologica*, **78**, 90–95.

Walker, L.C., Koliatsos, V.E., Kitt, C.A. Richardson, R.T., Rökaeus, Å. and Price, D.L. (1989). Peptidergic neurons in the basal forebrain magnocellular complex of the Rhesus monkey. *Journal of Comparative Neurology*, **280**, 272–282.

Yau, W.M., Dorsett, J.A. and Youther, M.L. (1986). Evidence for galanin as an inhibitory neuropeptide on myenteric cholinergic neurons in the guinea pig small intestine. *Neuroscience Letters*, **72**, 305–308.

Chapter 6

Galanin: distribution and function

A. Dresse and V. Seutin

6.1. *Introduction*

The mammalian encephalon expresses various neuropeptides localized in discrete brain regions. The neuroanatomical distribution of those peptides has been extensively studied during the last 10 years using morphological techniques such as immunohistochemistry and electron microscopy (see review in Bjorklund and Hökfelt, 1985). They are often co-localized with the classical neurotransmitters, acetylcholine (ACh), dopamine (DA), noradrenaline (NA), 5-hydroxytryptamine (5-HT) and γ-aminobutyric acid (GABA).

The functional role and importance of many neuropeptides remains the subject of debate and controversy. Furthermore, in spite of the numerous neuropeptides already discovered, it is clear that genes expressing brain-specific peptides which have not yet been fully sequenced and characterized are present in the brain of various species, (Sutcliffe, 1988), a conclusion derived from a molecular biology approach.

To develop our knowledge of the functional role of neuropeptides and to find new and potentially interesting brain-specific peptides, we are trying to combine electrophysiology with the powerful tool offered by molecular biology.

6.2. *Chemical structure of galanin*

As for many other brain peptides, galanin was first observed in the intestine. It is a 29-amino acid peptide first isolated from pig intestine by Tatemoto *et al.* in 1983; its name derives from the N-terminal and C-terminal residues which are, respectively glycine and *alanine*. As shown in Figure 6.1, taken from a review by Rökaeus (1987), galanin is part of a 123-amino acid protein called preprogalanin containing a signal peptide, a pregalanin message peptide formed by post-translational processing, galanin itself and a galanin-message-associated peptide.

By sequencing the mRNA coding for galanin in various species, it has been possible to deduce the amino acid sequence of porcine, rat and bovine

(A)

1 5 10 15
Gly-Trp-Thr-Leu-Asn-Ser-Ala-Gly-Tyr-Leu-Leu-Gly-Pro-His-Ala-

16 20 25
Ile-Asp-Asn-His-Arg-Ser-Phe-His-Asp-Lys-Tyr-Gly-Leu-Ala-NH_2

(B)

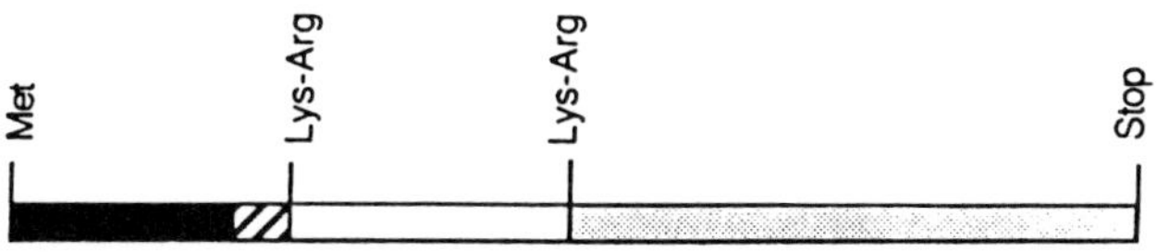

Figure 6.1. (A) Amino acid sequence of the porcine intestinal galanin molecule. (B) Schematic drawing of the 123-amino acid preprogalanin molecule: □, galanin part; ■, signal peptide; ▨, galanin message-associated peptide is represented by a stippled box. After Rökaeus *et al.*, 1987.

PORCINE GALANIN 1-29

GLY-TRP-THR-LEU-ASN-SER-ALA-GLY-TYR-LEU-
LEU-GLY-PRO-HIS-ALA-ILE-ASP-ASN-HIS-ARG-
SER-PHE-HIS-ASP-LYS-TYR-GLY-LEU-ALA-NH2

RAT GALANIN 1-29

GLY-TRP-THR-LEU-ASN-SER-ALA-GLY-TYR-LEU-
LEU-GLY-PRO-HIS-ALA-ILE-ASP-ASN-HIS-ARG-
SER-PHE-SER-ASP-LYS-HIS-GLY-LEU-THR-NH2

BOVINE GALANIN 1-29

GLY-TRP-THR-LEU-ASN-SER-ALA-GLY-TYR-LEU-
LEU-GLY-PRO-HIS-ALA-LEU-ASP-SER-HIS-ARG-
SER-PHE-GLN-ASP-LYS-HIS-GLY-LEU-ALA-NH2

Figure 6.2. Amino acid sequence of porcine, rat and bovine galanin 1–29. After Crawley and Wenk, 1989; Rökaeus and Carlquist, 1988.

galanin (Figure 6.2). Some variations may be observed in their composition which are sufficient to produce differences in immunological reactivity and which may have influenced the results of some immunohistochemical experiments.

6.3. *Peripheral localization of galanin*

6.3.1. **Respiratory tract**

Fine varicose galanin-like immunoreactivity (GAL-LI) has been observed beneath the epithelium, around seromucous glands and in the adventitia of the blood vessels in the nasal mucosa, the trachea and the major bronchi. The function of galanin in the respiratory system remains to be determined.

6.3.2. **Gastrointestinal tract**

Galanin was originally isolated from the upper small intestine of pigs. It is present from the oesophagus to the rectum as an intrinsic system, mainly localized in the submucosal and myenteric plexi of the upper part of the small intestine. Galanin appears to be a modulator of gastrointestinal function able to influence motility, absorption, secretion and blood flow.

6.3.3. **Pancreas**

A dense network of GAL-LI containing nerve fibres has been shown to surround the islets of Langerhans. At that level, galanin exerts a strong inhibitory action on glucose-induced insulin release. This effect has important physiological implications in the regulation of insulin and has allowed a better understanding of the molecular mechanisms involved in galanin action.

Indeed, it has been shown (Figure 6.3) that galanin activates ATP-dependent K^+ channels in insulin-secreting cells via a pertussis toxin-sensitive G-protein. This effect is shared by somatostatin. In contrast, hypoglycaemia-inducing sulphonylureas inhibit ATP-sensitive K^+ channels (De Weille *et al.*, 1988; Ahrén *et al.*, 1989; Dunne *et al.*, 1989; Nilsson *et al.*, 1989).

6.3.4. **Urogenital tract**

In the urogenital tract GAL-LI has been detected in the human prostate, vas deferens, corpus cavernosum and spongiosum. Lower amounts were found in the epididymis and testis as well as in the female tract (vagina, cervix, uterus, fallopian tubes and ovaries).

Galanin facilitates the contractions of the vas deferens, vesicula seminalis and cervix induced by electrical stimulation.

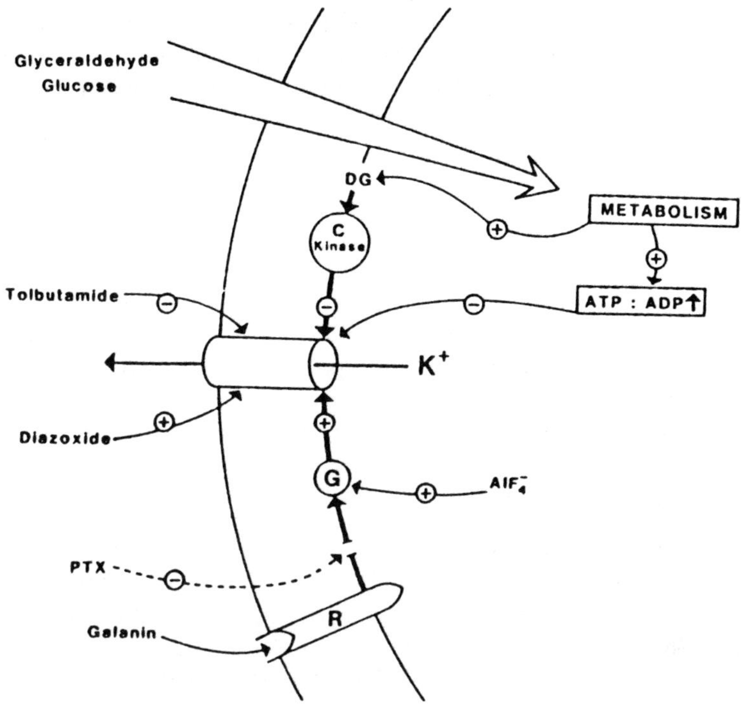

Figure 6.3. The K_{ATP} channel and its physiological regulation in insulin secreting cells. Channel activation, resulting in a membrane hyperpolarization, evoked by galanin is mediated by the receptor (R) activating a pertussis toxin (PTX)-sensitive G-protein (G) coupled to the K_{ATP} channel. Conversely, K^+ channel inhibition resulting in a membrane depolarization, evoked by either glucose or glyceraldehyde, is mediated either by a metabolic increase in the ATP : ADP ratio and/or through the activation of a C-kinase protein, coupled to the channel, via the metabolic generation of 1,2 diacylglycerol (DG).
After Dunne *et al.*, 1989.

6.3.5. **Adrenal gland**

GAL-LI is present in the medullary part of the adrenal gland in various species. The pig adrenal medulla was chosen as the source of mRNA to construct the cDNA library leading to the sequencing of preprogalanin.

6.4. *Localization of galanin in the central nervous system*

The distribution of galanin-containing cell bodies and fibre systems has been studied in various species including rat, pig, cow, monkey and human. In rat brain, the highest concentrations are found in the median eminence (943 pmol g^{-1}) and hypothalamus (160 pmol g^{-1}) (Köhler *et al.*, 1986; Beal *et al.*, 1988b; Gentleman *et al.*, 1989).

GAL-LI has been demonstrated in the cell bodies of paraventricular and supraoptic magnocellular nuclei where it coexists with vasopressin, in cell bodies of the nucleus arcuatus (together with tyrosine hydroxylase), in the locus coeruleus (with noradrenaline) and in the raphe nuclei (with 5-HT) (Skofitsch and Jacobowitz, 1985, 1986; Skofitsch *et al.*, 1986; Levine *et al.*, 1987; Meister and Hokfelt, 1988; Ceccatelli *et al.*, 1989).

An important coexistence of GAL-LI with choline acetyltransferase (ChAT) has been noted in cholinergic structures such as the medial septal nucleus, the nucleus of the diagonal band of Broca and the nucleus basalis (Chan-Palay, 1988b; Wenk and Rökaeus, 1988; Crawley and Wenk, 1989; Senut *et al.*, 1989).

Due to its important functional role, special attention has been drawn to galanin in the hippocampus. Retrograde staining techniques have revealed galanin- and ChAT-immunoreactive neurones projecting to the hippocampus. GAL-LI-containing neurones from the locus coeruleus also project to the hippocampus. Important functional effects of galanin have been studied in these structures. They will be reviewed in this chapter.

Finally, GAL-LI has been demonstrated in the spinal cord of pig and rats. GAL-LI containing cell bodies are present in the superficial layers of the dorsal horn (laminae I and II) and in dorsal root ganglia at the lumbosacral level (coexistence with substance P and calcitonin gene-related peptide). They are occasionally seen in the ventral horn. Fibres have been observed in the superficial layers of the spinal cord, Lissauer's tract and around the central canal. The galanin-like substance may therefore function as a neurotransmitter in primary afferents. This hypothesis is reinforced by the fact that a capsaicin treatment of the rats, known to cause a selective degeneration of primary sensory neurones of the C-fibre type, markedly decreases GAL-LI in the medulla.

6.5. *Functional role of galanin in the central nervous system*

Although only a recently discovered peptide, numerous papers are devoted to the functional role of galanin. Therefore, galanin represents a good example of the possible relationships between neuropeptides and classical neurotransmitters. It is not possible, in this short review, to quote all the papers related to this topic. The various facets of galanin properties are therefore illustrated by appropriate examples from the literature and from work performed in our own laboratory.

6.5.1. **Action of galanin on noradrenergic neurones**

In experiments using an indirect immunofluorescence technique combined with retrograde transport of Fast Blue, Holets *et al.* (1988) studied the efferent projections of locus coeruleus (LC) neurones containing neuropeptide Y, tyrosine hydroxylase and GAL-LI (Figure 6.4). It appears that

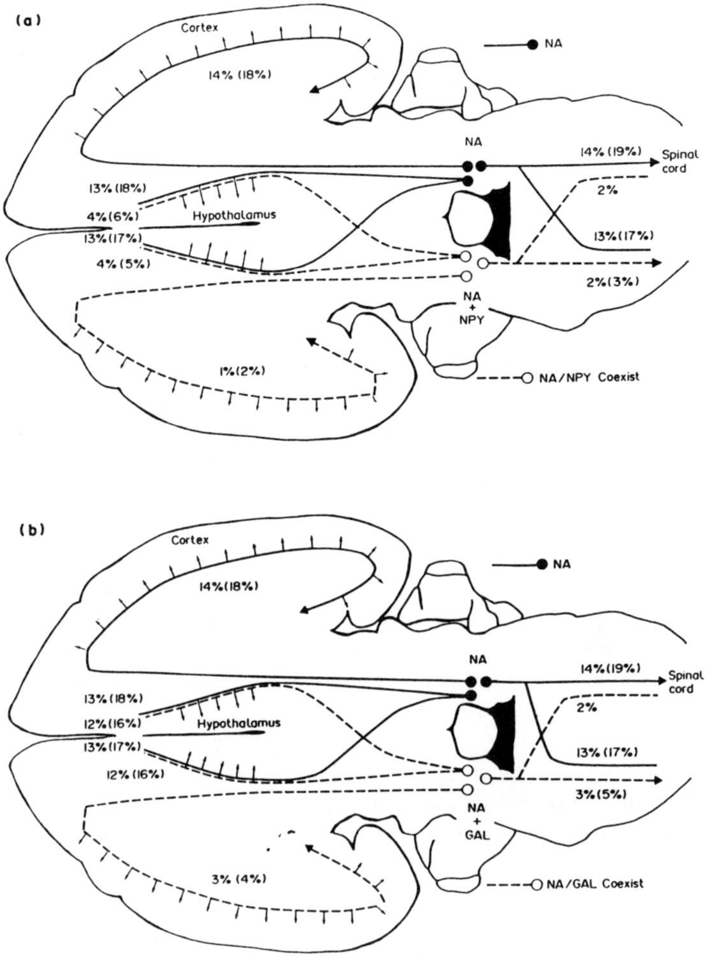

Figure 6.4. Schematic illustration of the percentages of noradrenergic and noradrenergic–peptidergic locus coeruleus projections to the cerebral cortex, hypothalamus and spinal cord. NA. Noradrenaline; NPY, neuropeptide Y, GAL, galanin. Solid line, ipsilateral projections; broken line, contralateral projections.
After Holets *et al.*, 1988.

most of the cells containing GAL-LI also contain the enzyme necessary for the synthesis of noradrenaline. LC cells also contain galanin receptors as shown by Köhler during this symposium (see also Köhler *et al.*, 1986, 1989).

a. *Effect of galanin on the spontaneous firing locus coeruleus cells recorded extracellularly*

We studied the effect of galanin on the spontaneous firing rate of locus coeruleus cells in rat brain slices. A concentration-dependent inhibition of the activity was observed between 10^{-9} and 10^{-7} M. The inhibitory effect was also present in low-Ca^{2+} high Mg^{2+} medium, suggesting a direct inhibitory effect of the peptide (Seutin *et al.*, 1989).

b. *Intracellular recording*

These results have been extended by intracellular recording using micropipettes filled with KCl (2 M) having a tip resistance between 80 and 150 MΩ (Seutin *et al.*, unpublished results). Under these conditions, presumed noradrenergic neurones of LC presented a typical firing rate between 1 and 4 Hz. Spike duration was about 1·5 ms and spike amplitude was above 60 mV from the threshold. Resting potentials were close to −60 mV. In several neurones, spontaneous oscillations of membrane potential were observed when the firing was prevented by injecting negative current. This effect was amplified when the slice was superfused with tetrodotoxin (TTX) and abolished by galanin and α_2 agonists such as clonidine (Figures 6.5 and 6.6).

Galanin (10^{-7} M) produced a hyperpolarization of the membrane (Figure 6.7) without modification of the input resistance. This contrasts with α_2 agonists which produce a large decrease in output resistance in these neurones (Figure 6.8). The results show that galanin is able to modulate the activity of noradrenergic neurones which is compatible with the opening of the ATP-dependent potassium channels described in pancreatic cells.

c. *Effect of galanin at the terminal level*

Nishibori *et al.* (1988) studied the effect of galanin on the cAMP response to NA in the rat cortex. They showed that galanin is able to inhibit in a concentration-dependent manner (from 10^{-8} to 10^{-5} M) the increase in cAMP formation produced by NA (10^{-4} M) (Figure 6.9).

It is known that terminals coming from the LC and innervating the paraventricular nucleus of the hypothalamus contain both NA and galanin (Levine *et al.*, 1987). At that level, galanin is able to inhibit the NA release produced by electrical stimulation in a slice preparation (Tsuda *et al.*, 1989). These results suggest that galanin may act partly by interacting with presynaptic α_2 receptors and inhibitory GTP-binding proteins. Interactions between galanin and NA have also been shown in cardiovascular regulatory centres (Harfstrand *et al.*, 1987).

6.5.2. **Action of galanin on cholinergic neurones**

The hippocampus is innervated by noradrenergic and cholinergic neurones co-containing galanin (Melander *et al.*, 1985, 1986a,b); Figure 6.10). Fisone *et al.* (1987) showed that galanin is able to reduce the ACh-evoked release both *in vivo* and *in vitro* in the ventral, but not in the dorsal, hippocampus.

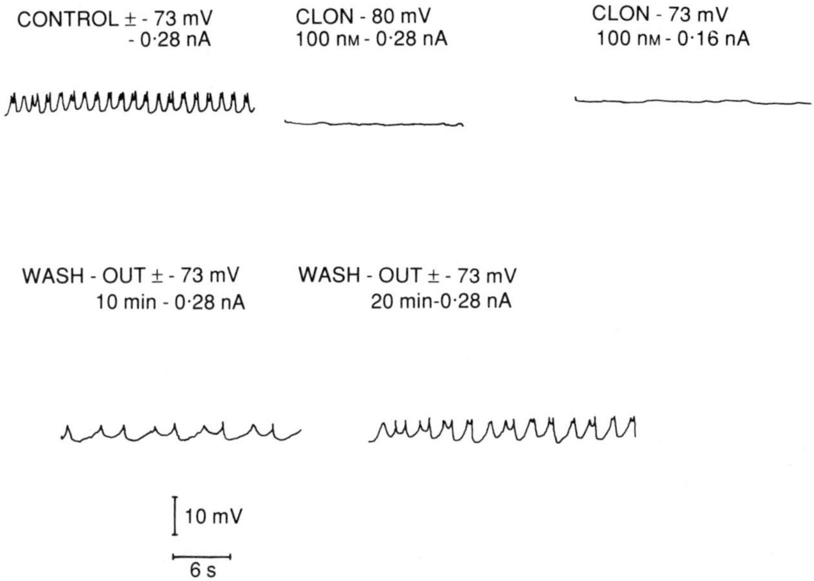

Figure 6.5. The trace is a voltage recording of a locus coeruleus (LC) neurone. The level of membrane potential and the amount of current injected are indicated. The spontaneous α_2 agonist clonidine (CLON) abolishes oscillations of membrane potential in LC neurones.

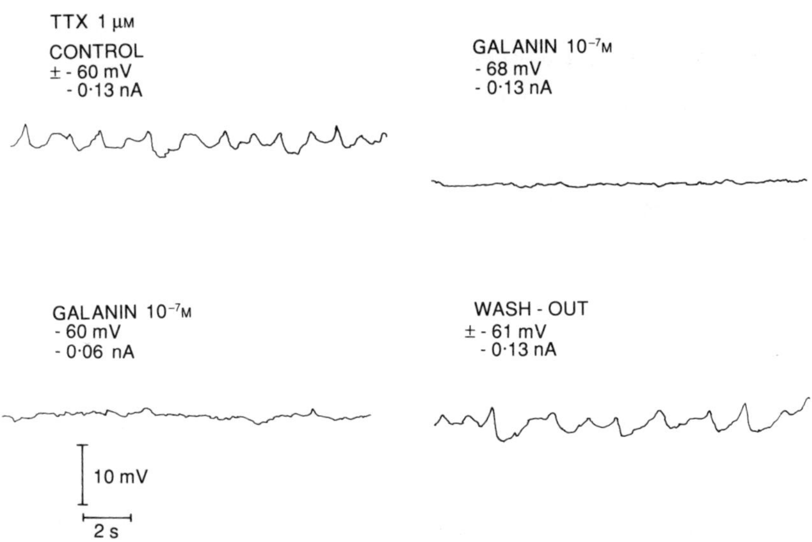

Figure 6.6. Galanin decreases oscillations of membrane potential in locus coeruleus neurones. This experiment was performed in the presence of TTX. Note that the effect of galanin is completely reversible.

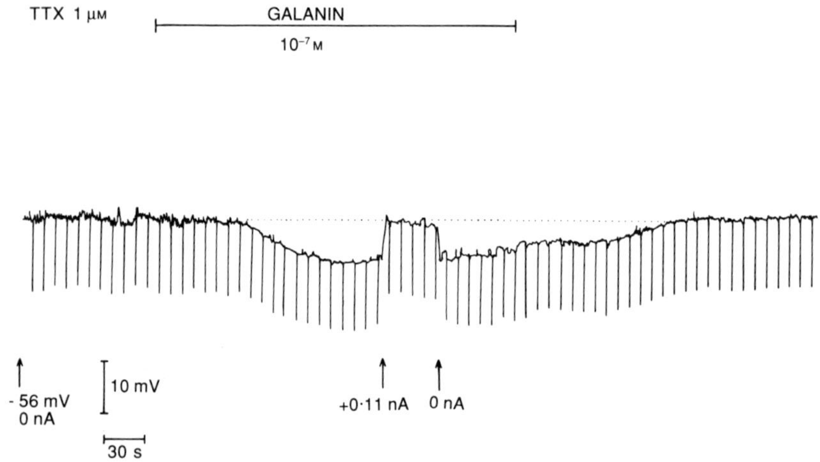

Figure 6.7. Effect of galanin on the membrane potential and input resistance of a locus coeruleus neurone. Input resistance was estimated by injecting 500 ms pulses of −0·1 nA. Note the reversible hyperpolarization and the lack of noticeable change in input resistance.

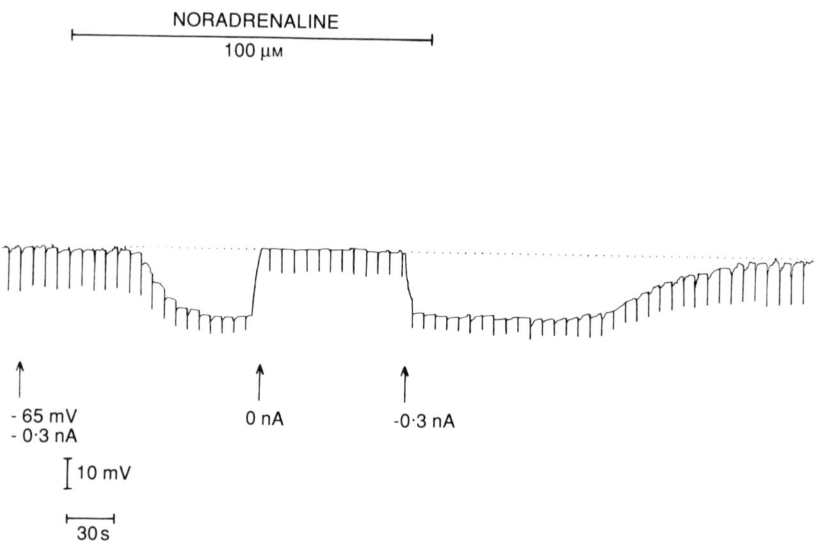

Figure 6.8. Effect of noradrenaline on the membrane potential and input resistance of a locus coeruleus neurone in the same conditions. Note the marked decrease (−40%) in input resistance.

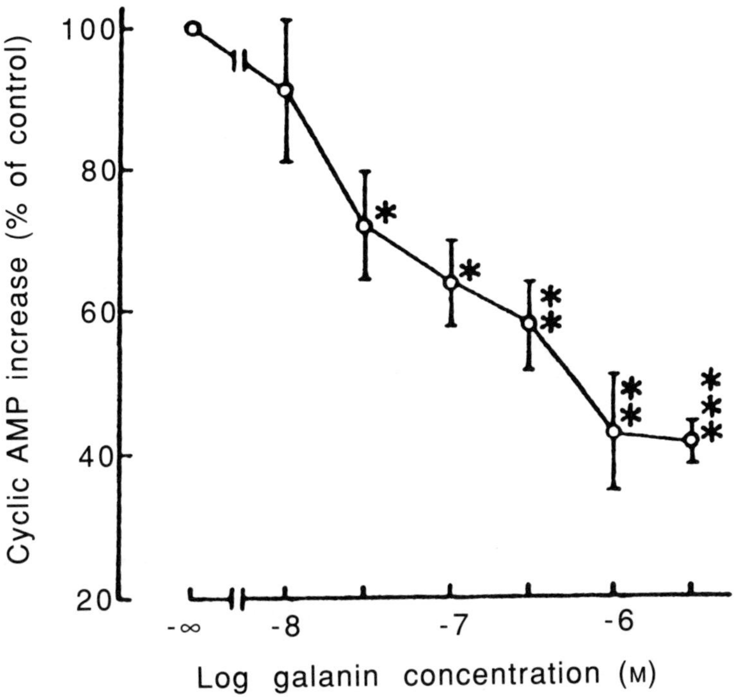

Figure 6.9. Time course of the effect of noradrenaline on the cyclic AMP levels in slices of rat cerebral cortex in the presence or absence of galanin which produced an inhibitory action. After Nishibori *et al.*, 1988.

Similarly, galanin inhibits the muscarinic stimulation of phosphoinositide turnover in the rat ventral hippocampus without effect in the dorsal hippocampus (Palazzi *et al.*, 1988; Figure 6.11). These observations may have important repercussions as it is known that ACh in the hippocampal formation is implicated in cognitive functions (Mastropaolo *et al.*, 1988). Interestingly, galanin protects hippocampal neurones against anoxia (Ben Ari and Lazdunski, 1989).

It is noteworthy that galanin hyperinnervated surviving neurones of the human basal nucleus of Meynert in dementia of the Alzheimer type (Chan-Palay, 1988; Beal *et al.*, 1988a). This hyperinnervation may aggravate the cholinergic deficit well documented in Alzheimer's disease (Crawley and Wenk, 1989).

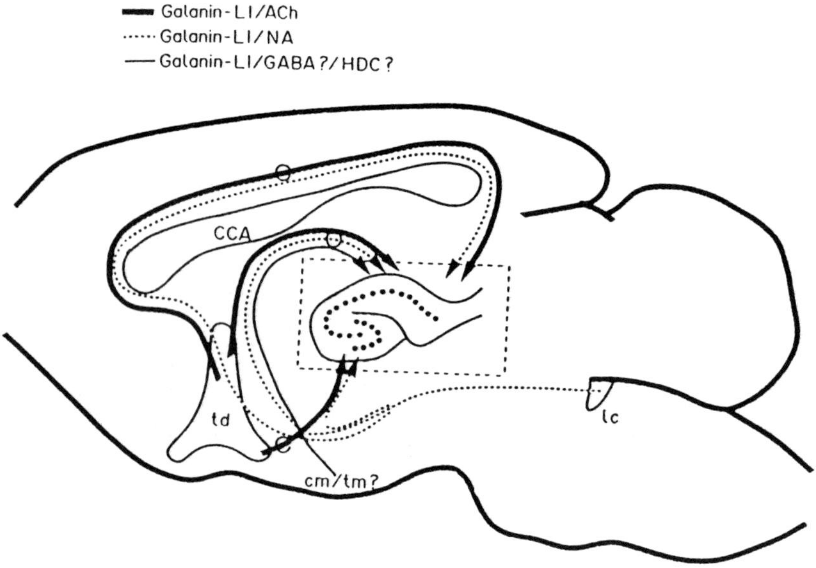

Figure 6.10. Schematic drawing of GAL-LI containing hippocampal afferents and their routes of entry. Contributions to GAL-IR hippocampal fibres are circled. ACh, acetylcholine; NA, noradrenaline; GABA, γ-aminobutyric acid;
After Melander *et al.*, 1986.

6.6. *Molecular biology in the study of brain peptides and proteins*

To determine the amino acid sequence of galanin, the techniques of molecular biology were used. It is also possible to discover new peptides and proteins acting as neuromodulators or receptors using these methods. Although numerous neuropeptides have already been discovered, the mammalian brain still contains undescribed genes coding for potential transmitters or modulators. For these reasons, we decided to use molecular biological techniques to look for brain-specific peptides and to study their potential transmitter or modulator functions by the electrophysiological methods in use in our laboratory.

As described in detail in Marechal *et al.* (1988) and Dresse and Marechal (1989), a rat brain cDNA library was established and screened for brain-specific clones. After appropriate controls, a few brain-specific cDNAs coding for proteins expressed only in the brain were found.

The sequencing of the first of them gave an open reading frame coding for 1821 amino acids. A strong homology was found between this nucleotide sequence in the rat brain and the gene coding for Microtubule Associated Protein (MAP 2) described in the mouse brain. After *in situ* hybridization and immunohistochemistry, a high concentration of MAP 2 mRNA and

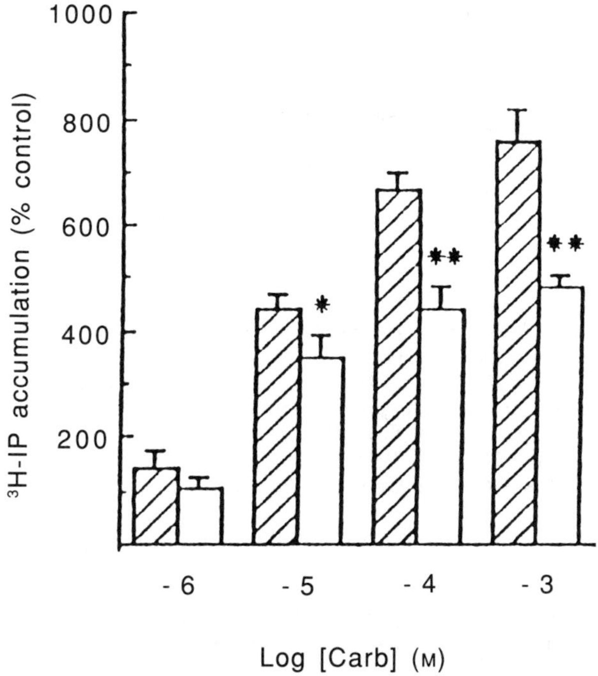

Figure 6.11. Concentration–response curve for the carbachol-stimulated accumulation of [^{3}H]-phosphoinosites (IP) in the ventral hippocampus, in the absence or presence of galanin 1 μM, added to the incubation medium 2 min before carbachol (Carb). Carbachol significantly ($P < 0{\cdot}01$) stimulated [^{3}H]IP accumulation at all concentrations. Galanin did not significantly influence basal [^{3}H]IP accumulation but reduced the carbachol effect.
After Palazzi *et al.*, 1988.

protein was found in the rat cortex and hippocampus (Marechal *et al.*, 1990).

Interestingly, a second clone has been found presenting a strong homology with the $GABA_A$ receptor. Other clones without any known homology are in the sequencing process. These results illustrate the power of the molecular tools applied to neurobiology. In the future, we intend to use our electrophysiological methods investigate the new brain-specific peptides presently sequenced.

6.7. *Summary*

Galanin is an interesting peptide of 29 amino acids found centrally and in various peripheral organs. In the brain, galanin is distributed in numerous functionally important structures such as brain-stem, hypothalamus, hippocampus and cortex. Galanin is often co-localized with classical transmitters (mainly acetylcholine and noradrenaline).

Using biochemical and electrophysiological methods, important inhibitory modulatory effects have been shown. They are partly described in this chapter.

Galanin has been discovered by the use of molecular biology methods. The interest and power of such techniques to study potentially active brain-specific peptides and proteins is also considered.

References

Ahrén, B., Berggren, P.O., Bokvist, K. and Rorsman, P. (1989). Does galanin inhibit insulin secretion by opening of the ATP-regulated K^+ channel in the B-cell? *Peptides*, **10**, 453–457.

Beal, M.F., Clevens, R.A., Chattha, G.K., MacGarvey, U.M., Mazurek, M.F. and Gabriel, S.M. (1988a). Galanin-like immunoreactivity is unchanged in Alzheimer's disease and Parkinson's disease dementia cerebral cortex. *Journal of Neurochemistry*, **51**, 1935–1941.

Beal, M.F., Gabriel, S.M., Swartz, K.J. and MacGarvey, U.M. (1988b). Distribution of galanin-like immunoreactivity in baboon brain. *Peptides*, **9**, 847–851.

Ben Ari, Y. and Lazdunski, M. (1989). Galanin protects hippocampal neurons from the functional effects of anoxia. *European Journal of Pharmacology*, **165**, 331–332.

Björklund, A. and Hökfelt, T. (1985). *Handbook of Chemical Neuroanatomy*, Vol. 4, GABA and neuropeptides in the CNS, Part I. Amsterdam: Elsevier.

Ceccatelli, S. Eriksson, M. and Hökfelt, T. (1989). Distribution and coexistence of corticotropin-releasing factor-, neurotensin-, enkephalin-, cholecystokinin-, galanin- and vasoactive intestinal polypeptide/peptide histidine isoleucine-like peptides in the parvocellular part of the paraventricular nucleus. *Neuroendocrinology*, **49**, 309–323.

Chan-Palay, V. (1988a). Galanin hyperinnervates surviving neurons of the human basal nucleus of Meynert in dementias of Alzheimer's and Parkinson's disease: a hypothesis for the role of galanin in accentuating cholinergic dysfunction in dementia. *Journal of Comparative Neurology*, **273**, 543–557.

Chan-Palay, V. (1988b). Neurons with galanin innervate cholinergic cells in the human basal forebrain and galanin and acetylcholine coexist. *Brain Research Bulletin*, **21**, 465–472.

Crawley, J. and Wenk, G. (1989). Co-existence of galanin and acetylcholine: is galanin involved in memory processes and dementia? *Trends in Neuroscience*, **12**, 278–282.

De Weille, J., Schmid-Antomarchi, H., Fosset, M. and Lazdunski, M. (1988). ATP-sensitive K^+ channels that are blocked by hypoglycemia-inducing sulfonylureas in insulin-secreting cells are activated by galanin, a hyperglycemia-inducing hormone. *Proceedings of the National Academy of Sciences USA*, **85**, 1312–1316.

Dresse, A. and Marechal, D. (1989). Recherche de nouveaux peptides cérébraux par les méthodes du génie génétique. *Bulletin et Mémoires de l'Académie Royale de Médecine de Belgique*, **144** (5–7), 325–334.

Dunne, M., Bullet, M., Li, G., Wollheim, C. and Petersen, O. (1989). Galanin activates nucleotide-dependent K^+ channels in insulin-secreting cells via a pertussis toxin-sensitive G-protein. *EMBO Journal*, **8**, 413–420.

Dutar, P., Lamour, Y. and Nicoll, R. (1989). Galanin blocks the slow cholinergic EPSP in CA1 pyramidal neurons from ventral hippocampus. *European Journal of Pharmacology*, **164**, 355–360.

Fisone, G., Wu, C., Consolo, S., Nordström, Ö, Brynne, N., Bartfai, T., Melander, T. and Hökfelt, T. (1987). Galanin inhibits acetylcholine release in the ventral hippocampus of the rat: histochemical, autoradiographic *in vivo*, and *in vitro* studies. *Proceedings of the National Academy of Sciences USA*, **84**, 7339–7343.

Gentleman, S.M., Falkai, P., Bogerts, B., Herrero, M.T., Polak, J.M. and Roberts, G.W. (1989). Distribution of galanin-like immunoreactivity in the human brain. *Brain Research*, **505**, 311–315.

Harfstrand, A., Fuxe, K., Melander, T., Hökfelt, T. and Agnati, L.F. (1987). Evidence for a cardiovascular role of central galanin neurons: focus on interactions with α_2-adrenergic and neuropeptide Y mechanisms. *Journal of Cardiovascular Pharmacology,* **12**, S199–S204.

Holets, V.R., Hökfelt, T. and Rökaeus, Å. (1988). Locus coeruleus neurons in the rat containing neuropeptide Y, tyrosine hydroxylase or galanin and their efferent projections to the spinal cord, cerebral cortex and hypothalamus. *Neuroscience*, **24**, 893–906.

Köhler, C., Persson, A., Melander, T., Theodorsson, E., Sedvall, G. and Hökfelt, T. (1989). Distribution of galanin-binding sites in the monkey and human telencephalon: preliminary observations. *Experimental Brain Research*, **75**, 375–380.

Köhler, C., Ericson, H., Watanabe, T., Polak, J., Palay, S.L., Palay, V. and Chan-Palay, V. (1986). Galanin immunoreactivity in hypothalamic histamine neurons: further evidence for multiple chemical messengers in the tuberomammillary nucleus. *Journal of Comparative Neurology*, **250**, 58–64.

Levine, M.C., Sawchenko, P.E., Howe, P.R.C., Bloom, S.R. and Polak, J.M. (1987). Organization of galanin-immunoreactive inputs to the paraventricular nucleus with special reference to their relationship to catecholaminergic afferents. *Journal of Comparative Neurology*, **261**, 562–582.

Marechal, D., Delapierre, D. and Dresse, A. (1988). Cloning and partial sequencing of a new rat brain specific cDNA. *Archives Internationales de Physiologie et de Biochimie*, **96**, 231–236.

Marechal, D., Kimura, H., Maeda, T. and Dresse, A. (1990). Cloning, sequencing and localization by *in situ* hybridization and immunohistochemistry of a rat brain cDNA coding for MAP 2. 17th CINP Meeting, Kyoto (Japan). Abstract, p. 216.

Mastropaolo, J., Nadi, N.S., Ostrowski, N.L. and Crawley, J.N. (1988). Galanin antagonizes acetylcholine on a memory task in basal forebrain-lesioned rats. *Proceedings of the National Academy of Sciences USA*, **85**, 9841–9845.

Meister, B. and Hökfelt, T. (1988). Peptide- and transmitter-containing neurons in the mediobasal hypothalamus and their relation to GABAergic systems: possible roles in control of prolactin and growth hormone secretion. *Synapse*, **2**, 585–605.

Melander, T., Staines, W.A., Hökfelt, T., Rökaeus, Å., Eckenstein, F., Salvaterra, P.M. and Wainer, B.H. (1985). Galanin-like immunoreactivity in cholinergic neurons of the septum–basal forebrain complex projecting to the hippocampus of the rat. *Brain Research*, **360**, 130–138.

Melander, T., Hökfelt, T. and Rökaeus, Å. (1986a). Distribution of galanin-like immunoreactivity in the rat central nervous system. *Journal of Comparative Neurology*, **248**, 475–517.

Melander, T., Staines, W.A. and Rökaeus, A. (1986b). Galanin-like immunoreactivity in hippocampal afferents in the rat, with special reference to cholinergic and noradrenergic inputs. *Neuroscience*, **19**, 223–240.

Nilsson, T., Arkhammar, P., Rorsman, P. and Berggren, P.O. (1989). Suppression of insulin release by galanin and somatostatin is mediated by a G-protein. *Journal of Biological Chemistry*, **264**, 973–980.

Nishibori, M., Oishi, R., Itoh, Y. and Saeki, K. (1988). Galanin inhibits noradrenaline-induced accumulation of cyclic AMP in the rat cerebral cortex. *Journal of Neurochemistry*, **51**, 1953–1955.

Palazzi, E., Fisone, G., Hökfelt, T., Bartfai, T. and Consolo, S. (1988). Galanin inhibits the muscarinic stimulation of phophoinositide turnover in rat ventral hippocampus. *European Journal of Pharmacology*, **148**, 479–480.

Rökaeus, Å. (1987). Galanin: a newly isolated biologically active neuropeptide. *Trends in Neuroscience*, **10**, 158–164.

Rökaeus, Å. and Carlquist, M. (1988). Nucleotide sequence analysis of cDNAs encoding a bovine galanin precursor protein in the adrenal medulla and chemical isolation of bovine gut galanin. *FEBS Letters*, **234**, 400–406.

Senut, M.C., Menetrey, D. and Lamour, Y. (1989). Cholinergic and peptidergic projections from the medial septum and the nucleus of the diagonal band of Broca to dorsal hippocampus, cingulate cortex and olfactory bulb: a combined wheatgerm agglutinin–apohorseradish peroxidase–gold immunohistochemical study. *Neuroscience* **30**, 385–403.

Seutin, V., Verbanck, P., Massotte, L. and Dresse, A. (1989). Galanin decreases the activity of locus coeruleus neurons *in vitro*. *European Journal of Pharmacology*, **164**, 373–376.

Skofitsch, G. and Jacobowitz, D. (1985). Immunohistochemical mapping of galanin-like neurons in the rat central nervous system. *Peptides*, **6**, 509–546.

Skofitsch, G. and Jacobowitz, D. (1986). Quantitative distribution of galanin-like immunoreactivity in the rat central nervous system. *Peptides*, **7**, 609–613.

Skofitsch, G., Sills, M. and Jacobowitz, D. (1986). Autoradiographic distribution of ^{125}I-galanin binding sites in the rat central nervous system. *Peptides*, **7**, 1029–1042.

Sutcliffe, J.G. (1988). mRNA in the mammalian central nervous system. *Annual Review of Neuroscience*, **11**, 157–198.

Tatemoto, K., Rökaeus, Å., Jornvall, H., McDonald, T.J. and Mutt, V. (1983). Galanin — a novel biologically active peptide from porcine intestine. *FEBS Letters*, **164**, 124–128.

Tsuda, K., Yokoo, H. and Goldstein, M. (1989). Neuropeptide Y and galanin in norepinephrine release in hypothalamic slices. *Hypertension*, **14**, 81–86.

Wenk, G. and Rökaeus, Å. (1988). Basal forebrain lesions differentially alter galanin levels and acetylcholinergic receptors in the hippocampus and neocortex. *Brain Research*, **460**, 17–21.

Part III

Opioids

Chapter 7

Opioid receptors

Stewart James Paterson

7.1. *Introduction*

The first evidence that morphine was producing a specific effect came from the observation that *N*-allylnorcodeine could block the respiratory depressant effect of morphine (Pohl, 1915). By the 1950s, the idea that narcotic alkaloids produce their effects by interacting with specific receptors had evolved from the study of the structure–activity relationships found in antinociceptive tests (Beckett and Casy, 1954; Beckett *et al.*, 1956). The proof that morphine acted on specific receptors came with the development of pure antagonists, the first of which was naloxone (*N*-allylnoroxymorphone) (Blumberg *et al.*, 1961).

The fact that morphine had *in vitro* effects was first demonstrated by Trendelenburg (1917) who showed that morphine inhibited the peristaltic reflex in the isolated guinea-pig ileum. Much later, morphine was shown to inhibit the electrically-evoked twitches in the guinea-pig ileum by decreasing the release of acetylcholine (Paton, 1957). This effect was blocked by naloxone (Kosterlitz and Watt, 1968). Furthermore, since there was a good correlation between inhibitory activity in the guinea-pig ileum and analgesic potency in humans (Kosterlitz and Waterfield, 1975), it would appear that the same receptors are involved in mediating both responses.

Following the identification of specific opioid receptors, it was speculated that these receptors had evolved to interact with an endogenous humoral substance. This was supported by the observation that naloxone partially blocked the antinociception produced in rats by stimulation of the periaqueductal grey (Akil *et al.*, 1972). Indeed, extracts of brain tissue were subsequently shown to inhibit the electrically-evoked twitches in the mouse vas deferens (Hughes, 1975) and to inhibit the binding of tritiated opioids (Terenius and Wahlstrom, 1975). The opioid material in the pig brain was identified as two pentapeptides, Tyr-Gly-Gly-Phe-Leu ([Leu^5]enkephalin) and Tyr-Gly-Gly-Phe-Met ([Met^5]enkephalin) (Hughes *et al.*, 1975b). A second endogenous opioid peptide, different from the pentapeptides, was reported to be present in the bovine pituitary (Teschemacher *et al.*, 1975). This material was shown to be a 31-amino acid polypeptide called β-endorphin (Li and Chung, 1976) which corresponded to the carboxy terminus of the pituitary hormone β-lipotrophin (Li *et al.*, 1965). A further opioid peptide, which had [Leu^5]enkephalin at the amino terminal, was isolated from the porcine pituitary (Lowney *et al.*, 1979). This peptide was called dynorphin and is a heptadecapeptide (Goldstein *et al.*, 1979). However, the complexity of the endogenous opioid peptide system has become apparent with the elucidation of the structures of the three opioid precursor molecules, pro-opiomelanocortin (Nakanishi *et al.*, 1979), proenkephalin (Noda *et al.*, 1982) and prodynorphin (Kakidani *et al.*, 1982). Each of these precursors can give rise to a number of biologically active opioid peptides.

The idea that opioids interact with more than one type of receptor was first proposed by Martin (1967). In subsequent experiments in the dog, Martin and co-workers carried out a detailed analysis of the effects of a number of opioids (Gilbert and Martin, 1976; Martin *et al.*, 1976). In these experiments they were able to identify three patterns of activity of opioids. It was proposed that opioids activated three different receptors for which the prototype agonists were morphine for the μ-receptor, ketazocine for the κ-receptor and *N*-allynormetazocine (SKF 10047) for the σ-receptor. However, more recent work has demonstrated that the σ-effects of opioids were due to activation of non-opioid receptors since the effects were not blocked by naloxone or naltrexone (Vaupel, 1983; Campbell *et al.*, 1989; Holtzman, 1989). Therefore, the σ-receptor is not an opioid receptor.

Following the identification of the endogenous opioid peptides, [Met^5]-enkephalin and [Leu^5]enkephalin, the peptides were found to be more active in the mouse vas deferens than in the guinea-pig ileum, whereas the converse was true with the alkaloid morphine (Lord *et al.*, 1977). It was proposed that the peptides interacted with a δ-receptor which was different from both the μ-and κ-receptors.

Thus, the endogenous opioid system consists of three families of peptides, derived from the three precursor molecules, which can interact with at least three types of opioid receptor, μ, δ and κ. In this chapter, the evidence that these three receptor types are separate entities is discussed.

7.2. *Heterogeneity of opioid receptors*

7.2.1. **Evidence from binding assays**

The characterization of binding sites is usually approached in one of two ways. In the first, the equilibrium dissociation constant (K_d) and the maximal number of binding sites of labelled ligands are estimated from saturation experiments. In the second approach, the binding characteristics of unlabelled ligands are determined by their competitive displacement of labelled compounds of known binding characteristics. The theoretical and practical problems associated with the investigation of opioid binding have been reviewed by Leslie (1987).

In homogenates of guinea-pig and rat brain, [Met^5]enkephalin and [Leu^5]enkephalin displaced the binding of tritiated enkephalins more readily than that of tritiated alkaloid opioids, whereas the converse was found with non-peptide opioids (Lord *et al.*, 1977; Chang *et al.*, 1979). These findings, together with observation of the relative potencies of morphine and the peptides in the guinea-pig ileum and mouse vas deferens bioassays, led to the suggestion that morphine interacted preferentially with the μ-binding site, whereas the opioid peptides interacted preferentially with a different site, which was termed the δ-binding site (Lord *et al.*, 1977).

In view of the pharmacological evidence that the ketazocine-like compounds activated κ-receptors (Martin, 1967; Hutchinson *et al.*, 1975; Martin *et al.*, 1976), the existence of κ-binding sites seemed probable. However, the demonstration of such a site proved difficult because the ketazocine-like compounds, in addition to their κ-affinity, also had high affinity for the μ- and δ-binding sites (Kosterlitz and Leslie; 1978; Magnan *et al.*, 1982). The κ-binding site was first characterized in displacement assays in homogenates of guinea-pig and rat brains as the site from which [^{3}H]-(±)-ethylketazocine and [^{3}H]-diprenorphine could not readily be displaced by selective μ- and δ-compounds (Chang *et al.*, 1981; Kosterlitz *et al.*, 1981; Gillan and Kosterlitz, 1982). In these circumstances, it was necessary to block the μ- and δ-binding sites with selective unlabelled ligands before the κ-binding sites could be characterized (Gillan and Kosterlitz, 1982; Magnan *et al.*, 1982). Similarly, the binding of the relatively selective δ-ligand [^{3}H]-[D-Ala^2, D-Leu^5]enkephalin was restricted to the δ-binding sites by the presence of unlabelled μ-ligand (Gillan and Kosterlitz, 1982). This approach has been superceded by the availability of highly selective δ-ligands such as [^{3}H]-[D-Pen^2,D-Pen^5]enkephalin (Cotton *et al.*, 1985) and κ-ligands such as [^{3}H]-U-69593 (Lahti *et al.*, 1985).

The view that μ-, δ- and κ-binding sites are separate entities is supported by the observation that the apparent binding capacities at saturation in the brain are different with compounds with differing selectivities for the three binding sites. Thus, the total number of opioid binding sites varied from $8{\cdot}3\,\text{pmol}\,g^{-1}$ in the dog cortex to $15{\cdot}8\,\text{pmol}\,g^{-1}$ in rat brain (Table 7.1). In guinea-pig brain, the opioid sites consisted of 24% μ, 32% δ and 44% κ. In contrast, in the rat brain the number of κ-sites was low and the corresponding values were 46% μ, 42% δ and 12% κ. On the other hand, in the rabbit brain the number of δ-sites was low and the proportions were 43% μ, 19% δ and 38% κ. Yet another pattern was seen in the dog cortex, where the proportion of μ-sites was low, 6% μ, 39% δ and 55% κ. Similar variations in the proportions of the three binding sites have been obtained from computer analysis of displacement assays in homogenates of the brain of the guinea-pig, the rat, the mouse, the monkey and humans (Pfeiffer and Herz, 1982; Maurer, 1982; Pfeiffer *et al.*, 1982; Neil, 1984; Neil *et al.*, 1986).

As in the whole brain, there are marked differences in the regional distribution of the three binding sites. In homogenates, the ratio of μ- to δ-

Table 7.1. Species distribution of opioid binding sites.

	Binding capacity (pmol/ g^{-1})		
	μ-site	δ-site	κ-site
Guinea-pig brain[a]	3·0	3·9	5·4
Human cortex[b]	2·2	3·2	3·6
Rat brain[a]	7·3	6·7	1·8
C57BL/10 mouse brain[a]	6·0	4·7	2·9
Californian rabbit brain[a]	5·2	2·3	4·5
Dog cortex[c]	0·5	3·2[d]	4·6[e]

The μ-sites were labelled with [^{3}H]-[D-Ala^2,MePhe^4,Gly-ol^5]enkephalin, the δ-sites with [d][^{3}H]-[D-Pen^2,D-Pen^5]enkephalin or with [^{3}H]-[D-Ala^2,D-Leu^5]enkephalin in the presence of unlabelled [D-Ala^2,MePhe^4,Gly-ol^5]enkephalin and the κ-sites with [^{3}H]-(−)-bremazocine or [e][^{3}H]-etorphine in the presence of unlabelled [D-Ala^2,MePhe^4,Gly-ol^5]enkephalin and [D-Ala^2,D-Leu^5]enkephalin. [a]Robson *et al.*, 1985; [b]Hiller *et al.*, 1987; [c]Sharif *et al.*, 1990.

to κ-sites varied across brain regions of the rat, guinea-pig, rabbit, cow and human (Chang *et al.*, 1981; Ninkovic *et al.*, 1981; Pfeiffer *et al.*, 1982; Robson *et al.*, 1985; Petrillo *et al.*, 1989). There are also marked interspecies variations in the distribution of the binding sites. A particularly striking example is the cerebellum. Although the rat cerebellum was devoid of opioid binding sites (Pert and Snyder, 1973), the guinea-pig cerebellum contained opioid binding sites mainly of the κ-type (Robson *et al.*, 1984), whereas the rabbit cerebellum contained mainly μ-sites (Meunier *et al.*, 1983). In both the guinea-pig and the rabbit, the density of opioid sites in the cerebellum was comparable to that found in the whole brain.

The distribution of opioid binding sites has also been analysed in the spinal cord of several species. In whole guinea-pig cord, the proportions of the three sites were 30% μ-sites, 59% κ-sites and 10% δ-sites (Zarr *et al.*, 1986). When the binding of [^{3}H]-bremazocine was measured in lumbosacral cord from the guinea-pig, pig and rat, the proportion of κ-binding sites was 42%, 31% and 35%, respectively (Traynor and Wood, 1987). Other studies of opioid binding in rat lumbosacral cord found the proportion of μ-sites to be 30–51%, of κ-sites to be 35–56% and of δ-sites to be 14% (Czlonkowski *et al.*, 1983; Traynor and Rance, 1984). Similarly, in six regions of human spinal cord, the proportions of the three sites varied between 33 and 68% for μ-sites, between 31 and 59% for κ-sites and between 1% and 15% for δ-sites (Czlonkowski *et al.*, 1983). In dog spinal cord, κ-sites were found to predominate with μ-binding sites also being present (Hunter *et al.*, 1989). Thus, in spinal cord from all the species studied, there are high levels of μ- and κ-sites and relatively low levels of δ-sites.

Another tissue of interest is the placenta in which opioid binding sites were found in tissue from human but not from mouse, hamster, rabbit or sheep (Valette *et al.*, 1979). Characterization of these opioid sites has shown that they were only of the κ-type (Porthe *et al.*, 1981).

A number of cell lines have been found to express opioid receptors. One of particular interest is the neuroblastoma × glioma hybrid cell line, NG108–15, which had only δ-binding sites (Klee and Nirenberg, 1974; Chang and Cuatrecasas, 1979).

The use of selective labelling techniques combined with autoradiography has further defined the differences in the distribution of the three binding sites in brain and spinal cord. In sections of rat brain, the μ-binding sites were discretely distributed in patches with high levels in the caudate-putamen, nucleus accumbens, amygdala, various thalamic nuclei and lamina IV of the cerebral cortex (Goodman *et al.*, 1980; Herkenham and Pert, 1981; Mansour *et al.*, 1986; Hawkins *et al.*, 1987, 1988). In contrast, the δ-binding sites were more evenly distributed with high levels found in the striatum, amygdala and lamina III, V and VI of the cerebral cortex (Goodman *et al.*, 1980; Gulya *et al.*, 1985; Mansour *et al.*, 1986; Blackburn *et al.*, 1988). Although the overall levels of κ-binding sites in rat brain were low, they had a distinct distribution with high levels in the amygdala, nucleus accumbens, caudate-putamen and thalamus (Quirion *et al.*, 1983; Mansour *et al.*, 1986; Morris and Herz, 1986; Jomary *et al.*, 1988). In contrast, in sections of guinea-pig brain, κ-binding sites were widely distributed with high levels in the olfactory bulb, substantia nigra, molecular layer of the hippocampus and cerebellum and lamina V and VI of the cerebral cortex (Foote and Maurer, 1982; Goodman and Snyder, 1982; Lewis *et al.*, 1984; Clark *et al.*, 1988; Jomary *et al.*, 1988; Sharif *et al.*, 1988). High levels of μ-binding sites were found in the medial thalamus, nucleus accumbens and periform cortex, whereas high levels of δ-binding sites were found in the caudate nucleus, hippocampus and lamina V and VI of the cerebral cortex (Goodman and Snyder, 1982).

In humans, μ-binding sites were predominant in the ventral tegmental area, whereas κ-binding sites were predominant in the substantia nigra. As in the guinea-pig, the deeper layers of the cerebral cortex had high levels of κ-binding sites, but the molecular layer of the cerebellum contained mainly μ-binding sites. In the hippocampus, the dentate gyrus contained mainly δ-binding sites, whereas the molecular layer contained mainly κ-binding sites (Maurer *et al.*, 1983; Cross *et al.*, 1987; Delay-Goyet *et al.*, 1987; Blackburn *et al.*, 1988).

The ontogeny of opioid binding sites has been studied in the rat (Spain *et al.*, 1985; Kornblum *et al.*, 1987; McDowell and Kitchen, 1987; Petrillo *et al.*, 1987; Kitchen *et al.*, 1990), the mouse (Tavani *et al.*, 1985) and man (Magnan and Tiberi, 1989). In rat brain, μ- and κ-binding sites were present in significant amounts during the early neonatal stages, whereas the δ-sites appeared much later. After birth, there was a marked increase in the number of μ- and δ-binding sites, but the number of κ-binding sites increased less than two-fold. Similarly, in human foetal brain, μ- and κ-binding sites were detected, but not δ-binding sites (Magnan and Tiberi, 1989). Thus, the three binding sites display a different pattern of ontogeny which is further evidence of separate sites.

Direct evidence for the existence of distinct μ-, δ- and κ-binding sites has been obtained from observations that each type of binding site can be selectively protected from irreversible inactivation by phenoxybenzamine (Robson and Kosterlitz, 1979; Kosterlitz *et al.*, 1981). *N*-ethylmaleimide (Smith and Simon, 1980) or β-chlornaltrexamine (James *et al.*, 1982) by preincubation with appropriate unlabelled ligands. The ability of the unlabelled ligands to protect each of the three binding sites reflected their relative potencies in displacement assays. This procedure has been used in homogenates of guinea-pig brain to obtain preparations which were enriched in each of the three binding sites (James *et al.*, 1982).

Therefore, there is considerable evidence from binding studies that the three opioid binding sites exist as separate entities. However, there is now considerable debate as to whether there are subtypes of these binding sites. A number of years ago, Pasternak and collegues first identified a high affinity site for which all opioids had high affinity. This site has been termed the μ_1-site, whereas the classical μ-site is referred to as the μ_2-site (Wolozin and Pasternak, 1981). More recently, there have been a number of reports that, in some tissues, the selective μ-ligand [^{3}H]-U-69593 labelled fewer sites than did not-selective tritiated ligands after supression of μ- and δ-binding. This has led to suggestion that there are subtypes of κ-binding sites (Lahti *et al.*, 1985; Zukin *et al.*, 1988; Hunter *et al.*, 1989). To prove that subtypes do exist, it will be necessary to develop a selective ligand for each subtype.

7.2.2. Evidence from pharmacological assays

Although the μ-, κ- and σ-receptors were first characterized in the spinal dog (Gilbert and Martin, 1976; Martin *et al.*, 1976), the use of opioids in a large number of *in vivo* tests have resulted in the identification of μ-, κ- and σ-receptors in the rat, mouse, pigeon and monkey (Teal and Holtzman, 1980; Tyers, 1980; Woods *et al.*, 1982).

In drug discrimination studies, it was found that animals trained to discriminate between saline and *N*-allylnormetazocine or related benzomorphan opioids, also responded to the non-opioids ketamine and phencyclidine (Holtzman, 1980). Furthermore, the use of stereo-isomers showed that the (+)-isomers were much more potent at producing σ-effects than were the (−)-isomers, whereas the converse was found for the opioid effects (Brady *et al.*, 1982; Khazan *et al.*, 1984). In addition, these effects were not blocked by the opioid antagonists, naloxone or naltrexone (Vaupel, 1983). Thus, although the σ-receptor was first characterized with opioid compounds, subsequent work has proved that the σ-receptor is a non-opioid receptor (see Johnson and Jones, 1990).

Other investigations with selective μ-, δ- and κ-agonists and antagonists have confirmed that these compounds produce distinct effects in *in vivo* tests (Porreca *et al.*, 1984; 1987; Schmauss and Yaksh, 1984).

However, our understanding of the mode of action of opioids has been facilitated by the use of *in vitro* bioassays using tissues in which neurotransmission is sensitive to inhibition by opioids. The most widely used tissues have been the electrically stimulated guinea-pig ileum (Kosterlitz and Watt, 1968), mouse vas deferens (Hughes *et al.*, 1975a), rat vas deferens (Lemaire *et al.*, 1978), rabbit vas deferens (Oka *et al.*, 1981) and hamster vas deferens (McKnight *et al.*, 1985).

Evidence for the presence of separate μ- and κ-receptors in isolated tissues was first obtained from a comparison of the agonist activity of normorphine and certain benzomorphan opioids in the guinea-pig ileum and mouse vas deferens bioassays (Hutchinson *et al.*, 1975). In the mouse vas deferens, relative to normorphine, the agonist activity of the ketazocine-like compounds was only 25% of that found in the guinea-pig ileum. Furthermore, three to seven times more naloxone was required to antagonize the inhibitory effects of the ketazocine-like compounds than those of normorphine.

In the mouse vas deferens, [Met^5]enkephalin and [Leu^5]enkephalin were found to be more active than morphine, whereas the converse was found in the guinea-pig ileum (Lord *et al.*, 1977). Furthermore, ten times more naloxone was required to antagonize the effect of the peptides in the mouse vas deferens than those of morphine. In contrast, the effects of the peptides and morphine were antagonized by the same low dose of naloxone in the guinea-pig ileum, suggesting that in this preparation the three compounds are all acting on the same receptors. These findings led to the suggestion that morphine interacted preferentially with μ-receptors whilst [Met^5]-enkephalin and [Leu^5]enkephalin interacted preferentially with δ-receptors which were different from μ- or κ-receptors (Lord *et al.*, 1977).

Further evidence for opioid receptor heterogeneity has been obtained in bioassay preparations which appear to contain a single type of opioid receptor. Since the electrically-evoked contractions of the rabbit vas deferens were inhibited by the κ-agonists bremazocine, ethylketazocine and ketazocine, but not by morphine, β-endorphin or [Leu^5]enkephalin, it was proposed that this preparation contained only κ-receptors (Oka *et al.*, 1981). The absence of μ- and δ-receptors was confirmed by the finding that neither the μ-agonist, [D-Ala^2,MePhe^4,Gly-ol^5]enkephalin, nor the δ-agonist, [D-Ala^2,D-Leu^5]enkephalin, had any agonist activity in the rabbit vas deferens (Corbett *et al.*, 1984).

In contrast, the electrically-evoked contractions of the hamster vas deferens were inhibited by the δ-agonist [D-Ala^2,D-Leu^5]enkephalin but not by the μ-agonists [D-Ala^2,MePhe^4,Gly-ol^5]enkephalin or morphine, nor by the κ-agonists bremazocine or ethylketazocine. The inhibitory effects of the agonists were inhibited by the δ-antagonist ICI 174864 and by relatively high concentrations of naloxone. Unexpectedly, the κ-agonists bremazocine and ethylketazocine were pure antagonists in the hamster vas deferens. Therefore, the hamster vas deferens appears to contain only δ-receptors (McKnight *et al.*, 1985).

The electrically-evoked contractions of the rat vas deferens displayed a different pattern of sensitivity to opioids (Lemaire *et al.*, 1978; Wuster *et al.*, 1979). Although β-endorphin was an agonist with a potency similar to that in the guinea-pig ileum and mouse vas deferens, other opioids were considerably less active in the rat vas deferens than in the other bioassays. Indeed, morphine, [Leu^5]enkephalin and [Met^5]enkephalin were almost inactive. This led to the suggestion that the effects of β-endorphin were mediated by a fourth type of opioid receptor which was termed ϵ (Wuster *et al.*, 1979; Schulz *et al.* 1981). However, the μ-agonist [D-Ala^2,MePhe^4,Gly-ol^5]enkephalin was an agonist in this preparation and its effects were blocked by low concentrations of naloxone (Gillan *et al.*, 1981). The low agonist potency of [Leu^5]enkephalin and [Met^5]enkephalin was found to be due to rapid breakdown of the peptides by tissue peptidases (McKnight *et al.*, 1983). Furthermore, the ketazocine-like compounds, bremazocine and ethylketazocine, had no agonist activity but were potent antagonists of the μ-agonist [D-Ala^2,MePhe^4,Gly-ol^5]enkephalin (Gillan *et al.*, 1981). Therefore, it appears likely that the rat vas deferens contains μ-receptors. Although the exact nature of the opioid receptor(s) in the rat vas deferens remains unclear, there is no unequivocal evidence for the presence of a separate ϵ-receptor (Sheehan *et al.*, 1988).

Although the finding that the hamster vas deferens contained only δ-receptors and that the rabbit vas deferens contained only κ-receptors, suggested that the different opioid receptors are separate entities; another approach involved the selective inactivation of each receptor type. β-Funaltrexamine, the fumaramate methyl ester of naltrexone, can be used to inactive μ-receptors. When the guinea-pig ileum is exposed to β-funaltrexamine followed by extensive washing, the potency of μ-agonists is decreased, whereas the potency of κ-agonists is not altered (Corbett *et al.*, 1985b). This is further evidence for separate μ- and κ-receptors.

Another approach was to use the non-selective opioid alkylating agent β-chlornaltrexamine (Portoghese *et al.*, 1980) together with selective protection of the different receptors. Preincubation of the guinea-pig ileum with β-chlornaltrexamine caused an irreversible decrease in the potency of μ- and κ-agonists. However, when [D-Ala^2,MePhe^4,Gly-ol^5]enkephalin, normorphine or [D-Ala^2,D-Leu^5]enkephalin was present during exposure to β-chlornaltrexamine, the IC_{50} of μ-agonists were little altered whereas those of κ-agonists were still increased (Chavkin and Goldstein, 1981; Corbett and Kosterlitz, 1986). Similarly, if dynorphin A(1–13) was present during the preincubation, the IC_{50} of κ-agonist were little affected, but those of μ-agonists were increased (Chavkin and Goldstein, 1981). Therefore, the κ-receptors are different from the μ-receptors. In the mouse vas deferens, the same technique has been used to show that μ-, δ- and κ-agonists each interact with a separate receptor (Cox and Chavkin, 1983; Goldstein and James, 1984).

One of the characteristic properties of opioids is that tolerance develops to their agonist action following prolonged exposure. This property has also been used to demonstrate heterogeneity of opioid receptors. When mice were infused with the μ-agonist sufentanyl or the δ-agonist [D-Ala^2, D-Leu^5)enkephalin for six days, the sensitivity of the vas deferens to μ- or δ-agonists was selectively reduced, whereas the sensitivity to ketazocine-like compounds was not altered. This indicated that ketazocine-like compounds were acting on κ-receptors which were different from either the μ- or δ-receptors (Schulz *et al.*, 1980a,b). The same experimental design has been used in the guinea-pig to demonstrate the presence of separate μ- and κ-receptors in the guinea-pig ileum (Schulz *et al.*, 1982; Yoshimura *et al.*, 1982).

Thus, there is considerable evidence available from both *in vivo* and *in vitro* experiments that there are separate μ-, δ- and κ-receptors.

7.3. *Selective μ-, δ- and κ-agonists and antagonists*

7.3.1. **Binding assays**

It is now possible to selectively label the three types of opioid binding sites in homogenates of brain tissue. The μ-binding sites can be labelled with [^{3}H]-[D-Ala^2,MePhe^4,Gly-ol^5]enkephalin (Kosterlitz and Paterson, 1981), the δ-sites with [^{3}H]-[D-Pen^2,D-Pen^5]enkephalin (Cotton *et al.*, 1985) and the κ-sites with [^{3}H]-U-69593 (Lahti *et al.*, 1985). Using these selective labelling techniques the most selective ligands for each of the three sites is discussed.

a. *The μ-binding site*

The prototype μ-ligand morphine is a relatively selective μ-ligand (Table 7.2). However, the most selective μ-ligands are the peptides [D-Ala^2, MePhe^4,Gly-ol^5]enkephalin, Tyr-D-Arg-Phe-Lys-NH_2 and Tyr-Pro-MePhe-D-Pro-NH_2. As far as antagonists are concerned, naloxone has a preference for the μ-binding site, but has a high degree of cross-reactivity to the κ-binding site and a little to the δ-binding site (Table 7.2). In contrast, the cyclic peptide D-Phe-Cys-Tyr-D-Trp-Orn-Thr-Pen-Thr-NH_2(CTOP) is a highly selective ligand for the μ-sites in binding assays.

b. *The δ-binding site*

The prototype δ-ligand [D-Ala^2,D-Leu^5]enkephalin is a relatively selective δ-ligand but has a significant affinity for the μ-binding site (Table 7.3). However, the cyclic peptide [D-Pen^2,D-Pen^5]enkephalin has a much improved selectivity for the δ-binding site. Recently, [D-Pen^2,*p*-ClPhe^4, D-Pen^5]enkephalin has been shown to have an even greater selectivity for the δ-binding site. A number of linear enkephalin analogues have also

Table 7.2. The relative affinity of opioids with a preference for the μ-binding site in homogenates of guinea-pig brain at 25°C.

	Affinity (K_i, nM)$^{-1}$ at μ-site	Relative affinity at		
		μ-site	δ-site	κ-site
Agonists				
[D-Ala^2,MePhe^4,Gly-ol^5]enkephalin	0·64	0·998	0·002	0
Tyr-D-Arg-Phe-Lys-NH_2	0·28	0·998	0	0·002
Tyr-Pro-MePhe-D-Pro-NH_2 (PL 017)	0·087	0·998	0·001	0·001[a]
Morphine	0·56	0·983	0·011	0·006[a]
Antagonists				
D-Phe-Cys-Tyr-D-Trp-Orn-Thr-Pen-Thr-NH_2 (CTOP)	0·59	0·998	0·001	0·001[a]
Naloxone	0·57	0·69	0·05	0·26

The μ-sites were labelled with [^{3}H]-[D-Ala^2,MePhe^4,Gly-ol^5]enkephalin (1 nM), the δ-sites with [^{3}H]-[D-Pen^2,D-Pen^5]enkephalin (1·5 nM) and the κ-sites with [^{3}H]-U-69593 (1·5 nM) or with [a][^{3}H]-(−)-bremazocine (0·1 nM) in the presence of 100 nM each of unlabelled [D-Ala^2, MePhe^4,Gly-ol^5]enkephalin and [D-Ala^2,D-Leu^5]enkephalin. Relative affinity is K_i^{-1} at μ, δ or κ/K_i^{-1} at μ + K_i^{-1} at δ + K_i^{-1} at κ.

Table 7.3. The relative affinity of opioids with a preference for the δ-binding site in homogenates of guinea-pig or rat brain.

	Affinity (K_i,nM)$^{-1}$ at δ-site	Relative affinity at		
		μ-site	δ-site	κ-site
Rat brain				
Agonists				
[D-Pen^2,*p*-ClPhe^4,D-Pen^5] enkephalin[a]	0·64	0·002[c]	0·998	ND
[D-Ser^2(*O-tert*-butyl),Leu^5] enkephalyl-Thr(*O-tert*-butyl)[b]	0·59	0·004	0·996[d]	ND
[D-Ser^2(*O-tert*-butyl)Leu^5] enkephalyl-Thr[b]	0·36	0·007	0·993[d]	ND
[D-Pen^2,D-Pen^5]enkephalin[b]	0·11	0·009	0·991[d]	ND
Guinea-pig brain				
Agonists				
[D-Pen^2,D-Pen^5]enkephalin	0·39	0·004	0·996	0
[D-Ala^2,D-Leu^5]enkephalin	0·74	0·101	0·899	0
Antagonists				
Naltrindole	8·30	0·011	0·983	0·006
ICI 174864	0·006	<0·033	>0·967	0

The μ-sites were labelled with [^{3}H]-[D-Ala^2,MePhe^4,Gly-ol^5]enkephalin (1 nM) or [c][^{3}H]-CTOP (0·5 nM), the δ-sites with [^{3}H]-[D-Pen^2,D-Pen^5]enkephalin (1·5 nM) or [d][^{3}H]-[D-Ser^2(*O-tert*-butyl),Leu^5]enkephalyl-Thr (2 nM) and the κ-sites with [^{3}H]-U-69593 (1·5 nM). Relative affinity is K_i^{-1} at μ, δ or κ/K_i^{-1} at μ + K_i^{-1} at δ + K_i^{-1} at κ.
ICI 174864, *N,N*-diallyl-Tyr-Aib-Aib-Phe-Leu; Aib, α-aminoisobutyric acid; Pen, β,β-dimethylcysteine. ND, not determined.
[a] Toth *et al.*, 1989; [b] Delay-Goyet *et al.*, 1988.

Table 7.4. The relative affinity of opioids with a preference for the κ-binding site in homogenates of guinea-pig brain at 25°C.

	Affinity (K_i, nM)$^{-1}$ at κ-site	Relative affinity at		
		μ-site	δ-site	κ-site
Agonists				
ICI 197067	5·9	0·001	0	0·999
U-69593	0·74	0·001	0	0·999
PD 117302	1·72	0·003	0	0·997
[D-Pro^{10}]Dynorphin A(1–11)	34·7	0·05	0·01	0·94
Dynorphin A(1–9)	12·7	0·03	0·04	0·93
(−)-Bremazocine	13·3	0·10	0·08	0·82
Antagonists				
Norbinaltorphimine	2·9	0·02	0·03	0·95
Mr 2266	3·6	0·16	0·08	0·76
(−)-Win 44441	1·4	0·48	0·05	0·47[a]

The μ-sites were labelled with [^{3}H]-[D-Ala^2,MePhe^4,Gly-ol^5]enkephalin (1 nM), the δ-sites with [^{3}H]-[D-Pen^2,D-Pen^5]enkephalin (1·5 nM) and the κ-sites with [^{3}H]-U-69593 (1·5 nM) or with [a][^{3}H]-(−)-bremazocine (0·1 nM) in the presence of 100 nM each of unlabelled [D-Ala^2,MePhe^4,Gly-ol^5]enkephalin and [D-Ala^2,D-Leu^5]enkephalin. Relative affinity is K_i^{-1} at μ, δ or κ/K_i^{-1} at μ + K_i^{-1} at δ + K_i^{-1} at κ.
U-69593, (5α,7α,8β)-(+)-*N*-methyl-*N*-(7-(1-pyrrolidinyl)-1-oxaspiro[4,5]dec-8-yl)-benzeneacetamide; PD 117302, (±)-trans-*N*-methyl-*N*-(2-(1-pyrrolidinyl)-cyclohexyl)-benzo[b]tiophene-4-acetamide; ICI 197067, (2S)-*N*-(2-(*N*-methyl-3,4-dichloro-phenylacetamido)-2-methylbutyl)pyrrolidine; Mr 2266, (−)-α-5,9-diethyl-2-(3-furylmethyl)-2′-hydroxy-6,7-benzomorphan; Win 44441, α-2,5,9-trimethyl-2-(cyclopropyl-3-pentanyl)-2′-hydroxy-6,7 benzomorphan.

been synthesized. Of these peptides, [D-Ser^2(*O-tert*-butyl),Leu^5]enkephalyl-Thr(*O-tert*-butyl) and [D-Ser^2(*O-tert*-butyl),Leu^5]enkephalyl-Thr display the highest degree of selectivity for the δ-binding site.

The peptide antagonist ICI 174864 is a highly selective ligand for the δ-binding site, but has a rather low potency (Table 7.3). However, the non-peptide antagonist naltrindole, which is also a highly selective δ-ligand, is over 1000 times more potent at the δ-binding site.

c. *The κ-binding site*

The prototype κ-ligand bremazocine is a highly potent, but relatively non-selective ligand, with a particularly high degree of cross-reactivity to the μ-binding sites (Table 7.4). The peptide dynorphin A(1–9) has a similar potency, but has an enhanced κ-selectivity. The stabilized dynorphin analogue [D-Pro^{10}]dynorphin A(1–11) displays a further enhancement of potency without any improvement in selectivity.

The first highly selective non-peptide κ-ligand was U-50488H (Von Voigtlander *et al.*, 1985). Since then a number of related analogues, ICI 197067, U-69593 and PD 117302, have been developed which have similarly high degrees of selectivity for the κ-binding site (Table 7.4).

Table 7.5. The agonist potencies (IC_{50}, nM) of opioids with a preference for the μ-binding site in *in vitro* bioassays at 37°C.

Opioid	Guinea-pig ileum	Mouse vas deferens
[D-Ala^2,MePhe^4,Gly-ol^5]enkephalin	4·5[a]	33[a]
Tyr-D-Arg-Phe-Lys-NH_2	254[b]	781[b]
Tyr-Pro-MePhe-D-Pro-NH_2(PL 017)	34[c]	240[c]
Morphine	68[d]	492[e]

[a] Corbett *et al.*, 1984; [b] Schiller *et al.*, 1989; [c] Chang *et al.*, 1983; [d] Kosterlitz and Watt, 1968; [e] Hughes *et al.*, 1975a.

Although Win 44441 is a κ-antagonist, it is important to realize that this compound has similar affinity for both the κ- and μ-binding sites (Table 7.4). On the other hand, the benzomorphan κ-antagonist Mr 2266 has a profile similar to that of bremazocine. Thus, neither compound can be considered to be a selective compound. In contrast, norbinaltorphimine is a highly selective ligand for the κ-binding site.

7.3.2. **Pharmacological assays**

The unequivocal characterization of the receptor involved in mediating the physiological actions of the opioid peptides requires the identification of this receptor with highly selective opioid ligands. Since binding assays do not provide information as to whether a selective ligand will interact with the receptor to produce an agonist response or will be an antagonist at this receptor, it is necessary to compare the results obtained in binding assays with those obtained in pharmacological assays.

a. *μ-Selective agonists*

The selective μ-agonists [D-Ala^2,MePhe^4,Gly-ol^5]enkephalin and Tyr-Pro-MePhe-D-Pro-NH_2 are potent agonists in the guinea-pig ileum and mouse vas deferens whereas morphine is a less potent agonist in both these tissues (Table 7.5).

[D-Ala^2,MePhe^4,Gly-ol^5]enkephalin, but not morphine, is also an agonist in the rat vas deferens (Gillan *et al.*, 1981; Magnan *et al.*, 1982). However, neither compound has any agonist action in the vasa deferentia of the hamster or the rabbit (Oka *et al.*, 1981; Corbett *et al.*, 1984; McKnight *et al.*, 1985).

b. *δ-Selective agonists*

The δ-selective peptides [DPen^2,*p*-ClPhe^4,D-Pen^5]enkephalin, [D-Ser^2(*O-tert*-butyl),Leu^5]enkephalyl-Thr(*O-tert*-butyl), [D-Ser^2(*O-tert*-butyl),Leu^5]-enkephalyl-Thr,[D-Pen^2,D-Pen^5]enkephalin and [D-Ala^2,D-Leu^5]enkephalin

Table 7.6. The agonist potencies (IC_{50}, nM) of opioids with a preference for the δ-binding site in *in vitro* bioassays at 37°C.

Opioid	Guinea-pig ileum	Mouse vas deferens	Hamster vas deferens
[D-Pen^2,*p*-ClPhe^4,D-Pen^5] enkephalin	8304[a]	0·89[a]	ND
[D-Ser^2(*O-tert*-butyl),Leu^5] enkephalyl-Thr(*O-tert*-butyl)	2790[b]	0·60[b]	ND
[D-Ser^2(*O-tert*-butyl),Leu^5] enkephalyl-Thr(*O-tert*-butyl)	1795[b]	1·07[b]	ND
[D-Pen^2,D-Pen^5]enkephalin	3000[c]	4·14[c]	81[d]
[D-Ala^2,D-Leu^5]enkephalin	8·9[c]	0·73[c]	21[d]

ND, not determined; Pen, β,β-dimethylcysteine.
[a] Toth *et al.*, 1989; [b] Gacel *et al.*, 1988; [c] Corbett *et al.*, 1984; [d] McKnight *et al.*, 1985.

are all potent agonists in the mouse vas deferens and, with the exception of [D-Ala^2,D-Leu^5]enkephalin, are weak agonists in the guinea-pig ileum (Table 7.6). The agonist effect of all these peptides in the guinea-pig ileum is due to activation of μ-receptors since the K_e for antagonism by naloxone is 2–3 nM (Kosterlitz *et al.*, 1980; Mosberg *et al.*, 1983). [D-Pen^2,D-Pen^5]-enkephalin and [D-Ala^2,D-Leu^5]enkephalin are also potent agonists in the hamster vas deferens (Table 7.6), but have no agonist activity in the rabbit vas deferens (Corbett *et al.*, 1984). In the rat vas deferens, [D-Pen^2,D-Pen^5]-enkephalin is devoid of agonist activity whereas [D-Ala^2,D-Leu^5]enkephalin is a potent agonist with an IC_{50} value of 134 nM (McKnight *et al.*, 1983).

c. *κ-Selective agonists*

The κ-selective compounds ICI 197067, U-69593, PD 117302, [D-Pro^{10}]-dynorphin A(1–11), dynorphin A(1–9) and (−)-bremazocine are potent agonists in the guinea-pig ileum, rabbit vas deferens and mouse vas deferens. In the vas deferens of the hamster, these compounds have little or no agonist activity (Table 7.7). These compounds are also devoid of agonist activity in the rat vas deferens (Gillan *et al.*, 1981; Corbett *et al.*, 1985a; Meecham *et al.*, 1989). However, the ketazocine-like compounds, such as bremazocine, but not the other κ-selective compounds, are antagonists at the μ- and δ-receptors in the vasa deferentia of the rat and hamster, respectively (Gillan *et al.*, 1981; Corbett *et al.*, 1985a; McKnight *et al.*, 1985; Meecham *et al.*, 1989). Bremazocine has also been shown to be an antagonist at the μ-receptors in the guinea-pig ileum (Corbett and Kosterlitz, 1986).

d. *Antagonists*

The lack of selectivity of the μ-antagonist naloxone is highlighted by the fact that it is a potent antagonist in all the *in vitro* bioassays. In the guinea-pig

Table 7.7. The agonist potencies (IC_{50}, nM) of opioids with a preference for the κ-binding site in *in vitro* bioassays at 37°C.

Opioid	Guinea-pig ileum	Mouse vas deferens	Rabbit vas deferens	Hamster vas deferens
ICI 197067	0·18[a]	15[a]	ND	ND
U-69593	1·3[b]	ND	50[b]	Inactive[c]
PD 117302	1·1[d]	ND	58[d]	ND
[D-Pro[10]]Dynorphin A(1–11)	3·3[e]	ND	12[e]	929[e]
Dynorphin A(1–9)	2·3[f]	6·5[f]	6·1[f]	1040[g]
(−)-Bremazocine	0·13[h]	2·0[h]	5·5[i]	Inactive[g]

ND, not determined.
[a] Costello *et al.*, 1988; [b] Traynor *et al.*, 1987; [c] Corbett *et al.*, 1985a; [d] Meecham *et al.*, 1989; [e] Gairin *et al.*, 1986, [f] Corbett *et al.*, 1982; [g] McKnight *et al.*, 1985; [h] Magnan *et al.*, 1982; [i] Hayes and Kelly, 1985.

Table 7.8. The potencies (K_e, nM) of selective opioid antagonists in *in vitro* bioassays.

Antagonist	K_e(nM) μ-receptor	δ-receptor	κ-receptor
Naloxone	1·9[a]	46[b]	16[c]
D-Phe-Cys-Tyr-D-Trp-Orn-Thr-Pen-Thr-NH_2 (CTOP)	16[d]	Inactive at 1 μM[e]	444[d]
ICI 174864	Inactive at 2 μM[f]	22[g]	ND
Naltrindole	22[h]	0·27[h]	100[h]
Mr 2266	1·9[i]	34[i]	2·5[i]
Norbinaltorphimine	25[j]	16[j]	0·05[j]

The antagonist potencies were determined at μ-receptors in the guinea-pig myenteric plexus, at δ-receptors in mouse vas deferens and at κ-receptors in the guinea-pig myenteric plexus.
ND, not determined.
[a] Corbett *et al.*, 1985b; [b] Mosberg *et al.*, 1983; [c] Meecham *et al.*, 1989; [d] Kosterlitz and Paterson, 1990; [e] Kramer *et al.*, 1989; [f] Takemori and Portoghese, 1985; [g] Cotton *et al.*, 1984; [h] Portoghese *et al.*, 1988; [i] Lord *et al.*, 1977; [j] Birch *et al.*, 1987.

ileum, naloxone readily antagonizes the μ-agonist [D-Ala^2,MePhe^4,Gly-ol^5]enkephalin with a K_e value of 1·9 nM, whereas it is a less effective antagonist of the κ-agonist U-69593 with a K_e value of 16 nM (Table 7.8). In the mouse vas deferens, naloxone antagonizes the μ-agonists [D-Ala^2, MePhe^4,Gly-ol^5]enkephalin and Tyr-Pro-MePhe-D-Pro-NH_2 with K_e values less than 3 nM (Handa *et al.*, 1981; Gillan *et al.*, 1981; Chang *et al.*, 1983), whereas it is less effective against the δ-agonist [D-Pen^2,D-Pen^5]enkephalin (Table 7.8). In the hamster vas deferens, naloxone antagonizes the agonist action of [D-Pen^2,D-Pen^5]enkephalin with a K_e value of 51 nM (McKnight *et al.*, 1985). In addition, in the rabbit vas deferens, naloxone antagonizes the inhibitory effect of the κ-agonist U-50488H with a K_e value of 30 nM (Hayes and Kelly, 1985). Thus, as in binding assays, naloxone has highest affinity for μ-receptors and is less effective at both δ- and κ-receptors.

On the other hand, D-Phe-Cys-Tyr-D-Trp-Orn-Thr-Pen-Thr-NH_2 (CTOP), which is a highly selective μ-ligand in the binding assays (Table 7.2) and is a highly potent μ-antagonist *in vivo* (Kramer *et al.*, 1989), was found to be a much less selective μ-compound in *in vitro* bioassays. In the guinea-pig ileum CTOP is a competitive antagonist at both μ- and κ-receptors (Table 7.8). However, because of its low potency at the μ-receptors in this tissue, it is no more selective for the μ-receptor than is naloxone.

The peptide ICI 174864 is a highly selective δ-antagonist. The K_e value in the mouse vas deferens against the δ-ligand [D-Thr^2,Leu^5]enkephalyl-Thr is 22 nM (Table 7.8) and in the hamster vas deferens against the δ-ligand [D-Pen^2,D-Pen^5]enkephalin is 44 nM (McKnight *et al.*, 1985). No antagonism of the agonist actions of the μ-ligand [D-Ala^2,MePhe^4,Gly-ol^5]enkephalin or the κ-ligand tifluadom were seen in the mouse vas deferens (Cotton *et al.*, 1984). Furthermore, ICI 174894 had no effect on the μ-activity of [D-Ala^2,D-Leu^5]enkephalin in the guinea-pig ileum (Table 7.8). The non-peptide antagonist, naltrindole has a K_e value of 0·27 nM against [D-Pen^2, D-Pen^5]enkephalin in the mouse vas deferens (Table 7.8). It is 500 times more potent than ICI 174864 as an antagonist of [D-Ala^2,D-Leu^5]enkephalin in the mouse vas deferens (Portoghese *et al.*, 1988). In the guinea-pig ileum, naltrindole has a K_e of 22 nM against the μ-ligand [D-Ala^2,MePhe^4, Gly-ol^5]enkephalin and 100 nM against the κ-ligand U-50488H (Table 7.8). In the rat vas deferens, naltrindole antagonizes β-endorphin with a K_e of 111 nM (Portoghese *et al.*, 1988).

Mr 2266 is not a selective antagonist and has equal affinity for the κ- and μ-receptors, but is a relatively weak antagonist at δ-receptors (Table 7.8). The μ- and κ-antagonism was measured in the guinea-pig with normorphine as the μ-ligand and ethylketazocine as the κ-ligand. δ-Antagonism was measured in the mouse vas deferens with [Leu^5]enkephalin as the δ-ligand (Lord *et al.*, 1977). In contrast, norbinaltorphimine is both a much more potent and a much more selective κ-antagonist than Mr 2266 (Table 7.8). In this case, the μ-ligand was [D-Ala^2,MePhe^4,Gly-ol^5]enkephalin and the κ-ligand was U-50488H. δ-Antagonism was measured in the vasa deferentia of the mouse and hamster with either [D-Ala^2,D-Leu^5]enkephalin or [D-Pen^2,D-Pen^5]enkephalin as the δ-ligand (Birch *et al.*, 1987).

7.4. *Conclusion*

In summary, there are now a number of highly selective ligands available for each of the three types of opioid receptors. At the μ-site, [D-Ala^2,MePhe^4,Gly-ol^5]enkephalin is a selective agonist and naloxone is a somewhat selective antagonist. Although CTOP has been shown to be a highly selective μ-ligand in binding and in *in vivo* tests, this high degree of selectivity was not found in *in vitro* bioassays. At the δ-site, [D-Pen^2,D-Pen^5]enkephalin is a highly selective agonist and naltrindole is a highly selective antagonist. At the κ-site, U-69593 is a highly selective agonist and norbinaltorphimine is a highly selective antagonist. There are also selective assay tissues available which contain only one type of opioid receptor. Thus, the hamster vas deferens contains δ-receptors and the rabbit vas deferens κ-receptors. Furthermore, the guinea-pig ileum can be used as a selective assay tissue for κ-receptors or μ-receptors, after either pretreatment with β-funaltrexamine or with β-chlornaltrexamine with μ-receptor protection, respectively.

It is also possible to selectively label the three binding sites. The selective agonists are all available as tritiated ligands as are naloxone and CTOP. The selective antagonists naltrindole and norbinaltorphimine should be available soon as tritiated ligands. Furthermore, there a number of tissues which appear to have largely one type of binding site. Thus, the rabbit cerebellum has μ-sites, the NG 108–15 cell line has δ-sites and the guinea-pig cerebellum or human placenta has κ-sites.

Through the use of these techniques and with the development of more selective opioid ligands, it should soon be possible to resolve the question as to whether there are subtypes of the μ-, δ- and κ-receptors and binding sites. This may provide more insight into why there are so many endogenous opioid peptides.

References

Akil, H., Mayer, D.J. and Liebeskind, J.C. (1972). Comparaison chez le rat entre l'analgésie induite par stimulation de la substance grise péri-aqueducale et l'analgésie morphinique. *Comptes Rendus de l'Académie des Sciences de Paris Serie D*, **274**, 3603–3605.

Beckett, A.H. and Casy, A.F. (1954). Synthetic analgesics: stereochemical considerations. *Journal of Pharmacy and Pharmacology*, **6**, 989–999.

Beckett, A.H., Casy, A.F. and Harper, N.J. (1956). Analgesics and their antagonists: some steric and chemical considerations, part III. The influence of the basic group on the biological response. *Journal of Pharmaceutical Science*, **8**, 874–884.

Birch, P.J., Hayes, A.G., Sheehan, M.J. and Tyres, M.B. (1987). Norbinaltorphimine: antagonist profile at κ-opioid receptors. *European Journal of Pharmacology*, **144** 405–408.

Blackburn, T.P., Cross, A.J., Hille, C. and Slater, P. (1988). Autoradiographic localization of delta opiate receptors in rat and human brain. *Neuroscience*, **2**, 497–506.

Blumberg, H., Dayton, H.B., George, M. and Rapaport, D.N. (1961). *N*-allylnoroxymorphone: a potent narcotic antagonist. *Federation Proceedings*, **20**, 311.

Brady, K.T., Balster, R.L. and May, E.L. (1982). Stereoisomers of *N*-allylnormetazocine: phencyclidine-like behavioural effects in squirrel monkeys and rats. *Science*, **215**, 178–180.

Campbell, B.G., Scherz, M.W., Keana, J.F.W. and Weber, E. (1989). Sigma receptors regulate contractions of the guinea-pig ileum longitudinal/myenteric plexus preparation elicited by both electrical stimulation and exogenous serotonin. *Journal of Neuroscience*, **9**, 3380–3391.

Chang, K.-J. and Cuatrecasas, P. (1979). Multiple opiate receptors. Enkephalins and morphine bind to receptors of different specificity. *Journal of Biological Chemistry*, **254**, 2610–2618.

Chang, K.-J., Hazum, E. and Cuatrecasas, P. (1981). Novel opiate binding sites selective for benzomorphan drugs. *Proceedings of the National Academy of Sciences USA*, **78**, 4141–4145.

Chang, K.-J., Cooper, B.R., Hazum, E. and Cuatrecasas, P. (1979). Multiple opiate receptors: different regional distribution in the brain and differential binding of opiates and opioid peptides. *Molecular Pharmacology*, **16**, 91–104.

Chang, K.-J., Wei, E.T., Killian, A. and Chang, J.K. (1983). Potent morphiceptin analogs: structure activity relationships and morphine like activities. *Journal of Pharmacology and Experimental Therapeutics*, **227**, 403–408.

Chavkin, C. and Goldstein, A. (1981). Demonstration of a specific dynorphin receptor in guinea pig ileum myenteric plexus. *Nature*, **29**, 591–593.

Clark, C.R., Birchmore, B., Sharif, N.A., Hunter, J.C., Hill, R.G. and Hughes, J. (1988). PD117302: a selective agonist for the κ-opioid receptor. *British Journal of Pharmacology*, **93**, 618–626.

Corbett, A.D. and Kosterlitz, H.W. (1986). Bremazocine is an agonist at κ-opioid receptors and an antagonist at μ-opioid receptors in the guinea-pig myenteric plexus. *British Journal of Pharmacology*, **89**, 245–249.

Corbett, A.D., Gillan, M.G.G., Kosterlitz, H.W. and Paterson, S.J. (1985a). Binding and pharmacological profile of a highly selective ligand for the κ-opioid receptor — U-69,593. *British Journal of Pharmacology*, **86**, 704P.

Corbett, A.D., Kosterlitz, H.W., McKnight, A.T. and Paterson, S.J. (1985b). Preincubation of guinea-pig myenteric plexus with β-funaltrexamine: discrepancy between binding assays and bioassays. *British Journal of Pharmacology*, **85**, 665–673.

Corbett. A.D., Paterson, S.J., McKnight, A.T., Magnan, J. and Kosterlitz, H.W. (1982). Dynorphin (1–8) and dynorphin (1–9) are ligands for the κ-subtype of opiate receptor. *Nature*, **299**, 79–81.

Corbett, A.D., Gillan, M.G.C., Kosterlitz, H.W., McKnight, A.T., Paterson, S.J. and Robson, L.E. (1984). Selectivities of opioid peptide analogues as agonists and antagonists at the δ-receptor. *British Journal of Pharmacology*, **83**, 271–279.

Costello, G.F., Main, B.G., Barlow, J.J., Carroll, J.A. and Shaw, J.S. (1988). A novel series of potent and selective agonists at opioid κ-receptors. *European Journal of Pharmacology*, **151**, 475–478.

Cotton, R., Giles, M.G., Miller, L., Shaw, J.S. and Timms, D. (1984). ICI 174864: a highly selective antagonist for the opioid δ-receptor. *European Journal of Pharmacology*, **97**, 331–332.

Cotton, R., Kosterlitz, H.W., Paterson, S.J., Rance, M.J. and Traynor, J.R. (1985). The use of [^{3}H]-[D-Pen^2,D-Pen^5]enkephalin as a highly selective ligand for the δ-binding site. *British Journal of Pharmacology*, **84**, 927–932.

Cox, B.M. and Chavkin, C. (1983). Comparison of dynorphin-selective kappa receptors in mouse vas deferens and guinea-pig ileum. *Molecular Pharmacology*, **23**, 36–43.

Cross, A.J., Hille, C. and Slater, P. (1987). Subtraction autoradiography of opiate receptor subtypes in human brain. *Brain Research*, **418**, 343–348.

Czlonkowski, A., Costa, T., Przewlocki, R., Pasi, A. and Herz, A. (1983). Opiate binding sites in human spinal cord. *Brain Research*, **267**, 392–396.

Delay-Goyet, P., Seguin, C., Gacel, G. and Roques, B.P. (1988). [^{3}H]-[D-Ser^2-(*O-tert*-butyl),Leu^5]enkephalyl-Thr^6 and [D-Ser^2(*O-tert*-butyl),Leu^5]enkephalyl-Thr^6(*O-tert*-butyl). *Journal of Biological Chemistry*, **263**, 4124–4130.

Delay-Goyet, P., Zajac, J.-M., Javoy-Agid, F., Agid, Y. and Roques, B.P. (1987). Regional distribution of μ, δ and κ opioid receptors in human brains from controls and Parkinsonian subjects. *Brain Research*, **414**, 8–14.

Foote, R.W. and Maurer, R. (1982). Autoradiographic localization of opiate κ-receptors in the guinea-pig brain. *European Journal of Pharmacology*, **85**, 99–103.

Gacel, G., Dauge, V., Breuze, P., Delay-Goyet, P. and Roques, B.P. (1988). Development of conformationally constrained linear peptides exhibiting a high affinity and pronounced selectivity for δ opioid receptors. *Journal of Medical Chemistry*, **31**, 1891–1897.

Gairin, J.E., Mazarguil, H., Alvinerie, P., Saint-Pierre, S., Meunier, J.-C. and Cros, J. (1986). Synthesis and biological activities of dynorphin A analogues with opioid antagonist properties. *Journal of Medical Chemistry*, **29**, 1913–1917.

Gilbert, P.E. and Martin, W.R. (1976). The effects of morphine- and nalorphine-like drugs in the non-dependent, morphine-dependent and cyclazocine-dependent chronic spinal dog. *Journal of Pharmacology and Experimental Therapeutics*, **198**, 66–82.

Gillan, M.G.C. and Kosterlitz, H.W. (1982). Spectrum of the μ-, δ- and κ-binding sites in homogenates of rat brain. *British Journal of Pharmacology*, **70**, 481–469.

Gillan, M.G.C., Kosterlitz, H.W. and Magnan, J. (1981). Unexpected antagonism in the rat vas deferens by benzomorphans which are agonists in other pharmacological tests. *British Journal of Pharmacology*, **72**, 13–15.

Goldstein, A. and James, I.F. (1984). Site-directed alkylation of multiple opioid receptors. II. Pharmacological selectivity. *Molecular Pharmacology*, **25**, 343–348.

Goldstein, A., Tachibana, S., Lowney, L.I., Hunkapiller, M. and Hood, L.E. (1979). Dynorphin (1–13), an extraordinary potent opioid peptide. *Proceedings of the National Academy of Sciences USA*, **76**, 6666–6670.

Goodman, R.R. and Snyder, S.H. (1982). κ-Opiate receptors localised by autoradiography to deep layers of cerebral cortex: relation to sedative effects. *Proceedings of the National Academy of Sciences USA*, **79**, 5703–5707.

Goodman, R.R., Snyder, S.H., Kuhar, M.J. and Young, W.S. (1980). Differentiation of delta and mu opiate receptor localizations by light microscopic autoradiography. *Proceedings of the National Academy of Sciences USA*, **77**, 6239–6243.

Gulya, K., Gehlert, D.R., Wamsley, J.K., Mosberg, H.I., Hruby, V.J., Duckles, S.P. and Yamamura, H.I. (1985). Autoradiographic localization of δ opioid receptors in the rat brain using a highly selective *bis*-penacillamine cyclic enkephalin analog. *European Journal of Pharmacology*, **111**, 285–286.

Handa, B.K., Lane, A.C., Lord, J.A.H., Rance, M.J. and Smith, C.F.C. (1981). Analogues of βLPH_{61-64} possessing selective agonist activity at μ-opiate receptors. *European Journal of Pharmacology*, **70**, 531–540.

Hawkins, K.N., Morelli, M., Gulya, K., Chang, K.-J. and Yamamura, H.I. (1987). Autoradiographic localization of [^{3}H][MePhe^3,D-Pro^4]morphiceptin ([^{3}H]PL017) to μ opioid receptors in rat brain. *European Journal of Pharmacology*, **133**, 351–352.

Hawkins, K.N., Knapp, R.J., Gehlert, D.R., Lui, G.K., Yamamura, M.S., Roeske, L.C., Hruby, V.J. and Yamamura, H.I. (1988). Quantitative autoradiography of [^{3}H]CTOP binding to mu opioid receptors in rat brain. *Life Sciences*, **42**, 2541–2551.

Hayes, A. and Kelly, A. (1985). Profile of activity of κ receptor agonists in the rabbit vas deferens. *European Journal of Pharmacology*, **110**, 317–322.

Herkenham, M. and Pert, C.B. (1981). Mosaic distribution of opiate receptors, parafascicular projections and acetylcholinesterase in rat striatum. *Nature*, **291**, 415–418.

Hiller, J.M., Itzhak, Y. and Simon, E.J. (1987). Selective changes in μ,δ and κ opioid receptor binding in certain limbic regions of the brain in Alzheimer's disease patients. *Brain Research*, **406**, 17–23.

Holtzman, S.G. (1980). Phencyclidine-like discriminative effects of opioids in the rat. *Journal of Pharmacology and Experimental Therapeutics*, **214**, 614–619.

Holtzman, S.G. (1989). Opioid- and phencyclidine-like discriminative effects of ditollyguanidine, a selective sigma agonist. *Journal of Pharmacology and Experimental Therapeutics*, **248**, 1054–1062.

Hughes, J. (1975). Isolation of an endogenous compound from the brain with pharmacological properties similar to morphine. *Brain Research*, **88**, 295–306.

Hughes, J., Kosterlitz, H.W. and Leslie, F.M. (1975a). Effect of morphine on adrenergic transmission in the mouse vas deferens. Assessment of agonist and antagonist potencies of narcotic analgesics. *British Journal of Pharmacology*, **53**, 371–381.

Hughes, J., Smith,T.W., Kosterlitz, H.W., Fothergill, L.A., Morgan, B.A. and Morris, H.R. (1975a). Identification of two related pentapeptides from the brain with potent opiate agonist activity. *Nature*, **258**, 577–579.

Hughes, J., Smith, T.W., Kosterlitz, H.W., Fothergill, L.A., Morgan, B.A. and Morris, H.R. (1975b). Identification of two related pentapeptides from the brain with potent opiate agonist activity. *Nature*. **258**, 577–579.

Hutchinson, M., Kosterlitz, H.W., Leslie, F.M., Waterfield, A.A. and Terenius, L. (1975). Assessment in the guinea-pig ileum and mouse vas deferens of benzomorphans which have strong antinociceptive activity but do not substitute for morphine in the dependent monkey. *British Journal of Pharmacology*, **55**, 541–546.

James, I.F., Chavkin, C. and Goldstein, A. (1982). Preparation of brain membranes containing a single type of opioid receptor highly selective for dynorphin. *Proceedings of the National Academy of Sciences USA*, **79**, 7570–7574.

Johnson, K.M. and Jones, S.M. (1990). Neuropharmacology of phencyclidine: basic mechanisms and therapeutic potential. *Annual Review of Pharmacology and Toxicology*, **30**, 707–750.

Jomary, C., Gairin, J.E., Cros, J. and Meunier, J.-C. (1988). Autoradiographic localization of supraspinal κ-opioid receptors with [^{125}I-Tyr^{1},D-Pro^{10}]dynorphin A(1–11). *Proceedings of the National Academy of Sciences USA*, **85**, 627–631.

Kakidani, H., Furutani, Y., Takahashi, H., Noda, M., Morimoto, Y., Hirose, T., Asai, M., Inayama, S., Nakanishi, S. and Numa, S. (1982). Cloning and sequence analysis of cDNA for porcine β-neo-endorphin/dynorphin precursor. *Nature*, **298**, 245–249.

Khazan, N., Young, G.A., El-Fakary, E.S., Hong, O. and Calligaro, D. (1984). Sigma receptors mediate the psychotomimetic effects of *N*-allylnormetazocine (SKF 10,047), but not its opioid agonistic-antagonistic properties. *Neuropharmacology*, **23**, 983–987.

Kitchen, I., Kelly, M. and Viveros, M.P. (1990). Ontogenesis of κ-opioid receptors in rat brain using [^{3}H]U-69593 as a binding ligand. *European Journal of Pharmacology,* **175**, 93–96.

Klee, W.A. and Nirenberg, M. (1974). A neuroblastoma × glioma hybrid cell line with morphine receptors. *Proceedings of the National Academy of Sciences USA*, **71**, 3474–3477.

Kornblum, H.I., Hurlbut, D.E. and Leslie, F.M. (1987). Postnatal development of multiple opioid receptors in rat brain. *Developmental Brain Research*, **37**, 21–41.

Kosterlitz, H.W. and Leslie, F.M. (1978). Comparison of the receptor binding characteristics of opiate agonists acting with μ or κ receptors. *British Journal of Pharmacology*, **64**, 607–614.

Kosterlitz, H.W. and Paterson, S.J. (1981). Tyr-D-Ala-Gly-MePhe-NH$(CH_2)_2$OH is a selective ligand for the μ-opiate binding site. *British Journal of Pharmacology*, **73**, 299P.

Kosterlitz, H.W. and Paterson, S.J. (1990). D-Phe-Cys-Tyr-D-Trp-Orn-Thr-Pen-Thr-NH_2 is a highly selective μ-ligand with low *in vitro* antagonist activity. *British Journal of Pharmacology*, **99**, 291P.

Kosterlitz, H.W. and Waterfield, A.A. (1975). *In vitro* models in the study of structure activity relationships of narcotic analgesics. *Annual Review of Pharmacology*, **15**, 29–48.

Kosterlitz, H.W. and Watt, A.J. (1968). Kinetic parameters of narcotic agonists and antagonists with particular reference to *N*-allylnoroxy-morphone (naloxone). *British Journal of Pharmacology*, **33**, 327–329.

Kosterlitz, H.W., Paterson, S.J. and Robson, L.E. (1981). Characterisation of the κ-subtype of the opiate receptor in the guinea-pig brain. *British Journal of Pharmacology*, **73**, 939–949.

Kosterlitz, H.W., Lord, J.A.H., Paterson, S.J. and Waterfield, A.A. (1980). Effects of changes in the structure of enkephalins and of narcotic analgesic drugs on their interaction with μ- and δ-receptors. *British Journal of Pharmacology*, **68**, 333–342.

Kramer, T.H., Shook, J.E., Kazmierski, W., Ayres, E.A., Wire, W.S., Hruby, V.J. and Burks, T.F. (1989). Novel peptidic mu opioid antagonists: pharmacologic characterization *in vitro* and *in vivo*. *Journal of Pharmacology and Experimental Therapeutics*, **249**, 544–551.

Lahti, R.A., Michelson, M.M., McCall, J.M. and Von Voigtlander, P.F. (1985). [^{3}H]-U-69,593 a highly selective ligand for the opioid κ-receptor. *European Journal of Pharmacology*, **109**, 281–284.

Lemaire, S., Magnan, J. and Regoli, D. (1978). Rat vas deferens: a specific bioassay for endogenous opioid peptides. *British Journal of Pharmacology*, **64**, 327–329.

Leslie, F.M. (1987). Methods used for the study of opioid receptors. *Pharmacological Reviews*, **39**, 197–249.

Lewis, M.E., Young, E.A., Houghton, R.A., Akil, A. and Watson, S.J. (1984). Binding of [^{3}H]dynorphin A to apparent κ-opioid receptors in deep layers of guinea pig cerebral cortex. *European Journal of Pharmacology*, **98**, 149–150.

Li, C.H. and Chung, D. (1976). Isolation and structure of an untriakontapeptide with opioid activity from camel pituitary gland. *Proceedings of the National Academy of Sciences USA*, **73**, 1145–1148.

Li, C.H., Barnafi, L., Chretien, M. and Chung, D. (1965). Isolation and amino-acid sequence of β-LPH from sheep pituitary gland. *Nature*, **208**, 1093–1094.

Lord, J.A.H., Waterfield, A.A., Hughes, J. and Kosterlitz, H.W. (1977). Endogenous opioid peptides: multiple agonists and receptors. *Nature*, **267**, 495–499.

Lowney, L.I., Gentleman, S.B. and Goldstein, A. (1979). A pituitary endorphin with novel properties. *Life Sciences*, **24**, 2377–2384.

McDowell, J. and Kitchen, I. (1987). Development of opioid systems: peptides, receptors and pharmacology. *Brain Research Reviews*, **12**, 397–421.

McKnight, A.T., Corbett, A.D. and Kosterlitz, H.W. (1983). Increase in potencies of opioid peptides after peptidase inhibition. *European Journal of Pharmacology*, **86**, 393–402.

McKnight, A.T., Corbett, A.D., Marcoli, M. and Kosterlitz, H.W. (1985). The opioid receptors in the hamster vas deferens are of the δ-type. *Neuropharmacology*, **24**, 1011–1017.

Magnan, J. and Tiberi, M. (1989) Evidence for the presence of μ- and κ- but not

δ-opioid sites in the human fetal brain. *Developmental Brain Research*, **45**, 275–281.
Magnan, J., Paterson, S.J., Tavani, A. and Kosterlitz, H.W. (1982). The binding spectrum of narcotic analgesic drugs with different agonist and antagonist properties. *Naunyn-Schmiedeberg's Archives of Pharmacology*, **319**, 197–205.
Mansour, A., Lewis, M.E., Khachaturian, H., Akil, A. and Watson, S.J. (1986). Pharmacological and anatomical evidence of selective μ, δ and κ opioid receptor binding in rat brain. *Brain Research*, **399**, 69–79.
Martin, W.R. (1967). Opioid antagonists. *Pharmacological Reviews*, **19**, 463–521.
Martin, W.R., Eades, C.G., Thompson, J.A., Huppler, R.E. and Gilbert, P.E. (1976). The effects of morphine- and nalorphine-like drugs in the nondependent and morphine-dependent chronic spinal dog. *Journal of Pharmacology and Experimental Therapeutics*, **197**, 517–532.
Maurer, R. (1982). Multiplicity of opiate receptors in different species. *Neuroscience Letters*, **30**, 303–307.
Maurer, R., Cortes, R., Probot, A. and Palacios, J.M. (1983). Multiple opiate receptors in human brain: an autoradiographic investigation. *Life Sciences*, **33**, Suppl I, 231–234.
Meecham, K.G., Boyle, S.J., Hunter, J.C. and Hughes, J. (1989). An *in vitro* profile of activity for the (+) and (−) enantiomers of spiradoline and PD117302. *European Journal of Pharmacology*, **173**, 151–157.
Meunier, J.-C., Kouakou, Y., Puget, A. and Moisand, C. (1983). Multiple opiate binding sites in the central nervous system of the rabbit. Large predominance of a mu subtype in the cerebellum and characterisation of a kappa subtype in the thalamus. *Molecular Pharmacology*, **24**, 23–29.
Mosberg, H.I., Hurst, R., Hruby, V.J., Gee, K., Yamamura, H.I., Galligan, J.J. and Burks, T.F. (1983). *Bis*-penacillamine enkephalins possess highly improved specificity towards δ-opioid receptors. *Proceedings of the National Academy of Sciences USA*, **80**, 5871–5874.
Morris, B.J. and Herz, A. (1986). Autoradiographic localization in rat brain of κ opiate binding sites labelled by [^{3}H]bremazocine. *Neuroscience*, **19**, 839–846.
Nakanishi, S., Inoue, A., Kita, T., Nakamura, M., Chang, A.C.Y., Cohen, S.N. and Numa, S. (1979). Nucleotide sequence of cloned cDNA for bovine corticotropin-β-lipotropin precursor. *Nature*, **278**, 423–427.
Neil, A. (1984). Affinities of some common opioid analgesics towards four binding sites in mouse brain. *Naunyn-Schmiedeberg's Archives of Pharmacology*, **328**, 24–29.
Neil, A., Terenius, L., Ternes, J.W., Ehrman, R.N. and O'Brien, C.P. (1986). Opiate receptors, neuropeptides in CNS and CSF of two *Macaca* species with different responsiveness to opiates. *European Journal of Pharmacology*, **122**, 143–147.
Ninkovic, M., Hunt, S.P., Emson, P.C. and Iversen, L.L. (1981). The distribution of multiple opiate receptors in bovine brain. *Brain Research*, **214**, 163–167.
Noda, M., Furutani, Y., Takahashi, H., Toyosato, M., Hirose, T., Inayama, S., Nakanishi, S. and Numa, S. (1982). Cloning and sequence analysis of cDNA for bovine adrenal preproenkephalin. *Nature*, **295**, 202–206.
Oka, T., Negishi, K., Suda, M., Matsumiya, T. and Ueki, M. (1981). Rabbit vas deferens: a specific bioassay for opioid κ-receptor agonists. *European Journal of Pharmacology*, **73**, 235–236.
Paton, W.D.M. (1957). The action of morphine and related substances on contraction and on acetylcholine output of coaxially stimulated guinea-pig ileum. *British Journal of Pharmacology and Chemotherapy*, **12**, 119–127.
Pert, C.B. and Snyder, S.H. (1973). Opiate receptor: demonstration in nervous tissue. *Science*, **179**, 1011–1014.

Petrillo, P., Tavani, A., Verotta, D., Robson, L.E. and Kosterlitz, H.W. (1987). Differential postnatal development of μ-, δ- and κ-opioid binding sites in rat brain. *Brain Research*, **428**, 53–58.

Petrillo, P., La Regina, A., Sbacchi, M., Tavani, A., Robson, L.E. and Kosterlitz, H.W. (1989). Regional variations in binding capacities at μ-, δ- and κ-opioid sites in membrane suspensions from rabbit brain. *European Journal of Pharmacology*, **166**, 213–217.

Pfeiffer, A. and Herz, A. (1982). Discrimination of three opiate receptor binding sites with the use of a computerised curve fitting technique. *Molecular Pharmacology*, **21**, 266–271.

Pfeiffer, A., Pasi, A., Mehraein, P. and Herz, A. (1982). Opiate receptor binding sites in human brain. *Brain Research*, **248**, 87–96.

Pohl, J. (1915). Uber das *N*-allylnorcodein, einen antagonisten des morphins. *Zeitschrift für Experimentalle Pathologie und Therapie*, **17**, 370–382.

Porreca, F., Mosberg, H.I., Hurst, R., Hruby, V.J. and Burks, T.F. (1984). Roles of mu, delta and kappa opioid receptors in spinal and supraspinal mediation of gastrointestinal transit effects and hot-plate analgesia in the mouse. *Journal of Pharmacology and Experimental Therapeutics*, **230**, 341–348.

Porreca, F., Mosberg, H.I., Omnass, J.R., Burks, T.F. and Cowan, A. (1987). Supraspinal and spinal potency of selective opioid agonists in the mouse writhing test. *Journal of Pharmacology and Experimental Therapeutics*, **240**, 890–894.

Porthe, G., Valette, A. and Cros, J. (1981). Kappa opiate binding sites in human placenta. *Biochemical and Biophysical Research Communications*, **101**, 1–6.

Portoghese, P.S., Sultana, M. and Takemori, A.E. (1988). Naltrindole, a highly selective and potent non-peptide δ opioid receptor antagonist. *European Journal of Pharmacology*, **146**, 185–186.

Portoghese, P.S., Larson, D.L., Sayre, L.M., Fries, D.S. and Takemori, A.E. (1980). A novel opioid receptor site directed alkylating agent with irreversible antagonistic and reversible agonistic activities. *Journal of Medical Chemistry*, **26**, 1341–1343.

Quirion, R., Weiss, A.S. and Pert, C.B. (1983). Comparative pharmacological properties and autoradiographic distribution of (3H)-ethylketazocine binding sites in rat and guinea-pig brain. *Life Sciences*, **33** (Suppl. I), 183–186.

Robson, L.E. and Kosterlitz, H.W. (1979). Specific protection of the binding sites of D-Ala^2-D-Leu^5-enkephalin (δ-receptors) and dihydromorphine (μ-receptors). *Proceedings of the Royal Society of London, B*, **205**, 424–432.

Robson, L.E., Gillan, M.G.C. and Kosterlitz, H.W. (1985). Species differences in the concentrations and distributions of opioid binding sites. *European Journal of Pharmacology*, **112**, 65–71.

Robson, L.E., Foote, R.W., Maurer, R. and Kosterlitz, H.W. (1984). Opioid binding sites of the κ-type in guinea-pig cerebellum. *Neuroscience*, **12**, 621–627.

Schmauss, C. and Yaksh, T.L. (1984). *In vivo* studies on spinal opiate receptor systems mediating antinociception. II. Pharmacological profiles suggesting a differential association of mu, delta and kappa receptors with visceral chemical and cutaneous thermal stimuli in the rat. *Journal of Pharmacology and Experimental Therapy*, **228**, 1–12.

Schiller, P.W., Nguyen, T.M.-D., Chung, N.N. and Lemieux, C. (1989). Dermorphin analogues carrying an increased positive charge in their "message" domain display extremely high μ opioid receptor selectivity. *Journal of Medical Chemistry*, **32**, 698–703.

Schulz, R., Seidl, E., Wuster, M. and Herz, A. (1982). Opioid dependence and cross-dependence in the isolated guinea-pig ileum. *European Journal of Pharmacology*, **84**, 33–40.

Schulz, R., Wuster, M. and Herz, A. (1981). Pharmacological characterisation of the ϵ-opiate receptor. *Journal of Phamacology and Experimental Therapy*, **216**, 604–606.

Schulz, R., Wuster, M., Krenss, H. and Herz, A. (1980a). Lack of cross-tolerance on multiple opiate receptors in the mouse vas deferens. *Molecular Pharmacology*, **18**, 395–401.

Shculz, R., Wuster, M., Krenss, H. and Herz, A. (1980b). Selective development of tolerance without dependence in multiple opiate receptors of mouse vas deferens. *Nature*, **285**, 242–243.

Sharif, N.A., Hunter, J.C., Hill, R.G. and Hughes, J. (1988). [^{125}I]Dynorphin(1–8) produces a similar pattern of κ-opioid receptor labelling to [^{3}H]dynorphin(1–8) and [^{3}H]etorphine in guinea-pig brain: a quantitative autoradiographic study. *Neuroscience Letters*, **86**, 272–278.

Sharif, N.A., Durie, E., Michel, A.D. and Whiting, R.L. (1990). Dog cerebral cortex contains μ-, δ- and κ-opioid receptors at different densities: apparent lack of evidence for subtypes of the κ-receptor using selective radioligands. *Brain Research*, **510**, 108–114.

Sheehan, M.J., Hayes, A.G. and Tyers, M.B. (1988). Lack of evidence for ϵ-opioid receptors in the rat vas deferens. *European Journal of Pharmacology*, **154**, 237–245.

Smith, J.R. and Simon, E.J. (1980). Selective protection of stereospecific enkephalin and opiate binding against inactivation by *N*-ethylmaleimide: evidence for two classes of opiate receptors. *Proceedings of the National Academy of Sciences USA*, **77**, 281–284.

Spain, J.W., Roth, B.L. and Coscia, C.J. (1985). Differential ontogeny of multiple opioid receptors (μ, δ and κ). *Journal of Neuroscience*, **5**, 584–588.

Takemori, A.E. and Portoghese, P.S. (1985). Receptors for opioid peptides in the guinea-pig ileum. *Journal of Pharmacology and Experimental Therapeutics*, **92**, 269–274.

Tavani, A., Robson, L.E. and Kosterlitz, H.W. (1985). Differential postnatal development of μ-, δ- and κ-opioid binding sites in mouse brain. *Developmental Brain Research*, **23**, 306–309.

Teal, J.J. and Holtzman, S.G. (1980). Discriminative stimulus effects of prototype opiate receptor agonists in monkeys. *European Journal of Pharmacology*, **68**, 1–10.

Terenius, L. and Wahlstrom, A. (1975). Search for an endogenous ligand for opiate receptors. *Acta Physiologica Scandinavica*, **94**, 74–81.

Teschemacher, H., Opheim, K.E., Cox, B.M. and Goldstein, A. (1975). A peptide like substance from pituitary that acts like morphine. I. Isolation. *Life Sciences*, **16**, 1771–1775.

Toth, G., Kramer, T.H., Knapp, R., Lui, G., Davis, P., Burks, T.F., Yamamura, H.I. and Hruby, V.J. (1989). [D-Pen^{2},D-Pen^{5}]enkephalin analogues with increased affinity and selectivity for δ opioid receptors. *Journal of Medical Chemistry*, **33**, 249–253.

Traynor, J.R. and Rance, M.J. (1984). Opiate binding in the rat spinal cord: evidence for mu and delta sites. *Neuropeptides*, **5**, 81–84.

Traynor, J.R. and Wood, M.S. (1987). Distribution of opioid binding sites in spinal cord. *Neuropeptides*, **10**, 313–320.

Traynor, J.R., Corbett, A.D. and Kosterlitz, H.W. (1987). Diprenorphine has agonist activity at opioid κ-receptors in the myenteric plexus of the guinea-pig ileum. *European Journal of Pharmacology*, **137**, 85–89.

Trendelenburg, P. (1917). Physiologische und pharmacologische versuche uber die dunndarmperistaltik. *Archive für Experimentelle Pathologie und Pharmacologie*, **81**, 55–129.

Tyers, M.B. (1980). A classification of opiate receptors that mediate antinociception in animals. *British Journal of Pharmacology*, **69**, 503–512.
Valette, A., Pontonnier, G. and Cros, J. (1979). Evidence for a stereospecific [^{3}H]etorphine binding in human placenta.*FEBS Letters*, **103**, 362–365.
Vaupel, D.B. (1983). Naltrexone fails to antagonise the σ-effects of PCP and SKF 10,047 in the dog. *European Journal of Pharmacology*, **92**, 269–274.
Von Voigtlander, D.H., Lahti, R.A. and Ludens, J.H. (1983). U-50,488: A selective and structurally novel non-mu (kappa) opioid agonist. *Journal of Pharmacology and Experimental Therapeutics*, **224**, 7–12.
Wolozin, B.L. and Pasternak, G.W. (1981). Classification of multiple morphine and enkephalin binding sites in the central nervous system. *Proceedings of the National Academy of Sciences USA*, **78**, 6181–6185.
Woods, H.J, Young, A.M. and Herling, S. (1982). Classification of narcotics on the basis of their reinforcing, discriminative and antagonist effects in rhesus monkeys. *Federation Proceedings*, **41**, 221–227.
Wuster, M., Schulz, R. and Herz, A. (1979). Selectivity of opioids towards the μ-, δ- and ϵ-opiate receptors. *Neuroscience Letters*, **15**, 193–198.
Yoshimura, K., Huidobro-Toro, J.P. and Way, E.L. (1982). Kappa opioid properties of dynorphin and its peptide fragments on the guinea-pig ileum. *Journal of Pharmacology and Experimental Therapeutics*, **222**, 71–79.
Zarr, G.D., Werling, L.L., Brown, S.R. and Cox, B.M. (1986). Opioid ligand binding in the spinal cord of the guinea-pig. *Neuropharmacology*, **25**, 471–480.
Zukin, R.S., Eghbali, M., Olive, D., Unterwald, E.M. and Tempel, A. (1988). Characterization and visualization of rat and guinea pig brain κ opioid receptors: evidence for κ_1 and κ_2 opioid receptors. *Proceedings of the National Academy of Sciences USA*, **85**, 4061–4065.

Chapter 8

Type-selective receptor and post-receptor regulation in the opioid system: studies with neuronal cultures

Rabi Simantov

8.1. *Chronic morphine application and selective receptor regulation*

Though short-term treatment with opiates, including morphine, increases opiate receptor binding (Pert and Snyder, 1976), it has been established that chronic application of morphine to experimental animals does not change receptor density (Klee and Streaty, 1974; Hollt *et al.*, 1975; Dum *et al.*, 1979). Yet, more potent and long-lasting opiates like etorphine do decrease the number of μ-opioid receptors in defined brain regions (Tao *et al.*, 1987). Considering the complexity and multiplicity of opioid receptors in the brain, it was useful to use more defined systems, like the neuroblastoma-glioma NG108-15 cells that express only δ-type receptors. Indeed, these and similar cell cultures were valuable to demonstrate that enkephalins and potent opiates induce down-regulation of δ-receptors. However morphine, which binds to the δ-receptors of these cells and blocks prostaglandin-induced adenylate cyclase activity (Sharma *et al.*, 1975), does not down-regulate the opioid receptors (Simantov *et al.*, 1982). Similarly, morphine does not induce receptor regulation in aggregating rat brain cell cultures (Lenoir *et al.*, 1984). Yet, μ-selective peptides like morphiceptin (R. Simantov and R. Levy, unpublished results) or Tyr-D-Ala-Gly-MePhe-NH(CH_2)OH (DAGO) (Vogel *et al.*, 1990) can induce down-regulation of μ-opioid receptors. These observations are in line with the notion that different opioid peptides and alkaloids possess selective regulatory effects on various opioid receptor subtypes.

8.2. *A differential effect of chronic membrane depolarization on various receptor subtypes*

Synaptic and neurotransmitter plasticity are widespread phenomena, in the developing as well as the mature nervous system. Among the environmental factors that induce plasticity in the brain, the activation state of the neurone has been drawing much attention, and experiments *in vivo* or with cultured cells have shown that long-lasting neuronal activation regulates structural pattern formation (Fawcett and O'Leary, 1985; Frank, 1987), trans-synaptic gene activation (Greenberg *et al.*, 1986) and the biosynthesis of neurotransmitters (Patterson, 1978; Black *et al.*, 1984) and neuropeptides (Kessler and Black, 1982; Black *et al.*, 1984; LaGamma *et al.*, 1985). Some of these processes, like the innervation of the optic tectum by retinal neurones or the expression of various neurotransmitters and neuropeptides, were extensively analysed. Less is known, however, of the role of chronic neuronal activation on the expression of the receptors for these neurotransmitter/neuropeptides, except the muscle nicotinic cholinergic receptor (Kuffler *et al.*, 1971; Schuetze and Role, 1987). As receptors in the central nervous system are often the target site of various drugs, some of them being used for weeks or months, it is valuable to investigate whether chronic activation of neuronal cells modulates the expression of such receptors. Moreover, the existence of multiple receptors for the same neurotransmitter, so-called receptor families, raises questions about the relationship between the transmembrane signalling system coupled to each receptor subtype, and its response to chronic activation. Recent studies, summarized here, indicate that chronic membrane depolarization of cultured neurones has a characteristic and subtype-specific effect on the expression of various muscarinic and opioid receptors. It is suggested that induction of receptor plasticity upon chronic excitation of neurones that exhibit different opioid, muscarinic and possibly other receptors, depends on the post-receptor signalling GTP-binding proteins and ion channels that are coupled to each receptor subtype.

8.2.1. **Plasticity in the expression of opioid receptors**

For the three opioid receptors μ, δ and κ, the first set of studies, conducted with aggregating fetal brain cells (Simantov and Levy, 1986), have shown that chronic membrane depolarization with potassium chloride decreases the expression of μ-receptors. This was observed with cultures of the rat forebrain as well as the hindbrain. However, in forebrain cultures the effect of potassium chloride on the rest of the opioid binding sites, namely the 'non-μ'-receptors, was different from that of hindbrain cells (Simantov and Levy, 1986). This was in line with studies indicating receptor heterogeneity in the two cultures (Lenoir *et al.*, 1984; Barg *et al.*, 1989), and the widely documented observation that the rat forebrain is rich with δ-receptors (Mansour *et al.*, 1988, and references therein). More unambiguous analysis of the effect of depolarization on the other two receptors, δ and κ, therefore became worthwhile.

Experiments with a subclone of the neuroblastoma–glioma NG108-15 cells that possess only δ-receptors have shown that treatment with 20 or 40 mM potassium chloride for 18–48 h increases the number of δ-receptors (Simantov and Levy, 1989a), a result similar to the effect of depolarization on the non-μ receptors of forebrain aggregates (Simantov and Levy, 1986).

For κ-receptors, 30–45% of the total opioid binding sites in adult guinea-pig brain are of this type (Kosterlitz *et al.*, 1981; Mansour *et al.*, 1988; Zukin *et al.*, 1988; Barg *et al.*, 1989), whereas in brain cell cultures of embryonic guinea-pig these receptors account for 75–80% of the total receptors (Barg *et al.*, 1989). These cultures were therefore suitable for investigating the effect of neuronal activation on the expression of κ-receptors. Experiments conducted recently (Barg and Simantov, 1990) have shown that chronic depolarization of such guinea-pig cultures with potassium chloride or veratridine decreases the binding of both [^{3}H]-diprenorphine (a universal opioid ligand) and [^{3}H]-U-69593 (a κ-selective ligand). In this study with κ-receptors, and in the previous study (Simantov and Levy, 1989a) with δ-receptors, chronic depolarization decreased or increased, respectively, the B_{max} of the radioligand, determined by the Rosental–Scatchard analysis, and had no effect on the receptor affinity. Collectively, the findings with the rat and guinea-pig brain cell cultures and the NG108-15 subclone cell line indicate that chronic membrane depolarization has a differential effect on the expression of the three opioid receptors, with δ-receptors responding in a clearly different way to μ- and κ-receptors.

8.2.2. **Effect of chronic neuronal activation on muscarinic receptors**

The question of whether such a differential effect of depolarization is unique to opioid receptors was tested with cultured neuronal cells expressing different muscarinic receptors. Three cell lines that bind the muscarinic receptor antagonist 1-quinuclidinyl [pheny1-4-^{3}H] benzylate ([^{3}H]-QNB) were treated acutely or chronically with potassium chloride, but chronic depolarization increased receptor density in only one of them (Simantov and Levy, 1989b). That this differential effect is also associated with subtype heterogeneity of the receptors was indicated in a displacement experiment with pirenzepine, a pharmacologically selective m1 antagonist (Hammer *et al.*, 1980); the two cell lines SC9 and WC5, in which depolarization does not increase receptor density, exhibit much higher affinity to pirenzepine than the third cell line (the above-mentioned subclone of NG108-15 cells). Moreover, characterization of the muscarinic receptor subtypes in hybridization experiments, using selective molecular probes for the various muscarinic receptors, have indicated that SC9 and WC5 cells express m3 (and possibly some m2) receptors, whereas the NG108-15 subclone possess m4 receptors, as previously indicated (R. Pinkas-Kramarski, R. Stein, R. Levy, R. Simantov and M. Sokolovsky unpublished results). It was therefore concluded that chronic membrane depolarization with KCl increases selectively the number of m4, but not m3, muscarinic receptors.

The differential regulatory effect of chronic membrane depolarization on the expression of muscarinic receptors was also studied in serum-free monolayer cultures of neuronal cells, prepared from defined rat brain structures. The neuroanatomical organization of cholinergic neurones in the septum–hippocampus pathway made these two regions very suitable for such analysis. Chronic depolarization of cultured septal neurones with potassium chloride increases the binding of [^{3}H]-QNB (1-quinuclidinyl [phenyl-4-^{3}H] benzylate), whereas hippocampal neurones have no such response (Simantov and Levy, 1989c). Experiments with pirenzepine have shown that the muscarinic receptors in the adult rat brain septum have three to five times lower affinity to this compound than the rat hippocampal tissue. Assuming that septal and hippocampal cholinergic neurones in culture maintain the same muscarinic receptor profile as in the adult tissues, the results suggest that chronic depolarization increases the number of presynaptic muscarinic receptors of septal neurones, whereas the hippocampal postsynaptic receptors have no such response (Simantov and Levy, 1989c). Whether these pre- and postsynaptic receptors are of m4 and m3 receptors subtypes, respectively, needs further analysis at the functional and molecular levels.

8.3. *Differential regulation of G-proteins*

Adenylate cyclase inhibition by opioids was observed in brain homogenates (Collier and Roy, 1974; Cooper *et al.*, 1982) and NG108-15 cells (Sharma *et al.*, 1975). These findings were followed with studies on the effect of opioids on GTPase activity (Koski and Klee, 1981) and pertussis toxin inhibition of opioids effect on adenylate cyclase (Kurose *et al.*, 1983). The interaction of G-protein α-subunits with purified μ-receptors (Ueda *et al.*, 1988) and the interaction of κ-opiate receptors with α-subunits of the G-protein (Attali *et al.*, 1989) have established the notion that the second messenger system that mediates opioid action in the nervous system involves G-protein subunits.

Recent experiments with rat and guinea-pig embryonic cell cultures have shown that μ-, δ- and κ-opioids have a differential effect on G-protein α-subunits (Vogel *et al.*, 1990). Furthermore, cells from different parts of the brain respond differently to the ligands. Thus, a μ-ligand like DAGO decreases the level of membrane-bound α_i and α_o G-proteins in hindbrain aggregating cells, but has an opposite effect on forebrain cultures. Under the same conditions the δ-selective opioid Try-D-Pen-Gly-Phe-D-Pen (DPDPE) increases the level of the two α-subunits in hindbrain cultures (Vogel *et al.*, 1990). It appears therefore that opioid agonists induce multiple changes in the level of membrane-bound G-protein subunits.

8.4. *Summary*

The post-receptor mechanisms of opioid as well as muscarinic receptors are still under investigation. A series of studies by Sharma *et al.* (1975) established that activation of δ-opioid receptors in NG108-15 cells decreases adenylate cyclase activity. Similarly, there are more recent observations that m4 muscarinic receptors use the same second messenger pathway (Evans *et al.*, 1984; Peralta *et al.*, 1988; Bonner, 1989). It is interesting, therefore, that in these two neurotransmitter systems, both operating via the inhibition of adenylate cyclase, and thus using α_i GTP-binding proteins, chronic depolarization increases the receptor number. It is of interest also that chronic membrane depolarization of neuroblastoma cells alters the amount of some membrane-bound GTP-binding proteins (Luetje and Nathanson, 1988). As depolarization increases the number of muscarinic receptors in these cells (Liles and Nathanson, 1987; Simantov and Levy, 1989b), the possibility that the changes in receptor density are coupled to alterations in the amount or the intracellular compartmentation of GTP-binding proteins should be considered.

Though the nature of the second messenger system of μ- and κ-receptors is less clear, the involvement of potassium and calcium ion channels seems certain (North, 1986; Hescheler *et al.*, 1987; Attali *et al.*, 1989). Interestingly, the post-receptor machinery of the muscarinic m3 (and m1) receptors also involves the activation of potassium channels (Bonner, 1989; Bujo *et al.*, 1988) as well as phosphatidyl inositol (Brown and Brown, 1983; Peralta *et al.*, 1988; Bonner, 1989 and references therein). Thus, it is tempting to hypothesize that receptors coupled to the adenylate cyclase system via $G\alpha_i$ are under a different regulatory mechanism than receptors coupled to potassium or calcium ion channels; a continuous membrane activation induces an apparent up-regulation of the first group of receptors, but not of the latter. Chronic activation of muscarinic or opioid receptors may therefore impose selective regulatory changes on neuronal pathways that use different receptor subtypes. The *in vivo* implications of these observations, and the possibility that plasticity of receptors for other neurotransmitters and neuropeptides use similar selective pathways, is worth further analysis.

References

Attali, B., Saya, D., Nah, S.Y. and Vogel, Z. (1989). *Journal of Biological Chemistry*, **264**, 347–353.

Barg, J. and Simantov, R. (1990). *Neuroscience Letters*, **111**, 222–227.

Barg, J., Levy, R. and Simantov, R. (1989). *International Journal of Developmental Neuroscience*, **7**, 173–180.

Black, I.B., Adler, J.E., Dreyfus, C.F., Jonakait, G.M., Katz, D.M., LaGamma, E.F. and Markey, K.M. (1984). *Science*, **225**, 1266–1270.

Bonner, T.I. (1989). *Trends in Neuroscience*, **12**, 148–151.
Brown, S.L. and Brown, J.H. (1983). *Molecular Pharmacology*, **24**, 351–356.
Bujo, H., Nakai, J., Kubo, T., Fukuda, K., Akiba, I., Maeda, A., Mishina, M. and Numa, S. (1988). *FEBS Letters*, **240**, 95–100.
Collier, H.O.J. and Roy, A.C. (1974). *Nature*, **248**, 24–27.
Cooper, D.M.C., Londons, C., Gill, D.L. and Rodbell, M. (1982). *Journal of Neurochemistry*, **38**, 1164–1167.
Dum, J., Meyer, G., Hollt, V. and Herz, A. (1979). *European Journal of Pharmacology*, **58**, 453–460.
Evans, J., Smith, M.M., Tanner, L.I. and Harden, T.K. (1984). *Molecular Pharmacology*, **26**, 395–404.
Fawcett, J.W. and O'Leary, D.D.M. (1985). *Trends in Neuroscience*, **8**, 201–206.
Frank, E. (1987) *Trends in Neuroscience*, **10**, 188–190.
Greenberg, M.E., Ziff, E.B. and Greene, L.A. (1986). *Science*, **234**, 80–83.
Hammer, R., Berrie, C.P., Birdsall, N.J.M., Burgen, A.S.V. and Hulme, E.C. (1980). *Nature*, **283**, 90–92.
Hescheler, J., Rosenthal, W., Trautwein, W. and Schultz, G. (1987). *Nature*, **325**, 445–447.
Hollt, V., Dum, J., Blasig, J., Schubert, P. and Herz, A. (1975). *Life Sciences*, **16**, 1823–1828.
Kessler, J.A. and Black I.B. (1982). *Brain Research*, **234**, 182–187.
Klee, W.A. and Streaty, R.A. (1974). *Nature*, **248**, 61–63.
Koski, G. and Klee, W.A. (1981). *Proceedings of the National Academy of Sciences USA*, **78**, 4185–4189.
Kosterlitz, H.W., Paterson, S.J. and Robson, L.E. (1981). *British Journal of Pharmacology*, **73**, 939–949.
Kuffler, S.W., Dennis, M.J. and Harris, A.J. (1971). *Proceedings of the Royal Society of London, B*, **177**, 555–563.
Kurose, H., Katada, T., Amano, T. and Ui, M. (1983). *Journal of Biological Chemistry*, **258**, 4870–4875.
LaGamma, E.F., White, J.D., Adler, J.E., Krause, J.E., McKelvy, J.F. and Black, I.B. (1985). *Proceedings of the National Academy of Sciences USA*, **82**, 8252–8255.
Lenoir, D., Barg, J. and Simantov, R. (1984). *Brain Research*, **304**, 285–290.
Liles, W.C. and Nathanson, N.M. (1987). *Journal of Neuroscience*, **7**, 2556–2563.
Luetje, C.W. and Nathanson, N.M. (1988). *Journal of Neurochemistry*, **50**, 1775–1782.
Mansour, A., Khachaturian, H., Lewis, M.E., Huda, A. and Watson, S.J. (1988). *Trends in Neuroscience*, **11**, 308–314.
North, R.A. (1986). *Trends in Neuroscience*, **9**, 114–117.
Patterson, P. (1978). *Annual Review of Neuroscience*, **1**, 1–17.
Peralta, E.G., Ashkenazi, A., Winslow, J.W., Ramachandran, J. and Capon D.J. (1988). *Nature*, **334**, 434–437.
Pert, C.B. and Snyder, S.H. (1976). *Biochemical Pharmacology*, **25**, 847–853.
Schuetze, S.M. and Role, L.W. (1987). *Annual Review of Neuroscience*, **10**, 403–457.
Sharma, S.K., Nirenberg, M. and Klee, W.A. (1975). *Proceedings of the National Academy of Sciences USA*, **72**, 590–594.
Simantov, R. and Levy, R. (1986). *Developmental Brain Research*, **26**, 301–304.
Simantov, R. and Levy, R. (1989a). *Journal of Neurochemistry*, **52**, 305–309.
Simantov, R. and Levy, R. (1989b). *Cellular and Molecular Neurobiology*, **9**, 87–94.
Simantov, R. and Levy, R. (1989c). *Brain Research*, **505**, 160–162.
Simantov, R. Levy, R. and Baram, D. (1982). *Biochimica et Biophysica Acta*, **721**, 478–484.

Tao, P.L., Law, P.Y. and Loh, H.H. (1987). *Journal of Pharmacology and Experimental Therapy,* **240**, 809–816.
Ueda, H., Harada, H., Nozaki, M., Katada, T., Ui, M., Satoh, M. and Takagi, H. (1988). *Proceedings of the National Academy of Sciences USA*, **85**, 7013–7017.
Vogel, Z., Barg, J. Attali, B. and Simantov, R. (1990). *Journal of Neuroscience Research*, in press.
Zukin, R.S., Eghbali, M., Olive, D., Unterwald, E.M. and Tempel, A. (1988). *Proceedings of the National Academy of Sciences USA*, **85**, 4061–4065.

Chapter 9

The pathophysiological functions of β-casomorphins

Krishnaswami Ramabadran, Vidya Kumar Shukla and Mylarrao Bansinath*

9.1. *Introduction*

Milk is a mammal-specific biological fluid secreted by the mammary gland. It is the first and sole food of newborn mammals for a certain period of time. The constituents of milk are of great importance and have evolved differently both in quality and in quantity to meet the specific requirements of neonatal development in various mammals. Cow's milk proteins constitute up to 30% of the total dietary protein intake. On the basis of nitrogen balance techniques and amino acid scoring procedures, it is clear that milk proteins serve as a high quality source of both nitrogen and indispensable amino acids in the nutrition of newborn and young children. Milk is a complex oil-in-water emulsion containing protein, fat, lactose, vitamins and minerals as well as other biologic products such as enzymes, cells, hormones and immunoglobulins, and contains, among other things, a heterogeneous mixture of proteins, classified into two major components, specifically, caseins and whey proteins. A number of hormones have also been found in milk (Koldovsky, 1980, 1989). Generally, casein is defined as that group of proteins precipitated from raw milk at a pH of 4·6 and 20°C. In milk, casein is present in the form of micelles made up of the various components bonded together as calcium caseinate complex and further associated with phosphate, magnesium and citrate ions. Casein constitutes 78–80% of the total protein in cow's milk and 20–30% of the total protein in human milk. Casein occurs in milk as a genetically controlled compositional variant. The linear casein molecule possesses remarkable emulsification properties due to the presence of bipolar lipophilic and hydrophilic amino acid sequences. The interaction between casein, calcium, and phosphate in the casein micelles gives the white appearance in milk. The casein micelles have been divided further into four major families: α-, β-, κ- and γ-caseins. While α-casein is the predominant sub-class of bovine milk, it is generally absent in human milk. From the α- and β-casein fractions, some opioid peptides called

* Author for correspondence.

Table 9.1. Amino acid sequences of various β-casomorphins.

	Amino acid sequence
Naturally occurring casomorphins	
β-Casomorphin (1–11)	Tyr-Pro-Phe-Pro-Gly-Pro-Ile-Pro-Asn-Ser-Leu
Bovine β-casomorphin (1–8)	Tyr-Pro-Phe-**Pro-Gly**-Pro-Ile-Pro
Human β-casomorphin (1–8)	Tyr-Pro-Phe-**Val-Glu**-Pro-Ile-Pro
Bovine β-casomorphin (1–7)	Tyr-Pro-Phe-Pro-Gly-Pro-Ile
Human β-casomorphin (1–7)	Tyr-Pro-Phe-Val-Glu-Pro-Ile
Bovine β-casomorphin (1–6)	Tyr-Pro-Phe-Pro-Gly-Pro
Bovine β-casomorphin (1–5)	Tyr-Pro-Phe-Pro-Gly
Bovine β-casomorphin (1–4)	Tyr-Pro-Phe-Pro
Bovine β-casomorphin (1–4) amide (morphiceptin)	Tyr-Pro-Phe-Pro-NH_2
Synthetic casomorphins:	
D-Phe^3-casomorphin (1–5)	Tyr-Pro-D-Phe-Pro-Gly
D-Pip^4-casomorphin (1–5) (Deprolorphin)[a]	Tyr-Pro-Phe-D-Pip-Gly
D-Pro^4-casomorphin (1–5) (Deprolorphin)	Tyr-Pro-Phe-D-Pro-Gly
Deproceptin	Tyr-Pro-Phe-D-Pro-NH_2
Valmuceptin	Tyr-Pro-Phe-Val-NH_2
Devalmuceptin	Tyr-Pro-Phe-D-Val-NH_2

[a] D-Pip, D-pipecolic acid.

α-casomorphins and β-casomorphins, respectively, have been identified and isolated. The pharmacological effects of β-casomorphins have been studied more than those of the α-casomorphins. In the bovine β-casein, opioid fragments are represented at positions 60–63, 60–64, and 60–66.

β-Casomorphins are short-chain opioid peptides of varying length. The peptide chain of seven amino acids in the sequence, Tyr-Pro-Phe-Pro-Gly-Pro-Ile, is the principal opioid peptide in bovine milk and is called β-casomorphin (1–7) (Henschen *et al.*, 1979; Chang *et al.*, 1985). All peptides larger than the tripeptide up to a chain length of 11 amino acids display at least some degree of opioid activity. β-Casomorphins (1–6), (1–5) and (1–4) can be derived from stepwise hydrolysis of β-casomorphin (1–7) or by chemical synthesis. The human β-casomorphin (1–7) is similar to bovine β-casomorphin (1–7) except for two amino acid residues (Table 9.1). β-Casomorphins have also been isolated from commercial baby formula (Brantl *et al.*, 1979). Furthermore, β-casomorphins can be formed as a digested product from the milk-derived β-casein. β-Casomorphins buried in the casein structure are biologically inactive until they are released from the β-casein by the action of intestinal microflora and/or the enzymes of digestive tract secretions. It is possible that the β-casomorphins so released are susceptible to degradation by intestinal proteases during the digestive process. However, β-casomorphins are considered to be fairly resistant to enzymatic breakdown because of their proline-rich sequence. Pronase, pepsin, trypsin, chymotrypsin, carboxypeptidase A and B and leucine aminopeptidase are some of the enzymes that cannot degrade β-casomorphins.

Interestingly, enzymatic digestion of casein from baby formula as well as dried cow's milk has been shown to release β-casomorphins and/or their derivatives (Chang *et al.*, 1985). Both Gram-positive and Gram-negative bacteria can release β-casomorphins from milk (Hamel *et al.*, 1985). As it is well known that orally ingested simple proteins are capable of exerting biological actions at the level of both central and peripheral nervous systems, β-casomorphins formed in the intestines would be expected to exert systemic pharmacodynamic effects. Following absorption from the gastrointestinal tract, β-casomorphins cross the blood–brain barrier. A specific saturable transport system for passage of β-casomorphin across the blood–brain barrier has been identified and the same system is also involved in the transport of other opioid peptides such as enkephalin and dynorphin (1–8) (Banks and Kastin, 1987). Enzymatic degradation of the naturally occurring β-casomorphins in the cerebrospinal fluid occurs less rapidly than in plasma (Stark *et al.*, 1987). Furthermore, β-casomorphins have been shown to cross the blood–brain barrier after intracarotid administration.

9.2. *Pharmacology of β-Casomorphins*

The pharmacology of β-casomorphins closely resembles that of morphine and related drugs. Results of opiate receptor binding assays of human and bovine β-casomorphins indicate that these compounds bind with opiate receptors in the rat brain membranes. Based on the binding affinity of β-casomorphins to opiate receptor subtypes, they are more selective μ-ligands with little affinity for δ- and κ-receptor subtypes. The opioid receptor selectivity of β-casomorphins has also been determined using isolated tissue preparations such as guinea-pig ileum and mouse vas deferens. The guinea-pig ileum contains both the endogenous opioid ligands and opiate receptors. In the electrically stimulated myenteric plexus-longitudinal muscle from the guinea pig ileum, the contractions of the muscle are evoked indirectly through the ganglionic release of acetylcholine. Morphine-like substances depress the release of acetylcholine, which is reflected by the proportional diminution of muscle twitches. The relative inhibitory potency of both endogenous opioids and exogenous opiates in this preparation correlates closely with their analgesic potency (Kosterlitz and Waterfield, 1975). The predominant opiate receptor type in the myenteric plexus is mu (μ). However, the presence of κ-receptors has also been demonstrated. The isolated mouse vas deferens preparation is considered to be more selective for δ-opioid agonists (Lord *et al.*, 1977).

Bovine β-casomorphins exert greater opioid activity in the guinea-pig ileum than in the vas deferens preparation (Kromer *et al.*, 1981). Because β-casomorphins can be derived from the cleavage of β-casein by proteases in the gastrointestinal tract and by caseolytic micro-organisms after ingestion of milk, they might represent truly natural agonists for the μ-type opiate receptor identified in the intestine. This conclusion is supported further by the 60–80% inhibition by naloxone of β-casomorphin binding in specific receptor binding assays (Brantl *et al.*, 1981). Opioid activities as evaluated in the guinea-pig ileum assay parallel the relative affinities of the β-casomorphins for μ-receptors in the brain membrane binding assay. Both the human and bovine β-casomorphins have the highest affinity for μ-receptors. However, human β-casomorphins (1–4) and (1–5) have relatively higher affinities for δ-receptors than the corresponding bovine β-casomorphins. Therefore, it appears that the substitution of the amino acid residue Pro-Gly in the bovine β-casomorphin amino acid sequence by the residue Val-Glu in human β-casomorphin (Table 9.1) causes an affinity shift in favour of the δ-receptor. This might explain some of the differences in the pharmacodynamics of human and bovine β-casomorphins that have been reported in the literature. Because of the short chain length of amino acids that can readily be substituted, many synthetic derivatives of β-casomorphins have been screened for their opioid activity. In general, substitution of the L-amino acids by the D-amino acids increases the opioid potency and μ-receptor selectivity, which could be the result of a decrease in breakdown by proteolytic enzymes and/or greater ability to cross the blood–brain barrier.

Even though it is not clear how much of the β-casein from ingested milk eventually gives rise to the β-casomorphins and how these peptides are absorbed from the intestine to reach the various target organs, the evidence suggests many physiopathological actions.

9.2.1. **Gastrointestinal Effects**

A role for the opioid peptides in gastrointestinal physiology is well established (Manara and Bianchetti, 1985; Kromer, 1988; Ramabadran, 1990b). Breast milk and commercial baby formula have been shown to have a stimulatory effect on the development of the intestine in the early stages of life (Sheard and Walker, 1988). Because of poorly developed gastrointestinal barriers in premature infants, the rate of absorption of β-casomorphins and other casein-related products is usually high. Casein-derived peptides such as β-casomorphin (1–5) influence the peristaltic activity of the ileum (Kromer *et al.*, 1980). The opioid agonists decrease peristalsis, an effect that can be blocked by naloxone. Indeed, this property of μ-receptor agonists has been widely used in the bioassay of β-casomorphins. Electrophysiological studies have shown that β-casomorphin (1–5) and β-casomorphin (1–4) amide (morphiceptin) decrease short-circuit current and stimulate intestinal absorption of electrolytes by an opioid-dependent mechanism (Hautefeuille *et al.*, 1986; Tome *et al.*, 1987). Studies in young mice using intracerebroventricular (i.c.v.) administration (Clark *et al.*, 1968) of β-casomorphin (1–7), β-casomorphin (1–5), morphiceptin and morphine (Figure 9.1) indicate that these compounds significantly inhibit charcoal meal transit

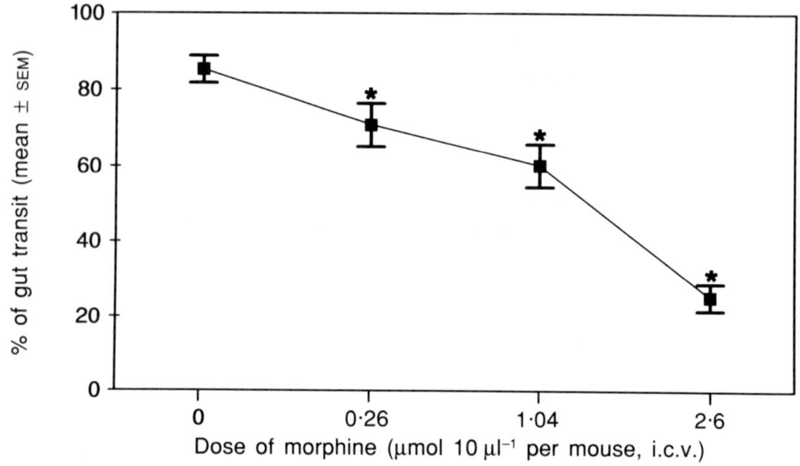

Figure 9.1. Effect of intracerebroventricular (i.c.v.) administration of morphine on charcoal meal transit in mice. Each vertical bar represents the mean ± SEM ($n > 10$ per dose). ANOVA: $F_{3,56} = 73{\cdot}5$, $P < 0{\cdot}00001$. *Post hoc* Newman–Keul's test indicate that the values obtained after morphine administration are significantly different ($P < 0{\cdot}05$) when compared to controls (0).

Table 9.2. Effect of i.c.v. administration of β-casomorphins on charcoal meal transit.[a]

Drug	Dose[b] (μmol)	*n*	Percentage of gut transit[c] (mean ± SEM)	Significance
Saline	0	29	83·24 ± 2·1	——
β-Casomorphin (1–7)	0·3	9	79·08 ± 2·6	NS
	1·0	11	81·67 ± 3·0	NS
	240	9	65·55 ± 4·4	$P < 0{\cdot}05$
β-Casomorphin (1–5)	37	10	76·87 ± 3·4	NS
	75	10	66·06 ± 4·7	$P < 0{\cdot}05$
	150	10	60·61 ± 4·8	$P < 0{\cdot}05$
β-Casomorphin (1–3)	110	11	82·74 ± 3·3	NS
	220	11	79·50 ± 3·2	NS
	440	10	74·48 ± 4·3	NS
Morphiceptin	60	11	70·44 ± 3·3	$P < 0{\cdot}05$
	120	11	68·44 ± 4·4	$P < 0{\cdot}05$
	240	12	62·36 ± 3·2	$P < 0{\cdot}05$

[a] ANOVA: Dose, $F_{3,280} = 67{\cdot}8$, $P < 0{\cdot}00001$; Drug, $F_{4,280} = 25{\cdot}8$, $P < 0{\cdot}00001$. Male mice (18–20 g) were used.
[b] Volume of injection, 10 μl; i.c.v. injection of saline or drugs was followed by charcoal meal.
[c] The animals were sacrificed 45 min later and length of the charcoal meal transit was measured and expressed as percentage of total distance of the small intestine. (Bansinath *et al.*, 1988; Ramabadran *et al.*, 1989)

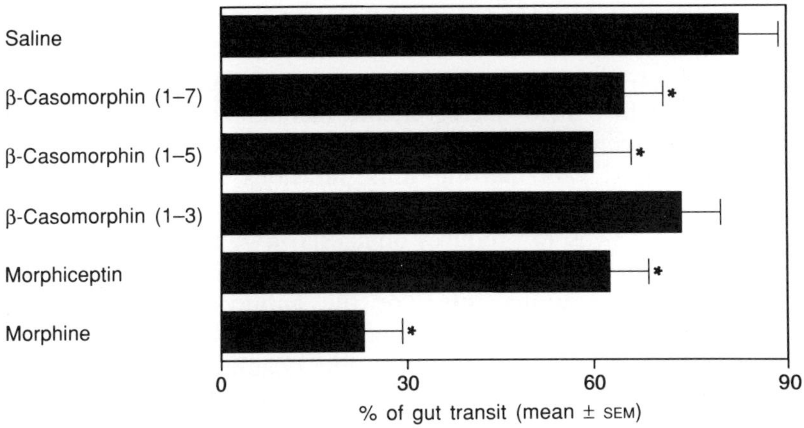

Figure 9.2. Effect of intracerebroventricular administration of β-casomorphins and morphine on charcoal meal transit in mice. Doses: β-casomorphin (1–7), 240 μmol per mouse; β-casomorphin (1–5), 150 μmol per mouse; β-casomorphin (1–3), 440 μmol per mouse; morphiceptin, 240 μmol per mouse; morphine, 26 μmol per mouse.
*, Statistical significance ($P < 0{\cdot}05$) when compared to saline controls.

(Bansinath *et al.*, 1988; Ramabadran *et al.*, 1989) by a central mechanism. However, β-casomorphin (1–3) does not modify the intestinal transit, indicating the minimum requirement of at least four amino acids in the structure of β-casomorphins (Table 9.2, Figure 9.2). Similarly, orally administered casein suspensions as well as D-Ala-β-casomorphin (1–4) and (1–5) significantly inhibit the gastrointestinal motility of a radioactive marker in rat pups (Daniel *et al.*, 1990) and inhibit intestinal propulsion in the guinea-pig colon (DePonti *et al.*, 1989). Thus the β-casomorphins act like the exogenous opiates in the inhibition of gastrointestinal motility and secretory functions by central as well as peripheral mechanisms. β-casomorphins are also implicated in the regulation of nutrient entry in the gastrointestinal tract (Meisel and Frister, 1989; Meisel *et al.*, 1989).

9.2.2. **Analgesic Effects**

A wide variety of experimental models are available for the evaluation of nociceptive responses (Ramabadran and Bansinath, 1986; Ramabadran *et al.*, 1989). The antinociceptive effects of β-casomorphins have been evaluated using thermonociceptive stimuli in the hot plate and tail flick tests and electrical nociceptive stimuli in the vocalization test. The antinociceptive responses in the hot plate and vocalization tests signify both spinal and supraspinal sites of actions, while the tail flick response is mainly due to the effects at the spinal level. In the hot plate and vocalization tests in rats, i.c.v. injection of β-casomorphin (1–5) has been shown to produce a dose-dependent analgesia and this effect is antagonized by i.c.v. naloxone (Grecksch *et al.*, 1981). The analgesic effect of morphiceptin following i.c.v.

injection has been reported in the tail flick test in rats (Chang *et al.*, 1982, 1983). Central administration of bovine β-casomorphins [(β-casomorphins (1–7), (1–6), (1–5) and (1–4)] increases the stimulus threshold in the vocalization test in a naloxone-reversible manner and the peak analgesic effect occurs between 5 and 30 min and lasts for 45–90 min. Interestingly, in 10-day-old neonatal rats, peroral milk infusions increases the paw lift latencies in the hot plate test (Blass and Fitzerald, 1988). Intraperitoneal administration of β-casein produces analgesia in 7- to 14-day-old rat pups (Giordano and Doescher, 1990). Taken together, these results implicate both spinal and supraspinal sites for the antinociceptive effects of β-casomorphins. Furthermore, early neonatal exposure of rats of morphiceptin results in a hyperalgesic state in later life (Zadina *et al.*, 1987). These findings suggest the possibility of a long-term modulation during the early neonatal period. However, extrapolation of these experimental data to human situations warrants further studies because of the wide differences in the developmental processes of human neonates.

The development of tolerance and physical dependence with repeated administration is a characteristic feature of all opioids including β-casomorphins. Tolerance and dependence have been demonstrated in rats following chronic infusion of morphiceptin into the brain using osmotic minipumps (Russell *et al.*, 1987) and, in the same animals, cross tolerance to δ-receptor agonists is minimal, confirming the μ-receptor selectivity of the former compound. Structural modifications of β-casomorphins by substitution with D-amino acids or cyclization of the peptides result in derivatives as potent as morphine in electrical stimulation of rat tail as a test model (Rüthrich *et al.*, 1990).

9.2.3. **Respiratory Effects**

Endogenous opioid systems are implicated in the control of central respiratory mechanisms at least during the early human prenatal phase (Santiago and Edelman, 1985; Lagercrantz, 1987; Ramabadran, 1990c). In addition, it is well known that μ-receptor agonists are potent respiratory depressants. Some infants with abnormal autonomic development and respiratory control mechanisms are predisposed to respiratory apnoea and are susceptible to sudden infant death syndrome (SIDS). In such infants, it has been hypothesized that β-casomorphins derived from milk may cause pronounced respiratory depression and could be implicated as one of the aetiological factors for SIDS and 'near-miss' SIDS (Ramabadran and Moore, 1988; Ramabadran and Bansinath, 1988, 1989). This hypothesis is compatible with reports indicating significant elevations in the cerebrospinal fluid levels of β-endorphin in infants suffering from prolonged apnoea of infancy (MacDonald *et al.*, 1986; Orlowski, 1986; Sankaran *et al.*, 1986; Southhall, 1987). Infants who need mechanical ventilation for allied conditions also show an increase in plasma β-endorphin levels. It is likely that in victims of SIDS and near-miss SIDS, hyperactivity of endogenous opioids in the central nervous system may exist, the tone of which could be augmented by the β-casomorphins derived from breast milk or infant formula (Ramabadran and Moore, 1988; Ramabadran and Bansinath, 1988, 1989). The developmental immaturity of the blood–brain barrier in neonates would greatly facilitate the entry of β-casomorphins (absorbed from the gastrointestinal tract) into the brain.

β-Casomorphins have been shown to have a potent respiratory depressant effect (Hedner and Hedner, 1987) when administered to newborn animals. Except for morphiceptin, all β-casomorphins are active following i.c.v. administration. Morphiceptin is the only compound shown to be effective following systemic injection. All ventilatory effects produced by β-casomorphins are readily reversible by naloxone. The depression of ventilatory pattern after the peripheral administration of morphiceptin might also arise from the activation of opiate receptors in the carotid body. However, further studies involving electrophysiological recordings of carotid sinus nerve activity following the administration of β-casomorphins are needed. These data are compatible with the notion that endogenous opioids may have a tonic influence on breathing, especially during early neonatal life. In this context, it is interesting to mention a case report where overproduction of endogenous opioids was shown to be responsible for recurrent episodes of respiratory failure in a young child who eventually died of apnoea (Brandt *et al.*, 1980). Administration of naloxone gave positive results on several occasions when the child was given artificial respiration, and β-endorphin levels in cerebrospinal fluid remained elevated particularly during apnoea. Compatible with our hypothesis, high levels of β-casomorphin (1–7) like immunoreactivity have been demonstrated in the plasma of newborn infants with apnoea (Spitzer *et al.*, 1988). These findings indicate that some respiratory disorders in newborn infants and children might be associated with hyperactivity of the endorphin system, superimposed by β-casomorphins. Administration of naloxone and other selective μ-antagonists under these circumstances might prevent apnoea and restore normal respiration. Indeed, a recent report indicates that oral administration of the long-acting opiate antagonist, naltrexone, prevented the occurrence of apnoea in children with elevated levels of β-endorphin in the cerebrospinal fluid (Myer *et al.*, 1990). However, the most striking adverse effect of antagonist treatment in these infants with a high level of endogenous opioid peptides is the precipitation of withdrawal syndrome. In addition, naltrezone has a much more developed morphinomimetic property which might interfere with its therapeutic action.

9.2.4. **Cardiovascular Effects**

Administration of opioid peptides intracerebrally, intravenously or applied directly upon the brain-stem, produces powerful cardiovascular responses

(Ramabadran, 1990a). In anaesthetized animals, the various types of β-casomorphins produce bradycardia, tachycardia, hypotension or hypertension depending on the site of administration and the dose of the compound used (Ramabadran and Bansinath, 1989). Electrophysiological studies conducted on the papillary muscles indicate prolongation of the fast-action potential (Nilius *et al.*, 1985). Furthermore, low concentrations of β-casomorphins enhance the specific binding of [H^3]-ouabain in myocardial membranes, implicating an action on the sodium pump (Liebmann *et al.*, 1986). β-casomorphin (1–5) has been shown to modulate the functional properties of the myocardial β-adrenoceptor-G-protein complex, presumably resulting in its desensitization through non-opoid mechanisms (Liebmann *et al.*, 1991).

9.2.5. **Endocrine Effects**

It is well accepted that endogenous opioid peptides modulate neuroendocrine functions both at the hypothalamic and pituitary levels. Following the administration of β-casomorphins, the plasma levels of prolactin, insulin and immunoreactive thyrotropin-releasing hormone are elevated (Mitsuma *et al.*, 1984). In conscious animals, β-casomorphin (1–7), morphiceptin and a casein peptone augment the release of postprandial insulin after a liver extract sucrose-test meal and this effect is antagonized by oral administration of naloxone (Schusdziarra *et al.*, 1983). β-Casomorphins may interact with the opiate receptors in the intestines, thereby influencing the hormonal and/or neural signal between the intestines and the islets of Langerhans. These effects may also be due to the actions of absorbed procasomorphins and/or β-casomorphins at the level of β-cells.

9.2.6. **Postpartum psychosis**

Outbursts of psychosis after childbirth in some women, defined as postpartum or lactation psychosis, is characterized by agitation, confusion, delusion or a sense of persecution, hallucinations and insomnia. Indeed, Hippocrates and the 19th century French pychiatrist, Louis Marcé both considered postpartum psychosis as a unique disorder. Because the incidence of psychosis during postpartum is low, being 1 in 500 to 1000 parturient women, only a limited number of studies have been done to identify the biological factors that could precipitate this disorder. One interesting report implicates β-casomorphins as one of the biological factors in the aetiology of postpartum psychosis (Lindstrom *et al.*, 1984). β-Casomorphin-like material has been identified in cerebrospinal fluid and plasma samples of women with severe postpartum psychosis. This finding is highly relevant to the clinical observations, suggesting a connection between milk production and outbursts of psychosis, which usually occurs after a few days to two weeks following delivery. High-performance liquid chromatography (HPLC) fractionation of the material from the cerebrospinal fluid of these patients showed that the active material eluted along with β-casomorphin (1–5) and (1–7) was partially inactivated by the post-proline cleaving enzyme (Terenius, 1988). The β-casomorphin-like compounds in women with postpartum psychosis might be related to abnormal fragmentation of β-casein and it can be postulated that these abnormal fragments might interact with κ-opiate receptors in the brain. Further work is needed to identify the nature of the proposed transformations and the mediating enzymes.

9.2.7. Plasma β-casomorphins during pregnancy and nursing

Opioid activity and opiate receptor concentrations in brain and plasma change as a function of pregnancy and lactation. β-Casomorphin-degrading enzymes have been identified in the human placenta (Puschel *et al.*, 1982). β-Casomorphin (1–8)-like immunoreactive materials were detected in the plasma of 26 out of 35 pregnant women and in the plasma of 100 out of 138 women after parturition (Koch *et al.*, 1987). β-Casomorphins from the postpartal plasma of women, when characterized by HPLC, indicate that these peptide fragments are not of uniform composition in various individuals and their susceptibility to enzymatic degradation also varies. β-Casomorphins and/or their precursors in pregnant women appear to play a physiological role during the various stages of pregnancy and also in the regulatory control of milk production and ejection. Presence of β-endomorphin and α-MSH-like immunoreactive has also been demonstrated in milk of lactating women (Ferrando *et al.*, 1990).

In one study, plasma samples of 24 newborn calves were analysed using a radioimmunoassay procedure for the presence of β-casomorphins before and after milk ingestion (Umbach *et al.*, 1985). In the plasma of 20 calves, a β-casomorphin (1–7)-like immunoreactive material was observed after, but not before, milk consumption. Chromatographic analyses and enzyme degradation studies revealed that this material was different from β-casomorphin (1–7) and therefore seemed to be a precursor. Because the intestinal mucosa of the newborn is known to be permeable to a variety of peptides and proteins (Thomson and Keelan, 1986), this protein precursor could easily be absorbed and cleaved at any site in the newborn to elicit appropriate effects. β-Casomorphin-like materials have also been isolated *in vivo* from duodenal chyme after feeding neonatal pigs with acid casein (Meisel, 1986), and also in the plasma of 2- to 4-week-od puppies following feeding with bovine casein-based milk formula or canine bitch's milk (Singh *et al.*, 1989). Interestingly, such compounds could not be detected in the plasma of puppies following the oral administration of soya protein-based non-casein formula.

9.2.8. **Immunomodulatory Effects**

Recent findings suggests that endogenous opioid peptides might play a role in immune functions; they enhance lymphocyte proliferative responses. As opiate receptors have been demonstrated on T lymphocytes (Wybran *et al.*, 1979) and human phagocytic leucocytes (Lopker *et al.*, 1980), it has been suggested that β-casomorphins with great affinity for μ-receptors have an endorphin-like activity on neonate immune cells, particularly with respect to the development of T cell functions and cellular immunity (Fiat and Jolles, 1989). The immunological properties of the various constituents of milk are well known. The immunomodulatory effects of β-casein may be of some physiological significance in pregnant and nursing women. Intravenous administration of the hexapeptide Val-Glu-Pro-Ile-Pro-Tyr obtained from the enzymatic digestion of human β-casein has been shown to enhance the resistance to infection with *Klebsiella pneumoniae* in mice (Parker *et al.*, 1984). This hexapeptide represents a fragment (4–9) of the human β-casomorphin (1–9). β-Casomorphins formed in the newborn's intestine may exert an anti-infective immunostimulating activity.

In patients with breast cancer, the precursor of β-casomorphins, β-casein, is detectable by radioimmunoassay in the plasma and is of diagnostic value. An assay of β-casein may also be of prognostic significance to follow-up treatment in certain types of breast cancer. Furthermore, casein has been identified in other types of cancers, including lung and intestinal carcinoma, suggesting an ectopic exocrine secretion of casein at least under some pathological conditions.

9.2.9. **Other Miscellaneous Effects**

Intrastriatal injections of β-casomorphins elicit rotation behaviour and muscular rigidity, an effect characteristic of the opioids injected by the same route (Havemann and Kuschinsky, 1981; Rauca and Matthies, 1986). Injection of morphiceptin into the hippocampus evokes epileptiform discharges and leads to generalized convulsions (Lee *et al.*, 1988; Ramabadran and Bansinath, 1990). Intracerebroventricular administration of β-casomorphins reduce separation-induced distress vocalizations in chicks (Panksepp *et al.*, 1984). Similarly, oral milk infusion reduces the separation-induced distress vocalization of rat pups (Blass and Fitzerald, 1988). This might be one of the mechanisms by which the mother could protect her infants from revealing their nest to predators. Thus, one of the physiological roles of β-casomorphin is to mediate the calming effect of milk.

Three potential opioid antagonist peptide sequences termed as Casoxin A (residues 35–41), Casoxin B (residues 57–60) and Casoxin C (residues 25–34) from bovine κ-casein have been isolated (Chiba *et al.*, 1989; Yoshikawa *et al.*, 1986, 1988). At present, the biological significance of the presence of both agonist and antagonist sequences in milk proteins is not clear.

9.3. *Conclusion*

Based upon the various findings described above, β-casomorphins can be considered to be milk-derived opioid peptides with potential physiological, pathophysiological and pharmacological implications. The amino acid sequence appears to be homologous in several species and minor changes result in compounds with varying opiate receptor selectivity. Therefore, the issue of interspecies differences in the ontogeny of sleep patterns, pain perception, gastrointestinal motility, respiration and other neonatal behaviours is of central importance, while extrapolating the functional significance of β-casomorphins. Demonstration of circulating β-casomorphins in pregnant and nursing women implicates a modulatory role in milk production and ejection. The pathophysiological functions of β-casomorphins in postpartal psychosis, neonatal apnoea and sudden infant death syndrome are some of the areas that need further study. Development of β-casomorphins and other casein derivatives might lead to pharmaceutical applications in dietary supplementation of desirable bioactive peptides and in the treatment of diarrhoea, inflammatory bowel diseases, dental and bone diseases, malabsorption and immune deficiency syndromes.

Acknowledgement

K.R. is grateful to Abbott Laboratories for their financial support and encouragement.

References

Banks, W.A. and Kastin, A.J. (1987). Saturable transport of peptides across the blood brain barrier. *Life Sciences*, **41**, 1319–1338.

Bansinath, M., Ramabadran, K., Turndorf, H. and Puig, M.M. (1988). Effects of acute and chronic hyperglycemia on morphine-induced gastrointestinal transit in mice. *Pharmacology*, **37**, 281–285.

Blass, E.M. and Fitzerald, E. (1988). Milk-induced analgesia and comforting in 10-day-old rats: opioid mediation. *Pharmacology Biochemistry and Behaviour*, **29**, 9–13.

Brandt, N.J., Terenius, L., Jacobson, B.B., Klinken, L., Nordius, A., Brandt, S., Blegvad, K. and Yssing, M. (1980). Hyperendorphin syndrome in a child with necrotizing encephalopathy. *New England Journal of Medicine*, **303**, 914–916.

Brantl, V., Teschemacher, H., Blaisig, J., Henschen, A. and Lottspeich, F. (1981). Opioid activities of β casomorphins. *Life Sciences*, **28**, 1903–1919.

Chang, K.J., Cuatrecasas, P., Wei, E.T. and Chang, J.K. (1982). Analgesic activity of intracerebroventricular administration of morphiceptin and β casomorphins, correlation with morphine (mu) receptor binding affinity. *Life Sciences*, **30**, 1547–1551.

Chang, K.J., Wei, E.T., Killian, A. and Chang, J.K. (1983). Potent morphiceptin analogs: structure activity relationships and morphine-like activities. *Journal of Pharmacology and Experimental Therapy*, **227**, 403–408.

Chang, K.J., Su, Y.F., Brent, D.A. and Chang, J.K. (1985). Isolation of a specific mu opiate receptor peptide, morphiceptin from an enzymatic digest of milk protein. *Journal of Biological Chemistry*, **260**, 9706–9712.

Chiba, H., Tani, F. and Yoshikawa, M. (1989). Opioid antagonist peptides derived from kappa casein. *Journal of Dairy Research*, **56**, 363–366.

Clark, W.G., Vivona, C.A. and Baxter, C.F. (1968). Accurate freehand injection into the lateral brain ventricle of the conscious mice. *Journal of Applied Physiology*, **25**, 319–321.

Daniel, H., Vohwinkel, M. and Rehner, G. (1990). Effect of casein and β casomorphins on gastrointestinal motility in rats. *Journal of Nutrition*, **120**, 252–257.

DePonti, F., Marcoli, M., Lecchini, S., Manzo, L., Frigo, G.M. and Crema, A. (1989). Effect of β-casomorphin on intestinal propulsion in the guinea pig colon. *Journal of Pharmacy and Pharmacology*, **41**, 302–305.

Fiat, A.-M. and Jolles, P. (1989). Caseins of various origins and biologically active casein peptides and oligosaccharides: structural and physiological aspects. *Molecular and Cellular Biochemistry*, **87**, 5–30.

Ferrando, T., Rainero, I., DeGannaro, T., Oggero, R., Mostert, M., Dattola, P. and Pinessi, L. (1990). β-endomorphin-like and α-MSH-like immunoreactivities in human milk. *Life Sciences*, **47**, 633–635.

Giordano, J. and Doescher, R. (1990). Multiple opioid receptors may mediate β-casein-induced analgesia in neonatal rats. *Progress in Clinical and Biological Research*, **328**, 457–460.

Grecksch, G., Schweigert, C. and Matthies, H. (1981). Evidence for analgesic activity of β casomorphin in rats. *Neuroscience Letters*, **27**, 325–328.

Hamel, U., Kielwein, G. and Teschemacher, H. (1985). β Casomorphin immunoreactive materials in cow's milk incubated with various bacterial species. *Journal of Dairy Research*, **52**, 139–148.

Hautefeuille, M., Brantl, V., Dumontier, A.M. and Desjeux, J.F. (1986). *In vitro* effects of β casomorphins on ion transport in rabbit illeum. *American Journal of Physiology*, **250**, G92–G97.

Havemann, U. and Kuschinsky, K. (1981). Further characterization of opioid receptors in the striatum mediating muscular rigidity in rats. *Naunyn-Schmiedeberg's Archives of Pharmacology*, **317**, 321–325.

Hedner, J. and Hedner, T. (1987). β Casomorphins induced apnea and irregular breathing in adult rats and newborn rabbits. *Life Sciences*, **41**, 2303–2312.

Henschen, A., Lottspeich, F., Brantl, V. and Teschemacher, H. (1979). Novel opioid peptides derived from casein (β casomorphins). *Hoppe-Seyler's Zeitschrift fur Physiologische Chemie*, **360**, 1217–1214.

Koch, G., Wiedemann, K., Drebes, E., Zimmermann, W., Link, G. and Teschemacher, H. (1987). Human β casomorphin-7 immunoreactive material in the plasma of women during pregnancy and after parturition. *Advances in Bioscience*, **65**, 35–40.

Koldovsky, O. (1980). Hormones in milk. *Life Sciences*, **26**, 1833–1836.

Koldovsky, O. (1989). Search for role of milk-borne biologically active peptides for the suckling. *Journal of Nutrition*, **119**, 1543–1551.

Kosterlitz, H.W. and Waterfield, A.A. (1975). *In vitro* models in the structure–

activity relationships of narcotic analgesics. *Annual Review of Pharmacology*, **15**, 29–47.

Kromer, W. (1988). Endogenous and exogenous opioids in the control of gastrointestinal motility and secretion. *Pharmacological Reviews*, **40**, 121–162.

Kromer, W., Pretzlaff, W. and Woinoff, R. (1980). Opioids modulate periodicity rather than efficay of peristaltic waves in the guinea pig ileum *in vitro*. *Life Sciences*, **26**, 1857–1865.

Kromer, W., Pretzlaff, W. and Woinoff, R. (1981). Regional distribution of an opioid mechanism in the guinea pig isolated intestine. *Journal of Pharmacy and Pharmacology*, **33**, 98–101.

Lagercrantz, H. (1987). Neuromodulators and respiratory control during development. *Trends in Neuroscience*, **10**, 368–372.

Lee, P.H.K., Obie, J. and Hong, J.-S. (1988). Intra-hippocampal injections of specific μ-receptor ligand PL017 produce generalized convulsions in rats. *Brain Research*, **441**, 381–385.

Liebmann, C., Barth, A., Neubert, K., Mentz, P. and Hoffmann, S. (1986). Effects of β casomorphin on H-ouabain binding to guinea-pig heart membranes. *Pharmazie*, **41**, 670–671.

Liebmann, C., Mentz, P., Schnittler, M., Schrader, U., Neubert, K. and Barth, A. (1991). Nonopoid effects of β-casomorphin-5 in guinea pig heart: Alterations to the β-adrenoceptor-G-Protein complex and inhibition of myocardial responses to Isoproterenol. *Peptides*, **12**, 265–270.

Lindstrom, L.H., Nyberg, F., Terenius, L., Bauer, K., Besev, G., Gunne, L.M., Lyrenas, S., Wildeck-Lund, G. and Lindberg, B. (1984). CSF and plasma β casomorphin-like opioid peptides in psychosis. *American Journal of Psychiatry*, **141**, 1059–1066.

Lopker, A., Abood, L.G., Hoss, W. and Lionetti, F.J. (1980). Stereoselective muscarinic acetylcholine and opiate receptors in human phagocytic leukocytes. *Biochemical Pharmacology*, **29**, 1361–1365.

Lord, J.A.H., Waterfield, A.A., Hughes, J. and Kosterlitz, H.W. (1977). Endogenous opioid peptides: Multiple agonists and receptors. *Nature*, **267**, 495–499.

MacDonald, M.G., Moss, I.R., Kefale, G.G., Ginsburg, H.M., Fink, R.J. and Chin, L. (1986). Effect of naltrexone on apnea of prematurity and on plasma β-endorphin-like immunoreactivity. *Developmental Pharmacology and Therapeutics*, **9**, 301–309.

Manara, L. and Bianchetti, A. (1985). The central and peripheral influences of opioids on gastrointestinal propulsion. *Annual Review of Pharmacology and Toxicology*, **25**, 249–273.

Meisel, H. (1986). Chemical characterization and opioid activity of an exorphin isolated from *in vivo* digests of casein. FEBS *Letters*, **196**, 223–227.

Meisel, H. and Frister, H. (1989). Chemical characterization of bioactive peptides from *in vivo* digests of casein. *Journal of Dairy Research*, **56**, 343–349.

Meisel, H., Frister, H. and Schlimme, E. (1989). Biologically active peptides in milk proteins. *Zeitschrift für Ernährungswissenschaft*, **28**, 267–278.

Mitsuma, T., Nogimori, T. and Chaya, M. (1984). β Casomorphin inhibits thytropin secretion in rats. *Experimental and Clinical Endocrinology*, **84**, 324–330.

Myer, E.C., Morris, B.L., Brase, D.A., Dewey, W.L. and Zimmerman, A.W. (1990). Naltrexone therapy of apnea in children with elevated cerebrospinal fluid β-endorphin. *Annals of Neurology*, **27**, 75–80.

Nilius, B., Neubert, K., Zett, L. and Barth, A. (1985). β Casomorphin affects fast and slow action potentials in ventricular myocardium. *Pharmazie*, **40**, 428–429.

Orlowski, J.P. (1986). Cerebrospinal fluid endorphins and the infant apnea syndrome. *Pediatrics*, **78**, 233–237.

Panksepp, J., Normansell, L., Siviy, S., Rossi, III., J. and Zolovick, A.J. (1984). Casomorphins reduce separation distress in chicks. *Peptides*, **5**, 829–831.

Parker, F., Migliore-Samour, D., Floc'h, F., Zerial, A., Werner, G.H., Jolles, J., Casaretto, M., Zahn, H. and Jolles, P. (1984). Immunostimulating heptapeptide from human casein: amino acid sequence, synthesis and biological properties. *European Journal of Biochemistry*, **145**, 677–682.

Puschel, G., Mentlein, R. and Heymann, E. (1982). Isolation and characterization of dipeptidyl peptidase IV from human placenta. *European Journal of Biochemistry*, **126**, 359–365.

Ramabadran, K. (1990a). Cardivascular effects of opioid peptides. In: *Opioid peptides*, Vol. IV, *Biochemistry and Applied Physiology*, edited by J.I. Szekely and K. Ramabadran. Boca Raton, FL: CRC Press, pp. 289–311.

Ramabadran, K. (1990b). Gastrointestinal effects of opioid peptides. In: *Opioid peptides, Vol. IV, Biochemistry and Applied Physiology*, edited by J.I. Szekely and K. Ramabadran. Boca Raton, FL: CRC Press, pp. 325–344.

Ramabadran, K. (1990c). Respiratory effects of opioid peptides. In: *Opioid peptides, Vol. IV, Biochemistry and Applied Physiology*, edited by J.I. Szekely and K. Ramabadran. Boca Raton, FL: CRC Press, pp. 313–324.

Ramabadran, K. and Bansinath, M. (1986). A critical analysis of the experimental evaluation of nociceptive reactions in animals. *Pharmaceutical Research*, **3**, 263–270.

Ramabadran, K. and Bansinath, M. (1988). Opioid peptides from milk as a possible cause of sudden infant death syndrome. *Medical Hypotheses*, **27**, 181–187.

Ramabadran, K. and Bansinath, M. (1989). Pharmacology of β casomorphins, opioid peptides derived from milk protein. *Asia Pacific Journal of Pharmacology*, **4**, 45–58.

Ramabadran, K. and Bansinath, M. (1990). Endogenous opioid peptides and epilepsy. *International Journal of Clinical and Pharmacology Therapy and Toxicology*, **28**, 47–62.

Ramabadran, K. and Moore, B.E. (1988). Sudden infant death syndrome and opioid peptides from milk. *American Journal Diseases of Children*, **142**, 12–13.

Ramabadran, K., Bansinath, M., Turndorf, H. and Puig, M.M. (1988) Stereospecific inhibition of the gastrointestinal transit by kappa opioid agonists in mice. *European Journal of Pharmacology*, **155**, 329–331.

Ramabadran, K., Bansinath, M., Turndorf, H. and Puig, M.M. (1989). Tail immersion for the evaluation of a nociceptive reaction in mice. *Journal of Pharmacological Methods*, **21**, 21–31.

Rauca, C. and Matthies, H. (1986). The effect of casomorphins on the apomorphine- and amphetamine-induced turning after nigral lesions in rats. *Neuropharmacology*, **25**, 1137–1140.

Russel, R.D., Leslie, J.B., Su, Y.F., Watkins, W.D. and Chang, K.J. (1987). Continuous intrathecal opioid analgesia: tolerance and cross-tolerance of mu and delta spinal opioid receptors. *Journal of Pharmacology and Experimental Therapeutics*, **240**, 150–158.

Rüthrich, H.-L., Grecksch, G. and Matthies, H. (1990). Structural modifications of analgesic efficacious β-casomorphin derivatives. *Naunyn-Schmiedeberg's Archives of Pharmacology*, **340**, Suppl., R34.

Sankaran, K., Hindmarsh, K.W., Wallace, S.M., McKay, R.J. and O'Donnell, M. (1986). Cerebrospinal fluid and plasma β endorphin concentrations in prolonged infant apnea (near miss sudden infant death syndrome). *Developmental Pharmacology and Therapeutics*, **9**, 224–230.

Santiago, T.V. and Edelman, N.H. (1985). Opioids and breathing. *Journal of Applied Physiology*, **59**, 1675–1685.

Schusdziarra, V., Schick, A., de la Fuente, A., Specht, J., Klien, M., Brantl, V. and

Pfeiffer, E.F. (1983). Effect of β casomorphins and analogs on insulin release in dogs. *Endocrinology*, **112**, 885–889.

Sheard, N.F. and Walker, W.A. (1988). The role of breast milk in the development of gastrointestinal tract. *Nutrition Review*, **46**, 1–8.

Singh, M., Rosen, C.L., Chang, K.J. and Haddad, G.G. (1989). Plasma β casomorphin-7 immunoreactive peptide increases after milk intake in newborn but not in adult dogs. *Pediatric Research*, **26**, 34–38.

Southall, D.P. (1987). Cerebrospinal fluid endorphins and the infant apnea syndrome. *Pediatrics*, **79**, 838.

Spitzer, A., Butler, S., Fox, W.W. and Chang, K.J. (1988). β Casomorphin-effects of opiate-like peptides from milk protein on apnea of infancy. *Pediatric Research*, **22**, 450A.

Stark, H., Lossner, B. and Matthies, H. (1987). Metabolism of β casomorphin and its derivatives in rat brain and liver homogenates. *Biomedica et Biochimica Acta*, **10**, 687–694.

Terenius, L. (1988). Milk-derived opioid peptides and their role in postpartum psychosis. In: *Molecular Mimicry in Health and Disease*, edited by A. Lernmark, T. Dyrberg, L. Terenius and B. Hökfelt. Amsterdam: Elsevier, pp. 15–22.

Thomson, K.B.R. and Keelan, M. (1986). The development of small intestine. *Canadian Journal of Physiology and Pharmacology,* **64**, 13–29.

Tome, D., Dumontier, A.M., Hautefeuille, M. and Desjeux, J.F. (1987). Opiate activity and transepithelial passage of intact β casomorphin in rabbit ileum. *American Journal of Physiology*, **253**, G737–G744.

Umbach, M., Teschemacher, H., Praetorius, K., Hirschhauser, R. and Bostedt, H. (1985). Demonstration of β casomorphin immunoreactive material in the plasma of newborn calves after milk intake. *Regulatory Peptides*, **12**, 223–230.

Wybran, J., Appelboom, T., Famacy, J.P. and Govaerts, A. (1979). Suggestive evidence for receptors for morphine and methionine enkephalin on normal human T lymphocytes. *Journal of Immunology*, **123**, 1068–1070.

Yoshikawa, M., Tani, F. and Chiba, H. (1988). Structure activity relationship of opioid antagonist peptides derived from milk proteins. In: *Peptide Chemistry*, edited by T. Shiba. Osaka: Protein Research Foundation, pp. 473–476.

Yoshikawa, M., Tani, F., Ashikaga, T., Yoshimara, T. and Chiba, H. (1986). Purification and characterization of an opioid antagonist from peptide digest of bovine κ-casein. *Agricultural and Biological Chemistry*, **50**, 2951–2954.

Zadina, J.E., Kastin, A.J., Manasco, P.K., Pignatiello, M.F. and Nastiuk, K.L. (1987). Long term hyperalgesia induced by neonatal β endorphin and morphiceptin is blocked by neonatal Tyr-MIF-1. *Brain Research*, **409**, 10–18.

Chapter 10

Opioids and memory

Ivan Izquierdo

10.1. *Introduction*

Humans probably noticed that opiates affect memory since they started using them as analgesics. However, systematic studies were scarce until 1978–79, and the nature of the effect was not understood until very recently. Most early studies were biased by the idea that, since humans acquire addiction to opioids, opioids must be rewarding and facilitate memory; which is clearly *non sequitur*. Alcohol is rewarding, humans have acquired addiction to alcohol for centuries, and alcohol certainly impairs memory. In fact, most drugs that facilitate memory are neither rewarding nor addictive (Izquierdo, 1989; McGaugh, 1989). Besides, several of the studies purportedly showing enhanced retention after opioid administration have employed aversive paradigms (e.g. Stein and Belluzzi, 1978; Mondadori and Waser, 1979). It is hard to see how a 'rewarding' agent could enhance avoidance behaviour when given after a footshock. It is far more likely that the enhancement results from an aversive effect of the post-training treatment, adding to that of the footshock: animals that receive toxic or otherwise aversive drugs after training learn to avoid both the footshock *and* the drug (see Izquierdo, 1989). Memory facilitation by morphine or the enkephalins has indeed been obtained using high — probably toxic — and presumably aversive doses (Izquierdo *et al.*, 1980a). For example, Mondadori and Waser (1979) observed memory facilitation using 40 or 100 $mg\,kg^{-1}$ of morphine, and Stein and Belluzzi (1978) observed it using intracerebroventricular (i.c.v.) doses of enkephalins several thousand times higher than the total brain content of these peptides (Izquierdo *et al.*, 1980a). Pre-1978 studies using lower, subtoxic doses of morphine showed, instead, that it impairs learning (Cook and Weidley, 1957; Castellano, 1975) or induces state dependency (i.e. Belleville, 1964).

10.2. *Naloxone facilitation of memory*

The influence of opioids on memory began to be understood only after the discovery of endogenous opioid peptides, and the subsequent verification that the opiate antagonist, naloxone, had effects of its own that could be explained by an antagonism to endogenous opioids.

Gallagher and Kapp (1978), Izquierdo (1979) and Messing *et al.* (1979) independently found that the administration of naloxone immediately after training enhances memory in rats. This obviously suggested that endogenous opioids are released during or immediately after training, and down-regulate memory. Messing *et al.* (1979) and Izquierdo (1979) used systemic injections of naloxone; Gallagher and Kapp (1978) injected it into the amygdala. Gallagher and Kapp (1978) and Messing *et al.* (1979) observed post-training facilitation of inhibitory avoidance behaviour; Izquierdo (1979) observed post-training facilitation of classical and avoidance conditioning in a shuttle box, and of habituation to a tone. The effect of naloxone is antagonized by low doses of morphine (Izquierdo, 1979; Messing *et al.*, 1979) or levorphanol (Gallagher and Kapp, 1978) given by the same route. Morphine and levorphanol on their own have effects opposite to that of naloxone. So it was clear from the beginning that: (a) post-training naloxone facilitates memory of very different behaviours regardless of the presence of pain during acquisition, so it could reasonably be considered an effect on memory in general; (b) endogenous opioids must, like morphine or levorphanol, have an effect opposite to that of naloxone; (c) the amygdala, which contains opioid peptides and opiate receptors, is a site of action for endogenous or exogenous opioid modulation of memory.

Memory facilitation by post-training naloxone was subsequently confirmed by many laboratories in over 50 different tasks regardless of their duration, aversiveness, complexity, response requirements or general nature, and involving a great variety of memory types in many species, including sophisticated cognitive tasks in monkeys and humans (see Martin *et al.*, 1984; Gallagher *et al.*, 1985; Izquierdo *et al.*, 1986; Izquierdo, 1989). The effect of naloxone was found to be shared by diprenorphine, naltrexone and other preferential blockers of opiate μ-receptors (Gallagher, 1982). The doses of naloxone used by different laboratories in rats or mice are comparable ($0{\cdot}2$–$2{\cdot}0\,\mathrm{mg\,kg^{-1}}$), although there is one report suggesting differential sensitivity of mice strains to naloxone (Castellano, 1981).

10.3. *The release of brain β-endorphin by novel training experiences*

As said, the effect of naloxone on its own suggested that it antagonizes endogenous opioids released in the brain during or after training.

We found that exposure to a very wide of training situations is followed by a decrease of brain β-endorphin immunoreactivity (Izquierdo *et al.*, 1980b, 1981, 1984; Netto *et al.*, 1985), but not pituitary or plasma β-endorphin (Izquierdo *et al.*, 1981, 1984) or brain Met-enkephalin (Carrasco *et al.*, 1982b) immunoreactivity, in rats. The decrease of brain β-endorphin immunoreactivity, like the effect of naloxone, occurs irrespective of the nature, duration, complexity, aversiveness or response requirement of the tasks, but is seen only when the tasks were presented for the first time, i.e. when they are novel experiences (Izquierdo *et al.*, 1984; Netto *et al.*, 1986; Netto and Maltchik, 1990). A second exposure to the tasks has no effect (Izquierdo *et al.*, 1980b, 1981, 1984). In contrast, only aversive tasks (Rossier *et al.*, 1977; Perry *et al.*, 1983) or electroconvulsive shock (Dias *et al.*, 1981; Carrasco *et al.*, 1982b), but not habituation tasks, are followed by a decrease of pituitary β-endorphin or of brain Met-enkephalin immunoreactivity. Therefore, the decrease of brain β-endorphin immunoreactivity seen after training correlates with the novelty, but not with the aversiveness or other characteristics of the learning experiences (Izquierdo *et al.*, 1984; Izquierdo and Netto, 1985).

The decrease of brain β-endorphin immunoreactivity seen after training experiences is interpreted as due to a release followed by diffusion and/or degradation of the substance, for various reasons. It cannot be explained by synthesis inhibition: β-endorphin biosynthesis takes hours whereas the training-induced depletion occurs in seconds (Izquierdo and Netto, 1985). Further, β-endorphin biosynthesis can only be blocked by a marked inhibition of protein synthesis, and the tasks that cause the depletion either enhance or have no effect on brain protein synthesis (see Izquierdo, 1989). The β-endorphin depletion is accompanied by naltrexone-reversible analgesia (Siegfried *et al.*, 1987); this argues against destruction without release, against the co-release of inactive or antagonistic cross-immunoreactive metabolites (Hammonds *et al.*, 1984), and in favour of a release of β-endorphin. There are no known intragranular endopeptidases that may cleave β-endorphin at its immunoreactive region (Lebouille *et al.*, 1985; Dalmaz *et al.*, 1986), which is a further argument against destruction without release. Post-training naloxone does not cause memory facilitation if the animals are prevented from releasing β-endorphin by a section of the fornix (Netto *et al.*, 1985), malnutrition (Perry *et al.*, 1990) or prior depletion of β-endorphin by exposure to another novel experience (Izquierdo and McGaugh, 1985). In addition, post-training naloxone does not induce memory facilitation in animals exposed to training experiences that are not novel and that therefore do not release brain β-endorphin (Netto *et al.*, 1986; Netto and Maltchik, 1990).

Thus, since novel training experiences are followed by a release of brain β-endorphin, but not of other endogenous opioids, and since post-training memory facilitation by naloxone depends very strictly on this release, it may be concluded that: (a) endogenous β-endorphin normally hinders memory storage; (b) post-training naloxone acts by interfering with this effect of β-endorphin.

10.4. *The effect of opioids on memory*

The first papers on memory facilitation by naloxone (Gallagher and Kapp, 1978; Izquierdo, 1979; Messing *et al.*, 1979; Izquierdo and Graudenz, 1980) were followed by a flurry of reports on enkephalin and endorphin effects on memory using low doses, comparable to the amounts of β-endorphin released in the brain during training (Izquierdo *et al.*, 1980b). Izquierdo *et al.* (1980a,b, 1981), Martinez and Rigter (1980) and Martinez *et al.* (1981) reported that the post-training systemic injection of 0·1–10·0 $\mu g\,kg^{-1}$ of β-endorphin to rats hinders retention of active (Izquierdo *et al.*, 1980a,b) and inhibitory avoidance (Martinez and Rigter, 1980; Martinez *et al.*, 1981), and of habituation to a tone (Izquierdo *et al.*, 1980a, 1981; Izquierdo and Graudenz, 1980), which suggests a generality of the effect across memory types. The effect of β-endorphin was found to be shared by Leu- (Izquierdo *et al.*, 1980a) and Met-enkephalin (Lucion *et al.*, 1982), but not by dynorphin A (Izquierdo *et al.*, 1985) except in some tasks in mice (Introini-Collison *et al.*, 1987). The β-endorphin effect is seen when β-endorphin is given prior to (Izquierdo, 1980a), or immediately after, training (Izquierdo *et al.*, 1980a,b; Martinez and Rigter, 1980), but not several minutes after training (Martinez and Rigter, 1980). These initial findings were replicated in many laboratories (i.e. Kovacs *et al.*, 1983; Introini and Baratti, 1984; Gallagher, 1985; Rodgers *et al.*, 1985; McGaugh, 1988). Dose–response curves varied between laboratories which suggested different sensitivity across rat strains (Izquierdo *et al.*, 1986); but the effect was nevertheless qualitatively similar across strains, species and tasks. At doses higher than those which produced amnesia, β-endorphin is in general ineffective (Martinez and Rigter, 1980); i.e. it has an inverted U dose–response curve, as is the case with most drugs that alter memory by an effect in the post-training period (McGaugh, 1988, 1989), including naloxone (Fulginiti and Cancela, 1983). The reasons for this inverted U dose–response curve are as unclear in the case of β-endorphin and naloxone as they are in the case of all other post-training drug treatments (Izquierdo, 1989; McGaugh, 1989). Toxicity, and the aversiveness that comes with toxicity (see above, and Izquierdo, 1989), may be a factor.

In a strain of rats that seems to be much more sensitive to opioids than those used by most other authors (see Izquierdo *et al.*, 1981), Kovacs *et al.* (1983) observed post-training facilitation by β-endorphin in animals submitted to a variant of the inhibitory avoidance procedure in which the animals were exposed to the apparatus several times before training. Interestingly, using this same procedure, γ-endorphin produced an amnesic effect (Kovacs *et al.*, 1983), which is also the opposite of that normally seen using more conventional, one-session training procedures (e.g. Dalmaz and Fin, 1989). The post-training amnesic effect of β-endorphin, like the facilitatory effect of naloxone, is seen only when animals are exposed for the first time to the training procedure and apparatus, i.e. they are novelty-dependent effects (Gallagher *et al.*, 1983; Netto *et al.*, 1986; Netto and Maltchik, 1990).

In our Wistar rat stock, the ED_{50} for the retrograde amnesic effect of β-endorphin in a shuttle avoidance task was found to be 140 ng per rat intraperitoneal (i.p.) (Izquierdo *et al.*, 1980b, 1981) and 25 ng per rat i.c.v. (Lucion *et al.*, 1982; Izquierdo *et al.*, 1982, 1986). This suggests that approximately one-fifth of the systemically given dose reaches brain receptors, presumably periventricular, in order to cause amnesia. The finding is consonant with the observation of Houghten *et al.* (1980) that 20% of a systemically injected dose of tritium-labelled β-endorphin reaches the brain ventricles, but penetrates very little into brain tissue in rats and rabbits. The dose of 25 ng per rat i.c.v. is approximately equal to the amount of hypothalamic/preoptic β-endorphin that is estimated to be released by diverse training procedures in the rat (Izquierdo *et al.*, 1980b, 1981, 1984; Netto *et al.*, 1985; Izquierdo, 1989).

The amnesic effect of β-endorphin is competitively antagonized by naloxone and naltrexone (for references see Bostock *et al.*, 1988; Izquierdo, 1989). In rats, the order of potency of opioid peptides to produce retrograde amnesia is β-endorphin > the enkephalins > α-endorphin > dynorphin A = 0 (for references see Izquierdo *et al.*, 1986). The order of potency of opiate receptor antagonists to produce retrograde memory facilitation is diprenorphin > naloxone, naltrexone > levallorphan > dextrallorphan = 0 (Gallagher, 1982). Both orders are partially, but not entirely, compatible with a decreasing order of affinity for opiate μ-receptors. Other factors (different rates of penetration into the appropriate brain regions after either i.p. or i.c.v. administration, for example) must play a role in addition to μ-receptor affinity; if not, dynorphin A would be expected to be more potent than Met-enkephalin and this, in turn, more potent than Leu-enkephalin (Watson and Abbott, 1990). Experiments using localized brain injections of specific synthetic μ-receptor agonists and antagonists are desirable (see below for possible sites of action for opioid effects on memory).

10.5. *Is the post-training effect of opioids related to their physiological role in memory regulation, and is it truly amnesic?*

The findings summarized above suggest that the primary effect of opioids is to induce retrograde amnesia by an action upon periventricular μ-receptors. β-endorphin, the most potent of these compounds, is released by all novel training procedures studied so far in amounts similar to doses that are effective when given i.c.v. (other opioids are not released by all forms of training). Systemic injections of β-endorphin reach the brain ventricular walls, the hypothalamic β-endorphin system projects to periventricular regions of the hypothalamus, thalamus, septum and brain-stem (Bloom and McGinty, 1981), and post-training naloxone has a facilitatory effect that depends on the β-endorphin release. Thus, it was suggested early on that there is an endogenous amnesic mechanism mediated by brain β-endorphin (Izquierdo *et al.*, 1980b, 1982). The suggestion was strengthened by the finding that the classic amnesic treatment, post-training electroconvulsive shock, releases large amounts of brain β-endorphin (Dias *et al.*, 1981), and that its amnesic effect is antagonized by naloxone (Carrasco *et al.*, 1982a).

It soon became apparent that this suggestion had to be substantially qualified. The amnesia caused by β-endorphin (Izquierdo, 1989), or by agents that release brain β-endorphin, such as electroconvulsive shock (Dias *et al.*, 1981), adrenocorticotrophic hormone (ACTH) or epinephrine (Carrasco *et al.*, 1982c), can be reversed by another injection of β-endorphin or by a repetition of the same or other treatments that release β-endorphin, given prior to testing (Izquierdo, 1984; Netto *et al.*, 1987). Rigter (1978) had reported early on that the pre-test administration of enkephalins reverts hypoxia-induced amnesia.

In addition, the administration of β-endorphin, or the presentation of a novel experience that releases β-endorphin prior to testing, produces a naloxone- or naltrexone-reversible enhancement of retrieval in untreated animals unless these are prevented from releasing β-endorphin at the time of training (Izquierdo and McGaugh, 1985, 1987). Retrieval enhancement by pre-test β-endorphin was first observed by De Wied *et al.* (1978) who described it as an 'increased resistance to extinction'.

The naltrexone-sensitive enhancement of retrieval by a novel experience given prior to testing is short-lasting (up to 3 h); it was seen first in mice (Izquierdo and McGaugh, 1985, 1987) and then in humans (Chaves and Izquierdo, 1986; Chaves *et al.*, 1988), including patients with amnesic syndromes of various aetiologies: depression, alcoholism, cerebrovascular accidents, brain tumours, Hakin–Adams syndrome, multi-infarct dementia, Alzheimer's disease (Chaves and Izquierdo, 1986). It depends on the activation of brain β-noradrenergic (Izquierdo and McGaugh, 1985) and cholinergic muscarinic systems (Netto *et al.*, 1990), and it might have a fleeting therapeutic value, too brief to be of any useful clinical potential (Chaves and Izquierdo, 1986; Izquierdo, 1989).

These findings suggested that β-endorphin installs a form of state-dependency in the post-training period, and that its retrograde amnesic effect is not in reality a true amnesia, but a temporary hindrance of retention that can be overcome by a second exposure to the drug at the time of testing (Izquierdo, 1984, 1989; Izquierdo and Netto, 1985). In physiological conditions, state-dependency to β-endorphin would become established in all novel training situations because of the release of brain β-endorphin in the post-training period (Izquierdo, 1984; Izquierdo *et al.*, 1984; Netto and Maltchik, 1990; Netto *et al.*, 1990). In animals treated with post-training naloxone this would not happen because naloxone would impede the effect of endogenous β-endorphin (Izquierdo and McGaugh, 1985). In animals treated with post-training β-endorphin or electroconvulsive shock the state-dependency would be greater than normal and therefore more difficult to ovecome by pre-test treatments (Izquierdo, 1984, 1989; Netto *et al.*, 1987; Netto and Maltchik, 1989).

Since a release of β-endorphin by another novel experience interpolated prior to testing enhances memories of previous novel experiences (Izquierdo and McGaugh, 1985, 1987; Chaves *et al.*, 1988), the system might be useful to 'bring to mind' memories of what to do in case of novelty (i.e. escape strategies, to freeze or not to freeze, etc.), or simply to better recall memories of things that once were new (Izquierdo *et al.*, 1984; Izquierdo and Netto, 1985).

It is likely that the retrograde effect of electroconvulsive shock or of relatively high doses of β-endorphin or other opioids includes a real amnesic component *in addition* to a state-dependency effect (Izquierdo, 1989; McGaugh, 1989). Some components of experiences previous to electroconvulsive shock or head trauma are indeed forever irrecoverable (Izquierdo, 1989). It is possible that this true amnesic effect may predominate when agonists other than β-endorphin are used. In mice (Introini-Collison *et al.*, 1987), but not in rats (Izquierdo *et al.*, 1985), the systemic post-training administration of dynorphin A hinders retention of some tasks but not others; the effect is not reversed by a second, pre-test, administration of the drug. Likewise, also in mice, post-training morphine given i.p. causes a retrograde amnesia for an inhibitory avoidance task that cannot be reversed by another pre-test injection of the drug (Castellano and McGaugh, 1989). Due to the peculiarities of different mouse strains in relation to opioid receptor subtypes and distribution (see Castellano, 1981), these findings are worthy of replication in other mouse strains and species.

Therefore, our original suggestion that the physiological role of brain opioids, particularly β-endorphin, is to mediate an endogenous amnesic mechanism (Izquierdo *et al.*, 1980b, 1981, 1982) must be substantially qualified. The *main* role of brain β-endorphin in memory would be to induce an endogenous state-dependency in the immediate post-training period for novel experiences, perhaps for most (if not all) significant novel experiences (Izquierdo, 1984, 1989; Izquierdo and Netto, 1985). An additional role of endogenous opioids, including β-endorphin when released in exaggerated amounts, and/or when acting on structures other than those involved in the generation of state-dependency (see below), might be to cause a real amnesia (Izquierdo, 1989).

10.6. *Is post-training memory facilitation by opioid antagonists a real facilitation?*

If the main endogenous opioid system involved in memory modulation is the brain β-endorphin system, and its major role is to induce a form of state-dependency for novel events, it does not necessarily follow that the post-training administration of opiate receptor antagonists should cause memory facilitation. Naloxone would be expected to cancel the β-endorphin-induced state-dependency, but not necessarily to facilitate. But this is precisely what happens, and it was this effect that led to the discovery of the effect and possible physiological role of β-endorphin and other opioids in memory modulation (see earlier).

Recent findings indicate that post-training naloxone has a dual effect on memory. At a low dose ($0{\cdot}2\,mg\,kg^{-1}$), naloxone does not facilitate memory, does not add to the facilitatory effect of post-training epinephrine or ACTH, but blocks the effect of post-training endogenous or injected β-endorphin. At a slightly higher dose ($0{\cdot}4\,mg\,kg^{-1}$), naloxone causes memory facilitation, adds to the facilitation caused by ACTH or epinephrine, and also blocks the instalment of state-dependency by post-training β-endorphin (Izquierdo and Netto, 1990).

Thus, it is likely that the facilitation caused by post-training naloxone is not the direct result of its antagonism to β-endorphin-induced state-dependency, but rather of an antagonism to other effects of β-endorphin on memory modulation; possibly the 'real' amnesia mentioned earlier. Opioids, including β-endorphin, inhibit the release of various transmitters from axon terminals, including acetylcholine, dopamine and norepinephrine (see Izquierdo, 1989, 1990). It has been known for some time that memory facilitation by post-training naloxone requires an intact noradrenergic transmission: it can be blocked by β-noradrenergic receptor antagonists given systemically (Izquierdo and Graudenz, 1980) or into the amygdala (McGaugh, 1988), or prevented by a pretreatment with α-methyl-tyrosine (Izquierdo *et al.*, 1981) or DSP-4 (Introini-Collison and Baratti, 1986; Bennett and Hock, 1990), or with 6-hydroxydopamine injected into the dorsal noradrenergic bundle (Gallagher *et al.*, 1985). Interactions of post-training β-endorphin and naloxone effects with cholinergic muscarinic (Baratti *et al.*, 1984) and dopaminergic systems (Izquierdo and Graudenz, 1980) have also been suggested. Cholinergic muscarinic, noradrenergic and dopaminergic systems in the brain have been proposed to play a role in memory (see Izquierdo, 1989; Netto *et al.*, 1990).

10.7. *Central sites of action of naloxone and opioids*

McGaugh and his colleagues (McGaugh *et al.*, 1987, 1988; McGaugh, 1988, 1989; Introini-Collison *et al.*, 1989) have presented convincing evidence suggesting that the amygdala is crucially involved in the influence of neuromodulatory systems on memory in the post-training period. The post-training intra-amygdala injection of norepinephrine (McGaugh, 1988) or naloxone (Gallagher and Kapp, 1978; Introini-Collison *et al.*, 1989) causes memory facilitation; in both cases, the effect is blocked by the concurrent intra-amygdala injection of β-noradrenergic receptor antagonists. The intra-amygdala injection of β-noradrenergic blockers attenuates the facilitatory effect of post-training systemic naloxone or epinephrine (McGaugh, 1988; McGaugh *et al.*, 1988; Introini-Collison *et al.*, 1989). Section of the stria terminalis, the main afferent/efferent pathway of the amygdala, attenuates post-training facilitation by systemic epinephrine (McGaugh, 1988) or naloxone administration (McGaugh *et al.*, 1987), as well as the effect of systemic β-endorphin administration (McGaugh *et al.*, 1987; McGaugh, 1989). Indeed, Gallagher and Kapp (1978) had shown that the post-training injection of levorphanol into the amygdala causes naloxone-reversible amnesia.

These findings suggest that: (a) post-training naloxone and epinephrine act via the reflex and/or indirect stimulation of a β-noradrenergic mechanism in the amygdala; (b) post-training β-endorphin effects may also be mediated by the amygdala and/or require an intact amygdala system in order to become manifest (Izquierdo, 1989); (c) at least some opioid effects on memory are mediated by the amygdala.

These studies do not detract from the suggestion that periventricular μ-receptors are involved in the induction of state-dependency by endogeneously released or injected β-endorphin. First, naloxone facilitation of memory may be, as suggested earlier, a phenomenon that requires, but is not mediated by, an antagonism to β-endorphin, and that could be mediated by the amygdala (Izquierdo and Netto, 1990). Second, as commented earlier, opioids, including β-endorphin, may also have a dual effect: a true amnesic effect (i.e. Introini-Collison *et al.*, 1987; Castellano and McGaugh, 1989) and a state-dependency effect (Izquierdo, 1989). It could well be that the former is mediated by the amygdala and the latter by periventricular receptors. Alternatively, as mentioned, the amygdala could be necessary for, but not the site of action of, β-endorphin.

Bostock *et al.* (1988) observed that the post-training injection of naloxone into the medial septal area of rats (a periventricular structure) facilitates, and that of β-endorphin depresses, retention of a radial maze task acquired in new spatial environments. This suggests that the medial septum is also a site of action for naloxone and β-endorphin. Whether this holds exclusively for spatial tasks, which depend on the medial septal–hippocampal system (Bostock *et al.*, 1988), or applies to other forms of memory as well, remains to be seen. The doses of β-endorphin that were effective when injected into the septum by Bostock and her colleagues (1988) were higher than those found by Lucion *et al.* (1982) to cause retrograde amnesia for shuttle avoidance behaviour upon i.c.v. administration, also in rats.

Further studies on the effect of localized brain microinjections of opioids and naloxone on memory modulation are clearly desirable. Among sites worth exploring are the locus coeruleus, in which β-endorphin fibres terminate on cell bodies of noradrenergic neurones that project to the amygdala, septum and elsewhere (Izquierdo, 1989), and the hypothalamus/preoptic region, where brain β-endorphin levels were actually found to decrease following training experiences (Izquierdo *et al.*, 1984, 1986).

10.8. *Peripherally mediated opioid regulation of memory?*

Martinez *et al.* (1988) have suggested that there are peripheral opioid mechanisms in memory modulation, probably mediated by Leu-enkephalin actions at δ-receptors, in addition to those mediated by β-endorphin actions at μ-receptors in the brain.

One major argument of Martinez *et al.* (1988) is that the preferential δ-agonists, Leu-enkephalin and D-Ala^2-D-Leu^5-enkephalin, affect learned behaviours when administered peripherally, but not when given into the amygdala (Gallagher *et al.*, 1982) or i.c.v. (Yamamoto *et al.*, 1982), in contrast to Met-enkephalin or β-endorphin, which are effective when given either systemically or i.c.v. (Izquierdo *et al.*, 1980a,b; Lucion *et al.*, 1982). The intra-amygdala injection of D-Ala^2-D-Met^5-enkephalin, unlike that of D-Ala^2-D-Leu^5-enkephalin, hinders memory (Gallagher *et al.*, 1982). The argument in favour of peripheral δ-, and central μ-receptor regulation of memory raised by these findings (Martinez *et al.*, 1988) is, however, somewhat weakened by the facts that: (a) Met- and Leu-enkephalin are equally potent at δ-receptors (Watson and Abbott, 1990); (b) dynorphin A, which is a more powerful μ-agonist than the enkephalins, but an extremely poor δ-receptor agonist (Watson and Abbott, 1990), has no effect on memory in rats when given either i.p. or i.c.v. over a very wide dose range in both active and inhibitory avoidance paradigms (Izquierdo *et al.*, 1985).

Unlike β-endorphin, which reaches the cerebrospinal fluid in significant amounts after peripheral injection (Houghten *et al.*, 1980; Izquierdo *et al.*, 1980b), the enkephalins penetrate much less readily (Rapoport *et al.*, 1980; Zlokovic *et al.*, 1985). It can, therefore, be assumed that their effect on learning and memory processes, when administered systemically, is exerted primarily at peripheral receptors (Martinez *et al.*, 1988). Part of this effect could be due to a reflex-induced release of brain β-endorphin: the i.p. injection of Met- or Leu-enkephalin, like that of the peripherally acting hormones, ACTH and epinephrine, causes a decrease of hypothalamic β-endorphin immunoreactivity (Carrasco *et al.*, 1982c). Part of the effect of systemically administered enkephalins could derive from other — β-endorphin-unrelated — peripherally mediated effects involving δ-opiate receptors. The systemic administration of Leu-enkephalin or of the selective δ-receptor agonist, D-Pen^2-D-Pen^5-enkephalin, impairs acquisition of one-way active avoidance in mice; the selective δ-receptor antagonist, ICI 154129 has an enhancing effect (Schulteis *et al.*, 1987). Naltrexone methyl bromide blocks the memory-impairing effect of peripherally administered post-training Met- or Leu-enkephalin, but not that of morphine or β-endorphin; unlike naltrexone, however, its methyl bromide derivative has no post-training effect of its own, which argues against a physiological influence of endogenously released peripherally acting opioids in post-training memory processes (Introini *et al.*, 1985). Martinez and his group have reported a weak antagonism of a very high dose of methylnaloxonium against the deleterious effect of Leu-enkephalin on acquisition of two different tasks in rats (Martinez *et al.*, 1985; Heinrichs and Martinez, 1986).

There have been suggestions that enkephalins present in the adrenal medulla could be co-secreted with epinephrine (Viveros *et al.*, 1979). It is possible that peripherally released enkephalins may influence learning acquired in circumstances that involve a release of epinephrine from the adrenal medulla, such as aversive tasks in general (Gold and Delanoy, 1981). This possibility, however, was examined by Dias *et al.* (1982), who concluded against it. At very low doses (50 ng per rat, i.p.), the enkephalins cause a severe impairment of two-way active avoidance in rats; if they were released in the periphery in comparable amounts during training they would make learning outright impossible. An endogenous physiological mechanism that modulates, or even hinders, memory is conceivable; one that makes learning inviable is not.

The adrenal medulla plays a role in the post-training effect of exogenously administered opioids on memory. The post-training effect of i.p. (Izquierdo *et al.*, 1982; Zhang *et al.*, 1987) or i.c.v. Met-enkephalin administration (Conte *et al.*, 1986) is abolished by adrenal medullectomy or adrenal denervation, but is reinstated by the concurrent administration of systemic epinephrine. This shows that Met-enkephalin does not act on the adrenal medulla, but needs the concomitant presence of epinephrine (which is secreted during training by the adrenal medulla; Gold and Delanoy, 1981) in order to be effective. Adrenal denervation also attenuates memory facilitation by naloxone (Zhang *et al.*, 1987).

10.9. *Final comment*

Opioids affect, and physiologically regulate, memory. The major physiological regulator is brain β-endorphin, which is released by exposure to novelty. It induces a post-training state-dependency, which is reversible by naloxone or other preferential μ-opiate receptor blockers. Unless β-endorphin is given or again released at the time of testing, amnesia occurs. The effect of β-endorphin is mimetized by the enkephalins and appears to be mediated by periventricular receptors, either in the septum (Bostock *et al.*, 1988) or elsewhere (Izquierdo, 1989); in addition, the amygdala is involved either as a site of action or as a co-participant in this effect. In addition to state-dependency, opioids may also induce some degree of true amnesia: post-training morphine or dynorphin in mice disrupts retention and this effect cannot be reversed by a second pre-test injection of the drugs. Whether this reflects or mimicks effects of endogenous brain opioids other than β-endorphin, is not known. Post-training naloxone or other μ-receptor antagonists block the effect of β-endorphin or other opioids, and produce, in addition, a facilitatory effect which is dependent on, but not mediated by, their antagonism to endogenously released β-endorphin and which appears to involve the disinhibition of β-noradrenergic mechanisms in the amygdala.

There may be, in addition, a parallel, peripheral regulation of memory in the post-training period preferentially involving δ-opiate receptors and using Leu-enkephalin as a mediator. It is not known whether this peripheral system is merely down-regulatory (i.e. amnesic), or involves the development of state-dependency effects as well; nor is it known whether it plays a physiological role at all.

10.10. *Summary*

Opioids affect memory, and endogenous opioid systems physiologically regulate memory. β-Endorphin appears to be the most important of the latter systems. It is released in the brain by all novel training experiences studied so far and induces a form of endogenous state-dependency, by which retrieval of such experiences is best when the animals are again submitted to the action of β-endorphin. The pre-test facilitation that derives from this can be obtained by interpolation of another novel experience, or by administration of another treatment that will release brain β-endorphin, prior to testing. In addition to this effect, β-endorphin and other opioid substances may also induce a degree of retrograde amnesia, at least at high doses. Naloxone and other opioid μ-receptor blockers antagonize these actions of opioids and, in addition, have a memory facilitatory effect on their own. The amygdala, as well as the septum and perhaps other periventricular structures, are possible sites of action for these effects of opioid μ-agonists and antagonists. In addition, there may be a peripherally mediated memory modulatory system involving δ-opioid receptors. The relation between this and the central β-endorphin-mediated mechanisms, is unclear.

Acknowledgements

This work was supported by Fundacao de Amparo a Pesquisa do Estado do Rio Grande do Sul and Conselho Nacional de Pesquisas e Desenvolvimento Tecnologico.

References

Baratti, C., Introini, I.B. and Huygens, P. (1984). Possible interaction between central cholinergic muscarinic and opioid peptidergic systems during memory consolidation in mice. *Behavioural and Neural Biology*, **40**, 155–169.

Belleville, R.E. (1964). Control of behavior by drug-produced internal stumuli. *Psychopharmacologia*, **5**, 95–105.

Bennett, M.C. and Hock, F.J. (1990). Interaction between catecholaminergic and

opioid systems in an active avoidance task. *Behavioural and Neural Biology*, **53**, 258–268.
Bloom, F.E. and McGinty, J. (1981). Cellular distribution and function of the endorphins. In: *Endogenous Peptides and Learning and Memory Processes*, edited by J.L. Martinez, Jr, R.A. Jensen, R.B. Messing, H. Rigter and J.L. McGaugh. New York: Academic Press, pp. 199–230.
Bostock, E., Gallagher, M. and King, R.A. (1988). Effects of opioid microinjections into the medial septal area on spatial memory in rats. *Behavioural Neuroscience*, **102**, 643–652.
Carrasco, M.A., Dias, R.D. and Izquierdo, I. (1982a). Naloxone reverses retrograde amnesia induced by electroconvulsive shock. *Behavioural and Neural Biology*, **34**, 352–357.
Carrasco, M.A., Perry, M.L.S., Dias, R.D., Wofchuck, S.T. and Izquierdo, I. (1982b). Effect of tones, footshocks, shuttle avoidance and electroconvulsive shock on Met-enkephalin immunoreactivity of rat brain. *Behavioural and Neural Biology*, **34**, 1–4.
Carrasco, M.A., Dias, R.D., Perry, M.L.S., Wofchuk, S.T., Souza, D.O. and Izquierdo, I. (1982c). Effect of morphine, ACTH, epinephrine, Met-, Leu-, and Des-Tyr-Met-enkephalin on β-endorphin-like immunoreactivity of rat brain. *Psychoneuroendocrinology*, **7**, 229–234.
Castellano, C. (1975). Effects of morphine and heroin on discrimination learning in mice. *Psychopharmacology*, **42**, 235–242.
Castellano, C. (1981). Strain-dependent effects of naloxone on discrimination learning in mice. *Psychopharmacology*, **73**, 152–156.
Castellano, C. and McGaugh, J.L. (1989). Effect of morphine on one-trial inhibitory avoidance in mice: lack of state-dependency. *Psychobiology*, **17**, 89–92.
Chaves, M.L.F. and Izquierdo, I. (1986). Previous exposure to a novel experience enhances performance in two simple memory tests in humans. *Brazilian Journal of Medical and Biological Research*, **19**, 211–219.
Chaves, M.L.F., Palmini, A.L., Bizzi, J.W.J. and Izquierdo, I. (1988). Naltrexone reverses the memory enhancing effect of novel experiences in memory tests in humans. *Neuropsychologia*, **26**, 491–494.
Conte, C.O., Rosito, G.B.A., Palmini, A.L., Lucion, A.B. and De Almeida, M.A.M.R. (1986). Pre-training adrenaline recovers the amnestic effect of Met-enkephalin in adrenal demedullated rats. *Behavioural Brain Research*, **21**, 163–166.
Cook, L. and Weidley, E. (1957). Behavioral effects of psychopharmacological agents. *Annals of the New York Academy of Sciences*, **66**, 740–752.
Dalmaz, C. and Fin, C. (1989). Gamma-endorphin affects retrieval of an inhibitory avoidance task. *Brazilian Journal of Medical and Biological Research*, **22**, 1121–1126.
Dalmaz, C., Netto, C.A., Volkmer, N., Dias, R.D. and Izquierdo, I. (1986). Distribution of proline endopeptidase in sub-synaptosomal fractions of rat hypothalamus. *Brazilian Journal of Medical and Biological Research*, **19**, 685–690.
De Wied, D., Bohus, B., van Ree, J.M. and Urban, I. (1978). Behavioral and electrophysiological effects of peptides related to lipotropin (β-LPH). *Journal of Pharmacology and Experimental Therapy*, **204**, 570–580.
Dias, R.D., Carrasco, M.A. and Izquierdo, I. (1982). Effect of the pre-training administration of β-endorphin, Met-, Leu-, and Des-Tyr-Met-enkephalin on acquisition and retention of a shuttle avoidance response in rats. *Brazilian Journal of Medical and Biological Research*, **15**, 55–60.
Dias, R.D., Perry, M.L., Carrasco, M.A. and Izquierdo, I. (1981). Effect of electro-

convulsive shock on β-endorphin immunoreactivity of rat brain, pituitary gland, and plasma. *Behavioural and Neural Biology*, **32**, 265–268.

Fulginiti, S. and Cancela, L.M. (1983). Effect of naloxone and amphetamine on acquisition and memory consolidation of active avoidance responses in rats. *Psychopharmacology*, **79**, 45–48.

Gallagher, M. (1982). Naloxone enhancement of memory processes: effects of other opiate antagonists. *Behavioural and Neural Biology*, **35**, 375–382.

Gallagher, M. (1985). Re-viewing modulation of learning and memory. In: *Memory Systems of the Brain*, edited by N.M. Weinberger, J.L. McGaugh and G. Lynch. London: Guilford, pp. 311–334.

Gallagher, M. and Kapp, B.S. (1978). Manipulation of opiate activity in the amygdala alters memory processes. *Life Sciences*, **23**, 1973–1978.

Gallagher, M., Kapp, B.S. and Pascoe, J.P. (1982). Enkephalin analogue effects in the amygdala central nucleus on conditioned heart rate. *Pharmacological and Biochemical Behaviour*, **17**, 217–222.

Gallagher, M., King, R.A. and Young, N.B. (1983). Opiate antagonists improve spatial memory. *Science*, **221**, 975–976.

Gallagher, M., Fanelli, R.J. and Bostock, E. (1985). Opioid peptides: their position among other neuroregulators of memory. In: *Contemporary Phsychology: Biological Processes and Theoretical Issues*, edited by J.L. McGaugh. Amsterdam: Elsevier, pp. 69–93.

Gold, P.E. and Delanoy, R. (1981). ACTH modulation of memory storage processing. In: *Endogenous Peptides and Learning and Memory Processes*, edited by J.L. Martinez, Jr, R.A. Jensen, R.B. Messing, H. Rigter and J.L. McGaugh. New York: Academic Press, pp. 79–98.

Hammonds, R.G., Nicholas, P. and Li, C.H. (1984). β-Endorphin-(1–27) is an antagonist of β-endorphin analgesia. *Proceedings of the National Academy of Sciences USA*, **71**, 1389–1390.

Heinrichs, S. and Martinez, J.L., Jr (1986). Modification of place preference conditioning in mice by systemically administered Leu-enkephalin. *Behavioural Brain Research*, **22**, 249–255.

Houghten, R.A., Swann, R.W. and Li, C.H. (1980). β-Endorphin: stability, clearance behavior, an entry into the central nervous system after injection of the tritiated peptide in rats or rabbits. *Proceedings of the National Academy of Sciences USA*, **77**, 4588–4591.

Introini, I.B. and Baratti, C.M. (1984). The impairment of retention induced by β-endorphin in mice may be mediated by a reduction of central cholinergic activity. *Behavioural and Neural Biology*, **41**, 152–163.

Introini, I.B., McGaugh, J.L. and Baratti, C.M. (1985). Pharmacological evidence of a central effect of naltrexone, morphine and β-endorphin and a peripheral effect of Met- and Leu-enkephalin on retention of an inhibitory avoidance response in mice. *Behavioural and Neural Biology*, **44**, 434–446.

Introini-Collison, I.B. and Baratti, C.M. (1986). Opioid peptidergic systems modulate the activity of β-adrenergic mechanisms during memory consolidation processes. *Behavioural and Neural Biology*, **46**, 227–241.

Introini-Collison, I.B., Nagahara, A. and McGaugh, J.L. (1989). Memory enhancement with intra-amygdala post-training naloxone is blocked by concurrent administration of propranolol. *Brain Research*, **476**, 94–101.

Introini-Collison, I.B., Cahill, L., Baratti, C.M. and McGaugh, J.L. (1987). Dynorphin induces task-specific impairment of memory. *Psychobiology*, **15**, 171–174.

Iquierdo, I. (1979). Effect of naloxone and morphine on various forms of memory in the rat: possible role of endogenous opiate mechanisms in memory consolidation. *Psychopharmacology*, **66**, 199–203.

Izquierdo, I. (1984). Endogenous state dependency: memory depends on the relation between the neurohumoral and hormonal states present after training and at the time of testing. In: *Neurobiology of Learning and Memory*, edited by G. Lynch, J.L. McGaugh and N.M. Weinberger. New York: Guilford, pp. 333–350.

Izquierdo, I. (1989). Different forms of post-training memory processing. *Behavioural and Neural Biology*, **51**, 171–202.

Izquierdo, I. (1990). Acetylcholine release is modulated by different opiate receptor types in different brain regions and species. *Trends in Pharmacological Sciences*, **11**, 179–180.

Izquierdo, I. and Graudenz, M. (1980). Memory facilitation by naloxone is due to release of dopaminergic and beta-adrenergic systems from tonic inhibition. *Psychopharmacology*, **67**, 265–268.

Izquierdo, I. and McGaugh, J.L. (1985). Effect of a novel experience prior to training or testing on retention of an inhibitory avoidance response in mice: involvement of an opioid system. *Behavioural and Neural Biology*, **44**, 228–238.

Izquierdo, I. and McGaugh, J.L. (1987). Effect of novel experiences on retention of inhibitory avoidance behavior in mice: the effect of previous exposure to the same or to another experience. *Behavioural and Neural Biology*, **47**, 109–116.

Izquierdo, I. and Netto, C.A. (1985). The role of β-endorphin in memory regulation. *Annals of the New York Academy of Sciences*, **444**, 162–167.

Izquierdo, I. and Netto, C.A. (1990). Dual action of post-training naloxone on memory. *Behavioural and Neural Biology*, **53**, 140–146.

Izquierdo, I., Paiva, A.C.M. and Elisabetsky, E. (1980a). Post-training intraperitoneal administration of Leu-enkephalin and β-endorphin causes retrograde amnesia for two different tasks in rats. *Behavioural and Neural Biology*, **28**, 246–250.

Izquierdo, I., De Almeida, M.A.M.R. and Emiliano, V.R. (1985). Unlike β-endorphin, dynorphin 1–13 does not cause retrograde amnesia for shuttle avoidance or inhibitory avoidance in rats. *Psychopharmacology*, **87**, 216–218.

Izquierdo, I., Netto, C.A. and Dias, R.D. (1986). Endorphins and memory regulation. In: *Opioid Peptides: Molecular Pharmacology, Biosynthesis and Analysis*, edited by R. Rapaka and S.L. Hawks, *National Institute of Drug Abuse and Research Monographs*, **70**, 237–254. Rockville: US Department of Health and Human Sciences.

Izquierdo, I., Dias, R.D., Perry, M.L., Souza, D.O. Elisabetsky, E. and Carrasco, M.A. (1982). A physiological amnestic mechanism mediated by endogenous opioid peptides, and its possible role in learning. In: *Neuronal Plasticity and Memory Formation*, edited by C. Ajmone Marsan and H. Matthies. New York: Raven Press, pp. 89–111.

Izquierdo, I., Souza, D.O., Dias, R.D., Carrasco, M.A., Volkmer, N., Perry, M.L.S. and Netto, C.A. (1984). Effect of various behavioral training and testing procedures on brain β-endorphin-like immunoreactivity, and the possible role of β-endorphin in behavioral regulation. *Psychoneuroendocrinology*, **9**, 381–389.

Izquierdo, I., Souza, D.O., Carrasco, M.A., Dias, R.D., Perry, M.L., Eisinger, S., Elisabetsky, E. and Vendite, D.A. (1980b). Beta-endorphin causes retrograde amnesia and is released from the rat brain by various forms of training and stimulation. *Psychopharmacology*, **70**, 173–177.

Izquierdo, I., Perry, M.L., Dias, R.D., Souza, D.O., Elisabetsky, E., Carrasco, M.A., Orsingher, O.A. and Netto, C.A. (1981). Endogenous opioids, memory modulation and state dependency. In: *Endogenous peptides and Learning and Memory Processes*, edited by J.L. Martinez, Jr, R.A. Jensen, R.B. Messing, H. Rigter and J.L. McGaugh. New York: Academic Press, pp. 269–290.

Kovacs, G.L., Bohus, B. and De Wied, D. (1983). Effects of β-endorphin and its fragments on inhibitory avoidance behavior in rats. *Psychoneuroendocrinology*, **8**, 411–420.

Lebouille, J.L.M., Burbach, P.H. and De Kloet, E.R. (1985). γ-Endorphin generating endopeptidase in rat brain: subcellular and regional distribution. *Biochemical and Biophysical Research Communications*, **127**, 44–48.

Lucion, A.B., Rosito, G., Sapper, D., Palmini, A. and Izquierdo, I. (1982). Intracerebroventricular administration of nanogram amounts of β-endorphin and Met-enkephalin causes retrograde amnesia in rats. *Behavioral Brain Research*, **4**, 111–115.

McGaugh, J.L. (1988). Modulation of memory storage processes. In: *Perspectives of Memory Research*, edited by P.R. Solomon, G.R. Goethals, C.M. Kelley and B.R. Stephens. New York: Springer, pp. 33–64.

McGaugh, J.L. (1989). Dissociating learning and performance: drug and hormone enhancement of memory storage. *Brain Research Bulletin*, **23**, 339–345.

McGaugh, J.L., Introini-Collison, I.B. and Nagahara, A. (1988). Memory-enhancing effects of post-training naloxone: involvement of β-noradrenergic influences in the amygdaloid complex. *Brain Research*, **446**, 37–49.

McGaugh, J.L., Introini-Collison, I.B., Juler, R.G. and Izquierdo, I. (1987). Stria terminalis lesion attenuates the effects of post-training naloxone and β-endorphin on retention. *Behavioural Neuroscience*, **100**, 839–844.

Martin, S., Aigner, T., Brown, M. and Mishkin, M. (1984). Effect of naloxone on recognition memory in monkeys. *Society of Neuroscience Abstracts*, **10**, 253.

Martinez, J.L., Jr and Rigter, H. (1980). Endorphins alter acquisition and consolidation of an inhibitory avoidance response in rats. *Neuroscience Letters*, **19**, 197–201.

Martinez, J.L., Jr, de Graaf, J., Chavkin, C. and Dana, R.C. (1985). Leu-enkephalin actions on avoidance conditioning are mediated by a peripheral opioid receptor. *Life Sciences*, **37**, 2345–2353.

Martinez, J.L., Jr, Weinberger, S.B. and Schulteis, G. (1988). Enkephalins and learning and memory: a review of the evidence for a site of action outside the blood–brain barrier. *Behavioural and Neural Biology*, **49**, 192–221.

Martinez, J.L., Jr, Rigter, H., Jensen, R.A., Messing, R.B., Vasquez, B.J. and McGaugh, J.L. (1981). Endorphin and enkephalin effects on avoidance conditioning: the other side of the pituitary–adrenal axis. In: *Endogenous Peptides and Learning and Memory Processes*, edited by J.L. Martinez, Jr, R.A. Jensen, R.B. Messing, H. Rigter and J.L. McGaugh. New York: Academic Press, pp. 305–324.

Messing, R.B., Jensen, R.A., Martinez, J.L., Jr, Spiehler, V., Vasquez, B.J., Soumireu-Mourat, B., Liang, K.C. and McGaugh, J.L. (1979). Naloxone enhancement of memory. *Behavioural and Neural Biology*, **27**, 266–275.

Mondadori, C. and Waser, P.G. (1979). Facilitation of memory processing by post-trial morphine: involvement of reinforcement mechanisms? *Psychopharmacology*, **63**, 297–300.

Netto, C.A. and Maltchik, M. (1990). Distinct mechanisms underlying memory modulation after the first and the second session of two avoidance tasks. *Behavioural and Neural Biology*, **53**, 29–38.

Netto, C.A., Dias, R.D. and Izquierdo, I. (1986). Differential effect of post-training naloxone, β-endorphin, Leu-enkephalin and electroconvulsive shock administration upon memory of an open-field habituation and a water-finding task. *Psychoneuroendocrinology*, **11**, 437–446.

Netto, C.A., Oliveira, C.B., Gianlupi, A., Quillfeldt, J. and Izquierdo, I. (1987). Reversal of the amnesia induced by electroconvulsive shock by pre-test adminis-

tration of another electroconvulsive shock, or of β-endorphin. *Peptides*, **8**, 605–608.
Netto, C.A., Oliveira, C.B., Gianlupi, A. and Quillfeldt, J. (1990). Effect of atropine and propranolol on retrieval enhancement by a novel experience or by
Netto, C.A., Cavalheiro, E.A., Carrasco, M.A., Volkmer, N., Dias, R.D. and Izquierdo, I. (1985). Response of the rat brain β-endorphin system to novelty: importance of the fornix connection. *Behavioural and Neural Biology*, **43**, 37–46.
Perry, M.L.S., Netto, C.A. and Izquierdo, I. (1990). Effects of ACTH, epinephrine and Met-enkephalin on brain β-endorphin-like immunoreactivity, and of ACTH, epinephrine, Met-enkephalin and naloxone on retention, in normal and protein-malnourished rats. *Brazilian Journal of Medical and Biological Research*, **23**, 65–72.
Perry, M.L.S., Dias, R.D., Carrasco, M.A. and Izquierdo, I. (1983). Effect of step-down inhibitory avoidance training on β-endorphin-like immunoreactivity of rat hypothalamus and plasma. *Brazilian Journal of Medical and Biological Research*, **16**, 339–343.
Rapoport, S.I., Klee, W.A., Pettigrew, K.D. and Ohno, K. (1980). Entry of opioid peptides into the central nervous system. *Science*, **207**, 84–86.
Rigter, H. (1978). Attenuation of amnesia in rats by systemically administered enkephalins. *Science*, **200**, 83–85.
Rodgers, R.J., Richards, C. and Precious, J.I. (1985). Naloxone administration following brief exposure to novelty reduces activity and rearing in mice upon 24 h-retest: a conditioned aversion. *Psychopharmacology*, **82**, 322–326.
Rossier, J., French, E.D., Rivier, C., Ling, N., Guillemin, R. and Bloom, F. (1977). Footshock induced stress increases β-endorphin levels in blood but not brain. *Nature*, **270**, 618–620.
Schulteis, G., Hruby, V.J. and Martinez, J.L., Jr (1987). Involvement of opioid delta receptors in active avoidance conditioning in mice. *Neuroscience Society Abstracts*, **13**, 845.
Siegfried, B., Netto, C.A. and Izquierdo, I. (1987). Exposure to novelty induces naltrexone-reversible analgesia in rats. *Behavioural Neuroscience*, **101**, 436–438.
Stein, L. and Belluzzi, J.D. (1978). Brain endorphins and the sense of well-being: a psychobiological hypothesis. In: *The Endorphins. Advances in Biochemical Pharmacology*, Vol. 18, edited by E. Costa and M. Trabucchi. New York: Raven Press, pp. 299–311.
Viveros, O.H., Diliberto, E.D., Jr, Hazum, E. and Chang, K.D. (1979). Opiate-like materials in the adrenal medulla: evidence for storage and secretion with catecholamines. *Molecular Pharmacology*, **16**, 1101–1108.
Watson, S. and Abbott, A. (1990). Receptor nomenclature supplement. *Trends in Pharmacological Science*, **10**, (Suppl.), 30 pp.
Yamamoto, M., Kawamuki, H., Satoh, M. and Takagi, H. (1982). Kyotorphin (L-Tyr-Arg) inhibits extinction of pole jumping avoidance response in the rat. *Neuroscience Letters*, **31**, 175–179.
Zhang, S.-Y., NcGaugh, J.L., Juler, R.G. and Introini-Collison, I.B. (1987). Naloxone ant [Met^5]-enkephalin effects on retention: attenuation by adrenal denervation. *European Journal of Pharmacology*, **138**, 37–44.
Zlokovic, B.V., Begley, D.J. and Chain-Eliash, D.G. (1985). Blood–brain barrier permeability to leucine-enkephalin, D-alanine^2-D-leucine^5-enkephalin and their *N*-terminal amino acid (tyrosine) *Brain Research*, **336**, 125–132.

Chapter 11

Opioid-induced respiratory depression in the management of acute pain: clinical aspects

Alan N. Sandler

11.1. *Introduction*

Respiratory depression has been known for centuries to be associated with opioid administration (Hickey and Severinghaus, 1981). From a pathophysiological point of view, respiration is depressed if the subject fails to respond adequately, on a moment-to-moment basis, to hypercapnia or hypoxia (Nunn, 1987). The detection and measurement of drug-induced respiratory depression is reviewed by Jordan (1982) and methods currently available are summarized in Table 11.1. Of the available methods, indirect measurement of ventilation and blood gas tensions, in combination, come closest to meeting the criteria required in the clinical setting.

11.2. *Investigation of respiratory depression in opioid-treated acute pain*

When opioids are used (especially postoperatively) with spontaneously breathing patients, respiratory depression has been assessed either by:

(1) carbon-dioxide ventilation response measurements using rebreathing techniques, or
(2) non-invasive monitoring of respiration, haemoglobin saturation and/or arterial blood gases.

The measurement of the carbon-dioxide ventilation response has provided important and useful data with regard to respiratory depression produced by opioids (Borison, 1977a).

Borison (1977b) emphasizes that studies using carbon dioxide forcing and/or making carbon dioxide measurements plus examining ventilation in terms of component changes in rate and depth, provide the most useful physiological information. He lists studies with various opioids in which

Table 11.1. Methods of detection and measurement of respiratory depression.

Measurement of resting breathing
Ventilation
Direct
(a) Spirometry
(b) Pneumotachograph
Indirect
(a) Canopy
(b) Strain gauge
(c) Respiratory inductive plethysmography (RIP)
Blood-gas tensions
Direct
(a) Arterial blood gases
Indirect
(a) Transcutaneous Po_2 or Pco_2
(b) End-tidal CO_2
(c) Oximetry
Tests of chemosensitivity
Response to hypercapnea
CO_2 response curve
Mouth occlusion pressure
Response to hypoxia
Measurement of response to added mechanical load

Adapted from Jordan, 1982.

respiratory depression was present mostly in pain-free situations (Borison, 1977b). From these studies it is generally agreed that a single excessive intravenous dose of an opioid causes, along with sedation, a depression in respiratory rate with little change in tidal volume. This may not be true for all conditions under which opioids are administered as ongoing research indicates little or no change in respiratory rate, but significant decreases in tidal volume (Etches *et al.*, 1989). In addition, it is important to note that while an altered carbon dioxide response may indicate depression of central respiratory control (Borison, 1977b), this may have little practical use in defining clinically significant respiratory depression in acute pain situations. For example, epidural fentanyl (a synthetic opioid) is administered by pulse injection or infusion to provide analgesia in postoperative patients with virtually no reports of severe postoperative respiratory complications (Etches *et al.*, 1989), and yet the carbon dioxide response has been shown to be depressed when equivalent doses of fentanyl are given by the epidural route (Renaud *et al.*, 1985).

Because of the interaction of sleep and respiration (Phillipson and Bowes, 1986), especially in older patients with systemic disease, Catley (1984) has recommended continuous assessment of the sleep stage. This may be difficult to achieve logistically, but these measurements are important in acute pain patients who may spend much of their time somnolent if good pain relief is achieved. However, standard sleep stage patterns may be altered by opioids (Moote *et al.*, 1989). In addition, the administration of opioids is synergistic with sleep in depressing the carbon dioxide-ventilation response (Forrest and Bellville, 1964).

11.3. *Clinical studies: respiratory depression and mode of administration*

Dissatisfaction with administration of opioids by conventional routes (primarily intramuscular bolus injection) for acute pain relief has led to the development of alternative highly effective techniques for opioid administration. These include continuous low-dose intravenous infusions of opioids (Catling *et al.*, 1980; Catley *et al.*, 1985; Owen *et al.*, 1987), patient-controlled analgesia (PCA) (Ferrante *et al.*, 1990), spinal opioid analgesia (Cousins *et al.*, 1988), and transdermal opioid administration (Caplan *et al.*, 1988; Duthie *et al.*, 1988; Gourley *et al.*, 1989).

11.3.1. **Intramuscular opioids**

Although intramuscular opioids have been the mainstay of acute pain relief for decades, there are few studies assessing the respiratory depressant effects in acute pain conditions. This results from the belief that it was not useful to measure respiratory depression related to opioids while a patient was in pain: almost all studies were performed in volunteers or patients not experiencing pain (Eckenhoff and Oech, 1960; Lasagna, 1964; Borison, 1977b; Hickey and Severinghaus, 1981).

We have recently performed a double-blind, randomized study comparing intramuscular morphine to epidural morphine in post-caesarean section patients in which the opioid was titrated to patient demand, analgesia was measured sequentially and respiration and haemoglobin saturation monitored continuously non-invasively for 24 h. In addition the non-invasive monitoring was repeated 3–4 days later overnight when the patients no longer required opioids for analgesia (Daley *et al.*, 1990). Although the epidural morphine group had significantly better analgesia than the intramuscular group there were no significant differences between the two groups in the incidence of apnoea, slow respiratory rate or haemoglobin desaturation. Haemoglobin saturation was neither significantly decreased during the opioid administration, nor significantly different from the later control measurements (Daley *et al.*, 1990).

11.3.2. **Intravenous opioids**

Intravenous opioid administration is the primary choice during anaesthesia, and thus many studies document postoperative opioid-induced respiratory depression. Owen *et al.* (1987) compared continuous infusions of morphine ($2\,mg\,h^{-1}$) and ketamine and found respiratory depression (respiratory rate less than 8 per min) only in the morphine group. Becker *et al.* (1976) demonstrated respiratory depression using carbon dioxide response measurements after fentanyl was used to supplement nitrous oxide anaesthesia. A biphasic recovery pattern of respiratory depression was seen in the postoperative period. Similar prolonged depression of ventilation using carbon dioxide response in the postoperative period when fentanyl is given by pulse injection intraoperatively has been demonstrated by others. Not surprisingly, respiratory depression has been noted 2–6 h postoperatively after high-dose fentanyl administration commonly used in anaesthesia for cardiopulmonary bypass procedures (Caspi *et al.*, 1988).

Although these studies illustrate opioid-induced respiratory depression postoperatively, they were not designed to measure postoperative ventilatory depression as a complication of postoperative analgesia. In particular, the measurement of pain is conspicuously absent in most of these studies, and thus dose response in terms of analgesia is unknown. Further criticism can be made of studies that have measured the respiratory depressant effects of continuous fentanyl or alfentanil infusions (Andrews *et al.*, 1983; O'Connor *et al.*, 1983) in which the opioid was utilized throughout the surgical procedure to provide analgesia. Although two of these studies (Andrews *et al.*, 1983; O'Connor *et al.*, 1983) measured postoperative pain and demonstrated a depressed carbon dioxide response, the fentanyl or alfentanil infusions were continued for only 1–2 h postoperatively. Other case reports have documented life threatening respiratory depression in the postoperative period after intraoperative alfentanil infusion.

Patients undergoing cholecystectomy were randomly given either intramuscular (i.m.) papaveretum or a continuous infusion of papaveretum in the postoperative period. Visual analogue pain scores (VAS) were measured daily for three days and arterial blood gases were measured 1·5 and 2·5 h after analgesia was achieved. The intravenous (i.v.) group had significantly less pain at 24 and 48 h than the i.m. group (Jordan *et al.*, 1979; Catling *et al.*, 1980). This study clearly demonstrated that the i.v. infusion group (four of seven subjects) developed apnoeic episodes (AP) and slow respiratory rates whereas the i.m. group was virtually free of these abnormal respiratory patterns (one of seven subjects). The i.v. group also demonstrated significantly greater $Paco_2$ and decreased Pao_2 after analgesia than the i.m. group. Whether the i.m. group would have developed similar abnormalities of respiratory pattern if further papaveretum had been given to improve analgesia is unknown.

In a more intensive study, Catley *et al.* (1985) have used non-invasive continuous monitoring to compare two different postoperative analgesic regimens in matched groups of patients undergoing either cholecystectomy or total hip replacement. One group received a continuous i.v. infusion of morphine whereas the other group received regional anaesthesia. While all patients received premedication (papaveretum and atrophine), no opioids were given intraoperatively. There were no differences in pain scores between the two groups, although no patient reported complete pain relief. Against this background of adequate, but not total, pain relief, 10 of 16 patients receiving the morphine infusion demonstrated a total of 456 episodes of pronounced desaturation (Sa_{O_2} < 80%) while breathing room air, analgesia and who developed numerous apnoeas and desaturations postoper-pronounced desaturation. In addition, respiratory pattern (RIP) monitoring demonstrated that ventilatory disturbances (central apnoea, obstructive apnoea, paradoxic breathing, slow respiratory rate, small tidal volume) were all more common in the patients receiving the morphine infusion. The incidence of respiratory disturbances increased with age especially in patients 66–75 years old. Pronounced oxygen desaturation and obstructive apnoeas only occurred when patients were asleep and most episodes of oxygen desaturation were associated with obstructive apnoea or paradoxic breathing. Central apnoea and slow respiratory rate were rarely associated with pronounced oxygen desaturation. Two patients receiving morphine analgesia and who developed numerous apnoeas and desaturations postoperatively were restudied on the 13th postoperative night while taking no opioid analgesics. No desaturations and very few apnoeas were seen. Jones *et al.* (1985) showed that administration of supplemental oxygen abolishes the pronounced episodes of desaturation with little change in the incidence of respiratory abnormalities. Measurements of carbon dioxide (PEt_{CO_2}, Pa_{CO_2}) were not made in either of these studies (Catley *et al.*, 1985; Jones *et al.*, 1985). Recently, Panos *et al.* (1990) and Stringer *et al.* (1990) compared in a double-blind, randomized design, the effects of bolus plus infusions of fentanyl given either by the i.v. or lumbar epidural route for the relief of post-thoracotomy pain. Continuous RIP, arterial blood gases (ABG), VAS and serum fentanyl concentration were measured for both groups for 24 h postoperatively. Control measurements of RIP and ABG were made during sleep the night prior to surgery. Both methods of fentanyl administration produced excellent and equivalent pain relief. Arterial P_{CO_2} was significantly elevated in both groups although this increase was not clinically significant. Arterial P_{O_2} was normal due to supplemental oxygen administration which is standard for this type of surgery. Respiratory pattern was abnormal in both groups with increased numbers of apnoeic episodes and slow respiratory rates. The postoperative RIP data were not significantly different to the preoperative data although large stochastic differences were present. This was related to the small sample size and the occurrence of a large number of episodes in a small number of patients. The data gathered from the i.v. infusion of fentanyl is in contrast to a similar study performed by our group comparing bolus dose i.v. morphine to bolus dose epidural morphine (Sandler *et al.*, 1986) in which there were virtually no respiratory pattern abnormalities in the i.v. group when equivalent high-quality analgesia was obtained.

11.3.3. **Patient-controlled analgesia**

Patient-controlled analgesia (PCA) with opioids has proved very effective in acute pain control. To date there are no studies assessing the effects of the PCA route on respiration using carbon dioxide response and only one study (Frater *et al*, 1989) used continuous non-invasive monitoring in post-operative patients in whom PCA was used for analgesia. These investigations need to be performed as opioid dosage can be very high under PCA conditions (Lehmann, 1990). Gillies *et al.* (1987) found significant increases in $Paco_2$ in post-abdominal surgery patients 24th after surgery which used PCA morphine compared to a comparison group given i.m. ketorolac (a non-steroidal, non-opioid analgesic) plus PCA morphine. Two other studies have documented decreased respiratory rates with PCA-administered buprenorphine (Gibbs *et al.*, 1982) or increases $Paco_2$ with PCA morphine, meperidine (pethidine) or ketobemidone (Tamsen *et al.*, 1982). In a study involving patients undergoing upper abdominal operations more PCA-treated patients had elevated capillary carbon dioxide levels (45·0–54·7 mmHg) than patients receiving i.m. or epidural narcotics (Rosenberg *et al.*, 1984). Respiratory depression requiring treatment with naloxone has been reported in a patient using PCA morphine to control post-cholecystectomy pain and who also had end-stage renal disease (Covington *et al.*, 1989). The respiratory depression was attributed to accumulation of morphine-6-glucuronide due to end-stage renal disease.

Frater *et al.* (1989) have compared meptazinol and morphine administered by PCA after hip replacement. Episodic hypoxaemia was seen in both groups associated with disturbances in ventilatory pattern (apnoeic episodes). There were no differences in hypoxic events or altered respiratory pattern between the two groups although pain scores were higher in the meptazinol group 8 h (but not later) after surgery. However, preoperative RIP monitoring was not undertaken in this study.

11.3.4. **Spinal analgesia**

The problem of respiratory depression and spinal opioids has been reviewed in depth by Etches *et al.* (1989).

a. *Morphine: Intrathecal*

There are numerous reports of severe respiratory depression after intrathecal morphine (Etches *et al.*, 1989). However, only one study has assessed chemosensitivity following intrathecal morphine in postoperative patients (Zhu *et al.*, 1987). Post-caesarean section patients were given either epidural morphine (5 mg), subarachnoid morphine (0·1–0·25 mg) or subcutaneous morphine (8 mg). Surprisingly, the carbon dioxide response over 24 h was not significantly altered in the intrathecal group, whereas it was significantly depressed in the epidural group.

b. *Morphine: Epidural*

There is general agreement that epidural morphine causes early respiratory depression (1–6 h post-dose) comparable to or greater than a similar parenteral dose (for example see Rawal and Wattwil, 1984). This is manifested as an increase in $P\text{Etco}_2$, a decrease in the slope of the carbon dioxide response curve, a decrease in the airway occlusion pressure response, or a decrease in minute ventilation in response to a $P\text{aco}_2$ of 55 mmHg.

There are few studies which consider the effects of epidural morphine on ventilatory control during the later phase of analgesia. Rawal and Wattwil (1984) found significant respiratory depression at 5 and 10 h postinjection which did not persist beyond this time. In particular, postoperative cholecystectomy patients given epidural morphine had respiratory rates greater than control despite the presence of significant respiratory depression. These studies demonstrate the inadequacy of monitoring respiratory rate as the sole indicator of respiratory depression.

Scheinin and Rosenberg (1982) compared epidural morphine (2 or 4 mg) to either epidural bupivicaine or parenteral narcotics following upper abdominal surgery. In this unblinded study, no clinically apparent respiratory depression was detected, but the $P\text{aco}_2$ measured at 4 h following anaesthesia was found to be significantly elevated in one to three out of ten patients in each group. Neither respiratory rate nor blood gases were monitored beyond 4 h. Asantila *et al.* (1986) compared thoracic epidural morphine (4–6 mg) with intercostal block or epidural bupivicaine in 51 patients undergoing thoracotomy. Fentanyl was given throughout the anaesthetic at a rate of $100\,\mu\text{g}\,\text{h}^{-1}$ and oxycodone was given postoperatively on a *pro re nata* (p.r.n.) basis. Blood gases and respiratory rate were measured at 1, 3 and 24 h postoperatively. However, differences between groups were minor. In contrast El-Baz *et al.* (1984) found severe respiratory depression (defined as loss of consciousness and a $P\text{aco}_2$ of greater than 60 mmHg) in eight of 30 post-thoracotomy patients given 5 mg doses of thoracic epidural morphine. Repeat doses were given as required (mean = 4 doses per 24 h). No other narcotics were administered. One of these eight patients suffered acute respiratory failure after a single dose. Allen *et al.* (1986) studied 70 patients given either 0, 2, 5 or 10 mg of epidural morphine for postoperative analgesia. These investigators found no differences in respiratory rate, but with a single blood gas done at 10 h postoperatively, they did find a higher $P\text{aco}_2$ in the patients given 10 mg. Four of 17 patients in this latter group had an elevated $P\text{aco}_2$ (50–54 mmHg). Parenteral narcotics were given on a p.r.n. basis during the study period. Lanz *et al.* (1985) gave 0, 1, 2, 3, 4 or 5 mg of epidural morphine for postoperative analgesia and monitored respiratory rate hourly for 24 h and in 27 of 139 patients measured blood gases at frequent intervals for the first 12 h postoperatively. No differences in respiratory rate were detected, but the $Pa\text{CO}_2$ was elevated by approximately 5 mmHg in the 5-mg group compared to the controls from 2·5 to 12 h postoperatively.

The studies cited above illustrate some of the problems which make any conclusions concerning the true incidence of significant respiratory depression after spinal opioids difficult. Patients are generally monitored intermittently rather than continuously. Pain scores may vary between groups given the same or different opioids by different routes (Catling *et al.*, 1980). In addition, the concomitant use of opioids administered by i.m. or i.v. routes when spinal opioids are being studied adds a major confounding variable to the aetiology of the respiratory depression.

The use of epidural morphine to provide analgesia following caesarean section deserves particular mention. Depressed carbon dioxide responsiveness may be present for up to 24 h following the administration of 5 mg of epidural morphine to post-caesarean section patients (Abboud *et al.*, 1987). However, the incidence of significant respiratory depression appears very low.

McMorland and Douglas (1986) claim that only two of 3000 post-caesarean section patients have developed a slow respiratory rate following epidural morphine, and in neither of these patients was there any suggestion of hypoxia or hypoventilation. In each case cited above, respiratory rate and/or somnolence was monitored intermittently, and periods of apnoea, hypoventilation or desaturation may have occurred.

Daley *et al.* (1990) have compared i.m. to epidural morphine in post-caesarian section patients using non-invasive techniques postoperatively. Although the epidural morphine group had significantly better analgesia than the i.m. group, there were no significant differences between the two groups in the incidence of apnoea, slow respiratory rate or haemoglobin desaturation.

Sandler *et al.* (1986) studied respiratory depression in 13 post-thoracotomy patients receiving either repeated doses of epidural or i.v. morphine for postoperative analgesia. In this randomized, double-blind clinical trial, patients were monitored continuously by a trained observer and RIP noted for 24 h after surgery. Patients also had ABG drawn from an indwelling arterial catheter at 2, 6, 12 and 24 h. Pain scores performed at the same time intervals were similar in both groups. The $Pa\text{CO}_2$ in the epidural group was elevated 2–12 h postoperatively, whereas it was elevated only at 2 h in the i.v. group. The respiratory rates were consistently lower in the epidural group. RIP monitoring revealed major differences between the groups. In the i.v. group, only one of five patients had an episode of slow respiratory rate (< 10 per min), and none had apnoeic episodes (15 s or longer). In the epidural group, however, five of eight patients had repeated episodes of slow respiratory rate and six of eight had numerous apnoeic episodes. All patients who demonstrated apnoea or hypoventilation had received at least 10 mg of epidural morphine per 24 h. Pulse oximetry was not used in this study and patients received supplemental oxygen throughout. Whether transient episodes of hypoxaemia occurred is unknown.

Epidural buprenorphine, a lipophilic, μ-receptor partial agonist, is associated with early and persistent respiratory depression in both patients (Gundersen *et al.*, 1986) and volunteers (Ravnborg *et al.*, 1987). Buprenorphine dissociates very slowly from μ-receptors; as a result, naloxone, even in large doses, may be ineffective in reversing respiratory depression once it develops. Abboud *et al.* (1987) measured the carbon dioxide response in post-caesarean section patients who received either epidural morphine or butorphanol. Carbon dioxide responsiveness was depressed for at least 12–16 h following 2–4 mg of butorphanol. Morphine had a greater depressant effect, but also provided more complete analgesia.

In addition to morphine itself there is a wealth of studies reporting changes of respiratory parameters following the administration of the highly potent opioids fentanyl, sufentanil, alfentanil and meperidine (pethidine), but space restrictions preclude considering these in detail.

Fentanyl in particular has the advantage of few cardiovascular- and sedation-related side-effects and these features, coupled with its lipid solubility allowing percutaneous absorption, make it an attractive candidate for a transdermal therapeutic system. In most cases the transdermal patches were applied 2 h prior to surgery. A lag time of 12–18 h was sometimes present before adequate analgesia was provided by the fentanyl patch alone. This was reflected in the increased requirement for supplemental opioids (morphine or pethidine). In those studies in which a large loading dose of fentanyl was given intraoperatively, this lag time was decreased (Holley and Van Stennis, 1988). In general, for major surgery (e.g. upper abdominal, thoracic or back surgery) a transdermal delivery rate of 75–100 $\mu g\ h^{-1}$ was required to provide adequate pain relief whereas in less traumatic surgery (e.g. lower abdominal, orthopaedic surgery) a lower transdermal delivery rate of 50–75 $\mu g\ h^{-1}$ was sufficient.

Respiratory depression after the use of fentanyl patches was present in a small number of patients in several studies (Duthie *et al.*, 1988; Gourlay *et al.*, 1989). Respiratory depression was based on the presence of bradynoea (< 10 breaths per min) and in some cases elevated $Pa\text{CO}_2$. In all the studies data were collected intermittently. In addition most of the patients had been given supplementary systemic opioids for inadequate analgesia. Although this produces a confounding variable when studying the respiratory effects of opiods administered by different routes (i.e. intravenously, epidurally) (Sandler, 1989) the administration of supplementary opioids may be unavoidable with patches when analgesia is inadequate.

11.4. *Conclusion*

Major advances in therapeutic regimens have been related to the introduction of new and effective techniques of administering established and newly developed opioids in acute pain states. The most severe side-effect of opioid administration, respiratory depression, has become a subject of intense investigation as the therapeutic advances have been introduced. The most striking recent development is the drive to document respiratory depressive changes in patients suffering from acute pain when satisfactory analgesia is achieved. In addition, the use of non-invasive continuous monitoring techniques has provided new information as to the respiratory effects and the safety of new methods of opioid administration.

References

Abboud, T.K., Moore, M. and Zhu, J. (1987). Epidural butorphanol or morphine for the relief of post-caesarean section pain: ventilatory response to carbon dioxide. *Anesthesia and Analgesia*, **66**, 887–893.

Allen, P.D., Walman, T. and Concepcion, M. (1986). Epidural morphine provides postoperative pain relief in peripheral vascular and orthopedic surgical patients: a dose response study. *Anesthesia and Analgesia*, **65**, 165–170.

Andrews C.H.J., Sinclair, M., Prys-Roberts, C. and Dye, A. (1983). Ventilatory effects during and after continuous infusion of fentanyl or alfentanil. *British Journal of Anaesthesia*, **55**, 211S–216S.

Asantila, R., Rosenberg, P.H. and Scheinin, B. (1986). Comparison of different methods of postoperative pain analgesia after thoracotomy. *Acta Anaesthesiologica Scandinavica*, **30**, 421–425.

Becker, L.D., Paulson, B.A. and Miller, R.D. (1976). Biphasic respiratory depression after fentanyl-droperidol or fentanyl alone used to supplement nitrous oxide anaesthesia. *Anesthesiology*, **44**, 291–296.

Borison, H.L. (1977a). Central nervous system respiratory depressants — control systems approach to respiratory depression. *Pharmacology and Therapeutics, Part B: General and Systematic Pharmacology*, **3**(2), 211–226.

Borison, H.L. (1977b). Central nervous system respiratory depressants — narcotic analgesics. *Pharmacology and Therapeutics, Part B: General and Systematic Pharmacology*, **3**, 227–237.

Caplan, R.A., Ready, L.B., Oden, R.V., Matsen, F.A., Nessly, M.L. and Olsson, G.L. (1988). Transdermal fentanyl for postoperative pain management. A double blind placebo study. *Journal of the American Medical Association*, **261**, 1036–1039.

Caspi, J., Klausner, J.M., Safadi, T., Amar, R., Rozin, R.R. and Merin, G. (1988). Delayed respiratory depression following fentanyl anesthesia for cardiac surgery. *Critical Care Medicine*, **16**, 238–240.

Catley, D.M. (1984). Postoperative analgesia and respiratory control. *International Anesthesiology Clinics*, **22**, 95–111.

Catley, D.M., Thornton, C., Jordan, C., Lehane, J.R., Royston, D. and Jones, J.G. (1985). Pronounced episodic oxygen desaturation in the postoperative period: its association with ventilatory pattern and analgesic regimen. *Anesthesiology*, **63**, 20–28.

Catling, J.A., Pinto, D.M. and Jordan, C. (1980). Respiratory effects of analgesia after cholecystectomy: comparison of continuous and intermittent papaveretum. *British Medical Journal*, **281**, 478–480.

Cousins, M.J., Cherry, D.A. and Gourlay, G.K. (1988). Acute and chronic pain: use of spinal opioids. In: *Neural Blockade. Clinical Anaesthesia and Management of Pain*, 2nd edn, edited by M.J. Cousins *et al.* Philadelphia: J.B. Lippincott, pp. 955–1029.

Covington, E.C., Ebrahim, L.G., Currie, K.O., Shepard, K.V. and Pippenger, C.E. (1989). Severe respiratory depression from patient-controlled analgesia in renal failure. *Psychosomatics*, **30**, 226–228.

Daley, M.D., Sandler, A.N., Turner, K.E., Vosu, H. and Slavchemko, P. (1990). A comparison of epidural and intramuscular morphine in patients following caesarean section. *Anesthesiology*, **72**, 289–294.

Duthie, D.J.R., Rowbotham, D.J., Wyld, R., Henderson, P.D. and Nimmo, W.S. (1988). Plasma fentanyl concentrations during transdermal delivery of fentanyl to surgical patients. *British Journal of Anaesthesia*, **60**, 614–618.

Eckenhoff, J.E. and Oech, S.R. (1960). The effects of narcotics and antagonists upon respiration and circulation in man. *Clinical Pharmacology*, **1**, 483–524.

El-Baz, N.M.I., Faber, P. and Jensik, R.J. (1984). Continuous epidural infusion of morphine for treatment of pain after thoracic surgery: a new technique. *Anesthesia and Analgesia*, **63**, 757–764.

Etches, R., Sandler, A.N. and Daley, D. (1989). Respiratory depression and spinal opioids. *Canadian Journal of Anaesthesia*, **36**, 165–185.

Ferrante, M.F., Ostheimer, G.W. and Covino, B.G. (Eds) (1990). *Patient Controlled Analgesia.* Cambridge MA: Blackwell.

Forrest, W.H. and Bellville, J.W. (1964). The effect of sleep plus morphine on the respiratory response to carbon dioxide. *Anesthesiology*, **25**, 137–141.

Frater, R.A.S., Moores, M.A., Parry, P. and Hanning, C.D. (1989). Analgesia-induced respiratory depression: comparison of meptazinol and morphine in the postoperative period. *British Journal of Anaesthesia*, **63**, 260–265.

Gibbs, J.M., Johnson, H.D. and Davis, F.M. (1982). Patient administration of i.v. buprenorphine for postoperative pain relief using the 'cardiff' demand analgesia apparatus. *British Journal of Anaesthesia*, **54**, 279–284.

Gillies, G.W.A., Kenny, G.N.C., Bullingham, R.E.S. and McCardle, C.S. (1987). The morphine sparing effect of ketorolac tromethamine. A study of a new, parenteral non-steroidal anti-inflammatory agent after abdominal surgery. *Anaesthesia*, **42**, 727–731.

Gourlay, G.K., Kowalski, S.R., Plummer, J.L., Cherry, D.A., Gaukroger, P. and Cousins, M.J. (1989). The transdermal administration of fentanyl in the treatment of postoperative pain: pharmacokinetics and pharmacodynamic effects. *Pain*, **37**, 193–202.

Gundersen, R.Y., Andersen, R. and Narverud, G. (1986). Postoperative pain relief with high dose epidural buprenorphine: a double blind study. *Acta Anaesthesiologica Scandinavica*, **30**, 664–667.

Hickey, R.F. and Severinghaus, J.W. (1981). Regulation of breathing: drug effects. In: *Lung Biology in Health and Disease: Regulation of Breathing*, Vol. 17, edited by T.F. Hornbein. New York: Decker, pp. 1251.

Holley, F.O. and van Stennis, I. (1988). Postoperative analgesia with fentanyl: pharmacokinetics and pharmacodynamics of constant rate i.v. and transdermal delivery. *British Journal of Anaesthesia*, **60**, 608–613.

Jones, J.G., Jordan, C. and Scudder, C. (1985). Episodic oxygen desaturation: the value of added oxygen. *Journal of the Royal Society of Medicine*, **78**, 1019–1022.

Jordan, C. (1982) Assessment of the effects of drugs on respiration. *British Journal of Anaesthesia*, **54**, 763–782.

Jordan, C., Jones, J.G. and Pinto, D.J. (1979). Postoperative respiratory monitoring. In: *Proceedings of the Third International Symposion of Ambulatory Monitoring*. London: Academic Press, pp. 373–379.

Lanz, E., Kehrberger, E. and Theiss, D. (1985). Epidural morphine: a clinical double blind study of dosage. *Anesthesia and Analgesia*, **64**, 786–791.

Lasagna, L. (1964). The clinical evaluation of morphine and its substitutes as analgesics. *Pharmacological Review*, **16**, 47–83.

Lehmann, K.A. (1990). Patient controlled analgesia for postoperative pain. *Advances in Pain Research and Therapeutics,* **14**, 297–324.

McMorland, G.H. and Douglas, J.D. (1986). Epidural morphine for postoperative analgesia. *Canadian Anaesthetists Society Journal*, **33**, 115–116.

Moote, C.A., Knill, R.L., Skinner, M.I. and Rose, E.A. (1989). Morphine disrupts nocturnal sleep in a dose dependent fashion. *Anesthesia and Analgesia*, **68**, S200.

Nunn, J.F. (1987). *Applied Respiratory Physiology*. 3rd edn. Cambridge: Butterworths.

O'Connor, M., Escarpa, A. and Prys-Roberts, C. (1983). Ventilatory depression during and after infusion of alfentanil in man. *British Journal of Anaesthesia*, **55**, 217S–222S.

Owen, H., Reekie, R.M., Clements, J.A., Watson, R. and Nimmo, W.S. (1987). Analgesia from morphine and ketamine. A comparison of infusions of morphine and ketamine for postoperative analgesia. *Anaesthesia*, **42**, 1051–1056.

Panos, L., Sandler, A.N., Stringer, D.G., Badner, N., Lawson, S. and Koren, G. (1990). Continuous infusions of lumbar epidural fentanyl and intravenous fentanyl for post-thoracotomy pain relief. I. Analgesic and pharmacokinetic effects. *Canadian Journal of Anaesthesia*, **37**, S66.

Phillipson, E.A. and Bowes, G. (1986). Control of breathing during sleep. In: *Handbook of Physiology*, Sect. 3, Vol. II, Part 2, edited by N.S. Cherniak and J.G. Widdicombe. Bethesda: American Physiological Society, pp. 649–689.

Ravnborg, M., Jensen, F.M., Jensen, N.H. and Holk, I.K. (1987). Pupillary diameter and ventilatory CO_2 sensitivity after epidural morphine and buprenorphine in volunteers. *Anesthesia and Analgesia*, **66**, 847–851.

Rawal, N. and Wattwil, M. (1984). Respiratory depression after epidural morphine — an experimental and clinical study. *Anesthesia and Analgesia*, **63**, 8–14.

Renaud, B., Brichant, J.F. and Clergue, F. (1985). Continuous epidural fentanyl: ventilatory effects and plasma kinetics. *Anaesthesiology*, **63**, A234.

Rosenberg, P.H., Heino, A. and Scheinin, B. (1984). Comparison of intramuscular analgesia, intercostal block, epidural morphine and on-demand i.v. fentanyl in the control of pain after upper abdominal surgery. *Acta Anaesthesiologica Scandinavica*, **28**, 603–607.

Sandler, A.N. (1989). Opioid induced respiratory depression in the postoperative period. *Anesthesiology Clinics of North America*, **7**, 193–210.

Sandler, A.N., Chovaz, P. and Whiting, W. (1986). Respiratory depression following epidural morphine: a clinical study. *Canadian Anaesthetists Society Journal*, **33**, 542–549.

Scheinin, B. and Rosenberg, P.H. (1982). Effect of prophylactic epidural morphine or bupivacaine on postoperative pain after abdominal surgery. *Acta Anaesthesiologica Scandinavica*, **26**, 474–478.

Stringer, D.G., Sandler, A.N., Panos, A.N., Lawson, S., Einarson, T.R. and Badner, N. (1990). Continuous infusions of lumbar epidural fentanyl and i.v. fentanyl for post-thoracotomy pain relief. II. Respiratory effects. *Canadian Journal of Anaesthesia*, **37**, S16.

Tamsen, A., Hartvig, P., Fagerlund, C., Dahlstrom, B. and Bondesson, U. (1982). Patient controlled analgesic therapy: clinical experience. *Acta Anaesthesiologica Scandinavica*, **74** (Suppl.), 157–160.

Zhu, J., Abboud, T.K. and Mantilla, M. (1987). Epidural, intrathecal or subcutaneous morphine for the relief of post-caesarean pain: ventilatory responses to CO_2. *Proceedings of the Annual Meeting of the Society for Obstetric Anesthesia and Perinatology*, p. 44.

Part IV

Autonomic transmission

Chapter 12

Neural regulation of vascular tone

John A. Bevan

12.1. *Introduction*

The heart continues to beat and the blood vessels still retain tone when the influence of the efferent innervation is abolished. In fact, in a mammal at rest, administration of a ganglionic blocking agent which interrupts the tonic motor activity of the autonomic nervous system has little effect on the blood pressure. If the kidneys are functional, there is 'whole body' autoregulation of the circulation. The body is able to maintain some degree of vascular integrity after its separation from the nervous system. Thus the immediate function of the innervation is not to initiate an adequate heart rate or blood pressure, but to modify an already functional circulation. It becomes active as part of the animal's adaptation to stress, or its implementation of changes essential for the normal function. This is not generally recognized. In the introduction to a recent article (Kawasaki *et al.*, 1988) the statement is made that 'The tone of peripheral blood vessels is primarily maintained by sympathetic vasoconstrictor nerves'.

The autonomic nervous system influences the circulation through its two divisions, the sympathetic and parasympathetic. The sympathetic system usually acts as a whole, although specialized effects on one part of the circulation or another have been documented. It acts in concert with the adrenal gland initiating the well-known classical response to stress. This includes a rise in arterial pressure and an increase in heart rate and redistribution of blood to organs of immediate importance to the threatened animal. The parasympathetic nervous system, on the other hand, seemingly a conglomerate of individual effector systems, possibly through a variety of transmitters, causes effects on more limited parts of the vascular system, resulting in specialized usually limited, but very essential, responses. To a considerable extent a number of these systems and their mechanisms in the circulation have yet to be charted and their efferent synaptic mechanisms described.

There are very real problems in generalizing about the nervous control of the vasculature. The first difficulty is that there is immense diversity of vascular neuroeffector mechanisms within an individual, and this is accentuated when the variation associated with development, ageing, different

Table 12.1. Characteristics of adrenergic receptors in large cerebral blood vessels.

	Adrenoceptor				
Species	α		β		Non-specific high threshold
Human	α_1	(+/+++)	β	+	?
Monkey	α_1	+++	β	+	?
Cat	Modified $\alpha_2 > \alpha_1$	++	β_1	++	0
Dog	α_2	+	β/0	+/0	?
Rabbit	Modified α_1	+	0	0	Present
Pig	0	0	β_1	+++	?
Guinea-pig	0	0	+	+++	?
Rat	0	0	β	+++	Present
Cow	α/0	+/0	?	?	?
Goat	α	?	0	?	?

α and β, α- and β-adrenoceptors, respectively. When the adrenoceptor has been subclassified, it is shown as α_1, α_2, β_1. 0, no receptor-mediated response present. ?, experiments do not permit a decision. +, ++, +++, relative magnitude of receptor-mediated response; +++ being the highest.

strains and species, environmental circumstances and disease are also considered. Most experimental laboratory studies are made with a single type of blood vessel selected by an investigator for a specific reason, for example, a skin vessel (referring to the rat tail artery), or because it doesn't have much collagen and is therefore good for electrophysiology (referring to the cerebral artery), and so on. For such reasons, our picture of the vasculature derived from *in vitro* investigation is very haphazard and piecemeal. For example, our views about the rat circulation are derived to a great extent from experiments with the tail, a mesenteric and cerebral resistance artery, and the aorta, and not a great deal more. The glimpse that we have of the circulation in one species is frequently limited and inadequate to allow us to form any general conclusions. This problem becomes unbelievably greater when we start comparing species, and the changes associated with other factors (see above) when the diversity almost seems to preclude logical conclusions.

Table 12.1 summarizes what is known about the adrenoceptors in a cerebral artery (the basilar) of a number of species (Bevan, 1984). There are differences in the absolute size of the α- and β-adrenoceptor-mediated response, and in their ratios and their subtypes. The diversification of the neuroeffector mechanism becomes even more complex when we superimpose upon this the variation that exists in cerebrovascular innervation. In the pig, for example, the innervation seems to be exclusively dilator. In the rabbit, the constrictor influences are dominant. In the dog, both constrictor and dilator mechanisms have been described, and so on. There are at least two ways of looking at these problems. First, that the differences do reflect important species specificity. Species are obviously different from each other, and this quite reasonably could include the mechanism of control of their cerebral circulation. But it is difficult to see why the nature of the vascular bed control should be so different — quantitatively yes, but why qualitatively? Secondly, (and this seems almost a more acceptable explanation), the characteristics we are measuring are not of primary, major, functional importance in the control of this vascular bed. It could be that other vascular parameters, e.g. pressure, flow and tissue metabolism, represent the essential major elements of cerebrovascular control. The postsynaptic receptor systems, and indeed the innervation, might be considered refinements of regulation of small importance. Indeed, there is some experimental support for this point of view (see below). The receptor population present in a blood vessel may represent unsuppressed characteristics of regional mesenchymal cells from which the blood vessels have developed (see below).

In this chapter we will attempt to describe a little of what is known about the neural regulation of vascular tone. The nervous system does not form synapses with vascular smooth muscle cells (except possibly in the very small arterioles). Rather the innervation is perivascular and is generally somewhat removed from individual effector cells. The neuromuscular cleft is greater than in other innervated smooth muscle systems. One gets the impression that the neural plexus is like a loosely fitting stocking or sleeve of axons drawn over a muscular tube. It is the whole artery that is innervated rather than individual vascular smooth muscle cells. Our emphasis will be on the control of the blood vessel wall tone, and particularly the synaptic and neuroeffector mechanisms whereby the transmitter regulates the function of the cells within the wall. This chapter will not examine the mode of action of transmitters on the effector cells. We will attempt to generalize from what has been established. However, it has been said that the only generalization that can be made with any confidence with respect to the vasculature is that none, or very few, can be made. The paucity of our knowledge, in particular the spotty nature of the information available, makes such an attempt very difficult. Only a certain degree of generalization can be expected, however, since diversification of blood vessel wall properties confers regional specialization. The process of generalization is further hampered by the fact that most investigators have studied middle-sized arteries. It is the small arteries and arterioles that control flow and these may have different properties from their parent vessels.

What is important in determining the tone of a blood vessel? Large blood vessels are relatively little contracted *in vivo*. The smaller resistance arteries, less than 400 μm down to 30 μm in diameter have a relatively high level of tone and may as much as double their diameter when exposed to vasodilator drugs *in vivo*. This tone is mainly derived from the physical forces associated with the pressure and the rate of flow within their lumena (Johnson, 1986; Bevan, 1991). Thus the innervation is not acting on a relaxed artery wall; it acts by modifying existing tone. It causes a change in diameter and this in turn influences pressure and flow, causing secondary changes in artery calibre (Figure 12.1). Thus the precise effect of the nerves is complicated by

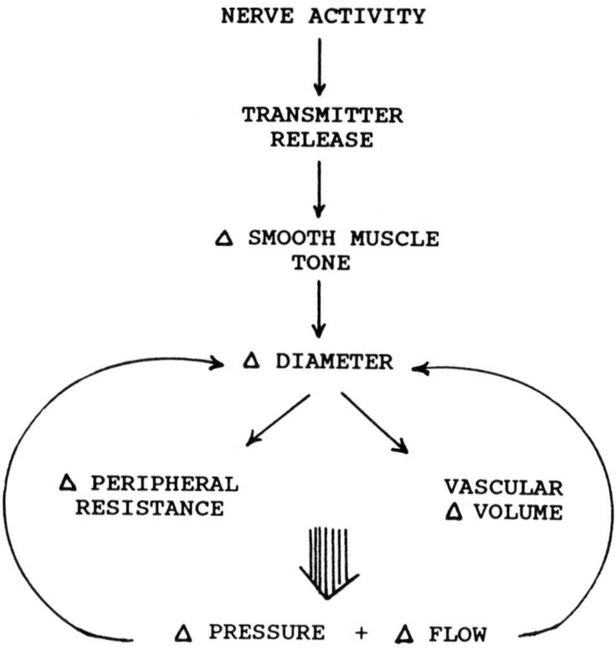

Figure 12.1. Illustration of secondary effects of nerve-induced changes in pressure and flow on vascular diameter.

concomitant changes in the circulation, both 'upstream' and 'downstream'. We know relatively little about these interactions, in particular their quantitative interrelationships.

Finally, it should be borne in mind that nervous regulation of vascular tone is a vast topic, with literally thousands of relevant references, which steadily increase every year. In a recent review on the electrophysiology of the sympathetic innervation of arteries and arterioles, 263 references were cited (Hirst and Edwards, 1989). In a review on non-adrenergic neuronal vasodilator mechanisms, there were 314 references (Bevan and Brayden, 1986). For this reason and because of the nature of this chapter, many current interesting lines of controversy must be omitted, and a number of statements made without reference. Further information, particularly of the sympathetic adrenergic innervation, can be found in a review on this topic (Bevan *et al.*, 1980).

12.2. *The sympathetic nervous outflow to the vasculature*

12.2.1. **Sympathetic neurones**

All blood vessels, including elastic arteries (with the puzzling exception of the rat) and probably excluding venules, receive an adrenergic innervation.

The relative density of innervation to the components of the arterial tree has not yet been made, although limited comparisons of vessels have been undertaken (Bevan *et al.*, 1980; Owen *et al.*, 1983; Appenzeller *et al.*, 1984). As the perivascular plexus of large arteries and veins contains innervating varicosities and also sympathetic axons *en passage* to the distal vascular bed, it is difficult to know just how to make the measurement. Density of histofluorescence, norepinephrine content and tritiated neuronal norepinephrine uptake have all been used as indices. What really matters is the concentration of the transmitter at the effector cells. Even this is difficult to define since the nerves are usually limited to the adventitio-medial junction, and because of this the transmitter is distributed unevenly across the vessel wall. What does seem clear is that sympathetic innervation density does not parallel patterns of postsynaptic adrenoceptors.

A few generalizations regarding the sympathetic innervation of the circulation can be made.

a. *Innervation density*

A number of general statements regarding innervation density can be made which, although negative, serve to refute previously made generalizations. Innervation density is not the same in all vessels of the same bed (Fuxe and Sedvall, 1965; Furness and Marshall, 1974); it can change dramatically along the course of a blood vessel (Bevan and Purdy, 1973). In any one species, it is not related to vessel diameter. Innervation density of the same anatomical vessel may be different in various species and in any one vessel tends to decline with advancing age (Shibata *et al.*, 1971; Waterson *et al.*, 1974). In a series of rabbit veins, the density of adrenergic innervation assessed by neural uptake of norepinephrine and catecholamine histofluorescence increased in the order: deep limb and muscle, kidney, skin (back), pulmonary, mesentery, skin, ear, head and paw (Bevan and Osher, 1965). A series of rabbit large- and middle-sized arteries and veins with similar α-receptor-mediated smooth muscle characteristics exhibited a positive correlation between innervation density and the size of the neurogenic response (Bevan, 1977).

b. *Innervation distribution (perivascular vs. intramedial)*

Although a ground terminal network limited to the adventitio-medial junction is the commonest pattern, in some blood vessels nerves penetrate and ramify within the muscle layer.

In both arteries and veins closely matched for characteristics other than nerve distribution, the frequency–response curve for the medially innervated vessel originates at a lower frequency and rises more steeply than that for the vessel with innervation at the adventitio-medial junction (Bevan, 1977). Transmitter effects are terminated in the medially innervated vessel primarily by neuronal uptake, in contast to a vessel with junctional innervation when diffusion and metabolism become more important (Ljung, 1976; Osswald, 1976). Thus, a medially innervated vessel would be expected to respond faster and to a greater extent to a change in sympathetic discharge pattern. Such a functional consequence is consistent with the presence of medial innervation in vessels where large responses would be physiologically desirable, e.g. in vascular sphincters (Hutchinson *et al.*, 1962; White *et al.*, 1973) and in subcutaneous arteries and veins of limbs where intense vasoconstriction resulting in temperature conservation may be critical (Keatinge, 1966).

c. *Cleft width*

The vascular neuromuscular cleft is commonly uncharacteristically large, belying the term synapse — 'intimate contact'. As the width is controlled or regulated, i.e. is reasonably consistent between individuals, it presumably represents an important biological characteristic. Generally speaking, cleft widths diminish as arteries get smaller. There have been attempts to relate cleft size to function. It has been found that the narrower the cleft the lower the threshold for neurogenic response, and the larger the response to a given frequency. Some representative widths in blood vessels are shown in Figure 12.2 and much of the existing literature has been reviewed (Rowan and Bevan, 1983). It can be strongly argued that cleft widths in excess of 1–2 μm are of little functional importance. In fact, the transmitter released from such varicosities may not reach the postsynaptic membrane in effective concentrations. That varicosity–smooth muscle separation is less in smaller blood vessels and that this is not related to the thinning out of *en passage* axons is illustrated in Figure 12.3. The distribution of cleft widths less than 1000 μm in the central ear artery of the rabbit, a muscular artery, dramatically increases in its first order branch which has a diameter only 50% of its parent (J. Dodge, personal communication).

Cleft width can influence neurotransmitter dynamics and the estimated transmitter concentrations at the postsynaptic membrane. The narrower the cleft, the higher the concentration of transmitter at the postsynaptic membrane (concentration falls off inversely with the cube of the radius), the greater the level of presynaptic α_2 inhibitory feedback on release, the more effective is uptake 1 in terminating nerve-induced responses and the less relevant is uptake 2 (Figure 12.4). In blood vessels with narrower synapses, there is less escape of the neurotransmitter into the blood stream; it is recaptured into the nerve terminal. The biological effect of released transmitter in small arteries and arterioles is more likely to be confined to the postsynaptic area. This is in contrast to the large arteries where the nerves almost act as a diffuse sprinkler system.

Why is neural control designed this way? Why do the neurones not form specific one-to-one relationships with individual smooth muscle cells? The

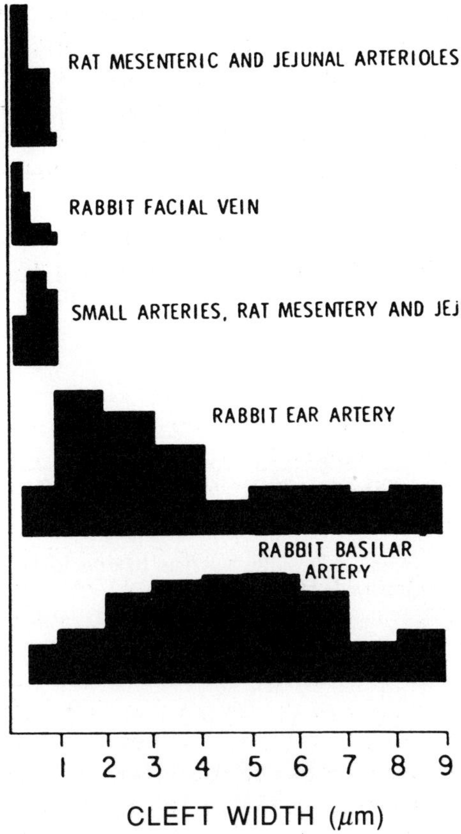

Figure 12.2. Examples of the variability of cleft width in different parts of the vascular system. From Rowan and Bevan, 1983; for data sources see original publication.

evidence is that in large- and middle-sized arteries, which usually have a respectable perivascular plexus (except possibly for the initial rapid transient phase of contraction), the smooth muscle cells act individually and independently of the local concentration of neurotransmitter. In smaller arteries when varicosity density is low, and there may be only one axon running along the length of the vessel, there is only localized transmitter release. This only becomes effective when propagated through the smooth muscle complex.

d. *Additional transmitters*

In certain arteries, α_1-adrenoceptor antagonists fail to block sympathetic nerve stimulation. This seems to be particularly a property of smaller vessels, but not exclusively so.

There is strong evidence that either neuropeptide-Y (NPY) or adenosine

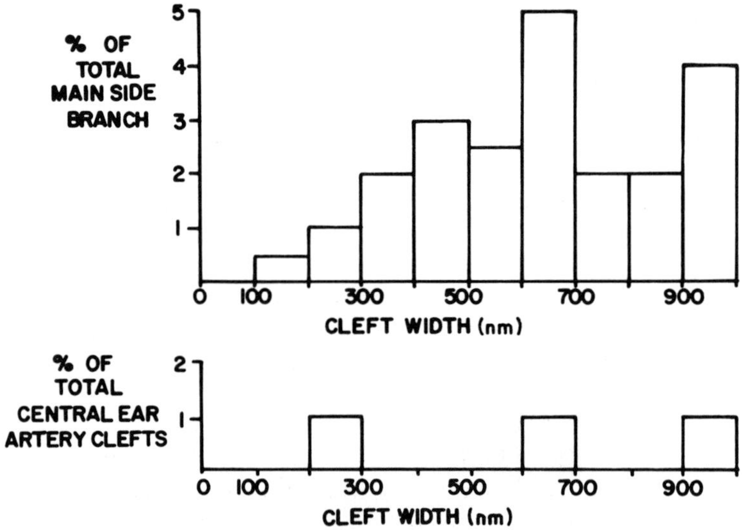

Figure 12.3. Distribution of synaptic cleft widths less than 1000 nm in the rabbit central ear artery and a first-order branch (main side branch).

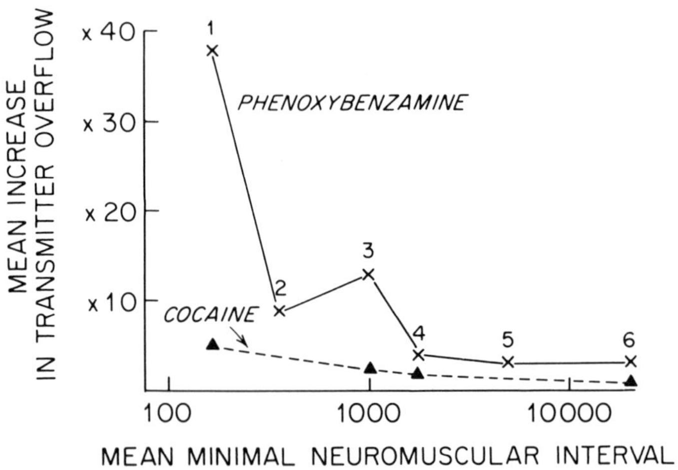

Figure 12.4. Mean increase in transmitter overflow after treatment with phenoxybenzamine and cocaine in relation to mean width of the neuromuscular interval. 1, Guinea-pig vas deferens; 2, rabbit atria; 3, portal vein; 4, guinea-pig uterine artery; 5, rabbit ear artery; 6, rabbit pulmonary artery.
From Bevan, 1977; for sources see original publication.

triphosphate (ATP) are released from some sympathetic nerves and act with norepinephrine to cause vasoconstriction. The evidence in support of each of these transmitters is strong, and not mutually exclusive. Burnstock has championed a role for ATP acting on postsynaptic P_{2x} purinoceptors. Strong support for this point of view has been published for the ear and saphenous artery of the rabbit (Kennedy *et al.*, 1986; Burnstock and Warland, 1987), the rat tail artery (Sneddon and Burnstock, 1985), guinea-pig mesenteric artery (Kügelgen and Starke, 1985), and dog cerebral artery (Muramatsu and Kogoshi, 1987). In these vessels the contribution of the purinergic component is inversely related to stimulation frequency. But this is not always the case in the rabbit hepatic artery, when a role for purinergic transmission was found only at higher frequencies (Brizzolara and Burnstock, 1990).

In a series of papers, Lundberg and colleagues (Lundberg *et al.*, 1986; Lundberg and Hökfelt, 1986; Duverger *et al.*, 1987) have provided support for the notion that this 36-amino acid peptide is a candidate co-transmitter with norepinephrine in the sympathetic control of some blood vessels. This peptide is co-released with norepinephrine, is subject to presynaptic regulation, and has a direct postsynaptic effect in some blood vessels, but not others. At some sites, at concentrations that are subthreshold when acting alone, NPY markedly potentiates responses to other agonists such as norepinephrine, whether mediated by α_1- or α_2-adrenoceptors (Hieble *et al.*, 1989). In contrast to most findings with ATP, the peptide component of transmission occurs at higher rather than lower frequencies. The role for NPY has been argued for the blood vessels of the nasal mucosa (Lacroix, 1989) and for rabbit cerebral arteries (Van Riper and Bevan, 1991a). Much more information regarding the distribution and role of these co-transmitters will have to be amassed before we can obtain a comprehensive picture.

12.3. *Postsynaptic sympathetic mechanism*

It is conventional wisdom that the net response of blood vessels to catecholamine stimulation depends on the absolute and relative magnitude of the α- and β-adrenoceptor components. There seems no reason to question this, except that the magnitude of the response to stimulation of either receptor population is influenced by the pre-existing level of vascular tone. Generally speaking, the higher the level of tone, the greater the magnitude of the dilator effect, and the lower the tone, the greater the size of the constriction. Relative size of α- and β-effects is altered by many drugs, hormones and biological circumstances, e.g. oestrogens, progesterone, thyroid, temperature and age.

The distribution of β_1- and β_2-adrenoceptors in blood vessels is not adequately known to allow generalization, and there are problems in identifying the α_2-adrenoceptor component *in vitro*. This essentially precludes any general statement regarding these receptors in the vascular neuroeffector complex. This is not the case for the α_1-adrenoceptor.

12.3.1. α_1-Adrenoceptor affinity

The primary vascular smooth muscle surface receptor mediating the effects of the sympathetic nervous system is the α_1-adrenoceptor. A systematic study of the sensitivity of a spectrum of large- and middle-sized rabbit arteries to norepinephrine mediated through α_1-adrenoceptors shows that it varies by considerably more than two orders of magnitude (Bevan *et al.*, 1986). There are two receptor-related phenomena that influence tissue sensitivity: receptor affinity and receptor number. In the case of rabbit vessels, sensitivity to catecholamines can be correlated with affinity (Figure 12.5) and not receptor reserve, which is the closest *in vitro* approximation to receptor number. The distribution of the cardiac output is directed by the resistance arteries. Receptor-related factors have not yet been measured in these blood vessels.

This receptor-related feature is specific to the α_1-adrenoceptor. It is not seen with α_1-adrenoceptor antagonists — prazosin affinity is the same in all blood vessels — nor to histamine acting on the H_1 receptor (Oriowo *et al.*, 1987). The same principle of relating sensitivity and affinity seems to be true for other comparisons: for arteries in other species, between the same artery in different species, and for the changes that occur with temperature and hypertension (Bevan *et al.*, 1989). It seems to apply across vascular beds and between species.

The basis of the variation of affinity of the receptor for norepinephrine remains to be defined. It may be that it results from the combination of varying ratios of different receptor subtypes with different affinities. Alternatively, there is strong evidence that the conformation of a receptor may be influenced by its lipid microenvironment (Shreeve, 1990). Variability could reflect different concentrations of a ternary molecule which reacts with the drug receptor complex, influencing its affinity (Mackay, 1990). Whatever the explanation, its biological significance is that it might explain the basis of some hormonal and agonist site selectivity. As it seems likely that transmitter spills out of the synapse diffusing into the surrounding cells to cause its effects, this variation in the postsynaptic receptor must be taken into account in attempts to describe sympathetic neural control.

12.3.2. Patterns of affinity variation

Blood vessels arise during development from primitive mesenchyme, as cords or clusters of angioblasts that form spaces lined by endothelial cells. By a process of coalescence, an irregular vascular plexus is formed. After a circulation is established by connection with a major vessel, the plexus

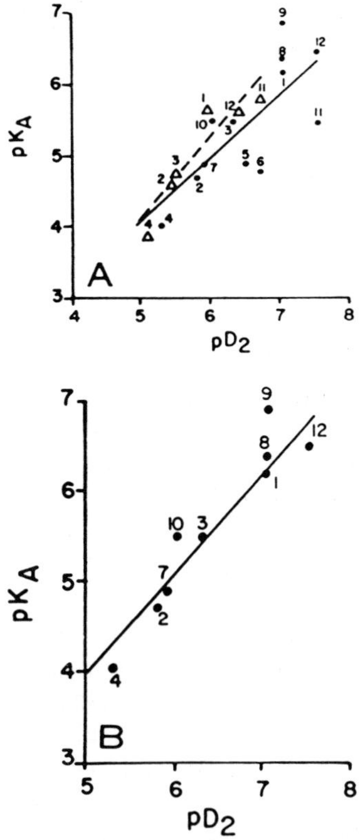

Figure 12.5. (A) Relationship between norepinephrine (•) negative log of ED_{50} (pD_2) and negative log of affinity constant (pK_A) for 12 rabbit arteries, and phenylephrine (△) pD_2 and pK_A for six rabbit arteries: 1, abdominal aorta; 2, superior mesenteric; 3, renal; 4, ovarian; 5, common iliac; 6 external iliac; 7, internal iliac; 8 large pulmonary; 9, medium pulmonary; 10, basilar; 11, ear; 12, thoracic-aorta. Each point is the mean of five to six experiments. (B) Relationship between norepinephrine pD_2 and pK_A for nine rabbit arteries after exclusion of three with a high-receptor reserve.
From Bevan *et al.*, 1986.

differentiates into a recognizable pattern of capillaries, arterial and venous primordia. The pattern of the vascular bed changes continue during the growth of the embryo until haemodynamic forces eventually establish a definitive pattern in the larger vessels.

The tunica intima, tunica media and adventitial connective tissue are of mesodermal origin (Bevan *et al.*, 1983). In the avian embryo, it has been shown that neural crest cells contribute to the medial smooth muscle layer in arteries derived from the branchial arch system. The endothelium of these arteries, however, is derived from mesenchyme, as in other vessels. Because the interaction of different cell types is important in the determination of tissue characteristics, particularly during early development, our hypothesis is that these same principles apply to the differentiation of arteries. Thus location of origin may account for some of the functional differences found in them (Bevan, 1979; Bevan *et al.*, 1983).

There is an abrupt change in the sensitivity of the α-adrenoceptor-mediated response of smooth muscle of the vertebral artery where the vessel runs medially along the lateral process of the atlas, i.e. at the upper level of the first cervical vertebra. This change in sensitivity is accounted for, at least in part, by a change of affinity. A similar change is seen where the internal carotid artery enters the bony carotid canal. These are sites where it is postulated that there is transition from arteries derived from the primitive aortae and branchial arch system with those that develop in and around the brain as the cerebral circulation.

Measurements of the responses of sequential segments to norepinephrine taken from the coeliac, superior and inferior mesenteric arteries a few millimetres from their origins in the aorta reveal an abrupt diminution in vascular smooth muscle sensitivity (Figure 12.6). The norepinephrine ED_{50} and affinity increase by a factor of 2 log units. There is a consistent change in the threshold concentration and a steepening of the concentration–response curves.

There sites seem to occur where there is a transition between smooth muscle cells exposed to different environmental influences. These changes in the vascular muscle are not reflected in changes in the sympathetic innervation pattern and density. They occur in vessels of varying diameter and wall thickness and, in the case of the internal carotid, in an artery that is not undergoing transition from an elastic to a muscular type. In one case, a vessel becomes modestly more sensitive, and in others it becomes markedly less sensitive. Thus junctions occur when arteries containing locally derived effector cells that have distinctive characteristics, probably originating from different regions, join together.

Shigei and colleagues (1983) have noted, in the dog venous system, marked correlations between regional differences in vascular characteristics and their embryological origin. They cite three examples (see Figure 12.7). (1) The veins of the body wall are highly sensitive to norepinephrine and serotonin, whilst those related to the digestive tube (the pulmonary, portal and mesenteric) are highly sensitive to histamine. During development the vertebrate embryo can be regarded as a double tube: the outer is the body wall and the inner, the digestive tube. These are connected only by the tissue of mesentery. The two groups of veins develop separately from the two layers. (2) It is well known that the inferior vena cava is an embryologically complex vessel. Its separately developing segments show differences in histological structure, responsiveness to vasoactive agents, and in their innervation. The middle segment of the inferior vena cava is similar in its functional characteristics to the portal and mesenteric veins, and this is consistent with the similarity of their origin. (3) The splenic vein has a complex genesis and during development forms a shunt between the spleen and the portal vein (Miki, 1983). In the adult the splenic vein has functional

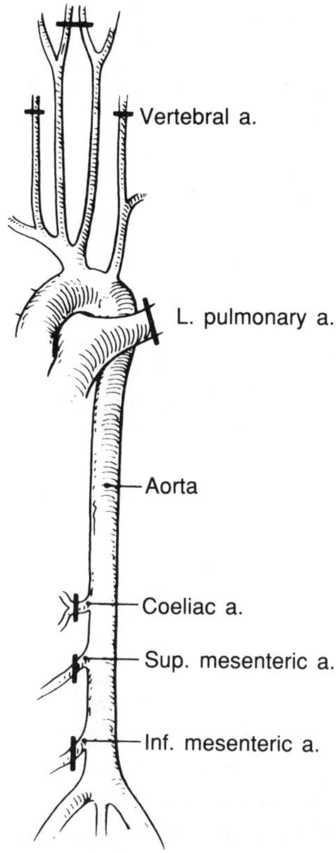

Figure 12.6. Representation of major arteries of the rabbit and sites (shown by *black bars*) of vascular transition zones.
From Bevan *et al.*, 1983.

characteristics quite different from other surrounding veins such as the gastrosplenic and gastroduodenal. These authors point out that just as in the arterial system, there are points of fusion in the venous system. Characteristics on either side of these sites of fusion can be abruptly and remarkably different.

12.3.3. α_1-Adrenoceptor reserve

The contractile response of some blood vessels to norepinephrine is less than their capacity to contract to other agonists. This has been particularly noted for cerebral arteries (Duckles and Bevan, 1976). Receptor analysis of the rabbit basilar artery has shown that the contraction of this artery is receptor number limited (Laher and Bevan, 1985). When the artery responds maximally to norepinephrine, an effect which may be no more than

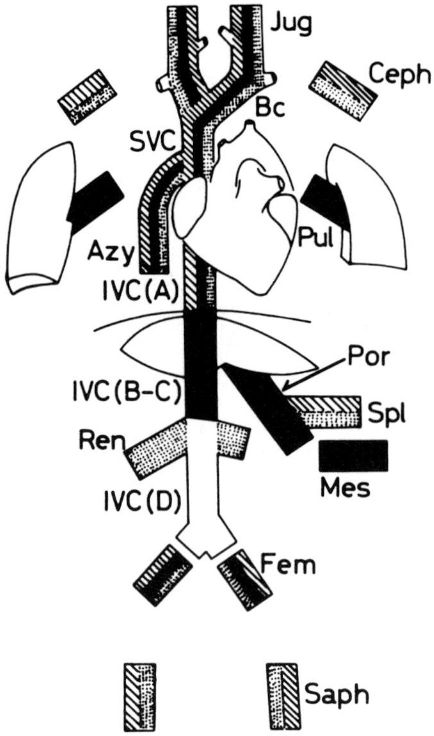

Figure 12.7. Schematic diagram showing distribution of sensitivities in the dog venous system. Marked veins are highly sensitive to norepinephrine (NE; hatched), 5-hydroxytrypramine (5-HT; stippled) and histamine (solid). Pul, pulmonary vein; Por, portal vein; Spl, splenic vein; Mes, mesenteric vein; IVC (A), IVC (B-C) and IVC (D), segments A, B-C and D of inferior vena cava, respectively. Jug, jugular; caph, caphalic; SVC, superior vena cava; Azy, azygos; ren, renal; fem, femoral; saph, sapherous.
From Ishikawa *et al.*, 1980.

10–15% of the maximum response, there is complete receptor occupation. This contrasts with what has been shown to occur in other arteries, such as the rabbit thoracic aorta and central ear artery, where maximum response is achieved only by the occupation of a relatively small percentage of the total available. Presumably, at the same junction where changes in affinity occur, there can be changes in receptor reserve. In the case of the cerebral arteries, this is a change from sizeable reserve to receptor limitation. This change *per se* has a relatively small consequence on sensitivity in the pharmacological sense, on the ED_{50}, but would serve to limit the magnitude of response to receptor activation. One explanation for these conclusions is that the vascular smooth muscle cell can limit the absolute number of receptors it expresses. Alternatively, the cells may regulate the effectiveness or efficiency of receptor coupling. This latter explanation seems more plausible after experiments which show that the contraction of the basilar artery to nor-

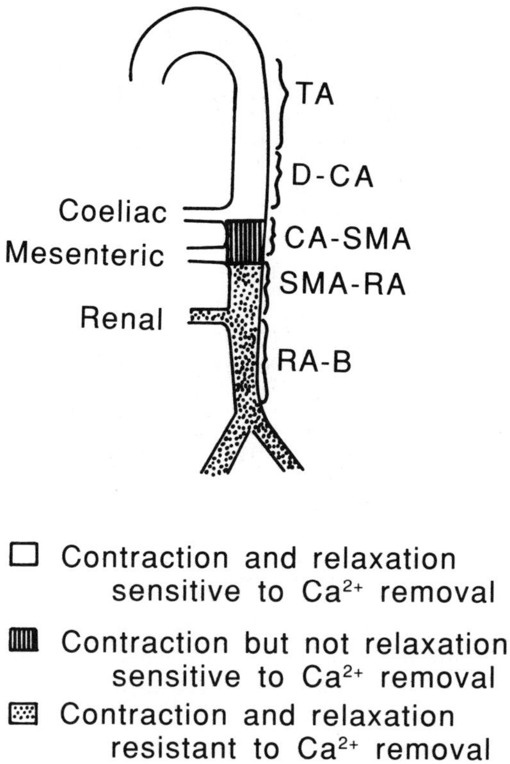

Figure 12.8. Diagrammatic representation of aorta and three of its branches, the coeliac artery (CA), the superior mesentery artery (SMA) and renal artery (RA). The aorta is divided into five segments: TA, D–CA, CA–SMA, SMA–RA, and to left RA and RA–B that between the left RA and the bifurcation. Localization of segments that contract and relax after exclusion of Ca^{2+} from the bath solution are shown. TA, thoracic aorta.
From Tayo and Bevan, 1986.

epinephrine is markedly potentiated by a calcium channel agonist (Laher *et al.*, 1989).

12.3.4. α_1-Adrenoceptor contraction; calcium dependence

That there is diversity in the calcium handling mechanism in different blood vessels is well known. Observations to date seem to show that these differences cannot be correlated with the pattern of α_1-adrenoceptor variation in affinity. One example will be described. The dependence on extracellular calcium of rabbit artery segments to norepinephrine contraction and relaxation to acetylcholine mediated through the endothelium have been systematically studied along the length of the aorta and its coeliac, superior mesenteric and renal arteries (Figure 12.8; Tayo and Bevan, 1986). Both responses in the thoracic and upper abdominal aorta were lost under nominal zero-calcium conditions. However, contractions of segments from the aorta below the origin of the renal artery and from the renal artery itself were resistant to the effect of calcium removal. The aorta between the superior mesenteric and the renal arteries was intermediate in its dependence. Relaxation of the aorta caudal to the origin of the coeliac artery and the renal artery was also resistant. Such a pattern was mirrored by changes in susceptibility to calcium channel blocking drugs. The transition of calcium-dependence of these effects does not correspond to sites of change in adrenoceptor affinity. The upper and lower parts of the abdominal aorta are not distinguishable from each other histologically; they have the typical appearance of elastic arteries, nor are these obvious changes in innervation based upon catecholamine histofluorescent microscopy.

12.3.5. **Low affinity sites for norepinephrine; γ or extraceptors**

When an adrenergic synaptic vesicle empties its content of norepinephrine by exocytosis, the concentration of norepinephrine at the postsynaptic membrane will vary with synaptic cleft width. Peak postsynaptic concentrations of norepinephrine have been determined in arteries of different cleft width by the method of Ljung (1969) and in the extrajunctional area by the transmitter gradient method. In vessels with wide clefts, at 8 Hz, junctional and extrajunctional norepinephrine concentrations were similar (0·15–0·55 μM) but in those with a separation of 100 nm, peak concentrations were of the order of 10 μM and extrajunctional levels were less than 10 nM. Extrapolation of this data to the narrower clefts, found in smaller blood vessels (Rowan and Bevan, 1983), suggests that postjunctional concentrations of transmitter in excess of 0·1 mM are achieved.

Reports of α-adrenoceptor antagonist-resistant vasoconstriction are now quite numerous. One explanation is that a co-transmitter is released and this is responsible for at least some of the pharmacological resistance. Another is that such high concentrations of norepinephrine occur within the cleft, that the concentrations of α-adrenoceptor antagonists that are α_1-adrenoceptor-selective, are not capable of effectively competing with norepinephrine at its receptor. A study of resistance arteries from the rabbit ear (75 μm unstretched lumen diameter) indicates that phentolamine (1·4 μM) at the highest concentration that does not have other effects, only antagonizes norepinephrine concentrations up to about 10^{-5} M (Owen *et al.*, 1983).

An additional explanation of α-adrenoceptor resistance is that in a narrow synapse, norepinephrine is acting on receptors other than the α-adrenoceptor to cause contraction and that these responses are resistant to pharmacological blockade. Hirst and Neild (1980) have proposed that α-adrenoceptor antagonist-resistant receptors, γ-adrenoceptors, are restricted to the postjunctional membrane and mediate the excitatory junctional potential (EJP) that occurs in response to norepinephrine released by electrical field stimulation. However, most rabbit arteries have a population of

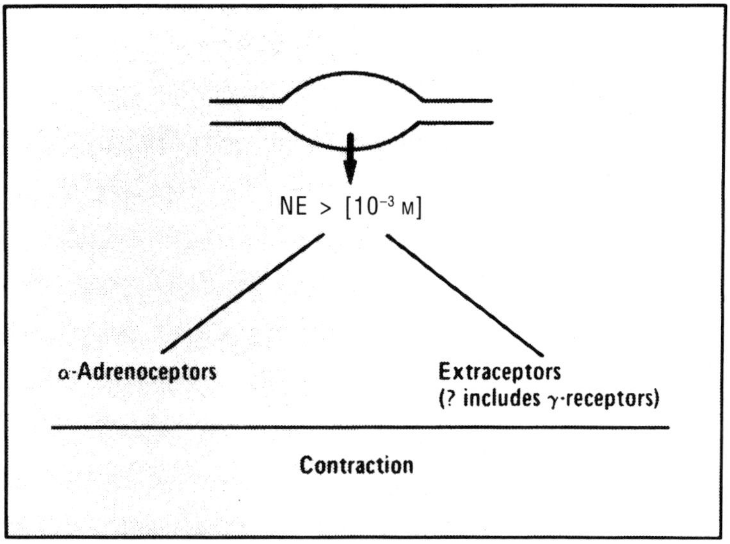

Figure 12.9. Possible mechanism of adrenergic transmission in resistance arteries. Norepinephrine (NE) achieves high concentrations at the postjunctional membrane when the neuromuscular separation is small, as is the case for resistant arteries. It may exert a postsynaptic effect leading to contraction through the α-adrenoceptor and also through the 'extraceptor'. The stimulation mediated through the α-adrenoceptor may be antagonist resistant because the effective concentration of NE is high. 'Extraceptors' are low-affinity sites that probably include the γ-receptor as a postjunctional α-adrenoceptor antagonist-resistant site associated with the excitatory junction potential.
From Bevan *et al.*, 1987.

low affinity sites outside the synapse (Bevan *et al.*, 1987) that are activated by high concentrations of norepinephrine. We have called these sites 'extraceptors' (Laher *et al.*, 1986a,b). These sites are not restricted to the postsynaptic junction, do not occur in veins, are relatively non-selective in their agonist structural requirements and can be responsible for contractions close to tissue maximum. Clearly, the narrower the cleft and the higher the stimulation frequency, the more such sites would be involved in and contribute to the resultant contraction (Figure 12.9). Piascik *et al.* (1988) have described binding sites for prazosin in the rabbit aorta that could represent such receptors.

12.3.6. **Branching Pattern**

Changes in α_1-adrenoceptor parameters with branching have only been studied in two vascular beds: the rabbit ear (Owen *et al.*, 1983) and the rabbit pial bed (Van Riper and Bevan, 1991b). The changes in the two vascular regions are completely different. In the former, the sensitivity of the response mediated through the α_1-adrenoceptor does not change over three branch orders. Maximum contractile effects are elicited in all three.

The implication is the α-adrenoceptor-linked response is not significantly different. In the brain circulation, on the other hand, comparisons of the α_1-adrenoceptor-mediated contraction within the middle cerebral artery and its branches reveal a progressive fall-off until in the smallest artery there is little or no response. This is paralleled by a decline in the contraction to serotonin, but not to the extraceptor activation nor to histamine. It is interesting that the field stimulation-elicited contraction falls off in parallel to the response to norepinephrine.

The basis of these regional changes in the blood vessels with branching is entirely unknown.

12.3.7. **Conclusions**

The sympathetic neural adrenergic outflow supplies most of the vasculature predominantly through a perivascular plexus. There is evidence for co-transmission by ATP and NPY in some blood vessels, but the extent of this in the circulation and its significance are not known. Amongst the parameters that lead to variation in vascular response are innervation density and distribution, cleft width, α_1-adrenoceptor affinity and number, and dependence on extracellular calcium. Particularly when the cleft is narrow, adrenoceptor number is low, or coupling is inefficient, the neurotransmitter might act through low affinity undifferentiated γ or extraceptors. There are very specific regional differences in the sympathetic neuroeffector upon branching. The fundamental basis of this variation is unknown except that in some instances there is a similar pattern between some receptor properties and vascular development.

12.4. *Parasympathetic (non-sympathetic) outflow to the vasculature*

In contrast to the sympathetic outflow which supplies most of the vasculature and is associated with postganglionic release of the same primary transmitter, the parasympathetic division outflow to the circulation is made up collectively of a number of relatively discrete outflow systems to limited vascular beds. These systems have been reported to depend on a variety of transmitters; the evidence is that there is a considerable species variation. Effective innervation commences at the level of middle-sized or muscular arteries, and in some instances veins of comparable size. This system is usually responsible for vasodilation. Thus, its influence starts at the level of circulation where the blood vessels exhibit significant intrinsic tone, i.e. are capable of dilating.

The experimental evidence for the transmitters of this division has been reviewed (Bevan and Brayden, 1986; see Figure 12.10). All classical criteria have been satisfied for acetylcholine (ACh), vasoactive intestinal polypeptide

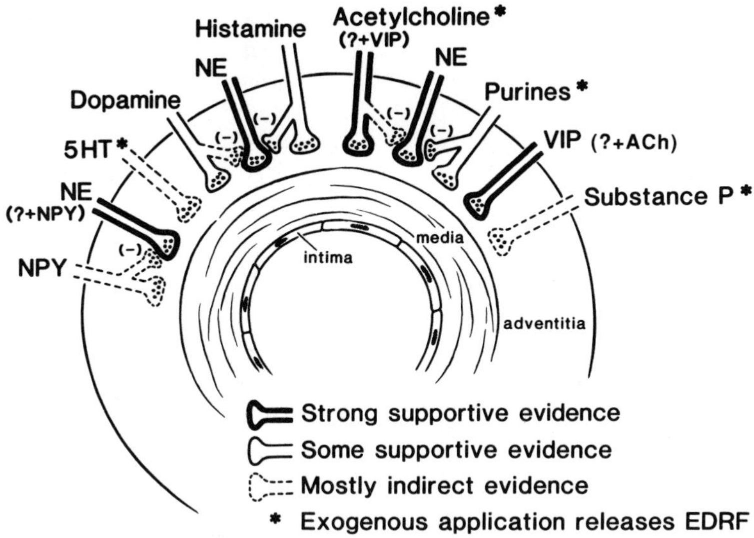

Figure 12.10. Putative vasodilator neurotransmitter mechanisms and the possible sites of interactions between the different neuronal systems. NPY, neuropeptide-Y; NE, norepinephrine; 5-HT, 5-hydroxytryptamine; VIP, vasoactive intestinal polypeptide; ACh, acetylcholine; EDRF, endothelial derived relaxing factor.
From Bevan and Brayden, 1986.

(VIP) and dopamine (DA). There is evidence in support of the purines, calcitonin gene-related peptide (CGRP) and histamine, and suggestive evidence (mostly indirect) for presynaptic effects of NPY, serotonin and norepinephrine on several of these putative transmitters, and also substance P. Finally, there have been claims for other transmitters, such as peptide histidine isoleucine (PHI) and the enkephalins. The experimental evidence for ACh and VIP is briefly reviewed. The reader is referred to a review by Bevan *et al.* (1980) for a discussion of the other possibilities. The impression based upon the present information is that ACh and VIP may be the most common and widespread of the parasympathetic mechanisms to the circulation; however, this may be an illusion based upon inadequate sampling of the entire system.

12.4.1. **Acetylcholine**

Choline acetyltransferase (ChAT) and high-affinity neuronal choline uptake systems have been used as indices for the presence of cholinergic neurones in blood vessels — although neither of these are considered to be completely reliable. Most studies have been made of the arteries of the head of the cat, rabbit and dog (Florence and Bevan, 1979). Based initially upon ChAT assays, arteries to the brain, face, eye, nose, mouth and tongue of the cat are considered to have a cholinergic supply. This distribution has been

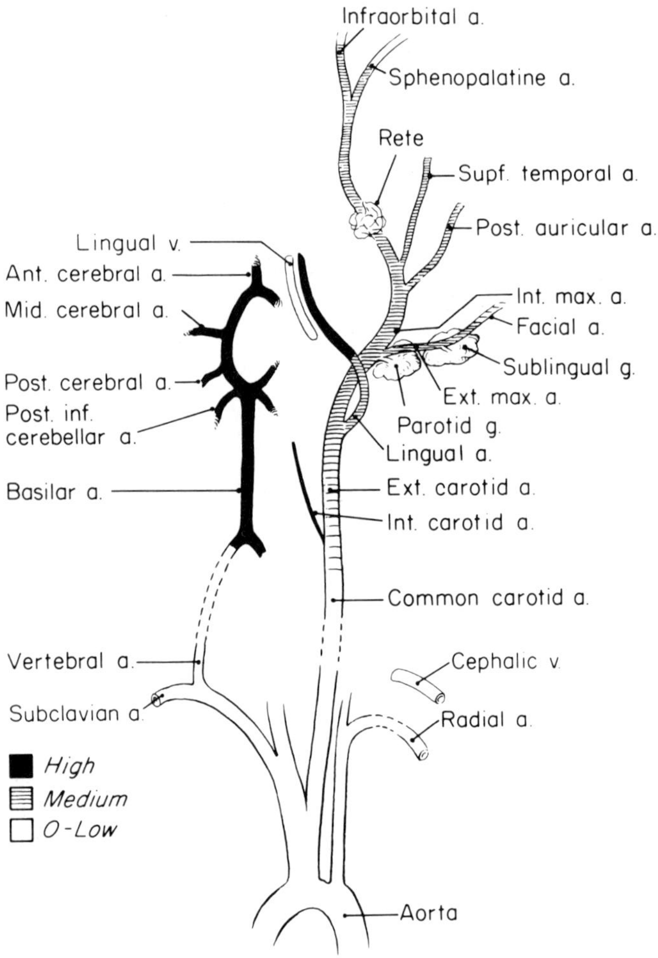

Figure 12.11. Anatomical representation of choline acetyltransferase levels in the cranial arterial system and some other blood vessels of the cat.
From Bevan *et al.*, 1982a.

confirmed by measurements of ACh content and by effects of atropine on the functional dilation that can be demonstrated *in vitro* in these arteries (Bevan *et al.*, 1982b; see Figure 12.11). Unpublished data suggests that a similar distribution of cholinergic neurones is present in the monkey. Significant levels of ChAT have not been found in the middle cerebral artery of man (unpublished data).

The distribution of cholinergic nerves to tissues in the head based on the indices mentioned above is complimented, and to a considerable extent confirmed, by *in vivo* studies that show an atropine-sensitive vasodilation in the choroid plexus, lachrymal gland, upper and lower eyelids, skin of the face, salivary glands, iris, ciliary body, nictitating membrane and the mucosa and muscle of the tongue (for references see Bevan and Brayden, 1986). The distribution of ChAT in the head is consistent with atrophine-sensitive vasodilation. It should be borne in mind that most *in vivo* studies are based upon a single intervention, specifically the effect of atropine. This drug, however, is known to be a local anaesthetic, and in some tissues has been reported to antagonize both serotonin and epinephrine. Thus more evidence than an effect of atropine is required to establish ACh as a neurotransmitter.

In a detailed systematic study, Wellman, Brayden and Bevan (1991) (in preparation) found that ChAT occurred in high concentrations in the inferior mesenteric and umbilical arteries of the cat, dog, rabbit and guinea-pig. This is consistent with findings of a limited study in the monkey (unpublished data). It can be seen from Figure 12.12 that there are additional distributions of this enzyme, representing species differences. Based largely upon the effect of atropine *in vivo*, cholinergic nerves have been described in lung, heart, uterus, skeletal muscle (but not of primates), kidney, liver, colon, rectum, part of the penile erectile system and in the paw (for references see Bevan and Brayden, 1986).

With regard to the mode of action of ACh on the blood vessels, it is well established that there are cholinergic dilator mechanisms that are independent of the endothelium (Brayden and Bevan, 1985). In veins, on the other hand, the cholinergic mechanisms reported have been entirely constrictor (Nakazato *et al.*, 1982). Only in one study (Van Riper and Bevan, 1991c) has an atropine-sensitive vasodilation been described as endothelium-dependent. This was found in a third-order branch of the rabbit middle cerebral artery; in this vessel the dilation was not exclusively atropine-sensitive, but there was a parallelism between atropine susceptibility and endothelium dependence.

12.4.2. **Vasoactive intestinal polypeptide**

VIP, the 28-amino acid polypeptide of the secretin-glucagon family on the basis of immunohistochemical study, has been observed at the adventitio-medial junction of blood vessels to the brain, gastrointestinal tract, the genitourinary tract, exocrine glands, lung, eyes, heart, kidney and skeletal muscle in a variety of species (see Bevan and Brayden, 1986). In many cases evidence is supported by the demonstration of cholinergic-resistant vasodilation.

VIP-immunoreactive nerve cell bodies are widely distributed. In a detailed and comprehensive study (Gibbins *et al.* 1984) in the cat, perivascular VIP-immunoreactive nerves were found to be widely distributed in arteries and arterioles supplying glands, muscles and mucous membranes of the fact (Figure 12.13). Within the cerebral circulation, perivascular VIP-immunoreactive nerves were most abundant in the circle of Willis and the proximal portions of the major cerebral arteries and their proximal branches supply-

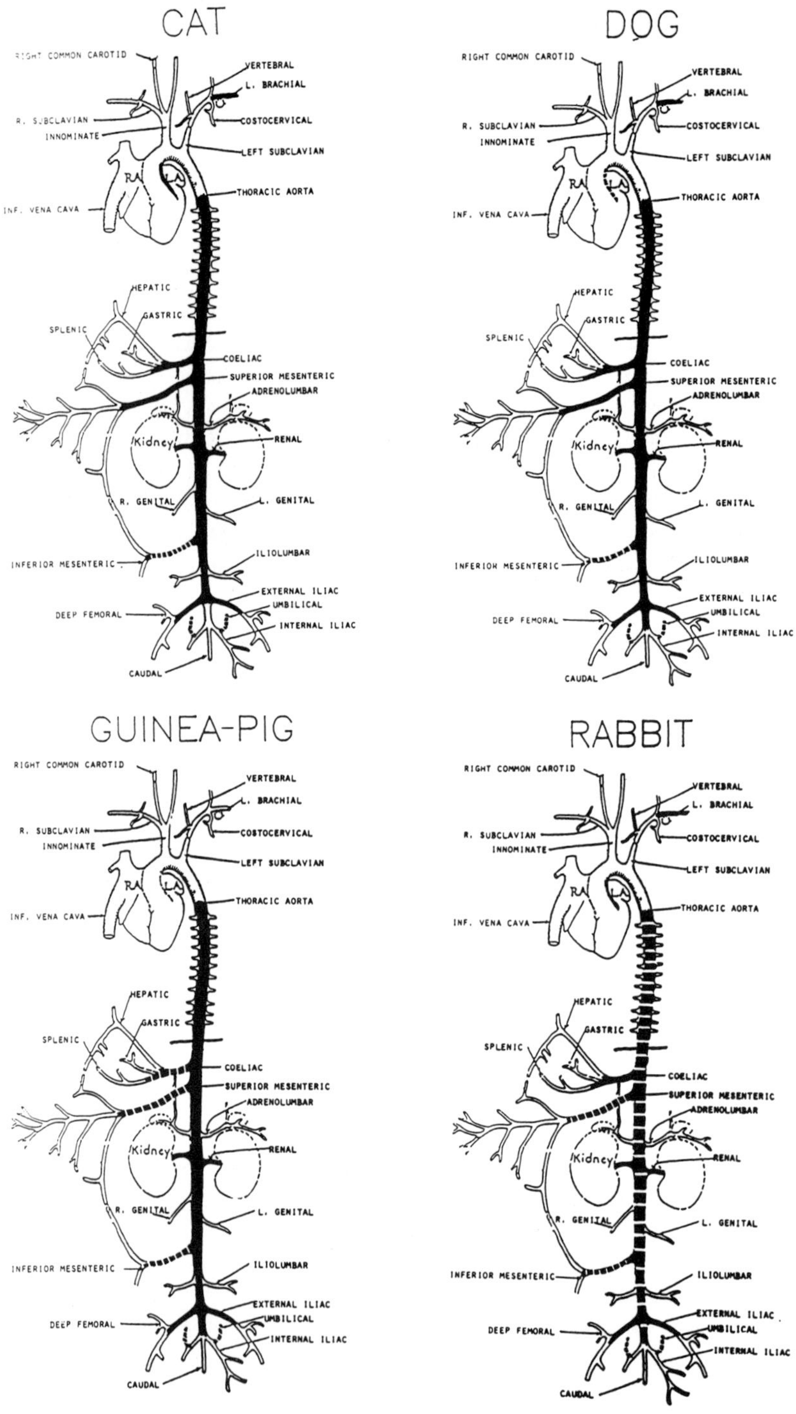

Figure 12.12. Distribution of choline acetyltransferase levels in the systemic arteries of the dog, cat, guinea-pig and rabbit. Interrupted artery fill, enzyme levels greater than 30 nM ACh g^{-1} h^{-1}; solid artery fill, activity below 30 nM ACh g^{-1} h^{-1}.

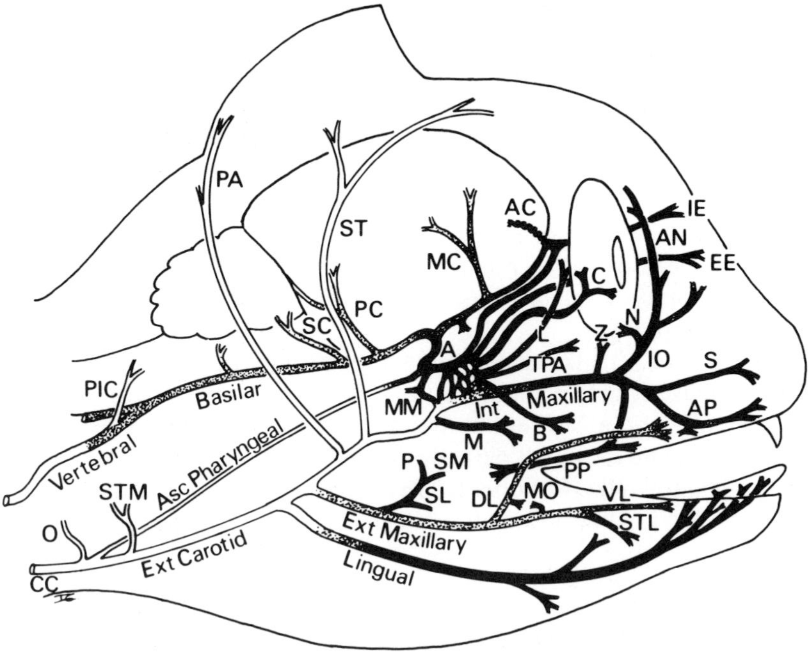

Figure 12.13. Relationships between the major extracerebral cephalic arteries of the cat, indicating the relative density of their perivascular vasoactive intestinal peptide-immunoreactive nerves. Stippling, light to moderate innervation. Solid fill, heavy innervation. Note the absence of an internal carotid artery. The external rete lies between the internal maxillary artery and the anastomosing artery (A). Other labelled arteries: AC, anterior cerebral; AN, angularis; AP, anterior palatine; B, buccinator; C, ciliary; CC, common carotid; DL, dorsal labial; EE, external ethmoid; IE, internal ethmoid: IO, intramorbital; L, lacrimal; M, masseteric; MC, middle cerebral; MM, middle meningeal; MO, molar gland; N, nictitating inferior cerebellar; O, occipital; P, parotid gland; PA, posterior auricular; PC, posterior cerebral; PIC, posterior inferior cerebellar; PP, posterior palatine; S, sphenopalatine; SC, superior cerebellar; SL, sublingual gland; SM, submandibular gland; ST, superficial temporal; STL, submental; STM, sternomastoid; TPA, deep anterior temporal; VL, ventral labial; Z, zygomatic gland. From Gibbins *et al.*, 1984.

ing the rostral brain-stem and ventral areas of the cerebral cortex. Nerves containing VIP-immunoreactive material were absent from distal portions of arteries supplying the posterior brain-stem, cerebellum and dorsal cerebral cortex. Cerebral perivascular VIP-immunoreactive nerves had extracerebral origins probably from VIP-immunoreactive perikarya within microganglia in the cavernous plexus and external rete. Extracerebral perivascular VIP-immunoreactive nerves probably arose from VIP-immunoreactive perikarya in microganglia associated with the tympanic plexus, chorda tympani, lingual nerve and Vidian nerve as well as from cells in the otic, sphenopalatine, submandibular and sublingual ganglia. Therefore, it seems likely that each major segment of the cephalic circulation is supplied by local VIP-immunoreactive neurones.

In a more recent systematic study in the rat, Suzuki *et al.* (1988) mapped the origin and pathway of several vascular VIP nerves, using not only immunofluorescent techniques, but denervation and retrograde axonal tracing methods. Interestingly, they found the VIP nerves to the rat cerebral blood vessels originate in the sphenopalatine and otic ganglia, but also arise from the internal carotid mini-ganglion. This contrasts with the cat, where the internal carotid artery is obliterated and where VIP fibres originate from several small aggregates of scattered ganglion cells. In many instances, VIP and ACh are associated in non-sympathetic control of blood vessels. They are both present in the perivascular plexus, but their distribution is not absolutely comparable.

All criteria for VIP transmission have been fulfilled in the feline cephalic arteries: release, postganglionic action, receptor characterization and specific antagonism by a VIP antibody have been demonstrated (Bevan *et al.*, 1984; Brayden and Bevan, 1986). Both mechanisms appear to be coupled in the cat salivary glands (Lundberg, 1981). The combination of ACh and VIP may be involved in thermoregulation, particularly of the head region.

12.4.3. **Dopamine**

DA is found in all adrenergic nerves. It is a precursor in the synthesis of norepinephrine. There is strong evidence that DA is likely to be found in specific nerves that regulate the calibre of small vessels of the dog kidney (Bell, 1988), the organ system where evidence for a role as a putative transmitter is strongest. In this species the classic criteria for a transmitter function have been satisfied, although the exact locus of DA release is debated. It may be that this substance also has a role in the kidney of the rat and the macaque monkey. The evidence supporting the role in these species is not found in other commonly used laboratory animals. The nerves are responsible for vasodilation and renin release (Bell and Lang, 1978). They may be involved in cutaneous vascular shunts and thus related to thermoregulation.

12.4.3. **Conclusions**

In general, there is a paucity of definitive information regarding the nature of the parasympathetic neurocontrol of the vasculature. The transmitters ACh and VIP are established and seem to be the most widespread and universal; together they may constitute the primary autonomic vascular dilator system. Only in a few arteries, however, from the head of the cat, is the experimental support complete. Suggestive as other observations are, they are at present not definitive. This outflow may play a role not only in cephalic vascular regulation and adaptation during salivation, and so on, but also in the maintenance of the temperature of the brain.

Although evidence for DA transmission is impressive in the dog kidney, this effect seems to be very species-specific.

12.5. *Final comments*

Unfortunately, the majority of the experiments carried out on the peripheral neural control mechanisms of the circulation are restricted to a small number of vessels. For this reason the information available is very piecemeal, haphazard and precludes species comparison. What is sadly needed are systematic studies of blood vessels in a species — at least in an entire vascular bed and also between species. Without this, a general view of a particular neural outflow, its distribution and the nature of the transmitter and the details of its postsynaptic system, cannot be charted and related to the functioning of the circulation. Only when this general view is achieved will we begin to obtain a comprehensive picture of what the regulatory and control mechanisms are in the circulation and what they do in support of the body's economy.

Acknowledgment

This work was supported by USPHS HL 32985 and 32383.

References

Appenzeller, O., Dhital, K., Cowen, T. and Burnstock, G. (1984). The nerves to blood vessels supplying blood to nerves: the innervation of vasa nervorum. *Brain Research*, **304**, 383–386.

Bell, C. (1988). Dopamine release from sympathetic nerve terminals. *Progress in Neurobiology*, **30**, 193–208.

Bell, C. and Lang, W. (1978). Effects of renal dopamine receptor and β-adrenoceptor blockade on rises in blood angiotensin after haemorrhage, renal ischaemia and frusemide diuresis in the dog. *Clinical Science and Molecular Medicine*, **54**, 17–23.

Bevan, J. (1977). Some functional consequences of variation in adrenergic synaptic cleft width and in nerve density and distribution. *Federation Proceedings*, **36**, 2439–2443.

Bevan, J. (1979). Sites and transition between functional systemic and cerebral arteries of rabbits occur at embryological junctional sites. *Science*, **204**, 635–637.

Bevan, J. (1984). Autonomic pharmacologist's guide to the cerebral circulation. *Trends in Pharmacological Science*, **5**, 234–236.

Bevan, J. (1990). Flow-dependent vascular tone. In: *The Resistance Vasculature*, in press.

Bevan, J. and Brayden, J. (1986). Nonadrenergic neural vasodilator mechanisms. *Circulation Research*, **60**, 309–326.

Bevan, J. and Osher, J. (1965). Relative sensitively of some large blood vessels of the rabbit to sympathomimetic amines. *Journal of Pharmacology and Experimental Therapy*, **150**, 370–374.

Bevan, J. and Purdy, R. (1973). Variations in adrenergic innervation and contractile responses of the rabbit saphenous artery. *Circulation Research*, **32**, 746–751.

Bevan, J., Bevan, R. and Duckles, S. (1980). Adrenergic regulation of vascular smooth muscle. In: *Handbook of Physiology*, Section 2: The Cardiovascular System, Vol. 2: Vascular Smooth Muscle, edited by D. Bohr, A. Somlyo and H. Sparks. Baltimore; American Physiological Society, pp. 515–566.

Bevan, R., Yang, J. and Bevan, J. (1983). Embryology and functional variation in the arterial system. In: *Vascular Neuroeffector Mechanisms — IV, 4th International Symposium on Vascular Neuroeffector Mechanisms*, 28–30 July 1981, Kyoto, Japan, edited by J. Bevan, R. Maxwell, M. Fujiwara, S. Shibata, N. Toda, and K. Mohri. New York: Raven Press, pp. 209–212.

Bevan, J., Oriowo, M. and Bevan, R. (1986). Physiological variation in α-adrenoceptor-mediated arterial sensitivity: relation to agonist affinity. *Science*, **234**, 196–197.

Bevan, J., Laher, I. and Rowan, R. (1987). Some implications of the high intrasynaptic norepinephrine concentrations in resistance arteries. *Blood Vessels*, **24**, 137–140.

Bevan, J., Bevan, R. and Shreeve, S. (1989). Variable receptor affinity hypothesis. *FASEB Journal*, **3**, 1696–1704.

Bevan, J., Moskowitz, M., Said, S. and Buga, G. (1984). Evidence that vasoactive intestinal polypeptide is a dilator transmitter to some cerebral and extracerebral cranial arteries. *Peptides*, **5**, 385–388.

Bevan, J., Buga, G., Florence, V., Gonsalves, A. and Snowden, A. (1982a). Distribution of choline acetyltransferase in cerebral and extracerebral cranial arteries of the cat. *Circulation Research*, **50**, 470–476.

Bevan, J., Buga, G., Jope, C., Jope, R. and Moritoki, H. (1982b). Further evidence for a muscarinic component to the neural vasodilator innervation of cerebral and cranial extracerebral arteries of the cat. *Circulation Research*, **51**, 421–429.

Brayden, J. and Bevan, J. (1985). Neurogenic muscarinic vasodilation in the cat. *Circulation Research*, **56**, 205–211.

Brayden, J. and Bevan, J. (1986). Evidence that vasoactive intestinal polypeptide (VIP) mediates neurogenic vasodilation of feline cerebral arteries. *Stroke*, **17**, 1189–1192.

Brizzolara, A. and Burnstock, G. (1990). Evidence for noradrenergic–purinergic cotransmission in the hepatic artery of the rabbit. *British Journal of Pharmacology*, **99**, 835–839.

Burnstock, G. and Warland, J. (1987). A pharmacological study of the rabbit saphenous artery *in vitro*: a vessel with a large purinergic contractile response to sympathetic nerve stimulation. *British Journal of Pharmacology*, **90**, 111–120.

Duckles, S. and Bevan, J. (1976). Pharmacological characterization of adrenergic receptors of a rabbit cerebral artery *in vitro*. *Journal of Pharmacology and Experimental Therapy*, **197**, 371–378.

Duverger, D., Edvinsson, L., McKenzie, E., Oblin, A., Rouquier, L., Scatton, B. and Zivkovic, B. (1987). Concentrations of putative neurovascular transmitters in major cerebral arteries and small pial vessels of various species. *Journal of Cerebral Blood Flow Metabolism*, **7**, 497–501.

Florence, V. and Bevan, J. (1979). Biochemical determination of cholinergic innervation in cerebral arteries. *Circulation Research*, **45**, 212–218.

Furness, J. and Marshall, J. (1974). Correlation of the directly observed responses of mesenteric vessels of the rat to nerve stimulation and noradrenaline with the distribution of adrenergic nerves. *Journal of Physiology (London)*, **239**, 75–88.

Fuxe, K. and Sedvall, G. (1965). The distribution of adrenergic nerve fibers to the blood vessels in skeletal muscle. *Acta Physiologica Scandinavica*, **64**, 75–86.

Gibbins, I., Brayden, J. and Bevan, J. (1984). Perivascular nerves with immunoreactivity to vasoactive intestinal polypeptide in cephalic arteries of the cat: distribution, possible origins and functional implications. *Neuroscience*, **13**, 1327–1346.

Hieble, J., Duesler, J. and Daly, R. (1989). Effects of neuropeptide Y on the response of isolated blood vessels to norepinephrine and sympathetic field stimulation. *Journal of Pharmacology and Experimental Therapy*, **250**, 523–528.

Hirst, G. and Edwards, F. (1989). Sympathetic neuroeffector transmission in arteries and arterioles. *Physiological Reviews*, **69**, 546–604.

Hirst, G. and Neild, T. (1980). Evidence for two populations of excitatory receptors on arterial smooth muscle. *Nature*, **283**, 767–768.

Hutchinson, E., Percival, C. and Young, I. (1962). Development of cardiovascular response in the kitten. *Quarterly Journal of Experimental Physiology*, **47**, 201–210.

Ishikawa, N., Ichikawa, T. and Shigei, T. (1980). Possible embryogenetical differences of the dog venous system in sensitivity to vasoactive substances. *Japanese Journal of Pharmacology*, **30**, 807–818.

Johnson, P. (1986). Autoregulation of blood flow. *Circulation Research*, **59**, 483–495.

Kawasaki, H., Takasaki, K., Saito, A. and Goto, K. (1988). Calcitonin gene-related peptide acts as a novel vasodilator neurotransmitter in mesenteric resistance vessels of the rat. *Nature*, **335**, 164–167.

Keatinge, W. (1966). Electrical and mechanical response of arteries to stimulation of sympathetic nerves. *Journal of Physiology* (*London*), **185**, 701–715.

Kennedy, C., Saville, V.L. and Burnstock, G. (1986). The contributions of noradrenaline and ATP to the responses of the rabbit central ear artery to sympathetic nerve stimulation depend on the parameters of stimulation. *European Journal of Pharmacology*, **122**, 291–300.

Kügelgen, I. and Starke, K. (1985). Noradrenaline and adenosine triphosphate as co-transmitters of neurogenic vasoconstriction in rabbit mesenteric artery. *Journal of Physiology*, **367**, 435–455.

Lacroix, J. (1989). Sympathetic vascular control of the pig nasal mucosa (III): co-release of noradrenaline and neuropeptide Y. *Acta Physiologica Scandinavica*, **135**, 17–28.

Laher, I. and Bevan, J. (1985). Alpha adrenoceptor number limits response of some rabbit arteries to norepinephrine. *Journal of Pharmacology and Experimental Therapy*, **233**, 290–297.

Laher, I., Khayal, M. and Bevan, J. (1986a). Norepinephrine sensitive, phenoxybenzamine-resistant receptor sites associated with contraction in rabbit arterial but not venous smooth muscle: possible role in adrenergic neurotransmission. *Journal of Pharmacology and Experimental Therapy*, **237**, 364–368.

Laher, I., Nishimura, S. and Bevan, J. (1986b). Prazosin selectively antagonized norepinephrine contractions at low-affinity, non-α adrenoceptor sites (extraceptors) in arterial muscle. *Journal of Pharmacology and Experimental Therapy*, **239**, 846–852.

Laher, I., Germann, P. and Bevan, J. (1989). The selective potentiation of noradrenaline-induced tone by Bay K 8644 in the rabbit basilar artery. *Journal of Cerebral Blood Flow and Metabolism*, **9**, 759–764.

Ljung, B. (1969). Local transmitter concentration in vascular smooth muscle during vasoconstrictor activity. *Acta Physiologica Scandinavica*, **77**, 212–223.

Ljung, B. (1976). Physiological patterns of neuroeffector control mechanisms. In: *Vascular Neuroeffector Mechanisms*, edited by J. Bevan, G. Burnstock, B. Johansson, R. Maxwell and O. Nedergaard. Basel: Karger, pp. 143–155.

Lundberg, J. (1981). Evidence for coexistence of vasoactive intestinal polypeptide (VIP) and acetylcholine in neurons of cat exocrine glands. Morphological, biochemical and functional aspects. *Acta Physiologica Scandinavica*, **112**, (Suppl. 496), 1–57.

Lundberg, J. and Hökfelt, T. (1986). Multiple coexistence of peptides and classical transmitters in peripheral autonomic and sensory neurons — functional and pharmacological implications. In: *Progress in Brain Research*, Vol. 68, edited by T. Hökfelt, K. Fuxe and B. Pernow. Amsterdam: Elsevier, pp. 241–261.

Lundberg, J., Fried, G., Pernow, J. and Theodorsson-Norheim, E. (1986). Corelease of neuropeptide Y and catecholamines upon adrenal activation in the cat. *Acta Physiologica Scandinavica*, **126**, 231–238.

Mackay, D. (1990). Interpretation of relative potencies, relative efficacies and apparent affinity constants of agonist drugs estimated from concentration–response curves. *Journal of Theoretical Biology*, **142**, 415–427.

Miki, S. (1983). The genesis of the splenic vein. In: *Vascular Neuroeffector Mechanisms*, edited by J. Bevan, R. Maxwell, M. Fujiwara, S. Shibata, N. Toda, and K. Mohri. New York: Raven Press, pp. 195–201.

Muramatsu, I. and Kogoshi, S. (1987). Purinergic and non-purinergic innervation in the cerebral arteries of the dog. *British Journal of Pharmacology*, **92**, 901–908.

Nakazato, Y., Ohga, A., Shigei, T. and Uematsu, T. (1982). Extrinsic innervation of the canine abdominal vena cava and the origin of cholinergic vasoconstrictor nerves. *Journal of Physiology*, **328**, 191–203.

Oriowo, M., Bevan, J. and Bevan, R. (1987). Variation in sensitivity of alpha adrenoceptor-mediated contraction of the vascular smooth muscle of rabbit elastic and muscular arteries is related to receptor affinity. *Journal of Pharmacology and Experimental Therapy*, **241**, 239–244.

Osswald, W. (1976). Transmitter disposition mechanisms. In: *Vascular Neuroeffector Mechanisms*, edited by J. Bevan, G. Burnstock, B. Johansson, R. Maxwell and O. Nedergaard. Basel: Karger, pp. 123–130.

Owen, M., Walmsley, J., Mason, M., Bevan, R. and Bevan, J. (1983). Adrenergic control in three artery segments of diminishing diameter in the rabbit ear. *American Journal of Physiology*, **245**, H320–H326.

Piascik, M., Kusiak, J., Pitha, J., Butler, B., Le, H. and Babich, M. (1988). Alkylation of alpha-1 receptors with a chemically reactive analog of prazosin reveals low affinity sites for norepinephrine in rabbit aorta. *Journal of Pharmacology and Experimental Therapy*, **246**, 1001–1011.

Rowan, R. and Bevan, J. (1983). Distribution of adrenergic synaptic cleft width in vascular and non-vascular smooth muscle. In: *Vascular Neuroeffector Mechanisms — IV, Proceedings of the 4th International Symposium on Vascular Neuroeffector Mechanisms*, 28–30 July 1981, Kyoto, Japan, edited by J. Bevan, R. Maxwell, M. Fujiwara, S. Shibata, N. Toda and K. Mohri. New York: Raven Press, pp. 75–84.

Shibata, S., Hattori, K., Sakurai, I., Mori, J. and Fujiwara, M. (1971). Adrenergic innervation and cocaine-induced potentiation of adrenergic responses of aortic strips from young and old rabbits. *Journal of Pharmacology and Experimental Therapy*, **177**, 621–632.

Shigei, T., Ichikawa, T., Ishikawa, N., Uematsu, T. and Tsuru, H. (1983). Functional venous characteristics in relation to embryology. In: *Vascular Neuroeffector Mechanisms — IV, 4th International Symposium on Vascular Neuroeffector Mechanisms*, 28–30 July 1981, Kyoto, Japan, edited by J. Bevan, R. Maxwell, M. Fujiwara, S. Shibata, N. Toda and K. Mohri. New York: Raven Press, pp. 203–208.

Shreeve, S. (1990). Effect of detergent solubilization on the affinity of some quinazoline derivatives for the α_1-adrenoceptor. *European Journal of Pharmacology*, **188**, 71–80.

Sneddon, P. and Burnstock, G. (1985). ATP as a co-transmitter in the rat tail artery. *European Journal of Pharmacology*, **106**, 149–152.

Suzuki, N., Hardebo, J. and Owman, C. (1988). Origins and pathways of cerebrovascular vasoactive intestinal polypeptide-positive nerves in rat. *Journal of Cerebral Blood Flow and Metabolism*, **8**, 697–712.

Tayo, F. and Bevan, J. (1986). Extracellular calcium dependence of contraction and endothelium-dependent relaxation varies along the length of the aorta and its branches. *Journal of Pharmacology and Experimental Therapy*, **240**, 594–601.

Van Riper, D. and Bevan, J. (1991a). Evidence that neuropeptide Y and norepinephrine mediate electrical stimulated vasoconstriction of rabbit middle cerebral artery. *Circulation Research*, in press.

Van Riper, D. and Bevan, J. (1991b). Selective variation of agonist and neurally-mediated vasoconstriction with rabbit middle cerebral artery branch order. *Journal of Pharmacology*, in press.

Van Riper, D. and Bevan, J. (1991c). Electrical field stimulation mediated relaxation of rabbit middle cerebral artery: evidence of a cholinergic endothelium-dependent component. In preparation.

Waterson, J., Frewin, D. and Soltys, J. (1974). Age-related differences in catecholamine fluorescence of human vascular tissue. *Blood Vessels*, **11**, 79–85.

Wellman, G., Brayden, J. and Bevan, J. (1991). Biochemical and functional evidence for a cholinergic neurodilator pathway in systemic arteries. In preparation.

White, F., Ikeda, M. and Elsner, R. (1973). Adrenergic innervation of large arteries in the seal. *Comparative General Pharmacology*, **4**, 271–276.

Chapter 13

Role and pharmacology of vascular pre- and postjunctional α_2-adrenoceptors

James R. Docherty and Sonia Connaughton

13.1. *Historical Perspective*

Following the subclassification of adrenoceptors into α- and β-subtypes by Ahlquist (1948), the α-adrenoceptors were thought of as receptors which mediate smooth muscle contraction and by implication to be receptors present on the vascular smooth muscle cells in the cardiovascular system. However, even in the 1950s, there was evidence to question this simple picture. As early as 1934 Bacq and Frederico found that α-adrenoceptor antagonists could potentiate the adrenergic stimulation-evoked contraction, and in 1957 Brown and Gillespie found that the α-adrenoceptor antagonists dibenamine and phenoxybenzamine increased the release of neurotransmitter from cat spleen. However, since phenoxybenzamine was shown to increase release of noradrenaline by blockade of neuronal uptake (Thoenen *et al.*, 1964), these results were largely overlooked until evidence accumulated that the α-adrenoceptor antagonist phentolamine increased stimulation-evoked release of noradrenaline by an action distinct from uptake blockade (Starke *et al.*, 1971) and that the α-agonists xylazine (Heise *et al.*, 1971) and clonidine (Starke *et al.*, 1972) decreased stimulation-evoked release of noradrenaline. This led to the concept of prejunctional or presynaptic receptors present on adrenergic nerve terminals (for reviews see Starke, 1977; Langer, 1977; Westfall, 1977), and differences between pre- and postjunctional α-adrenoceptors led to the subclassification of α-adrenoceptors into α_1-postjunctional and α_2-prejunctional (Langer, 1974) (see Figure 13.1).

13.2. *Vascular postjunctional α_2-adrenoceptors in vivo*

The anatomical subdivision of α-adrenoceptors into α_1-postjunctional and α_2-prejunctional did not stand for long. In the pithed rat preparation, Drew and Whiting (1979) reported that pressor responses to the α-adrenoceptor agonist phenylephrine were blocked by the α_1-adrenoceptor antagonist prazosin, but that the pressor response to noradrenaline was resistant to prazo-

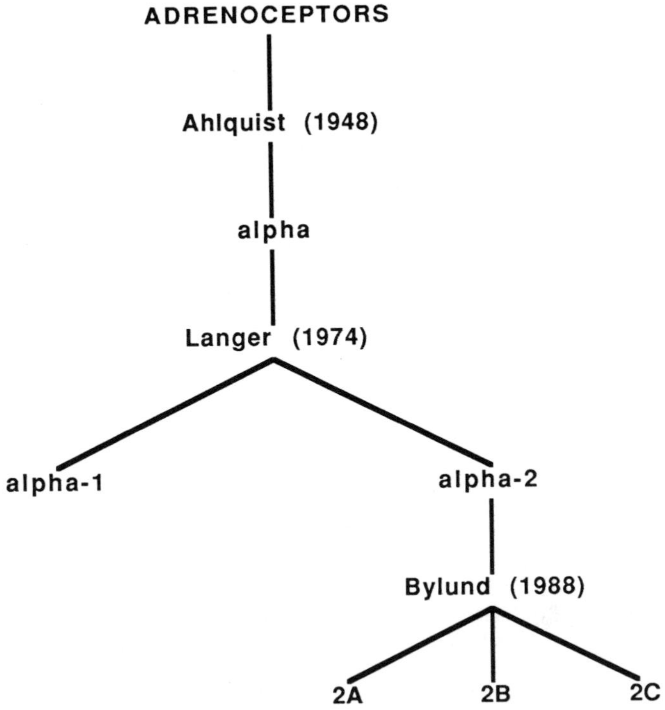

Figure 13.1. Historical developments in α_2-adrenoceptor pharmacology.

sin. This led Drew and Whiting to propose that two types of α-adrenoceptor were present on vascular smooth muscle in the pithed rat: the classical α_1-adrenoceptor and another as yet unidentified α-adrenoceptor.

Further work in the same year confirmed that this unidentified receptor in the pithed rat was indeed a postjunctional α_2-adrenoceptor, since the response was mimicked by α_2-adrenoceptor selective agonists and blocked by α_2-selective antagonists such as yohimbine (Docherty *et al.*, 1979; Timmermans *et al.*, 1979, Docherty and McGrath, 1980). Subsequently, vascular postjunctional α_2-adrenoceptors were also identified *in vivo* in the dog (Constantine and Lebel, 1980), rabbit (Madjar *et al.*, 1980), cat (Drew and Whiting, 1979) and man (Elliott and Reid, 1983).

These identifications of α_2-adrenoceptors postjunctionally on vascular smooth muscle *in vivo* were, at least initially, not matched by concomitant identification of α_2-adrenoceptors postjunctionally *in vitro* using isolated smooth muscle preparations. Vascular postjunctional α_2-adrenoceptors proved difficult to demonstrate *in vitro* (see Docherty and Starke, 1981), leading to the suggestion that either α_2-adrenoceptors were present on microvessels not yet examined *in vitro*, or that additional hormonal factors such as angiotensin were required for the expression of postjunctional α_2-

adrenoceptors. Both of these assumptions have proved to be at least partly correct, since α_2-adrenoceptors can be demonstrated in human microvessels (Nielsen *et al.*, 1990) and the addition of a contractile agent such as angiotensin can reveal α_2-adrenoceptor-mediated contractile responses in some tissues (Schumann and Lues, 1983). However, in some isolated, relatively large blood vessels, α_2-adrenoceptors can be demonstrated without the need to employ angiotensin, for instance, in the human saphenous vein.

13.3. *Vascular postjunctional α_2-adrenoceptors in the human saphenous vein*

Investigations of vascular postjunctional α-adrenoceptors in some human isolated blood vessels have produced results suggesting that a mixed population of α_1- and α_2-adrenoceptors may be present postjunctionally (Stevens and Moulds, 1981; Steel *et al.*, 1984). Evidence that nerve stimulation-evoked contractions can involve postjunctional α_2-adrenoceptors proved difficult to obtain in the early 1980s, and this led to the suggestion that, analogous to vascular β_2-adrenoceptors, vascular α_2-adrenoceptors may be mainly non-synaptic (Langer *et al.*, 1980; Wilffert *et al.*, 1982). However, vascular contractions to nerve stimulation in human saphenous vein appear to be mediated predominantly by α_2-adrenoceptors, since the α_2-adrenoceptor antagonist yohimbine was at least 10 times more potent than the α_1-adrenoceptors antagonist prazosin at inhibiting stimulation-evoked contractions (Docherty and Hyland, 1985, 1986). Contractions to exogenous agonists in the human saphenous vein also involve predominantly α_2-adrenoceptors since yohimbine has relatively high potency (pA_2 values in the range 7.40–8.27) and prazosin had low potency (pA_2 approximately 6.5) or acted non-competitively (Muller-Schweinitzer, 1984; Steen *et al.*, 1984; Docherty and Hyland, 1986; Beckeringh *et al.*, 1987; Connaughton and Docherty, 1988). Hence, vascular postjunctional α_2-adrenoceptors seem to be widely located throughout the body in both arteries and veins, in large and small vessels, and mediate both nerve stimulation and agonist-evoked responses. These receptors can be easily identified *in vitro* in some tissues such as human saphenous vein without the need to precontract the tissue with another agent.

13.4. *Subtypes of α_2-adrenoceptor*

Bylund (1985) subdivided α_2-adrenoceptors into α_{2A} and α_{2B} and subsequently α_{2C} (Bylund, 1988) from radioligand studies employing [^{3}H]-yohimbine. Yohimbine failed to distinguish between subtypes, but the α_1-adrenoceptor antagonist prazosin had surprising affinity for the α_{2B}, and

ORDER NUMBER
PO NYAATP08

BOOK NUMBER
5559341

BAY NUMBER
7196-8

AUTHOR	Stone T W
TITLE	Aspects of Synaptic Transmission: LTP,

to a lesser extent the α_{2C}, subtype, being five times less potent than yohimbine at the α_{2B}, 40 times less potent at the α_{2C} and 500 times less potent at the α_{2A} (Bylund, 1988). Functional correlates of these ligand binding sites have proved difficult to find, although based on the potency of prazosin, Bylund *et al.*, (1988) suggested that α_2-adrenoceptors of adrenergic nerve terminals may be α_{2B}, whereas α_2 of cholinergic nerves may be α_{2A}, since prazosin had high potency prejunctionally at the adrenergic nerve terminals of rat submandibular gland (Turner *et al.*, 1984), mouse vas deferens, rabbit pulmonary artery (Kapocsi *et al.*, 1987) and rat cerebral cortex (Nasseri and Minneman, 1987), but low potency at the α_2-receptors on the cholinergic nerve terminals of guinea-pig ileum (Kapocsi *et al.*, 1987). However, this interpretation relies solely on the prejunctional potency of prazosin in radioactive overflow experiments, and it should be noted that prazosin in concentrations above 0·3 μM increases the basal outflow of tritium in tissues preincubated with tritium-labelled noradrenaline (see Connaughton and Docherty, 1990a; Kapocsi *et al.*, 1987).

We have recently investigated the potencies of a series of 10 α-adrenoceptor antagonists at α_2-adrenoceptors in functional studies and compared potencies obtained with affinities of these antagonists for α_{2A} ligand binding sites in human platelet and for α_{2B} ligand binding sites in rat kidney. It is important to carry out both functional and ligand binding studies in the same laboratory to eliminate inter-laboratory differences in functional or ligand binding studies. Among the compounds employed, as well as prazosin, was ARC 239 which also shows selectivity for α_{2B} ligand binding sites over α_{2A} ligand binding sites (Bylund, 1985, 1988).

In overflow studies, in which the stimulation-evoked release of tritium in tissues preincubated with [^{3}H]-noradrenaline was taken as a measure of transmitter release, antagonist potency was expressed as an EC_{30} value (concentration of antagonist producing 30% potentiation of the stimulation-evoked release of tritium) in rat atrium, vas deferens and submandibular gland (see Table 13.1). Prazosin and ARC 239 both showed higher potency prejunctionally in rat atrium than prejunctionally in rat vas deferens and rat submandibular gland, suggesting that the prejunctional α_2-adrenoceptor on rat atrium differs from those of rat vas deferens and rat submandibular gland. In terms of correlation of functional and ligand binding data from 10 antagonists, the prejunctional α_2-adrenoceptor of rat atrium resembles the α_{2B} ligand binding site whereas the prejunctional α_2-adrenoceptor of rat vas deferens resembles the α_{2A} ligand binding site (Connaughton and Docherty, 1990b) (see Figure 13.2); and presumably the prejunctional α_2-adrenoceptor of rat submandibular gland also resembles the α_{2A} site (see Table 13.1). Table 13.2 lists the suggested interpretation of published results on prejunctional α_2-adrenoceptors, including the three tissues mentioned above. Note that we re-interpret the α_2-adrenoceptor of rat submandibular gland as α_{2A} due to the low potency of ARC 239 rather than relying on prazosin which raises the basal outflow of tritium at concentrations above 0·3 μM. If this

Table 13.1. EC_{30} values obtained to α-adrenoceptor antagonists prejunctionally in rat atrium, vas deferens and submandibular gland.

	EC_{30}		
Antagonist	Atrium	Vas deferens	Submandibular gland
Chlorpromazine	$6{\cdot}53 \pm 0{\cdot}36$	$<6{\cdot}0$	/
BDF 8933	$9{\cdot}18 \pm 0{\cdot}24$	$9{\cdot}26 \pm 0{\cdot}32$	$8{\cdot}88 \pm 1{\cdot}22$
Prazosin	$6{\cdot}97 \pm 0{\cdot}26$	$<6{\cdot}5$	$<6{\cdot}5$
ARC 239	$7{\cdot}40 \pm 0{\cdot}63$	$6{\cdot}17 \pm 0{\cdot}71$[a]	$5{\cdot}95 \pm 0{\cdot}75$[a]
Yohimbine	$7{\cdot}89 \pm 0{\cdot}14$	$7{\cdot}60 \pm 0{\cdot}04$	$7{\cdot}35 \pm 0{\cdot}88$

Values are mean and 95% confidence limits from at least three experiments.
[a] Potency in rat vas deferens or submandibular gland significantly different from potency in rat atrium (Student's *t*-test, [a] $P<0{\cdot}05$).

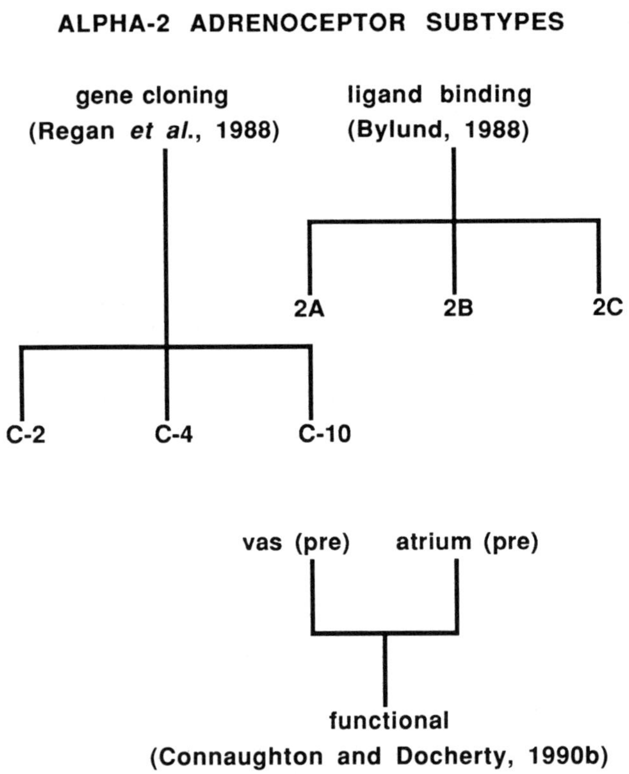

Figure 13.2. Possible relationship between gene cloning, ligand binding and functional subclassifications of α_2-adrenoceptor. The α_{2A} ligant binding site seems to be similar to the receptor cloned from the C-10 chromosome, and resembles the functional prejunctional α_2-adrenoceptor of rat deferens. The α_{2B} ligand binding site may resemble the functional prejunctional receptor of rat atrium. Other similarities between classifications remain to be established.

Table 13.2. Suggested classification of prejunctional α_2-adrenoceptors from published results.

Tissue	Receptor	Subtype	Reference
Rat vas deferens	2A		Connaughton and Docherty, 1990b
Rat submandibular	2A		Present data
Guinea-pig ileum (cholinergic)	2A		Kapocsi *et al.*, 1987
Rat atrium		2B	Connaughton and Docherty, 1990b
Rat cerebral cortex		2B	Nasseri and Minneman, 1987

classification is even partly true (e.g. for the tissues in Table 13.1), then it is clear that more than one subtype of α2-adrenoceptor can be present on adrenergic nerves.

13.5. *Prejunctional α_1-adrenoceptors or subtype of α_2-adrenoceptors*

In the light of evidence for a subtype of prejunctional α_2-adrenoceptor at which prazosin has relatively high potency (about 10 times less potent than yohimbine) it is worth re-examining evidence for prejunctional α_1-adrenoceptors, much of which is based on the relatively high potency of prazosin (see Starke, 1987; Docherty, 1989). For example, prazosin ($0.3\,mg\,kg^{-1}$) increases noradrenaline release *in situ* in dog heart (Cavero *et al.*, 1979), and has lower potency than yohimbine, suggesting that this prejunctional receptor resembles the α_{2B} ligand binding site. However, other studies in which α_1 selective agonists inhibit transmission, and the inhibition can be reversed by prazosin but not yohimbine, are difficult to explain in terms of α_2-adrenoceptor subtypes.

13.6. *Involvement of G-proteins in α_2-adrenoceptor-mediated responses*

Gene cloning techniques suggest that there are at least three genes coding for α_2-adrenoceptors, and the expressed receptors seem to belong to the G-protein linked superfamily of receptors (Kobilka *et al.*, 1987; Regan *et al.*, 1988) (see Figure 13.2). Pertussis toxin, which catalyses the adenosine 5′-diphosphate (ADP)-ribosylation of the guanine-nucleotide binding regulatory proteins G_o and G_i (Murayama and Ui, 1983; Dolphin, 1987), attenuates various responses including α_2-adrenoceptor-mediated vasoconstriction in vascular smooth muscle (Boyer *et al.*, 1983; Docherty, 1988; Nichols *et al.*, 1988). The α_{2A}, α_{2B} and α_{2C} ligand binding sites are all reported to be linked to inhibition of adenylate cyclase, presumably via G_i or G_o (Bylund, 1988). Since these ligand binding sites are presumably postjunctional, it would seem that there is good evidence for the involve-

Table 13.3. Published reports on the effects of pertussis toxin on prejunctional α_2-adrenoceptor-mediated responses.

Tissue	Effect	Reference
Rat hippocampus	Attenuate	Allgaier *et al.*, 1985
Rat vas deferens	Attenuate	Lai *et al.*, 1983
Pithed rat heart	NIL	Docherty, 1988 Nichols *et al.*, 1988
Rat vas deferens	NIL	Docherty, 1988
Rat atria	NIL	Docherty, 1990
Mouse atria	NIL	Musgrave *et al.*, 1987

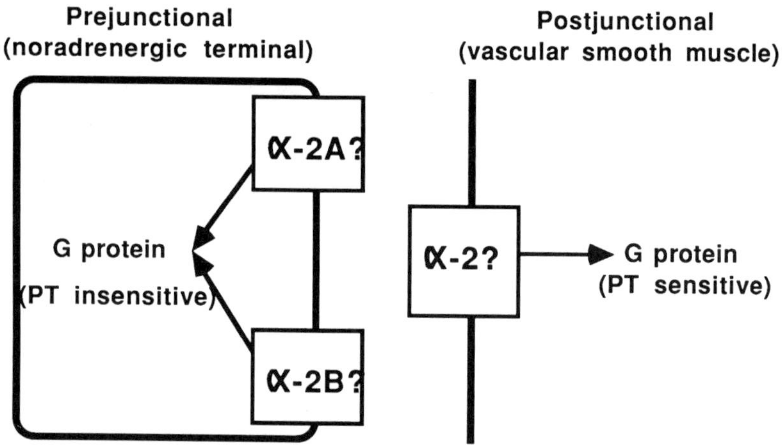

Figure 13.3. Diagramatic representation of pre- and postjunctional α_2-adrenoceptors and their linkage to G-proteins. Both α_{2A}- and α_{2B}-receptors may be present prejunctionally, and the postjunctional α_2-adrenoceptor of vascular smooth muscle has not yet been examined in enough detail for subtyping.

ment of pertussis toxin-sensitive G-proteins in responses mediated by postjunctional α_2-adrenoceptors. However, Table 13.3 shows the conflicting evidence on the possible involvement of pertussis toxin-sensitive G-proteins in prejunctional inhibitory responses mediated by α_2-adrenoceptors. The majority view would support the notion that at least some prejunctional α_2-adrenoceptors are linked to neuronal inhibition through pertussis toxin-insensitive G-proteins (Table 13.3 and Figure 13.3). Since prejunctional α_2-adrenoceptors of rat vas deferens and rat atrium are probably different subtypes of the α_2-adrenoceptor (see above), and yet mediate responses insensitive to pertussis toxin, it would seem that more than one subtype of α_2-adrenoceptor are linked to prejunctional responses via pertussis toxin-insensitive G-proteins (see Figure 13.3). The evidence is also not in favour of prejunctional α_2-adrenoceptors linked to inhibition of adenylate cyclase by a mechanism unaffected by pertussis toxin, since agents which affect cAMP in neurones do not influence the prejunctional response to α_2-adrenoceptor agonists and antagonists in mouse atria (Musgrave *et al.*, 1987). If the prejunctional α_2-adrenoceptors of rat vas deferens and rat atrium do indeed represent the α_{2A} and α_{2B} ligand binding sites, respectively, then it is rather baffling that the functional receptors do not appear to be linked via pertussis toxin-sensitive G-proteins to the inhibition of adenylate cyclase, whereas the ligand binding sites do. Is this evidence for receptor promiscuity with regard to G-proteins? Certainly, there is no clear evidence that the same α_2-adrenoceptor subtype can link to different G-proteins, depending on the tissue.

13.7. *Summary*

α_2-Adrenoceptors are widely located pre- and postjunctionally in the cardiovascular system, but evidence is emerging for subtypes of functional α_2-adrenoceptor in line with ligand binding and gene cloning evidence. Prejunctional and postjunctional α_2-adrenoceptors appear to be linked via different G-proteins to cellular responses, being linked to pertussis toxin-insensitive and -sensitive G-proteins, respectively.

References

Allgaier, C., Feuerstein, T.J., Jackisch, R. and Hertting, G. (1985). Islet-activating protein (pertussis toxin) diminishes α_2-adrenoceptor mediated effects on noradrenaline release. *Naunyn-Schmiedeberg's Archives of Pharmacology*, **331**, 235–239.

Ahlquist, R.P. (1948). A study of the adrenotropic receptors. *American Journal of Physiology*, **153**, 586–600.

Bacq, Z.M. and Frederico, H. (1934). Action adrenolytique d'un derive du dioxane (933F). *Comptes Rendus Societé Belge de Biologie*, **117**, 806–808.

Beckeringh, J.J., Zerkowski, H.-R., Rohm, N. and Brodde, O.-E. (1987). α-Adrenoceptors in preparations of the human saphenous vein. *Journal of Cardiovascular Pharmacology*, **10** (Suppl. 4), S91–S93.

Boyer, J.L., Cardenas, C., Posadas, C. and Garcia-Sainz, J.A. (1983). Pertussis toxin induces tachycardia and impairs the increase in blood pressure produced by alpha$_2$-adrenergic agonists. *Life Sciences*, **33**, 2627–2633.

Brown, G.L. and Gillespie, J.S. (1957). The output of sympathetic transmitter from the spleen of the cat. *Journal of Physiology*, **138**, 81–102.

Bylund, D.B. (1985). Heterogeneity of alpha-2 adrenergic receptors. *Pharmacology Biochemistry and Behaviour*, **22**, 835–843.

Bylund, D.B. (1988). Subtypes of α_2-adrenoceptors: pharmacological and molecular biological evidence converge. *Trends in Pharmacological Sciences*, **9**, 356–361.

Bylund, D.B. Ray-Prenger, C. and Murphy, T.J. (1988). Alpha-2A and alpha-2B adrenergic receptor subtypes: antagonist binding in tissues and cell lines containing only one subtype. *Journal of Pharmacology and Experimental Therapeutics*, **245**, 600–607.

Cavero, I., Dennis, T., Lefevre-Borg, F., Perrot, P., Roach, A.G. and Scatton, B.

(1979). Effects of clonidine, prazosin and phentolamine on heart rate and coronary sinus catecholamine concentration during cardioaccelerator nerve stimulation in spinal dogs. *British Journal of Pharmacology*, **67**, 283–292.

Connaughton, S. and Docherty, J.R. (1988). Evidence that SK&F 104078 does not differentiate between pre- and postjunctional α_2-adrenoceptors. *Naunyn-Schmiedeberg's Archives of Pharmacology*, **338**, 379–382.

Connaughton, S. and Docherty, J.R. (1990a). No evidence for differences between pre- and postjunctional α_2-adrenoceptors in the periphery. *British Journal of Pharmacology*, **99**, 97–102.

Connaughton, S. and Docherty, J.R. (1990b). Functional evidence for heterogeneit of peripheral prejunctional α_2-adrenoceptors. *British Journal of Pharmacology*, **101**, 285–290.

Constantine J.W. and Lebel, W. (1980). Complete blockade by phenoxybenzamine of α_1- but not α_2-vascular receptors in dogs and the effects of propranolol. *Naunyn-Schmiedeberg's Archives of Pharmacology*, **314**, 149–156.

Docherty, J.R. (1988). Pertussis toxin and prejunctional α_2-adrenoceptors in rat heart and vas deferens. *Journal of Autonomic Pharmacology*, **8**, 197–201.

Docherty, J.R. (1989). The pharmacology of α_1- and α_2-adrenoceptors: evidence for and against a further subdivision. *Pharmacology and Therapeutics*, **44**, 241–284.

Docherty, J.R. (1990). No effect of pertussis toxin on peripheral prejunctional α_2-adrenoceptor-mediated responses and on endothelium-dependent relaxations in the rat. *British Journal of Pharmacology*, **100**, 348–352.

Docherty, J.R. and Hyland, L. (1985). Evidence for neuro-effector transmission through postjunctional α_2-adrenoceptors in human saphenous vein. *British Journal of Pharmacology*, **84**, 573–576.

Docherty J.R. and Hyland L. (1986). An examination of 5-hydroxytryptamine receptors in human saphenous vein. *British Journal of Pharmacology*, **89**, 77–81.

Docherty, J.R. and McGrath, J.C. (1980). A comparison of pre- and postjunctional potencies of several alpha-adrenoceptor agonists in the cardiovascular system and anococcygeus muscle of the rat. *Naunyn-Schmiedeberg's Archives of Pharmacology*, **312**, 107–116.

Docherty J.R. and Starke, K. (1981). Postsynaptic α-adrenoceptor subtypes in rabbit blood vessels and rat anococcygeus *in vitro*. *Journal of Cardiovascular Pharmacology*, **3**, 854–866.

Docherty, J.R. MacDonald, A. and McGrath, J.C. (1979). Further subclassification of α-adrenoceptors in the cardiovascular system, vas deferens and anococcygeus of the rat. *British Journal of Pharmacology*, **67**, 421P–422P.

Dolphin, A.C. (1987). Nucleotide binding proteins in signal transduction and disease. *Trends in Neurosciences*, **10**, 53–57.

Drew, G.M. and Whiting, S.B. (1979). Evidence for two distinct types of postsynaptic α-adrenoceptor in vascular smooth muscle *in vivo*. *British Journal of Pharmacology*, **67**, 207–215.

Elliot, H.L. and Reid, J.L. (1983). Evidence for postjunctional vascular α_2-adrenoceptors in peripheral vascular regulation in man. *Clinical Science*, **65**, 237–241.

Heise, A., Kroneberg, G. and Schlossman, K. (1971). α-Sympathicomimetische eigenschaften als ursache der blutdrucksteigernden und blutdrucksenkenden wirkung von BAY 1470. *Naunyn-Schmiedeberg's Archives of Pharmacology*, **268**, 348–360.

Kapocsi, J., Somogyi, G.T., Ludvig, N., Serfozo, P., Harsing, L.G., Woods, R.J. and Vizi, E.S. (1987). Neurochemical evidence for two types of presynaptic alpha$_2$-adrenoceptors. *Neurochemical Research*, **12**, 141–147.

Kobilka, B.K., Matsui, H., Kobilka, T.S., Yang-Feng, T.L., Francke, U., Caron, M.G., Lefkowitz, R.J. and Regan, J.W. (1987). Cloning, sequencing and ex-

pression of the gene coding for the human platelet α_2-adrenergic receptor. *Science*, **238**, 650–656.
Lai, R.-T., Watanabe, Y. and Yoshida, H. (1983). Effect of islet-activating protein (IAP) on contractile responses of rat vas deferens: evidence for participation of Ni (inhibitory GTP binding regulating protein) in the α_2-adrenoceptor-mediated response. *European Journal of Pharmacology*, **90**, 453–456.
Langer, S.Z. (1974). Presynaptic regulation of catecholamine release. *Biochemical Pharmacology*, **23**, 1739–1800.
Langer, S.Z. (1977). Presynaptic receptors and their role in the regulation of transmitter release. *British Journal of Pharmacology*, **60**, 481–497.
Langer, S.Z., Massingham, R. and Shepperson, N.B. (1980). Presence of postsynaptic α_2-adrenoceptors of predominantly extrasynaptic location in the vascular smooth muscle of the dog hind limb. *Clinical Science*, **59** (Suppl. 6), 225s–228s.
Madjar, H. Docherty, J.R. and Starke, K. (1980). An examination of pre- and postsynaptic alpha-adrenoceptors in the autoperfused rabbit hind limb. *Journal of Cardiovascular Pharmacology*, **2**, 619–627.
Muller-Schweinitzer, E. (1984). Alpha-adrenoceptors, 5-hydroxytryptamine receptors and the action of dihydroergotamine in human venous preparations obtained during saphenectomy procedures for varicose veins. *Naunyn-Schmiedeberg's Archives of Pharmacology*, **327**, 299–303.
Murayama, T. and Ui, M. (1983). Loss of inhibitory function of the guanine nucleotide regulatory component of adenylate cyclase due to its ADP ribosylation by islet-activating protein pertussis toxin in adipocyte membranes. *Journal of Biological Chemistry*, **258**, 3319–3326.
Musgrave, I., Marley, P. and Majewski, J. (1987). Pertussis toxin does not attenuate α_2-adrenoceptor mediated inhibition of noradrenaline release in mouse atria. *Naunyn-Schmiedeberg's Archives of Pharmacology*, **336**, 280–286.
Nasseri, A. and Minneman, K.P. (1987). Relationship between α_2-adrenergic receptor binding sites and the functional receptors inhibiting norepinephrine release in rat cerebral cortex. *Molecular Pharmacology*, **32**, 655–662.
Nichols, A.J., Motley, E. and Ruffolo, R.R. (1988). Differential effect of pertussis toxin on pre- and postjunctional α_2-adrenoceptors in the cardiovascular system of the pithed rat. *European Journal of Pharmacology*, **145**, 345–349.
Nielsen, H., Mortensen, F.V. and Mulvany, M.J. (1990). Responses to noradrenaline in human subcutaneous resistance arteries are mediated by both α_1- and α_2-adrenoceptors. *British Journal of Pharmacology*, **99**, 31–34.
Regan, J.W., Kobilka, T.S., Yang-Feng, T.L., Caron, M.G., Lefkowitz, R.J. and Kobilka, B.K. (1988). Cloning and expression of a human kidney cDNA for an α-adrenergic receptor subtype. *Proceedings of the National Academy of Sciences USA*, **85**, 6301–6305.
Schumann, H.-J. and Lues, I. (1983). Postjunctional α-adrenoceptors in the isolated saphenous vein of the rabbit. *Naunyn-Schmiedeberg's Archives of Pharmacology*, **323**, 328–334.
Starke, K. (1977). Regulation of noradrenaline release by presynaptic receptor systems. *Reviews of Physiology, Biochemistry and Pharmacology*, **77**, 1–124.
Starke, K. (1987). Presynaptic α-autoreceptors. *Reviews of Physiology, Biochemistry and Pharmacology*, **107**, 73–146.
Starke, K., Montel, H. and Schumann, J.J. (1971). Influence of cocaine and phenoxybenzamine on noradrenalin uptake and release. *Naunyn-Schmiedeberg's Archives of Pharmacology*, **270**, 210–214.
Starke, K., Wagner, J. and Schumann, H.J. (1972). Adrenergic neurone blockade by clonidine: comparison with guanethidine and local anaesthetics. *Archives Internationales de Pharmacodynamie et de Therapie*, **195**, 291–308.
Steen, S., Sjoberg, T., Skarby, T., Norgren, L. and Andersson, K.-E. (1984). The

postjunctional α-adrenoceptors of the human saphenous vein. *Acta Pharmacologica et Toxicologica*, **55**, 351–357.

Stevens, M.J. and Moulds, R.F.W. (1981). Heterogeneity of postjunctional α-adrenoceptors in human vascular smooth muscle. *Archives Internationales de Pharmacodynamie et de Therapie*, **254**, 43–57.

Thoenen, H., Hurlimann, A. and Haefely, W. (1964). Wirkungen von phenoxybenzamin, phentolamine und azapetin auf adrenergische synapsen der katzenmilz. *Helvetica Physiologica Pharmacologica Acta*, **22**, 148–161.

Timmermans, P.B.M.W.M., Kwa, H.Y. and Van Zwieten, P.A. (1979). Possible subdivision of postsynaptic α-adrenoceptors mediating pressor responses in the pithed rat. *Naunyn-Schmiedeberg's Archives of Pharmacology*, **310**, 189–193.

Turner, J.T., Pierce, D.L. and Bylund, D.B. (1984). Alpha-2 adrenergic regulation of norepinephrine release in the rat submandibular gland as measured by HPLC-EC. *Life Sciences*, **35**, 1385–1394.

Westfall, T.C. (1977). Local regulation of adrenergic neurotransmission. *Physiological Reviews*, **57**, 659–728.

Wilffert, B., Timmermans, P.B.M.W.M. and Van Zweiten, P.A. (1982). Extrasynaptic location of alpha-2 and noninnervated beta-2 adrenoceptors in the vascular system of the pithed normotensive rat. *Journal of Pharmacology and Experimental Therapy*, **221**, 762–768.

Chapter 14

Synaptic transmission in airways

Peter J. Barnes

14.1. *Introduction*

Autonomic nerves regulate many aspects of airway function and influence the tone of airway smooth muscle, airway secretions, blood flow and microvascular permeability (Barnes, 1986e). Neural control of human airways is complex and the contribution of neurogenic mechanisms to the pathogenesis of airway disease is still uncertain (Kaliner and Barnes, 1988). Because changes in bronchomotor tone in asthma occur rapidly, it was suggested many years ago that there might be an abnormality in autonomic neural control in asthma with an imbalance between excitatory and inhibitory pathways, resulting in excessively 'twitchy' airways. Cholinergic and adrenergic mechanisms in airways have long been recognized, but in addition to these classical pathways non-adrenergic non-cholinergic (NANC) mechanisms have more recently been described (Figure 14.1). While originally these were conceptualized as separate neural pathways it is now apparent that NANC mechanisms describe co-transmitter release from nerves such as cholinergic and afferent nerves. The idea that autonomic control may be abnormal in asthma was first suggested by the observations of Alexander and Paddock (1921), who observed that wheezing was precipated in asthmatics, but not in normal subjects, by injection of the cholinergic agonist pilocarpine, and that this was reversed by injection of the β-adrenoceptor agonist adrenaline. This suggested an imbalance between cholinergic and adrenergic nervous systems. Several types of autonomic defect have been proposed in asthma, including enhanced cholinergic, α-adrenergic and excitatory NANC mechanisms, or reduced β-adrenergic and inhibitory NANC mechanisms. Various abnormalities in airway control have been described in asthma, although it now seems unlikely that these are primary defects, but are secondary to the disease or its treatment. Nevertheless, it is likely that neural mechanisms contribute to the symptoms of asthma and other airway diseases.

The recognition that inflammation plays a key role in asthma raises the possibility that there may be some interaction between neural and inflammatory mechanisms (Barnes, 1986a). Inflammatory mediators may modulate or facilitate the release of neurotransmitters from airway nerves, or may act on

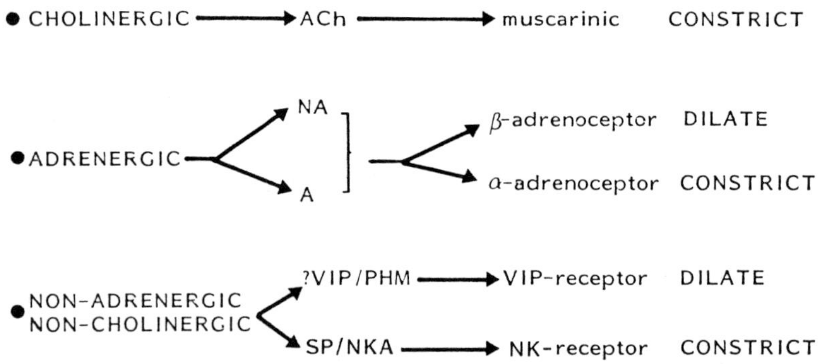

Figure 14.1. Neural control of airways. At least three types of neural mechanism are recognized. Cholinergic nerves release acetylcholine (ACh) which acts on muscarinic receptors (M), adrenergic nerves release noradrenaline (NA) and the adrenal medulla releases adrenaline (A) which act on adrenoceptors. Non-adrenergic non-cholinergic (NANC) nerves are also recognized, which may include several types of nerve, some bronchodilator and some bronchoconstrictor. The neurotransmitters of NANC nerves are likely to be peptides, such as vasoactive intestinal peptide (VIP), substance P (SP), peptide histidine methionine (PHM) and neurokinin A. (NKA).

autonomic receptors. Similarly, neural mechanisms may contribute to the inflammatory reaction in the airway wall, and the concept of neurogenic inflammation, which is well established in skin and gut, may also apply to the airways (Barnes, 1986b; Lundberg and Saria, 1987).

The purpose of this chapter is to review aspects of neurotransmission in airways, and particularly those mechanisms which may be relevant to asthma.

14.2. *Cholinergic mechanisms*

Cholinergic nerves are the dominant neural bronchoconstrictor pathway in animal and human airways (Richardson, 1979; Barnes, 1986e). Cholinergic pathways arise in the dorsal motor muscles of the vagus and travel down the vagus nerve to synapse in parasympathetic ganglia which are situated in the airway wall itself (Figure 14.2). Short postganglionic nerve fibres then pass to target cells in the airway which are predominantly airway smooth muscle and submucosal glands. Stimulation of cholinergic pathways results in bronchoconstriction and mucus secretion.

There has been considerable interest in whether cholinergic mechanisms are exaggerated in asthma or chronic obstructive airways disease (COAD). This idea is supported by the observation that many stimuli which produce bronchospasm (such as sulphur dioxide, prostaglandins, histamine and cold air) also stimulate afferent receptors and may therefore lead to reflex cholinergic bronchoconstriction (Nadel and Barnes, 1984; Nadel *et al.*, 1986). Anticholinergic drugs are effective bronchodilators in COAD and acute

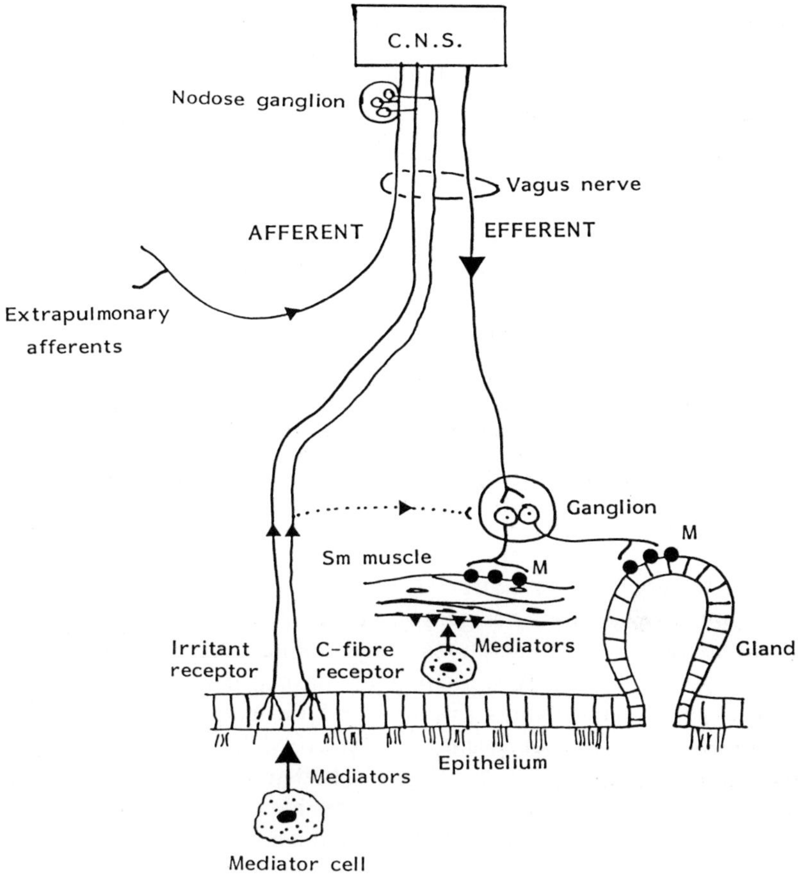

Figure 14.2. Cholinergic control of airways.

asthma, although they are usually less useful in chronic asthma. There are several mechanisms which might contribute to cholinergic bronchoconstriction in asthma (Barnes, 1987b).

14.2.1. **Increased vagal tone**

There is normally a certain degree of vagal tone which is demonstrated by the bronchodilation which follows vagus nerve secretion in animals and anticholinergic drugs in normal human subjects. There may be an increase in central vagal drive in asthmatic patients, although there is no direct evidence for this. Indirect evidence, which may suggest such an increase in vagal tone, is the enhanced vagal cardiac tone (as determined by the Valsalva manoeuvre and sinus arrhythmia) which has been demonstrated in asthma (Kallenbach *et al.*, 1985). There is also evidence that the increase in sinus arrhythmia gap increases at night as bronchoconstriction increases, suggesting that an increase in vagal cholinergic tone may contribute to nocturnal asthma (Postma *et al.*, 1985).

14.2.2. **Reflex bronchoconstriction**

There may be increased reflex bronchoconstriction due to stimulation of sensory receptors in the airway (irritant receptors and C-fibre endings) by inflammatory mediators. Several mediators, such as histamine, prostaglandins and bradykinin, have been shown to stimulate sensory receptors (Barnes, 1986e), and it is possible that these receptors may be more easily triggered in asthma, since airway epithelium may be damaged, or sensory endings 'sensitized' by inflammatory mediators such as bradykinin or prostaglandins (Kaufman *et al.*, 1980; Coleridge and Coleridge, 1984).

14.2.3. **Increased acetylcholine release**

There may be enhanced neurotransmission in cholinergic ganglia, perhaps because of release of other neurotransmitters or mediators, or facilitation of acetylcholine release from postganglionic nerve terminals. Thus, a thromboxane mimetic, U46619, facilitates acetylcholine release in canine airways (Chung *et al.*, 1985), whereas tachykinins have a similar action in rabbit, ferret and guinea-pig airways (Tanaka and Grunstein, 1986; Hall *et al.*, 1989). Since adrenergic nerves may inhibit acetylcholine release, either via β-adrenoceptros (Danser *et al.*, 1987; Rhoden *et al.*, 1988) or via α_2-receptors (Grundstrom *et al.*, 1981), it is possible that a defect in adrenergic mechanisms may be reflected by an increase in cholinergic tone. Neurotransmission through parasympathetic ganglia may be enhanced by inflammatory mediators, and there is evidence for facilitated transmission in sensitized animals exposed to allergen (McCaig, 1987). Histamine, surprisingly, has an inhibitory effect on ganglionic neurotransmission and on postganglionic nerves in guinea-pig and human airways, which is mediated through neuronal H3-receptors (Ichinose *et al.*, 1989; Ichinose and Barnes, 1989). These receptors are activated by low concentrations of histamine and may represent a safety device to inhibit reflex bronchoconstriction, whereas larger concentrations of histamine may override this mechanism and cause bronchoconstriction directly by acting on H1-receptors on airway smooth muscle.

14.2.4. **Muscarinic receptors**

There may be an increased effect of cholinergic stimulation of airway smooth muscle due to an increase in muscarinic receptor density or affinity, or due to increased efficacy of signal transduction (Barnes, 1987c, 1990a). Asthmatic patients show an exaggerated bronchoconstrictor response to cholinergic agonists, but this is not specific, since a similar increased responsiveness is observed with other spasmogens, such as histamine, leukotrienes or prostaglandins, suggesting that an isolated enhancement of muscarinic receptors is unlikely. There are conflicting reports about the response of asthmatic airways *in vitro* to cholinergic agonists and other spasmogens, and an exaggerated response to cholinergic agonists has not consistently been demonstrated. In guinea-pigs, which become hyper-responsive to acetylcholine after intravenous or inhaled platelet-activating factor (PAF), there is no increase in response of airways *in vitro* to acetylcholine, no change in muscarinic receptors as determined by direct receptor binding, nor any change in coupling or biochemical consequences of receptor activation as measured by cholinergic stimulation of phosphoinositide turnover (Robertson *et al.*, 1988). This indicates that the increased cholinergic responsiveness cannot be explained by enhancement of muscarinic receptors in airway smooth muscle, and perhaps is more likely to be explained by mechanical factors such as airway oedema induced by PAF.

14.2.5. **Cholinergic mechanisms in asthma**

Cholinergic antagonists are generally less effective as bronchodilators in asthma than are β-agonists, which reverse bronchoconstriction irrespective of the contractile stimulus (Gross and Skorodin, 1984). This implies that airway smooth muscle is contracted mainly by mechanisms additional to vagal tone, and presumably several mediators may act directly on airway smooth muscle, and against which cholinergic antagonists would not be effective. Thus, histamine bronchoconstriction is weakly affected by anticholinergic treatment in human subjects (whereas in dog, histamine bronchoconstriction is largely abolished by vagal nerve section or by atropine). Cholinergic mechanisms are likely to be more important in acute asthma exacerbations, since nebulized anticholinergics may be almost as effective as β-agonists as bronchodilators (Rebuck *et al.*, 1987).

14.2.6. **Cholinergic mechanisms in COAD**

Cholinergic mechanisms appear to play a more important role in COAD, and anticholinergics may be as effective as β-agonists (Gross and Skorodin, 1984). This indicates that vagal tone is the only reversible element in the airways obstruction of COAD. There is no direct evidence for increased vagal cholinergic tone in COAD and the bronchodilator response may be explained entirely by geometric factors since vagal tone will have a relatively greater effect on airway resistance if the airway is narrowed (Barnes, 1987b). Cholinergic stimulation may contribute to the increased mucus secretion in chronic bronchitis.

14.2.7. **Muscarinic receptor subtypes**

At least three subtypes of muscarinic receptor have been recognized pharmacologically, and five distinct receptor subtypes have now been cloned. Muscarinic receptor subtypes have recently been recognized in airways (Barnes *et al.*, 1988). Inhibitory muscarinic receptors (autoreceptors) have been demonstrated on cholinergic nerves of airways in animals *in vivo* (Fryer and Maclagan, 1984). Autoreceptors have also been demonstrated on human bronchi *in vitro* (Minette and Barnes, 1988). These receptors inhibit acetylcholine release and therefore may serve to limit vagal bronchoconstriction. These receptors are of the M2-subtype and clearly different pharmacologically from M3-receptors on airway smooth muscle. Drugs such as atropine and ipratropium bromide, which block both prejunctional receptors and those on smooth muscle with equal affinity, therefore increase acetylcholine release which may then overcome the postjunctional blockade. This means that such drugs will not be as effective against vagal bronchoconstriction as against cholinergic agonists, so it may be necessary to re-evaluate the contribution of cholinergic nerves when drugs which are selective for the muscarinic receptors on airway smooth muscle (M3-antagonists) are developed. Indeed, in animals low doses of ipratropium bromide increase vagally-mediated bronchoconstriction (Fryer and Maclagan, 1987).

Recently, the presence of muscarinic autoreceptors has been demonstrated in human subjects *in vivo*. A cholinergic agonist, pilocarpine, which selectively activates these M2-receptors, inhibits cholinergic reflex bronchoconstriction induced by sulphur dioxide in normal subjects, but such an inhibitory mechanism does not appear to operate in asthmatic subjects, suggesting that there may be dysfunction of these autoreceptors (Minette *et al.*, 1989). Such a defect in muscarinic autoreceptors may then result in exaggerated cholinergic reflexes in asthma, since the normal feedback inhibition of acetylcholine release may be lost. This might also explain the sometimes catastrophic bronchoconstriction which occurs with β-blockers in asthma which, at least in mild asthmatics, appears to be mediated by cholinergic pathways (Ind *et al.*, 1989). Antagonism of inhibitory β-receptors on cholinergic nerves would result in an increased release of acetylcholine which could not switch itself off in the asthmatic subject (Barnes, 1989) (Figure 14.3).

M1-receptors, which are excitatory, are present in airway ganglia of animals and may be inhibited by pirenzepine (Bloom *et al.*, 1988). The function of these M1-receptors in regulation of airway tone is not yet certain, but they may play an important role in the 'setting' of vagal tone, since these receptors appear to be important in the chronic regulation of ganglionic transmission, whereas the classic nicotinic receptors may be more important in rapid neurotransmission, as in reflexes. Similar receptors are also likely to be present in human parasympathetic ganglia, since pirenzepine inhibits reflex bronchoconstriction at doses which do not inhibit the direct effect of

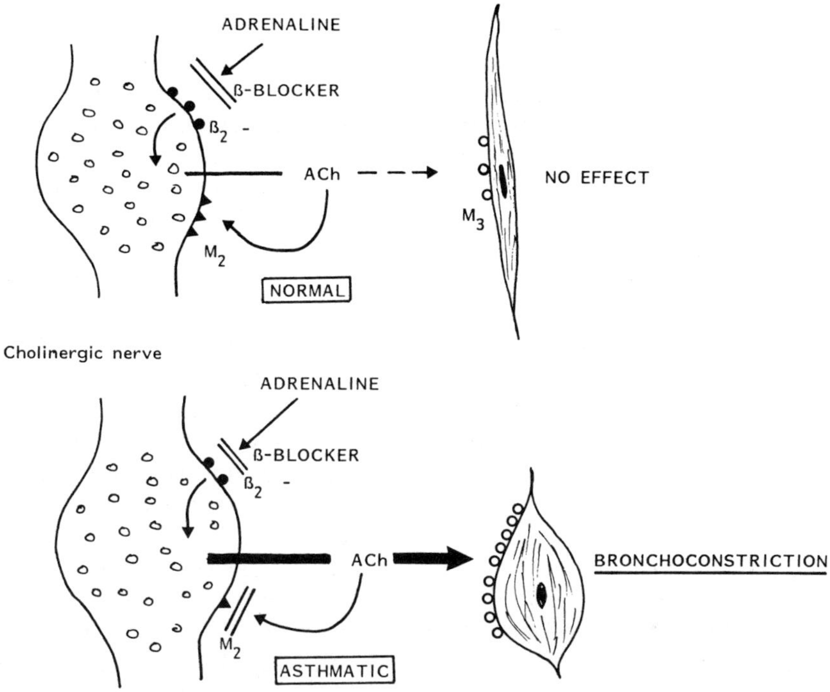

Figure 14.3. Possible mechanism of β-blocker induced bronchoconstriction. β-Blockers may inhibit the modulatory effect of circulating adrenaline on β_2-receptors of cholinergic nerves, thus increasing acetylcholine (ACh) release. In normal people this may act at M2 autoreceptors to inhibit further ACh release, so no effect on airway smooth muscle is seen. In asthmatic patients, if there is a defect in M2 autoreceptors the increased ACh cannot switch itself off. Released ACh also has a greater effect on airway smooth muscle because of bronchial hyper-reactivity.

cholinergic agonists in airway tone (Lammers *et al.*, 1989a). Muscarinic receptor subtypes have now been mapped out in human lung by autoradiographic technique (Mak and Barnes, 1990). M3-receptors are localized, as expected, to airway smooth muscle and submucosal glands, but M1-receptors are found on submucosal glands and on alveolar walls.

14.3. *Adrenergic mechanisms*

Since adrenergic agonists have a dramatic effect in relieving asthmatic bronchoconstriction, it was logical to suggest that there might be a defect in adrenergic control in asthma. Szentivanyi (1968) proposed that there was a fundamental defect in β-adrenoceptor function in asthma. Adrenergic mechanisms involve sympathetic nerves, circulating catecholamines and α- and β-adrenoceptors. Several defects might be present in asthma (Barnes, 1988).

14.3.1. **Adrenergic innervation**

Adrenergic nerves do not control human airway smooth muscle directly (Richardson, 1979; Barnes, 1986e), but could influence cholinergic neurotransmission via prejunctional adrenoceptors (Grundstrom *et al.*, 1981; Danser *et al.*, 1987; Rhoden *et al.*, 1988). There is no evidence to suggest that sympathetic neurotransmission may be abnormal in asthma, but it is possible that inflammatory mediators, such as histamine, might impair the release of noradrenaline from adrenergic nerves. Adrenergic neural control of the bronchial vasculature may also be important in asthma, particularly during exercise and cold air challenge, when conditioning of inspired air may be important.

14.3.2. **Circulating catecholamines**

Since adrenergic nerves do not directly control airway smooth muscle, it seems probable that circulating catecholamines may play a more important role in regulation of bronchomotor tone (Barnes, 1986c). Although the catecholamines noradrenaline, adrenaline and dopamine are present in the circulation, only adrenaline has physiological effects, and is secreted by the adrenal medulla. Since β-blockers cause bronchoconstriction in asthmatic patients, but not in normal subjects, this suggests that there is an increase in adrenergic drive to the airways and in the absence of adrenergic innervation this might be provided by circulating adrenaline. However, plasma adrenaline concentrations are not elevated in asthmatic patients (Barnes *et al.*, 1982a), even in those who bronchoconstrict with intravenous propranolol (Ind *et al.*, 1985). A degree of exercise sufficient to precipitate exercise-induced asthma fails to elevate plasma adrenaline, although such a rise is seen in normal subjects, who perform the same degree of exercise (Barnes *et al.*, 1981c). This suggests that there may be a problem in mobilization of adrenaline in asthma, but this is unlikely to be due to a defect in adrenal medullary secretion, since hypoglycaemia stimulates a large rise in plasma adrenaline, as in normal subjects. The nature of this impaired secretary response in asthma remains uncertain.

14.3.3. **β-adrenoceptors**

The possibility that β-receptors are abnormal in asthma has been extensively investigated. The original suggestion that there was a primary defect in β-receptor function in asthma (Szentivanyi, 1968) has not been substantiated (Tattersfield *et al.*, 1983) and any defect in β-receptors is likely to be secondary to the disease, perhaps as a result of inflammation or as a result of adrenergic therapy. Airways from asthmatic patients fail to relax normally to isoprenaline, suggesting a possible defect in β-receptor function in airway smooth muscle (Cerrina *et al.*, 1986; Goldie *et al.*, 1986). Whether this is due to a reduction in β-receptors, a defect in receptor coupling or some abnormality in the biochemical pathways leading to relaxation, is not yet known. However, the fact that asthmatic airways relax normally to theophylline suggests the defect may be specific for β-receptors (Goldie *et al.*, 1986).

It is possible that inflammation might lead to such abnormalities in β-receptor function. β-receptors are widely distributed in lung and are localized to many different types of cell (Barnes *et al.*, 1982b; 1983a; Carstairs *et al.*, 1985). Stimulation of phosphoinositide (PI) hydrolysis may lead to down-regulation and uncoupling of β-receptors in airway smooth muscle, probably via the activation of protein kinase C which occurs in response to diacylglycerol generated by PI hydrolysis (Grandordy *et al.*, 1990). Since many inflammatory mediators and spasmogens may stimulate PI hydrolysis in airway smooth muscle cells this may provide an explanation for impaired β-receptor function in asthma. Thus, stimulation of one type of receptor may affect another receptor (receptor transmodulation). Since such a defect would be proportional to the severity of inflammation it might only be relevant in more severe asthmatic patients.

14.3.4. **α-Adrenoceptors**

α-Receptors which mediate bronchoconstriction have been demonstrated in airways of several species, including humans, but α-adrenoceptor-mediated contraction may only be demonstrated under certain conditions (Kneussl and Richardson, 1978). In canine trachea histamine and serotonin facilitate α-adrenergic bronchoconstriction *in vitro* (Kneussl and Richardson, 1978; Barnes *et al.*, 1983b) and *in vivo* (Brown *et al.*, 1983), an effect which is not due to any change in α-receptor density or affinity (Barnes *et al.*, 1983b). In sensitized guinea-pigs exposed to allergen aerosol there is an increase in α-receptor density (Barnes *et al.*, 1980). If α-adrenergic facilitation were important in asthma then α-blocking drugs should be beneficial, yet specific α-blockers such as prazosin have little or no effect in asthma (Barnes *et al.*, 1981a,b; Baudouin *et al.*, 1988). It is difficult to understand how α-receptors on airway smooth muscle would be activated in the absence of direct adrenergic innervation, and in any case noradrenaline causes bronchodilation rather than bronchoconstriction in asthmatic patients (Larssen *et al.*, 1986).

The situation is complicated by the demonstration of inhibitory α_2-receptors on cholinergic nerves which would have the opposite effect to α-receptors on airway smooth muscle (Anderson *et al.*, 1986), and the demonstration that α-agonists reduce microvascular leakiness in airways (Boschetto *et al.*, 1989), and may therefore have a beneficial anti-inflammatory effect in asthma, by reducing airway mucosal oedema. Indeed, it is this property of adrenaline to blanch the skin which first suggested that it might be useful in asthma at the beginning of this century, when it was viewed as a disease of vascular instability.

14.4. *NANC nerves and neuropeptides*

The role of NANC nerves in regulation of airway calibre remains uncertain, since the neurotransmitters involved have not always been conclusively identified and potent specific blockers are not yet available (Barnes, 1986d). There is increasing evidence that neuropeptides may act as neurotransmitters of NANC nerves, and many neuropeptides, which have potent effects on many aspects of airway function, have now been identified in human airways (Barnes, 1987b,d,e; Lundberg and Saria, 1987; Uddman and Sundler, 1987).

14.4.1. **Inhibitory NANC nerves**

Electrical field stimulation of human airways results in a neural bronchodilator response which is not affected by adrenergic blockade. The neurotransmitter of this inhibitory NANC response is not yet certain, but circumstantial evidence has implicated vasoactive intestinal peptide (VIP). A defect in non-adrenergic inhibitory nerves has been proposed in asthma, since this is the only neural bronchodilator pathway in human airways (Richardson, 1979). This could arise from an intrinsic defect in these nerves (which seems unlikely), or could be due to a secondary abnormality such as increased breakdown of the neurotransmitter (which may be VIP) or a defect in the NANC inhibitory receptors. An absence of VIP-immunoreactive nerves has been described in asthmatic airways (Ollerenshaw *et al.*, 1989b). VIP is susceptible to enzymatic degradation by a variety of enzymes (Caughey *et al.*, 1988). Inflammatory cells release a variety of peptidases (including tryptase), which may lead to more rapid breakdown of VIP in asthmatic airways (Barnes, 1987a). Mast cell tryptase is able to block NANC inhibitory responses in canine airways *in vitro* and to increase airway responsiveness (Sekizawa *et al.*, 1989). NANC bronchodilation has been demonstrated in human airways *in vivo* (Michoud *et al.*, 1987; Ichinose *et al.*, 1988; Lammers *et al.*, 1988), but does not appear to be defective in mild asthma (Lammers *et al.*, 1989b). However, this does not preclude a secondary defect in more severe asthma, when inflammation is more pronounced. VIP is a potent dilator of human bronchi *in vitro* (Palmer *et al.*, 1986). VIP is a co-transmitter with acetylcholine in airway cholinergic nerves (Laitinen *et al.*, 1985) and may act as a 'braking' mechanism to cholinergic bronchoconstriction, since VIP acts as a functional antagonist to acetylcholine-induced contraction of airway smooth muscle. If VIP is more rapidly degraded in asthma, this may lead to exaggerated cholinergic bronchoconstriction (Figure 14.4).

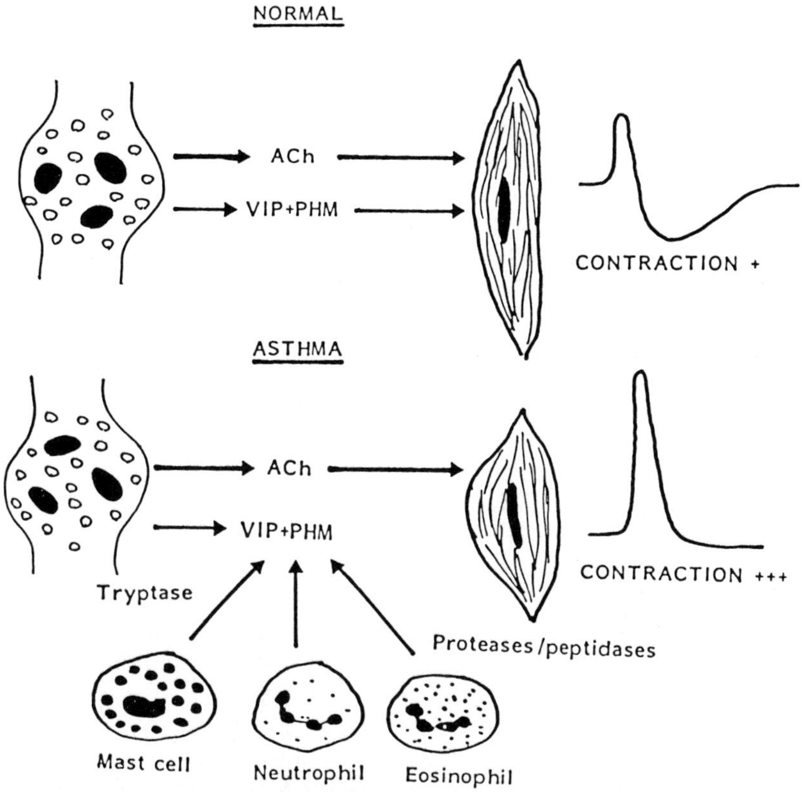

Figure 14.4. Vasoactive intestinal peptide (VIP) co-transmission in asthma. VIP acts as a co-transmitter with acetylcholine (ACh) in airway cholinergic nerves and may act as a functional 'brake' for cholinergic nerve bronchoconstriction. In asthma, peptidases from inflammatory cells (e.g. tryptase from mast cells) may rapidly degrade VIP, leading to unopposed cholinergic bronchoconstriction. PHM, peptide histidine methionine.

14.4.2. **Excitatory NANC nerves**

Electrical field stimulation of guinea-pig bronchi results in a biphasic contractile response. A brief cholinergic response is followed by a slow contractile response. Thus, circulating NANC response is inhibited by prior treatment with capsaicin to destroy unmyelinated sensory nerves which contain neuropeptides, and by a tachykinin antagonist (Lundberg *et al.*, 1988). This suggests that retrograde activation of sensory nerves may release constrictor peptides such as tachykinins. If these sensory endings are activated in asthma by exposure of epithelial nerve endings and release of mediators, such as bradykinin and prostaglandins, then an axon reflex may be triggered (Barnes, 1986b). Release of tachykinins would then lead to bronchoconstriction, microvascular leakage and mucus hypersecretion.

14.4.3. **Tachykinins**

Substance P (SP) has long been recognized as a bronchoconstrictor and also contracts human and animal airways *in vitro* (Lundberg *et al.*, 1983a). It also has a number of other effects on airway function which mimic asthma (Barnes, 1987e; Lundberg *et al.*, 1988). Other tachykinins have now been identified in airway nerves, including neuropeptide K and neurokinin A (NKA) (Martling *et al.*, 1987). SP constricts human airways *in vitro* (Lundberg *et al.*, 1983a), but has no effect when given by infusion or inhalation *in vivo* (Fuller *et al.*, 1987b). By contract, NKA is more potent as a constrictor of human bronchi *in vitro* (Martling *et al.*, 1987; Palmer and Barnes, 1987), and also causes bronchoconstriction *in vivo* either by infusion (Evans *et al.*, 1988) or by inhalation (Joos *et al.*, 1987).

Tachykinins are degraded predominantly by neutral metalloendopeptidase (enkephalinase, EC 3.4.24.11) (Skidgel *et al.*, 1984; Sekizawa *et al.*, 1987) which is localized predominantly to airway epithelium. Epithelium removal greatly exaggerates the constrictor effect of tachykinins (Grandordy *et al.*, 1988; Frossard *et al.*, 1989). Specific inhibitors of neutral endopeptidase, such as phosphoramidon and thiorphan, enhance the contractile response to NKA to the same extent as epithelial removal, and no further effect of epithelium removal can be demonstrated, suggesting that metabolism of NKA by epithelium enzymes accounts for this effect of epithelium (Frossard *et al.*, 1989). For SP it is slightly more complex, since it may in addition release prostaglandins and a relaxant factor from airway epithelium via SP-preferring (NK-1)receptors. These observations may be of relevance to asthma, since if epithelium is shed then tachykinins, if released from sensory nerves, would not be degraded as effectively and this would exaggerate their effects — such as bronchoconstriction, microvascular leakage and mucus secretion.

SP is a potent inducer of microvascular leakage in airways (Lundberg *et al.*, 1983b) and is more potent than NKA in this respect (Rogers *et al.*, 1988). SP also stimulates mucus secretion both in animal (Coles *et al.*, 1984) and human bronchi *in vitro* (Rogers *et al.*, 1989). SP is again more potent than NKA. These last two responses are therefore mediated by NK-1 receptors.

Recent studies suggest that SP-immunoreactive nerves may be increased in the airways of asthmatics (Ollerenshaw *et al.*, 1989a). This could be the result the chronic inflammation in the airways.

14.4.4. **Calcitonin gene-related peptide**

Calcitonin gene-related peptide (CGRP) is also localized to sensory nerves in airways (Uddman and Sundler, 1987), but perhaps its most striking effect is potent and long-lasting vasodilatation (Brain *et al.*, 1985). CGRP is a potent dilator of bronchial vessels *in vitro* (McCormack *et al.*, 1989), and causes a long-lasting increase in blood flow in canine trachea (Salonen *et al.*, 1988). Receptors for CGRP are localized predominantly to airway blood vessels in animal and human airways (Mak and Barnes, 1988), and this suggests that CGRP may account for some of the hyperaemia which is characteristic of asthmatic airways.

14.4.5. **Axon reflex mechanisms**

Shedding of airway epithelium may expose sensory nerve endings and these may be triggered or 'sensitized' by certain mediators. 'Hyperalgesia' of the airways may therefore develop in asthmatic airways (Barnes, 1990b). Bradykinin may be particularly effective in this respect and it induces a marked dyspnoea which is reminiscent of an asthma attack (Fuller *et al.*, 1987). Bradykinin would be formed from plasma which exudes into the asthmatic airway lumen as a result of microvascular leakage. Stimulation of these sensory nerves may then cause antidromic stimulation of these nerves, with release of their neuropeptides (Figure 14.5). Such neurogenic inflammation has also been demonstrated in rodent lung and mediators such as bradykinin release tachykinins from sensory nerves in lung (Saria *et al.*, 1988). In some animal models of hyper-reactivity, depletion of sensory neuropeptides by prior treatment with capsaicin results in a reduction in responsiveness (Thompson *et al.*, 1987). Whether such neurogenic inflammation is involved in human asthma has not yet been demonstrated, since there are no specific blockers of tachykinins available for clinical use. However, the increase in SP-immunoreactive nerves described in asthmatic airways (Ollerenshaw *et al.*, 1989a) may provide evidence that such local reflexes become important in disease. Axon reflex mechanisms, and possibly also local reflexes mediated by sensory nerve input to parasympathetic ganglia, provide a mechanism for amplifying the inflammatory response in asthmatic airways. These nerves would spread the inflammatory response from sites of epithelial damage, and therefore amplify the inflammatory process. It follows that drugs which reduce neurogenic inflammation might be useful in asthma therapy (Barnes *et al.*, 1990).

14.4.6. **Modulation of sensory neuropeptide release**

In the central nervous system opiates inhibit the release of SP, and enkephalins act as the endogenous modulators of SP-ergic neurones. Opiates are effective in inhibiting NANC constriction of guinea-pig airways *in vitro* (Frossard and Barnes, 1987) and *in vivo* (Belvisi *et al.*, 1988). This is mediated by μ-opioid receptors on sensory nerve endings which inhibit the release of tachykinins. Similarly, opioids inhibit neurogenic microvascular leak in guinea-pig airways (Belvisi *et al.*, 1989b), and mucus secretion induced by capsaicin in human bronchi (Rogers and Barnes, 1989). The central inhibitory neurotransmitter, γ-aminobutyric acid, is similarly effec-

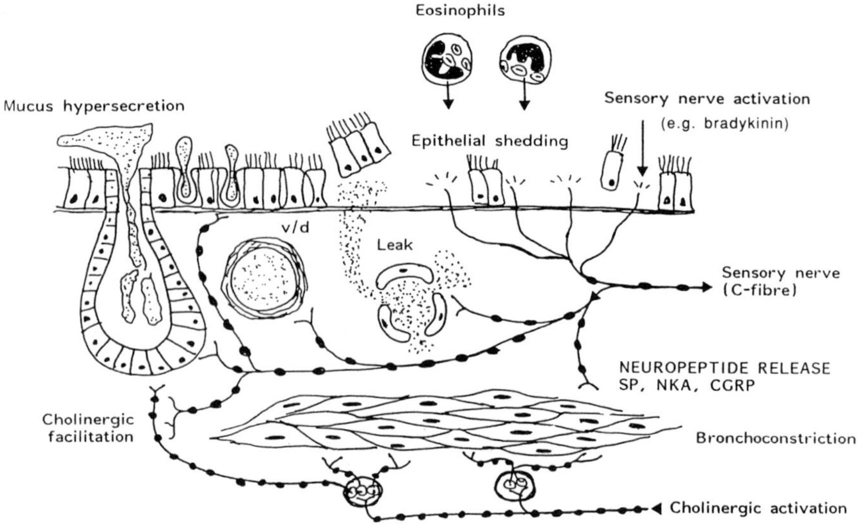

Figure 14.5. Axon reflex mechanisms in asthma. Neuropeptides in sensory nerves, such as substance P (SP), neurokinin A (NKA) and calcitonin gene-releated peptide (CGRP), may be released from collateral branches of sensory nerves to augment the inflammatory response. v/d, vasodilation.

tive on NANC bronchoconstriction (Belvisi *et al.*, 1989a). Several other agonists appear to inhibit sensory neuropeptides via activation of prejunctional receptors on sensory nerves (Barnes *et al.*, 1990), possibly via the activation of an ATP-sensitive potassium channel (Ichinose *et al.*, 1990).

14.4.7. **Other neuropeptides**

Several other neuropeptides have been localized to airway nerves, but their physiological role is far from certain. Neuropeptide-Y (NPY) is a co-transmitter with noradrenaline and appears to modulate cholinergic neuro-transmission (Stretton and Barnes, 1989), and the release of neuropeptides from sensory nerves (Matran *et al.*, 1989; Stretton and Barnes, 1988). Galanin, a co-transmitter with VIP in cholinergic nerves, also modulates sensory nerves (Giuliani *et al.*, 1989), whereas cholecystokinin octapeptide is a potent bronchoconstrictor without obvious neuromodulatory function (Stretton and Barnes, 1989).

14.5. *Conclusions*

Neural control of airway calibre is far from simple and it is likely to contribute to the airway narrowing and airway hyper-responsiveness in asthma. Complex interactions may occur between the different components of autonomic control and inflammatory mediators released from cells in the inflamed airway may profoundly alter the balance of neural control. Further elucidation of these interactions should shed light on the mechanisms of airway disease and may lead to therapeutic advances. The discovery of many potent neuropeptides in human airway nerves complicates matters further, but may lead to novel approaches to treatment in the future.

Acknowledgement

I am very grateful to Madeleine Wray for her careful preparation of this manuscript.

References

Alexander, H.L. and Paddock, R. (1921). Bronchial asthma: response to pilocarpine and epinepheine. *Archives of International Medicine*, **27**, 184–191.

Andersson, R.G.G., Fugner, A., Lundgren, B.R. and Muacevic, G. (1986). Inhibitory effects of clonidine on bronchospasm induced in guinea-pigs by vagal stimulation or antigen challenge. *European Journal of Pharmacology*, **123**, 181–185.

Barnes, P.J. (1986a). Airway inflammation and autonomic control. *European Journal of Respiratory Disease*, **69** (Suppl. 147), 80–87.

Barnes, P.J. (1986b). Asthma as an axon reflex. *Lancet*, **i**, 242–245.

Barnes, P.J. (1986c). Endogenous catecholamines and asthma. *Journal of Allergy and Clinical Immunology*, **77**, 791–795.

Barnes, P.J. (1986d). Non-adrenergic non-cholinergic neural control of human airways. *Archives International de Pharmacologie et de Therapie*, **280** (Suppl.), 208–228.

Barnes, P.J. (1986e). State of art. Neural control of human airways in health and disease. *American Review of Respiratory Disease*, **134**, 1289–1314.

Barnes, P.J. (1987a). Airway neuropeptides and asthma. *Trends in Pharmacological Science*, **8**, 24–27.

Barnes, P.J. (1987b). Cholinergic control of airway smooth muscle. *American Review of Respiratory Disease*, **136**, S42–S45.

Barnes, P.J. (1987c). Muscarinic receptors in lung. *Postgraduate Medical Journal*, **63** (Suppl.), 13–19.

Barnes, P.J. (1987d). Neuropeptides in human airways, function and clinical implications. *American Review of Respiratory Disease*, **136**, S77–S83.

Barnes, P.J. (1987e). Neuropeptides in the lung, localization, function and pathophysiologic implications. *Journal of Allergy and Clinical Immunology*, **79**, 285–295.

Barnes, P.J. (1988). Adrenergic regulation of airway function. In: *The Airways: Neural Control in Health and Disease*, edited by M.A. Kaliner and P.J. Barnes. New York: Dekker, pp. 57–85.

Barnes, P.J. (1989). Muscarinic receptor subtypes: implications for lung disease. *Thorax*, **44**, 161–167.

Barnes, P.J. (1990a). Muscarinic receptors in airways: recent developments. *Journal of Applied Physiology*, **68**, 1777–1785.

Barnes, P.J. (1990b). Neurogenic inflammation in airways and its modulation. *Archives International de Pharmacologie et de Therapie*, **303**, 67–82.

Barnes, P.J., Dollery, C.T. and MacDermot, J. (1980). Increased pulmonary α-adrenergic and reduced β-adrenergic receptors in experimental asthma. *Nature*, **285**, 569–571.

Barnes, P.J., Ind, P.W. and Dollery, C.T. (1981a). Inhaled prazosin in asthma. *Thorax*, **36**, 378–381.

Barnes, P.J., Wilson, N.M. and Vickers, H. (1981b). Prazosin, an α_1-adrenoceptor antagonist partially inhibits exercise-induced asthma. *Journal of Allergy and Clinical Immunology*, **68**, 411–419.

Barnes, P.J., Ind, P.W. and Brown, M.J. (1982a). Plasma histamine and catecholamines in stable asthmatic subjects. *Clinical Science*, **62**, 661–665.

Barnes, P.J., Basbaum, C.B. and Nadel, J.A. (1983a). Autoradiographic localization of autonomic receptors in airway smooth muscle: marked differences between large and small airways. *American Review of Respiratory Disease*, **127**, 758–762.

Barnes, P.J., Minette, P.A. and Maclagan, J. (1988). Muscarinic receptor subtypes in lung. *Trends in Pharmacological Science*, **9**, 412–416.

Barnes, P.J., Belvisi, M.G. and Rogers, D.F. (1990). Modulation of neurogenic inflammation: novel approaches to inflammatory diseases. *Trends in Pharmacological Science*, **11**, 185–189.

Barnes, P.J., Brown, M.J., Silverman, M. and Dollery, C.T. (1981c). Circulating catecholamines in exercise and hyperventilation-induced asthma. *Thorax*, **36**, 435–440.

Barnes, P.J., Basbaum, C.B., Nadel, J.A. and Roberts, J.M. (1982b). Localization of β-adrenoceptors in mammalian lung by light microscopic autoradiography. *Nature*, **299**, 444–447.

Barnes, P.J., Skoogh, B.-E., Brown, J.K. and Nadel, J.A. (1983b). Activation of α-adrenergic responses in tracheal smooth muscle: a post-receptor mechanism. *Journal of Applied Physiology*, **54**, 1469–1476.

Baudouin, S.V., Altman, T.J. and Johnson, A.J. (1988). Prazosin in the treatment of chronic asthma. *Thorax*, **43**, 385–387.

Belvisi, M.G., Ichinose, M. and Barnes, P.J. (1989a). Evidence for GABA β-receptors on non-adrenergic non-cholinergic nerves in guinea-pig airways. *British Journal of Pharmacology*, **97**, 1225–1231.

Belvisi, M.G., Rogers, D.F. and Barnes, P.J. (1989b). Neurogenic plasma extravasation: inhibition by morphine in guinea pig airways *in vivo*. *Journal of Applied Physiology*, **66**, 268–272.

Belvisi, M.G., Chung, K.F., Jackson, D.M. and Barnes, P.J. (1988). Opioid modulation of non-cholinergic neural bronchoconstriction in guinea-pig *in vivo*. *British Journal of Pharmacology*, **95**, 413–418.

Bloom, J.W., Baumgartener-Folkerts, C., Palmer, J.D., Yamamura, H.I. and Halonen, M. (1988). A muscarinic receptor subtype modulates vagally stimulated bronchial contraction. *Journal of Applied Physiology*, **85**, 2144–2150.

Boschetto, P., Roberts, N.M., Rogers, D.F. and Barnes, P.J. (1989). Effect of anti-asthma drugs on microvascular leakage in guinea-pig airways. *American Review of Respiratory Disease*, **139**, 416–421.

Brain, S.D., Williams, T.J., Tippins, J.R., Morris, H.R. and MacIntyre, I. (1985). Calcitonin gene-related peptide is a potent vasodilator. *Nature*, **313**, 54–56.

Brown, J.K., Shields, R., Jones, C. and Gold, W.M. (1983). Augmentation of alpha-adrenergic responsiveness in trachealis muscle of living dogs. *Journal of Applied Physiology*, **54**, 1558–1566.

Carstairs, J.R., Nimmo, A.J. and Barnes, P.J. (1985). Autoradiographic visualization of beta-adrenoceptor subtypes in human lung. *American Review of Respiratory Disease*, **132**, 541–547.

Caughey, G.H., Leidig, F., Viro, N.F. and Nadel, J.A. (1988). Substance P and vasoactive intestinal peptide degradation by mast cell tryptase and chymase. *Journal of Pharmacology and Experimental Therapeutics*, **244**, 133–137.

Cerrina, J., Ladurie, M.L., Labat, C., Raffestin, B., Bayol, A. and Brink, C. (1986). Comparison of human bronchial muscle responses to histamine *in vivo* with histamine and isoprotenerol agonists *in vitro*. *American Review of Respiratory Disease*, **134**, 57–61.

Chung, K.F., Evans, T.W., Graf, P.D. and Nadel, J.A. (1985). Modulation of cholinergic neurotransmission in canine airways by thromboxane-mimetic U 46619. *European Journal of Pharmacology*, **117**, 373–375.

Coleridge, J.C.G. and Coleridge, H.M. (1984). Afferent vagal C fibre innervation of the lung and airways and its functional significance. *Review of Physiology and Biochemical Pharmacology*, **99**, 1–110.

Coles, S.J., Neill, K.H. and Reid, L.M. (1984). Potent stimulation of glycoprotein secretion in canine trachea by substance P. *Journal of Applied Physiology*, **57**, 1323–1327.

Danser, A.H.J., van den Ende, R., Lorenz, R.R., Flavahan, N.A. and Vanhoutte, P.M. (1987). Prejunctional β_1-adrenoceptors inhibit cholinergic neurotransmission in canine bronchi. *Journal of Applied Physiology*, **62**, 785–790.

Evans, T.W., Dixon, C.M.S., Clarke, B., Conradson, T.-B. and Barnes, P.J. (1988). Comparison of neurokinin A and substance P on cardiovascular and airway function in man. *British Journal of Clinical Pharmacology*, **25**, 273–275.

Frossard, N. and Barnes, P.J. (1987). μ-Opioid receptors modulate non-cholinergic constrictor nerves in guinea-pig airways. *European Journal of Pharmacology*, **141**, 519–522.

Frossard, N., Rhoden, K.J. and Barnes, P.J. (1989). Influence of epithelium on guinea pig airway respones to tachykinins, role of endopeptidase and cyclooxygenase. *Journal of Pharmacology and Experimental Therapeutics*, **248**, 292–299.

Fryer, A.D. and MacLagan, J. (1984). Muscarinic inhibitory receptors in pulmonary parasympathetic nerves in the guinea-pig. *British Journal of Pharmacology*, **83**, 973–978.

Fryer, A.D. and Maclagan, J. (1987). Ipratropium bromide potentiates bronchoconstriction induced by vagal nerve stimulation in the guinea-pig. *European Journal of Pharmacology*, **139**, 187–191.

Fuller, R.W., Dixon, C.M.S., Cuss, F.M.C. and Barnes, P.J. (1987). Bradykinin-induced bronchoconstriction in man, mode of action. *American Review of Respiratory Disease*, **135**, 176–180.

Giuliani, S., Ammann, R., Papini, A.M., Maggi, C.A. and Meli, A. (1989). Modulatory action of galanin on responses due to antidromic activation of peripheral terminals of capsaicin-sensitive sensory nerve. *European Journal of Pharmacology*, **163**, 91–96.

Goldie, R.G., Spina, D., Henry, P.J., Luliich, K.M. and Paterson, J.W. (1986). *In vitro* responsiveness of human asthmatic blockers to carbachol, histamine, β-receptor agonists and theophylline. *British Journal of Clinical Pharmacology*, **22**, 669–676.

Grandordy, B., Rhoden, K. and Barnes, P.J. (1991). Effects of protein kinase C activation on adrenoceptors in airway smooth muscle. *Biochemical and Biophysical Research Communications*, in press.

Grandordy, B.M., Frossard, N., Rhoden, K.J. and Barnes, P.J. (1988). Tachykinin-induced phosphoinositide breakdown in airway smooth muscle and epithelium, relationship to contraction. *Molecular Pharmacology*, **33**, 515–519.

Gross, N.J. and Skorodin, M.S. (1984). Anticholinergic antimuscarinic bronchodilators. *American Review of Respiratory Disease*, **129**, 856–870.

Grundstrom, N., Andersson, R.G.G. and Wikberg, J.E.S. (1981). Prejunctional α_2-adrenoceptors inhibit contraction of tracheal smooth muscle by inhibiting cholinergic neurotransmission. *Life Sciences*, **28**, 2981–2986.

Hall, A.K., Barnes, P.J., Meldrum, L.A. and Maclagan, J. (1989). Facilitation by tachykinins of neurotransmission in guinea-pig pulmonary parasympathetic nerves. *British Journal of Pharmacology*, **97**, 274–280.

Ichinose, M. and Barnes, P.J. (1989). Inhibitory histamine H3-receptors on cholinergic nerves in human airways. *European Journal of Pharmacology*, **163**, 383–386.

Ichinose, M. and Barnes, P.J. (1990). A potassium channel activator modulates both non-cholinergic and cholinergic neurotransmission in guinea pig airways. *Journal of Pharmacology and Experimental Therapeutics*, **252**, 1207–1212.

Ichinose, M., Inoue, H., Miura, M. and Takishima, T. (1988). Nonadrenergic bronchodilation in normal subjects. *American Review of Respiratory Disease*, **138**, 31–34.

Ichinose, M., Stretton, C.D., Schwartz, J.-C. and Barnes, P.J. (1989). Histamine, H.3-receptors inhibit cholinergic neurotransmission in guinea pig airways. *British Journal of Pharmacology*, **97**, 13–15.

Ind, P.W., Barnes, P.J., Brown, M.J. and Dollery, C.T. (1985). Plasma histamine concentration during propranolol induced bronchoconstriction. *Thorax*, **40**, 903–909.

Ind, P.W., Dixon, C.M.S., Fuller, R.W. and Barnes, P.J. (1989). Anticholinergic blockade of beta-blocker induced bronchoconstriction. *American Review of Respiratory Disease*, **139**, 1390–1394.

Joos, G., Pauwels, R. and van der Straeten, M. (1987). Effect of inhaled substance P and neurokinin A on the airways of normal and asthmatic subjects. *Thorax*, **42**, 779–783.

Kaliner, M.A. and Barnes, P.J. (eds) (1988). *The Airways: Neural Control in Health and Disease*. (Lung Biology in Health and Disease Series, Vol. 33). New York: Marcel Dekker.

Kallenbach, J.M., Webster, T., Dowdeswell, R., Reinach, S.G., Scott Millar, R.N. and Zwi, S. (1985). Reflex heart rate control in asthma. *Chest*, **87**, 644–648.

Kaufman, M.P., Coleridge, H.M., Coleridge, J.C.G. and Baker, D.G. (1980). Bradykinin stimulates afferent vagal C-fibers in intrapulmonary airways of dogs. *Journal of Applied Physiology*, **48**, 511–517.

Kneussl, M.P. and Richardson, J.B. (1978). Alpha-adrenergic receptors in human and canine tracheal and bronchial smooth muscle. *Journal of Applied Physiology*, **45**, 307–311.

Laitinen, A., Partanen, M., Hervonen, A., Peto-Huikko, M. and Laitinen, L.A. (1985). VIP-like immunoreactive nerves in human respiratory tract. Light and electron microscopic study. *Histochemistry*, **82**, 313–319.

Lammers, J.-W., Minette, P., McCusker, M. and Barnes, P.J. (1989a). The role of pirenzepine-sensitive (M1) muscarinic receptors in vagally mediated bronchoconstriction in humans. *American Review of Respiratory Disease*, **139**, 446–449.

Lammers, J.-W., Minette, P., McCusker, M.T., Chung, K.F. and Barnes, P.J. (1988). Nonadrenergic bronchodilator mechanisms in normal human subjects *in vivo*. *Journal of Applied Physiology*, **64**, 1817–1822.

Lammers, J.-W., Minette, P., McCusker, M.T., Chung, K.F. and Barnes, P.J. (1989b). Capsaicin-induced bronchodilation in asthmatic patients: role of the nonadrenergic inhibitory system. *Journal of Applied Physiology*, **67**, 856–861.

Larssen, K., Martinsson, A. and Hjemdahl, P. (1986). Influence of circulating alpha-adrenoceptor agonists on pulmonary function and cardiovascular variables in patients with exercise induced asthma and healthy subjects. *Thorax*, **41**, 522–528.

Lundberg, J.M. and Saria, A. (1987). Polypeptide-containing neurons in airway smooth muscle. *Annual Review of Physiology*, **49**, 557–572.

Lundberg, J.M., Martling, C.-R. and Saria, A. (1983a). Substance P and capsaicin-induced contraction of human bronchi. *Acta Physiologica Scandinavica*, **119**, 49–53.

Lundberg, J.M., Saria, A., Brodin, E., Rusells, S. and Folkers, R. (1983b). A substance P antagonist inhibits vagally induced increase in vascular permeability and bronchial smooth muscle contraction in the guinea-pig. *Proceedings of the National Academy of Sciences USA*, **80**, 1120–1124.

Lundberg, J.M., Saria, A., Lundblad, L., Angaard, A., Martling, C.-R., Theodorsson-Norheim, E., Stjarne, P. and Hökfelt, T. (1988). Bioactive peptides in capsaicin-sensitive C-fiber afferents of the airways: functional and pathophysiological implications. In: *The Airways, Neural Control in Health and Disease*, edited by M.A. Kaliner and P.J. Barnes. New York: Marcel Dekker, pp. 417–445.

McCaig, D.J. (1987). Comparison of autonomic responses in the trachea isolated from normal and albumin sensitive guinea-pigs. *British Journal of Pharmacology*, **92**, 809–816.

McCormack, D.G., Salonen, R.O. and Barnes, P.J. (1989). Effect of sensory neuropeptides on canine bronchial and pulmonary vessels *in vitro*. *Life Sciences*, **45**, 2405–2412.

Mak, J.C.M. and Barnes, P.J. (1988). Autoradiographic localization of calcitonin gene-related peptide binding sites in human and guinea pig lung. *Peptides*, **9**, 957–964.

Mak, J.C.W. and Barnes, P.J. (1990). Autoradiographic visualization of muscarinic receptor subtypes in human and guinea pig lung. *American Review of Respiratory Disease*, **141**, 1559–1568.

Martling, C.-R., Theordorsson-Norheim, E. and Lundberg, J.M. (1987). Occurrence and effects of multiple tachykinins: substance P, neurokinin A, neuropeptide K in human lower airways. *Life Sciences*, **40**, 1633–1643.

Matran, R., Martling, C.-R. and Lundberg, J.M. (1989). Neuropeptide γ and α_2-receptor inhibition of cholinergic and non-adrenergic non-cholinergic bronchoconstriction. *European Journal of Pharmacology*, **163**, 15–23.

Michoud, M.-C., Amyot, R., Jeanneret-Grosjean, A. and Couture, J. (1987). Reflex decrease of histamine-induced bronchoconstriction after laryngeal stimulation in humans. *American Review of Respiratory Disease*, **136**, 618–622.

Minette, P.A. and Barnes, P.J. (1988). Prejunctional inhibitory muscarinic receptors on cholinergic nerve in human and guinea-pig airways. *Journal of Applied Physiology*, **64**, 2532–2537.

Minette, P.A.H., Lammers, J., Dixon, C.M.S., McCusker, M.T. and Barnes, P.J. (1989). A muscarinic agonist inhibits reflex bronchoconstriction in normal but not in asthmatic subjects. *Journal of Applied Physiology*, **67**, 2461–2465.

Nadel, J.A. and Barnes, P.J. (1984). Autonomic regulation of the airways. *Annual Review of Medicine*, **35**, 451–467.

Nadel, J.A., Barnes, P.J. and Holtzman, M.J. (1986). Autonomic factors in the hyper-reactivity of airway smooth muscle. In: *Handbook of Physiology: The Respiratory System III*. Bethesda, MD: American Physiological Society, pp. 693–702.

Ollerenshaw, S.L., Jarvis, D.L., Woolcock, A.J., Scheibner, T. and Sullivan, C.E. (1989a). Substance P immunoreactive nerve fibres in airways from patients with and without asthma. *American Review of Respiratory Disease*, **139**, A237.

Ollerenshaw, S., Jarvis, D., Woolcock, A., Sullivan, C. and Scheibner, T. (1989b). Absence of immunoreactive vasoactive intestinal polypeptide in tissue from the lungs of patients with asthma. *New England Journal of Medicine*, **320**, 1244–1248.

Palmer, J.B.D. and Barnes, P.J. (1987). Neuropeptides and airway smooth muscle function. *American Review of Respiratory Disease*, **136**, S50–S54.

Palmer, J.B., Cuss, F.M.C. and Barnes, P.J. (1986). VIP and PHM and their role in non-adrenergic inhibitory responses in isolated human airways. *Journal of Applied Physiology*, **61**, 1322–1328.

Postma, D.S., Keyzer, J.J., Koeter, G.H., Sluiter, H.J. and De Vries, K. (1985). Influence of the parasympathetic and sympathetic nervous systems on nocturnal bronchial obstruction. *Clinical Science*, **69**, 251–258.

Rebuck, A.S., Chapman, K.R., Abboud, R., Pare, P.D., Kreisman, H., Wolkove, N. and Vickerson, P. (1987). Nebulized anticholinergic and sympathomimetic treatment of asthma and chronic obstructive airways disease in the emergency room. *American Journal of Medicine*, **82**, 59–64.

Rhoden, K.J., Meldrum, L.A. and Barnes, P.J. (1988). Inhibition of cholinergic neurotransmission in human airways by β_2-adrenoceptors. *Journal of Applied Physiology*, **65**, 700–705.

Richardson, J.B. (1979). State of art. Nerve supply to the lungs. *American Review of Respiratory Disease*, **119**, 785–802.

Robertson *et al.* (1988). The effect of platelet activating factor on histidine and muscarine receptor function in guinea pig airways. *American Review of Respiratory Disease*, **137**, 1317–1322.

Rogers, D.F. and Barnes, P.J. (1989). Opioid inhibition of neurally mediated mucus secretion in human bronchi. *Lancet*, **i**, 930–932.

Rogers, D.F., Aursudkij, B. and Barnes, P.J. (1989). Effects of tachykinins on mucus secretion in human bronchi *in vitro*. *European Journal of Pharmacology*, **174**, 283–286.

Rogers, D.F., Belvisi, M.G., Aursudkij, B., Evans, T.W. and Barnes, P.J. (1988). Effects and interactions of sensory neuropeptides on airway microvascular leakage in guinea pig. *British Journal of Pharmacology*, **95**, 1109–1116.

Salonen, R.O., Webber, S.E. and Widdicombe, J.G. (1988). Effects of neuropeptides and capsaicin on the canine tracheal vasculature *in vivo*. *British Journal of Pharmacology*, **95**, 1262–1270.

Saria, A., Martling, C.-R., Yan, Z., Theordorsson-Norheim, E., Gamse, R. and Lundberg, J.M. (1988). Release of multiple tachykinins from capsaicin-sensitive sensory nerves in the lung by bradykinin, histamine, dimethylphenyl piperazinium and vagal nerve stimulation. *American Review of Respiratory Disease*, **137**, 1330–1335.

Sekizawa, K., Caughey, G.H., Lazarus, S.K., Gold, W.M. and Nadel, J.A. (1989). Mast cell tryptase causes airway smooth muscle hyper-responsiveness in dogs. *Journal of Clinical Investigation*, **83**, 175–179.

Sekizawa, K., Tamaoki, J., Nadel, J.A. and Borson, D.B. (1987). Enkephalinase inhibitor potentiates substance P and electrically induced contraction in ferret trachea. *Journal of Applied Physiology*, **63**, 1401–1405.

Skidgel, R.A., Engelbrecht, A., Johnson, A.R. and Erdos, E.G. (1984). Hydrolysis of substance P and neurokinins by converting enzyme and neutral endoproteinase. *Peptides*, **5**, 769–776.

Stretton, C.D. and Barnes, P.J. (1988). Modulation of cholinergic neurotransmission in guinea-pig trachea by neuropeptide Y. *British Journal of Pharmacology*, **93**, 672–678.

Stretton, C.D. and Barnes, P.J. (1989). Cholecystokinin octapeptide constricts guinea-pig and human airways. *British Journal of Pharmacology*, **97**, 675–682.

Stretton, C.D., Belvisi, M.G. and Barnes, P.J. (1989). Neuropeptide Y modulates non-adrenergic non-cholinergic neural bronchoconstriction *in vivo* and *in vitro*. *British Journal of Pharmacology*, **98**, 781P.

Szentivanyi, A. (1968). The beta-adrenergic theory of the atopic abnormality in bronchial asthma. *Journal of Allergy*, **42**, 203–232.

Tanaka, D.T. and Grunstein, M.M. (1986). Effect of substance P on neurally mediated contraction of rabbit airway smooth muscle. *Journal of Applied Physiology*, **60**, 458–463.

Tattersfield, A.E., Holgate, S.T., Harvey, J.E. and Gribbin, H.R. (1983). Is asthma due to partial beta-blockade of airways? *Agents and Actions*, **13**, 265–271.

Thompson, J.E., Scypinski, L.A., Gordon, T. and Sheppard, D. (1987). Tachykinins mediate the increase in airway responsiveness caused by toluene diisocyanate. *American Review of Respiratory Disease*, **136**, 43–49.

Uddman, R. and Sundler, F. (1987). Neuropeptides in the airways, a review. *American Review of Respiratory Disease*, **136**, S3–S8.

Chapter 15

Nitric oxide as a neurotransmitter in smooth muscle

William Martin, Ian F. Gibson, John S. Gillespie and Xiaorong Liu

15.1. *Introduction*

It is now widely accepted that the endothelium-derived relaxing factor (EDRF; Furchgott and Zawadzki, 1980) responsible for endothelium-dependent vasodilation is nitric oxide (Palmer *et al.*, 1987; Ignarro *et al.*, 1987; Furchgott, 1988), generated enzymically from the guanidino nitrogen(s) of the inactive precursor, L-arginine (Palmer *et al.*, 1988). Although originally discovered in the endothelial cell, it is now clear that the L-arginine–nitric oxide pathway is present and may serve important biological functions in other cell types, including macrophages (Hibbs *et al.*, 1987; Iyenger *et al.*, 1987) and neurones in the central nervous system (Garthwaite *et al.*, 1988). The latter study suggests that nitric oxide may operate as a neurotransmitter or neuromodulator in the central nervous system. This chapter reviews data obtained in our own and other laboratories, suggesting that the L-arginine–nitric oxide system represents a novel neurotransmission process present in the autonomic nervous system.

15.2. *Concept of Non-Adrenergic, Non-Cholinergic Nerves*

Although not appreciated at the time, examples of autonomic neurogenic responses mediated by neurotransmitters other than noradrenaline and acetylcholine appeared in the early literature. For example, Langley and Anderson (1895) described parasympathetic actions in the pelvic viscera, which uncharacteristically, were not blocked by atropine. Even subsequent to acetylcholine becoming accepted as the parasympathetic neurotransmitter, these anomalous 'atropine resistant' responses were not considered to arise from the action of a separate neurotransmitter. Instead, the favoured explanation was that of Dale and Gaddum (1930), in which atropine was proposed to form a 'barrier' through which acetylcholine could not pass. Blockade of the action of acetylcholine was envisaged only when it was released outside the barrier, and 'atropine resistance' occurred when release took place within the barrier. Early on, the only comparable drugs available which blocked adrenergic responses were ergot and its derivatives (Dale, 1906). However, the variability of the blockade produced by these agents (Jang, 1940), now explained by their ability to block α- but not β-adrenoceptors, prevented the early recognition of anomalous, sympathetic responses. It was only with the advent of selective adrenergic neurone blocking drugs, such as bretylium and guanethidine, that the existence of relaxant nerves to the gut that were not adrenergic was firmly established (Greeff *et al.*, 1962; Burnstock *et al.*, 1963; Paton and Vane, 1963). These studies together with those describing 'atropine-resistance' led to the concept that non-adrenergic, non-cholinergic (NANC) nerves formed part of the autonomic nervous system. The widespread distribution of NANC nerves in the gastrointestinal tract, lung, eye and cardiovascular and urogenital systems has been the subject of several reviews (Burnstock, 1972, 1979).

15.2.1. **Anococcygeus and retractor penis muscles**

The anococcygeus muscles, although originally described by Langley and Anderson (1896), only became popular as an isolated experimental tissue following the work of Gillespie and colleagues (Gillespie, 1972; Gillespie and McGrath, 1973, 1974). Unusually for smooth muscle, the paired anococcygeus takes a tendinous origin from the upper coccygeal vertebrae, and runs to form a bar on the ventral surface of the colon. In the male of certain species it extends to form a retractor penis muscle.

The anococcygeus and retractor penis together with the penile arteries receive two anatomically distinct sets of nerves: a sympathetic motor innervation from the lumbar region of the spinal cord and a parasympathetic inhibitory innervation from the sacral cord. Studies with adrenergic neurone blockers, adrenoceptor antagonists and 6-hydroxydopamine on isolated preparations indicate that the motor innervation is by conventional adrenergic nerves (Luduena and Grigas, 1966; Gillespie, 1972; Klinge and Sjöstrand, 1974), although in the retractor penis of pigs and sheep it may not be entirely adrenergic (Ambache and Killick, 1978). In the presence of tone, produced spontaneously in the retractor penis, or induced by drugs in the cases of the ancoccygeus and penile artery, electrical field stimulation results in relaxation (Luduena and Grigas, 1966; Gillespie, 1972; Klinge and Sjöstrand, 1974). These relaxant responses are undoubtedly neurogenic in origin since they are blocked by tetrodotoxin and can be elicited following electrical stimulation of the extrinsic nerves (Langley and Anderson, 1895; Gillespie, 1972; Gillespie and McGrath, 1972; Klinge and Sjöstrand, 1974). Treatment with 6-hydroxydopamine, which destroys adrenergic nerves, leaves these relaxant responses untouched (Gibson and Gillespie, 1973), demonstrating that they do not arise from a co-transmission process from sympathetic fibres. The separate spinal origin of the motor and inhibitory fibres supports the existence of two distinct sets of nerves (Langley and Anderson, 1895; Gillespie and McGrath, 1973).

Changes in membrane potential have been observed in association with relaxation induced by the NANC nerves (Creed *et al.*, 1975; Creed and Gillespie, 1977; Byrne and Muir, 1984). Following blockade of the adrenergic nerves in the anococcygeus of the rabbit and retractor penis of the bull, stimulation with single pulses leads to small hyperpolarizations, and these can rise to 20–30 mV following trains of stimuli at low frequencies. Hyperpolarization is associated with a rise in membrane conductance, probably due to potassium, since experiments in which passive membrane hyperpolarization was produced by current injection show a reversal potential close to the potassium equilibrium potential (−80 mV). In contrast, in the anococcygeus of the rat, repetitive stimulation induces a powerful relaxation, but only small (2 mV) hyperpolarizations and increases in conductance are observed. Clearly, therefore, some degree of smooth muscle membrane hyperpolarization is associated with activation of the NANC nerves, but this is unlikely to contribute significantly to the mechanisms by which relaxation takes place.

15.2.2. **Ultrastructural identification of NANC nerves**

Application of the fluorescence technique of Falck (1962) has revealed a dense network of adrenergic fibres in the anococcygeus and retractor penis of all species studied (Bell and McLean, 1970; Gillespie, 1972; Gillespie and McGrath, 1974; Creed *et al.*, 1977). Evidence for the localization of cholinergic fibres from acetylcholinesterase staining has been obtained in the anococcygeus of the cat and retractor penis of the dog and bull (Bell and McLean, 1970; Klinge *et al.*, 1970; Garrett *et al.*, 1972), but not in the anococcygeus of the rat (Gillespie, 1972). The existence of adrenergic and cholinergic varicosities, characterized by the presence of granular and agranular vesicles, respectively, has been demonstrated in the anococcygeus of the rat and the retractor penis of the bull (Gillespie and Lüllmann-Rauch, 1974; Eränkö *et al.*, 1976; Gibbins and Haller, 1979).

Identification of the NANC nerve fibres by electon microscopy has, however, proved more difficult: Gillespie and Lüllmann-Rauch (1974) failed to identify such fibres in the anococcygeus of the rat, but a later study on the same tissue avoiding the use of permanganate, which had been shown to destroy NANC nerves in the ureter (Hoyes and Barber, 1976), described a nerve profile that differed from adrenergic and cholinergic nerves (Gibbins and Haller, 1979). These fibres, which accounted for roughly 40% of the total present, were not lost following treatment with 6-hydroxydopamine, and contained a characteristically high proportion of electron-opaque, chromaffin-negative vesicles. At that time Gibbins and Haller (1979) suggested that this nerve profile, which closely resembled those of known peptidergic ‘p-type’ axons (Bargmann *et al.*, 1967; Baumgarten *et al.*, 1970), was that of the NANC nerve in the anococcygeus. In a subsequent publication, however, Gibbins (1982) revised his findings and described a range of varicosities with different proportions of clear and small p-type vesicles with no clear division into two classes corresponding to NANC and cholinergic nerves. Those varicosities containing small, clear vesicles appeared to be the most likely candidates for the NANC nerve. A separate study on the bovine retractor penis revealed three distinct nerve populations (Eränkö *et al.*, 1976): those containing granular and agranular vesicles, identified as adrenergic and cholinergic, respectively, but the third, containing numerous large and small granular vesicles, clearly differed from those found in the anococcygeus (Gibbins, 1982). The close anatomical relationship between the anococcygeus and retractor penis, makes it likely that they share a common neurotransmitter. It is unfortunate, therefore, that a single clearly identifiable profile representing the NANC nerves has failed to emerge in electron microscopic examinations of the two tissues.

15.2.3 **Identification of the NANC transmitter**

In the search for the identity of the NANC transmitter in the anococcygeus, retractor penis and penile artery, the effects of selective receptor blocking agents were examined: these included antagonists for noradrenaline, acetylcholine, histamine, 5-hydroxytryptamine and bradykinin (Gillespie, 1972; Luduena and Grigas, 1966, 1972; Klinge and Sjöstrand, 1974; Gillespie and McKnight, 1978), but none was effective. Ethanol was the only substance found early on which effectively and selectively inhibits NANC relaxation of the anococcygeus of the rat and rabbit and the retractor penis of the bull, but its mechanism of action is obscure (Gillespie *et al.*, 1982).

One of the fundamental criteria which must be satisfied in order to establish a substance as a neurotransmitter is that exogenous application of the substance in question should mimic the effects of nerve stimulation (Eccles, 1964). Specifically, the search was for a single substance which mimicked the effects of NANC nerve stimulation in all three tissues in all species. This approach led to the testing of a wide range of substances, many of which appeared to be promising candidates on individual tissues but not on others. For example, β-adrenoceptor agonists relax the anococcygeus of the rabbit and cat and the retractor penis of the bull (Gillespie and McGrath, 1974; Klinge and Sjöstrand, 1974; Creed *et al.*, 1977), but not the anococcygeus of the rat (Gillespie, 1972). In addition, muscarinic agonists relax the anococcygeus of the rabbit and cat but not the rat. The finding that very few substances relax the anococcygeus of the rat has proved useful in that this tissue represents the most stringent test for a potential NANC candidate. Substances discounted on this basis include histamine, 5-hydroxytryptamine, dopamine, amino acids and prostaglandins (Gillespie, 1972; Gillespie and McGrath, 1974).

Certain peptides, however, have appeared to represent potential candidates: bradykinin relaxes the anococcygeus of the rat, rabbit and cat (Gillespie and McKnight, 1978), but it too was discounted on its ability to contract the retractor penis of the bull (Klinge and Sjöstrand, 1974). Large amounts of vasoactive intestinal polypeptide (VIP) are present in the anococcygeus of the rat, cat and rabbit (Hunter *et al.*, 1984) and in these, as in the anococcygeus of the mouse, histochemical studies have revealed networks of varicose fibres characteristic of autonomic nerves (Gibson and Tucker, 1982). Furthermore, VIP relaxes the anococcygeus of the mouse, rat, cat and rabbit (Gibson and Tucker, 1982; Hunter *et al.*, 1984) and the retractor penis of the dog and bull (Sjöstrand *et al.*, 1981; Bowman *et al.*, 1982a). VIP is unlikely to be the NANC neurotransmitter, however, since its time course of action is inappropriately slow and tachyphylaxis readily develops to it but not to nerve stimulation (Bowman and Gillespie, 1983; Carvajal *et al.*, 1986). Moreover, VIP antiserum and chymotrypsin inhibit the actions of VIP but do not affect NANC nerve stimulation (Carvajal *et al.*, 1986). Other peptides which fail to mimic the actions of the NANC nerves include leucine- and methionine-enkephalin, neurotensin and somatostatin (Sjöstrand *et al.*, 1981; Bowman and Gillespie, 1983).

Extensive evidence now supports the existence of purinergic nerves, i.e. nerves that utilize ATP as their neurotransmitter (Burnstock, 1972, 1979), and for nerves utilizing ATP as a co-transmitter (Sneddon and Burnstock, 1984). Certain reports have proposed that the NANC nerves in the anococcygeus of the rat, rabbit and mouse are purinergic (Burnstock *et al.*, 1978; Gibson and Tucker, 1982). This proposal is supported by the existence of a network of non-adrenergic varicose fibres which, typical of purinergic nerves, are stained by quinacrine (Burnstock *et al.*, 1978; Olson and Alund, 1979; Iijima, 1983). Furthermore, electrical field stimulation induces release of ATP from the anococcygeus of the rat and rabbit even in tissues in which the adrenergic nerves are destroyed with 6-hydroxydopamine (Burnstock *et al.*, 1978).

Although ATP does relax the anococcygeus of the rabbit and cat (Gillespie and McGrath, 1974; Creed *et al.*, 1977), it contracts that of the rat (Gillespie, 1972) and also the retractor penis of the dog and bull (Luduena and Grigas, 1966; Klinge and Sjöstrand, 1974). Evidence was presented, however, that ATP has a biphasic action on the anococcygeus of the rat and mouse, consisting of a contractile effect, resulting from the production of prostanoids, and a relaxant effect which is only uncovered fully in the presence of a cyclo-oxygenase inhibitor, such as indomethacin (Burnstock *et al.*, 1978; Gibson and Tucker, 1982). The concentrations of ATP required to induce relaxation are high, however, and it is difficult to reconcile the requirement for indomethacin when NANC responses are produced in its absence.

The most compelling evidence against the NANC transmitter being ATP comes, however, from experiments utilizing the polypeptide from bee venom, apamin. This agent, which effectively blocks the relaxant effects of ATP and purinergic nerves in gastrointestinal muscle (Banks *et al.*, 1979; Sjöqvist *et al.*, 1980), has no effect on NANC relaxation in the anococcygeus of the rat or the retractor penis of the bull (Bowman and Gillespie, 1982). It is therefore unlikely that ATP functions as the neurotransmitter of the NANC nerves in the anococcygeus and retractor penis.

15.2.4. **Inhibitory factor**

Since pharmacological studies failed to produce a convincing candidate for the NANC neurotransmitter, it was logical to assume it was a novel substance. Consequently, two separate approaches were employed in attempts to elucidate its nature. The first of these was the 'overflow' technique of Loewi (1921) in which we attempted to bioassay on an unstimulated tissue transmitter released upon NANC nerve stimulation of a donor tissue upstream. This technique has repeatedly failed to demonstrate overflow of transmitter. The second approach of extracting anococcygeus muscle in phosphate buffer and looking for relaxant activity by bioassay was similarly unsuccessful in our laboratory. Ambache *et al.* (1975), however, reported the presence of activity in acid extracts of bovine retractor penis (BRP) that mimicked the actions of the NANC nerve in that tissue. This activity was stable on ice, but was thermolabile, being lost slowly at room temperature or quickly (within 1–2 min) in a boiling water bath. The substance responsible for this activity was not identified, but its inability to partition into ether ruled against it being a lipid such as a prostaglandin. We confirmed that a relaxant subtance mimicking the actions of the NANC nerves can be extracted from the BRP using dilute acid, and termed this substance inhibitory factor (Gillespie and Martin, 1980; Gillespie *et al.*, 1981).

15.2.5. **Physical properties of inhibitory factor**

As previously reported, inhibitory factor is thermolabile in solution (Ambache *et al.*, 1975), but we determined that it is stable indefinitely if freeze-dried and stored in the absence of moisture. We also confirmed the insolubility of inhibitory factor in ether and found that it is insoluble in acetone, but soluble in dilute methanol, although pure methanol destroys it. Undoubtedly, the most characteristic feature of inhibitory factor is that its activity is generated following acidification (Gillespie and Martin, 1980). This property, which we discovered accidentally, has proved invaluable in following inhibitory factor through a battery of extraction and purification steps. It also explained our initial failure to extract inhibitory factor using phosphate buffer and the success of Ambache *et al.* (1975) who employed dilute hydrochloric acid. If BRP is extracted in neutral buffer or methanol, no inhibitory activity is detected until the extract is acidified and subsequently neutralized: the activation process is rapid being complete within 2 min and has a threshold of pH 4 and an optimum at pH 2 (Gillespie and Martin,

1980). These findings indicate that inhibitory factor exists in two forms, a stable but inactive form, and biologically active but unstable form. Interconversion between these two forms is possible since, when activity is allowed to decay at room temperature, full activity can be regenerated upon renewed exposure to acid, although only partial recovery is obtained if activity has been lost by boiling.

Based on the ability to pass ultrafiltration membranes, the molecular weight of both the inactive and acid-activated forms of inhibitory factor appear to be less than 500 Da (Gillespie *et al.*, 1981). No evidence that the process of acid-activation occurs with a change in molecular weight has been obtained.

Investigation of the electrical charge on inhibitory factor was carried out by ion-exchange chromatography. We determined that both the inactive and acid-activated forms bound to, and could be subsequently eluted from, an anion exchange resin (AG1-X8, formate form). Neither form, however, bound to a cation exchange resin (AG50-W, sodium form). Based on these findings, we concluded that both the inactive and active form of inhibitory factor bear a negative, but no positive, charge (Gillespie *et al.*, 1981).

15.2.6. **Chemical nature of inhibitory factor**

In view of the proposal that the NANC innervation was purinergic (Burnstock *et al.*, 1978), we wished to establish if the activity of inhibitory factor was derived from ATP. Extracts of BRP do contain large amounts of adenine nucleotides, but these can be removed by adsorption on alkaline alumina with no loss of inhibitory factor activity (Bowman *et al.*, 1979).

A major effort was made to determine the class of compound to which inhibitory factor belonged. Its insolubility in ether (Ambache *et al.*, 1975; Gillespie *et al.*, 1981) suggested it was not a lipid. We therefore considered the possibility that it might be a peptide (Gillespie *et al.*, 1981). The solubility in methanol suggested that if it did belong to this class it had to be small since large peptides would have been denatured. Incubation of the inactive form of inhibitory factor with a range of proteases including trypsin, subtilisin, leucine aminopeptidase, pyroglutamate aminopeptidase and carboxypeptidase, led to no loss of inhibitory activity. The active form of inhibitory factor also was unaffected following incubation with pepsin at pH 2. Furthermore, neither the broad-spectrum protease inhibitor, trasylol, nor the specific inhibitor of angiotensin converting enzyme, SQ20881, had any effect on the activity of inhibition factor or the response to NANC stimulation (Gillespie *et al.*, 1981). It was therefore thought unlikely that inhibitory factor was a peptide.

We next considered the possibility that inhibitory factor was a carbohydrate. Monosaccarides exist in two forms: an open chain or, following interaction between the aldehyde and alcohol groups, a cyclic hemiacetal. It was possible, therefore, that if inhibitory factor was a sugar, acid-activation might represent the known ability of low pH to induce conversion from the enol form to the hemiacetal. Furthermore, the hemiacetal form of sugars are known to react with alcohols to form acetals (or glycosides), and we had previously found that pure methanol destroys inhibitory factor. Consistent with this possibility was our finding that periodic acid or sodium periodate, which selectively oxidize glycols, led to complete loss of activity when incubated with either the inactive or the acid-activated form of inhibitory factor (Gillespie *et al.*, 1981). Inconsistent with this idea, however, was the action of sodium borohydride (Gillespie *et al.*, 1981). This agent selectively reduces aldehyde and ketones, and was therefore predicted to react only with the inactive form where the aldehyde group would be available. Confusingly, however, it was the active form of inhibitory factor that was destroyed and the inactive form was either unaffected or in some experiments potentiated. We concluded, therefore, that if inhibitory factor was a sugar, the inactive form was the cyclic hemiacetal and the acid-activated form was the open chain form.

15.2.7. **Distribution of inhibitory factor**

Before a substance is accepted as a neurotransmitter it should be shown to be present in prejunctional nerve fibres (Eccles, 1964). We therefore wished to establish whether or not inhibitory factor was present only in tissues possessing an appropriate NANC innervation (Gillespie and Martin, 1980). In addition to BRP, inhibitory factor was found in extracts of rat anococcygeus which has the NANC nerve, but it was also found in skeletal muscle, cardiac muscle and liver where no NANC nerve has been reported. It was even recovered in the poorly innervated uterus and the uninnervated umbilical artery, although in these two tissues the activity recovered was substantially less than from BRP. It was necessary to postulate, therefore, that if inhibitory factor was the NANC neurotransmitter then it must be present also in non-nervous structures.

If inhibitory factor was the NANC neurotransmitter, it would be expected to be found contained within storage vesicles, and these can be isolated by subcellular fractionation. Homogenization of BRP proved difficult, but inhibitory factor activity was clearly concentrated in the high speed pellet containing vesicle-like structures (Gillespie and Hunter, 1982).

15.2.8. **Pharmacological actions of inhibitory factor**

The ability of inhibitory factor to mimic the actions of the NANC nerves in the BRP satisfies an important criterion for acceptance as a neurotransmitter (Eccles, 1964). This possibility was strengthened further by the finding that it also relaxes the penile artery (Bowman *et al.*, 1981) and the more discriminating rat anococcygeus (Gillespie and Martin, 1980), which is relaxed by very few stimuli. In addition to these effects on tissues possessing an appropriate NANC innervation, inhibitory factor was found to act on a variety of gastrointestinal and cardiovascular preparations. It relaxes spontaneous and carbachol-induced tone in the guinea-pig taenia coli, fundal strip, duodenum and colon, but has no effect on the ileum or gall bladder (Crossley and Gillespie, 1983). The relaxant action of inhibitory factor on the taenia coli, unlike NANC nerve stimulation, is not blocked by apamin, indicating that it is unlikely to act as a neurotransmitter in this tissue. This ability to relax smooth muscle is also reflected in its vasodilator action on a range of isolated, noradrenaline-constricted blood vessels including the bovine coronary artery, rat, rabbit and cat aorta and cat and rabbit pulmonary and renal artery (Bowman *et al.*, 1981). Two preparations containing resistance vessels, the rat perfused hindquarters and isolated perfused mesentery, are also dilated by inhibitory factor. Inhibitory factor has no effect, however, on rat spontaneously beating atria or paced right ventricular strips (Bowman *et al.*, 1981).

15.2.9. **Properties in common with endothelium-derived relaxing factor**

Inhibitory factor relaxes vascular smooth muscle by an endothelium-independent mechanism (Bowman *et al.*, 1986), but it and the NANC neurotransmitter have many properties in common with endothelium-derived relaxing factor (EDRF; Furchgott and Zawadzki, 1980). Both EDRF and inhibitory factor are destroyed by borohydride (Gillespie *et al.*, 1981; Griffith *et al.*, 1984), both display anionic properties (Gillespie *et al.*, 1981; Cocks *et al.*, 1985), and both are reported to be activated by acid (Gillespie and Martin, 1980; Murray *et al.*, 1986). The half-life of EDRF is between 6 and 40 s (Griffith *et al.*, 1984; Förstermann *et al.*, 1985) and, although this is shorter than that of inhibitory factor, the discrepancy is reduced considerably when destruction of EDRF by superoxide anions is reduced following treatment with superoxide dismutase (Gryglewski *et al.*, 1986; Rubanyi and Vanhoutte, 1986). Certain drugs including hydroquinone and pyrogallol, which destroy EDRF through production of superoxide anions (Moncada *et al.*, 1986), also block NANC relaxation of the rat anococcygeus in a superoxide dismutase-reversible manner (Gillespie and Sheng, 1990). Surprisingly, however, these two agents have no effect on NANC relaxation of the BRP, possibly reflecting a higher level of endogenous superoxide dismutase in this tissue (Gillespie and Sheng, 1990). Anoxia also reversibly blocks both endothelium-dependent relaxation of rabbit aorta (Furchgott and Zawadzki, 1980) and NANC relaxation of BRP (Bowman and McGrath, 1985).

One of the most intriguing links between EDRF, inhibitory factor and the NANC transmitter is that they all relax smooth muscle in association with an elevation in cyclic GMP content (Rapoport and Murad, 1983; Bowman and Drummond, 1984). The rise in cyclic GMP content precedes the onset of relaxation suggesting that it may control it. This concept is supported by the findings that the membrane permeant analogue, 8-bromo cyclic GMP, itself relaxes smooth muscle, and that the actions of EDRF, inhibitory factor and the NANC neurotransmitter are potentiated by M & B 22,948, a selective cyclic GMP phosphodiesterase inhibitor, and blocked by inhibitors of soluble guanylate cyclase, including methylene blue and *N*-methylhyroxylamine (Bowman and Drummond, 1984; Martin *et al.*, 1985; Bowman *et al.*, 1986; Gibson and Mirzazadeh, 1989). This latter finding indicates that all three agents stimulate the soluble, but not the particulate, form of guanylate cyclase, and for EDRF this has been confirmed directly by studies using the purified enzyme (Ignarro *et al.*, 1986; Mülsch *et al.*, 1987).

Another important inhibitor which we discovered is haemoglobin. This came to light when we determined that inhibitory factor relaxed every isolated vascular preparation tested yet had no vasodilator action in the anaesthetized rat (Bowman *et al.*, 1981). On further investigation, it became clear that inhibitory factor was inactivated rapidly when mixed with blood, haemolysate or purified haemoglobin, but not with plasma or washed erythrocyte ghosts (Bowman and Gillespie, 1982). Haemoglobin was soon shown to inhibit not only the action of inhibitory factor, but also that of the NANC neurotransmitter in the anococcygeus of the rat, the BRP and bovine and canine penile arteries (Bowman *et al.*, 1982b; Bowman and Gillespie, 1982, 1983), and of EDRF in the rabbit aorta (Martin *et al.*, 1985). The action of haemoglobin is reversible and highly selective; the relaxant effects of stimuli acting via soluble guanylate cyclase are blocked, but those acting through particulate guanylate cyclase or adenylate cyclase are not (Bowman and Drummond, 1984; Martin *et al.*, 1986b). Its mechanism of action is almost certainly through the binding and inactivation of stimulants of soluble guanylate cyclase (Martin *et al.*, 1985). Soluble guanylate cyclase contains a ferrous haem moiety with which stimulants interact (Craven and De Rubertis, 1978), and haemoglobin, by providing alternative haem-containing ligand binding sites, competitvely inhibits activation of the enzyme.

Although haemoglobin powerfully blocks NANC transmission in the anococcygeus, retractor penis and penile artery, it does not block the apamin-sensitive purinergic nerves typified by those in the guinea-pig taenia coli (Bowman and Gillespie, 1982). Haemoglobin and apamin can therefore be used to differentiate between these two types of nerve.

15.2.10 **Identity as nitric oxide**

Nitric oxide is now widely accepted as being the active principle generated by the nitrovasodilator drugs (Arnold *et al.*, 1977; Katsuki *et al.*, 1977). This substance, in common with EDRF, inhibitory factor and the NANC transmitter, relaxes smooth muscle by stimulating soluble guanylate cyclase, is labile, blocked by haemoglobin and methylene blue and potentiated by superoxide dismutase (for review see Furchgott, 1988). On the basis of these striking similarities, Furchgott (1988) proposed that EDRF, the active form of inhibitory factor, and the NANC transmitter were all nitric oxide. In addition, he speculated that the inactive form of inhibitory factor was inorganic nitrite from which nitric oxide was generated following exposure to acid. These proposals were all later confirmed. Palmer and co-workers (1987), using a sensitive chemiluminescence detection system, showed that nitric oxide can indeed be released by bovine aortic endothelial cells and, importantly, the amounts released can fully account for the biological activity of EDRF. Kelm and Schrader (1988), using a difference spectrophotometric technique, agreed that nitric oxide can account for the EDRF activity released from the guinea-pig isolated heart preparation.

The identity of EDRF as nitric oxide has, however, been challenged on the basis of differences in pharmacological activity on a range of tissues, and on possible differences in electrical charge (Dusting *et al.*, 1988; Long and Berkowitz, 1989). More recently, evidence has been presented that EDRF is not nitric oxide itself, but a substance which can readily release it such as a nitrosothiol (Myers *et al.*, 1989, 1990). Regardless of whether the substance released from the endothelium is native nitric oxide or a nitrosothiol compound, there is general agreement that the final mediator which activates soluble guanylate cyclase is nitric oxide.

In support of the proposal that the active form of inhibitory factor is nitric oxide is the rank order of effectiveness of these two substances on a range of different smooth muscles: both powerfully relax the rabbit aorta and BRP, are much less effective on the rat anococcygeus, and have no effect on the guinea-pig trachea (Gillespie and Sheng, 1988a).

The proposal that the inactive form of inhibitory factor is inorganic nitrite (Furchgott, 1988) was based on its known ability to generate nitric oxide when acidified, according to the following scheme (Sisler, 1956):

$$2HNO_2 \rightleftharpoons NO + NO_2 + H_2O \tag{1}$$

Once formed, nitric oxide decays through a series of reactions to form equal amounts of nitrate and nitrite thus:

$$2NO + O_2 \rightarrow 2NO_2 \tag{2}$$

$$2NO_2 \rightleftharpoons N_2O_4 \tag{3}$$

$$N_2O_4 + H_2O \rightleftharpoons HNO_2 + HNO_3 \tag{4}$$

In support of the proposal, Furchgott (1988) demonstrated that the weak dilator action of sodium nitrite is potentiated following acidification, and that in common with inhibitory factor, this occurs below pH 4 with an optimum of pH 2. Furthermore, by employing a diazotization reaction, we confirmed that extracts of BRP do contain nitrite in micromolar quantities (Martin *et al.*, 1988). In addition, we found that when extracts are acid activated at pH 2 for 10 min and neutralized, the generation of relaxant activity is associated with a 70% fall in nitrite content, consistent with Equation (1). The loss of relaxant activity observed when extracts are incubated at room temperature or boiled, and their re-activation following renewed exposure to acid is also consistent with the decay of nitric oxide to nitrite and nitrate (Equations (2)–(4)), and the regeneration of nitric oxide from the remaining nitrite.

There remained, however, several properties of inhibitory factor which could not be explained in terms of the above scheme. For example, the active form inhibitory factor binds to and can be eluted from an anion exchange resin (Gillespie *et al.*, 1981), but nitric oxide is not anionic. Furthermore, although inhibitory factor and nitric oxide both lose activity when mixed with free haemoglobin, only solutions of the latter lose activity when mixed with intact erythrocytes (Gillespie and Sheng, 1988b). The stability of solutions of nitric oxide and inhibitory factor are also different: the former decays within seconds, but the latter is stable for many hours when stored on ice (Gillespie *et al.*, 1981). The greatest impediment to accepting the above scheme, however, is that the nitrite content, measured by diazotization, is too low to account for the relaxant activity of inhibitory factor when compared to that of acidified solutions of nitrite.

Many of the apparent differences between inhibitory factor and nitric oxide could be explained, however, if extracts of BRP contained an additional substance which bound and stabilized the nitric oxide formed on acidification (Martin *et al.*, 1988). Our prediction was that such a substance would, by effectively taking nitric oxide out of solution, drive Equation (1) further to the right. In support of this hypothesis is the observation that acidification does lead to a greater loss in nitrite from extracts than from simple solutions of sodium nitrite. The greater and more stable relaxant activity of acidified extracts is also consistent with a binding substance. The most convincing evidence that nitrite is the source of inhibitory factor activity, however, is that if further nitrite is added to extracts prior to acidification, relaxant activity is enhanced *pro rata* (Martin *et al.*, 1988).

The nature of the proposed binding substance in extracts which stabilizes nitric oxide is as yet uncharacterized. Many substances of biological origin including proteins, sugars and thiols are known to bind and to stabilize nitric oxide (Braughler *et al.*, 1979), and these could potentially be present in extracts. Whether or not inhibitory factor bears any relationship to the nitrosothiols recently described by Myers *et al.* (1990) remains to be determined.

15.2.11. **The L-arginine–nitric oxide system and NANC transmission**

Following our demonstration that inhibitory factor activity can be explained by the generation of nitric oxide from nitrite (Martin *et al.*, 1988), we considered the possibility that the biological precursor of the NANC neurotransmitter and of EDRF was nitrite. We failed, however, to detect an enzyme in the BRP or bovine aortic endothelial cells that could generate nitric oxide from nitrite (unpublished data). This approach turned out to be incorrect, however, since a series of reports subsequently showed that the precursor is not nitrite, but L-arginine (Hibbs *et al.*, 1977; Iyengar *et al.*, 1987; Palmer *et al.*, 1988; Schmidt *et al.*, 1988). Studies using mass spectrometry indicate that it is the guanidino nitrogen(s) of L-arginine that are incorporated into nitric oxide (Iyengar *et al.*, 1987; Palmer *et al.*, 1988), and chemical substitution at this point has led to the development of N^G-monomethyl L-arginine (L-NMMA), an inhibitor of the enzymic formation of nitric oxide from L-arginine. Although L-NMMA inhibits endothelium-dependent relaxation through blockade of EDRF synthesis, the D-isomer (D-NMMA) is inactive (Rees *et al.*, 1989), thus providing a test of the selectivity of the drug. Furthermore, it acts as a competitive inhibitor, since its effects are reversed by excess L-arginine.

Following elucidation of the formation of nitric oxide from L-arginine in the endothelial cell and macrophage, Garthwaite and colleagues (1988) showed that this pathway is present in central neurones. It is possible, therefore, that nitric oxide functions as a neurotransmitter or neuromodulator in the central nervous system (CNS). This, and the similarity of the NANC neurotransmitter to nitric oxide, prompted us to investigate if it too was derived from L-arginine. Adding L-arginine to isolated strips of BRP fails, however, to potentiate NANC relaxation (Gillespie and Xiaorong, 1989). The possibility was considered, however, that nitric oxide might still be the NANC neurotransmitter, but that endogenous levels of L-arginine are high enough to saturate the nitric oxide synthesizing enzyme. Consequently, BRP was stored for up to 10 days in the cold in the hope that endogenous levels of L-arginine would fall. Over this period NANC relaxation is progressively lost, but addition of L-arginine does not potentiate responsiveness. Adopting a different approach, by attempting to inhibit the nitric oxide synthesizing enzyme with L-NMMA was also disappointing: in concentrations up to 100 μM it failed to produce a convincing inhibition of the NANC response. These two negative findings argued against the involvement of the L-arginine–nitric oxide system in the NANC transmission process in BRP. However, findings in the rat anococcygeus were quite different. In this tissue L-NMMA produces two effects, a modest rise in tone and a rapid inhibition of NANC relaxation (Gillespie *et al.*, 1989; Li and Rand, 1989). Blockade is not complete; at the highest concentration tested (300 μM) it rarely exceeds 60%. It is specific, however, since it is not produced by the D-isomer, and is reversed by addition of exogenous L-arginine. Furthermore, the ability to inhibit the NANC response without affecting the relaxation induced by exogenously applied nitric oxide shows that the locus of action is the nerve terminals.

The ability of L-NMMA to inhibit the NANC response in the rat anococcygeus, but not the BRP, was surprising. The anatomical continuity of the two muscles and the similarity of their innervation makes it likely that they share a common neurotransmitter. In a recent report on mouse anococcygeus, however, the effectiveness of L-NMMA in blocking the NANC relaxation was compared with that of another analogue of L-arginine, N^G-nitro-L-arginine (L-NOARG; Gibson *et al.*, 1990). In this tissue, L-NMMA produces, as in rat anococcygeus, about 50% inhibition of NANC relaxation, but L-NOARG is about 30 times more potent and blocks relaxation completely. As with L-NMMA, the action of L-NOARG is competitive in nature, since it is reversed by the addition of exogenous L-arginine. Following publication of this report, we examined the effects of L-NOARG on the NANC response in the BRP and rat anococcygeus and found that in these tissues also, complete blockade can be produced with concentrations of around 100 μM. In addition, we have recently found that NANC relaxation of the bovine penile artery is blocked by L-NOARG (unpublished observations). In all these tissues, the L-NOARG-induced blockade can be reversed using L-arginine, but the concentrations required are greater than with blockade induced by L-NMMA, reflecting the greater efficacy of L-NOARG. The blockade by L-NOARG is also highly selective since the relaxant actions of nitric oxide and a range of nitrovasodilators is unaffected (Gibson *et al.*, 1990).

The effectiveness of L-NOARG on the rat and mouse anococcygeus and on the BRP and bovine penile artery strongly implicates the L-arginine–nitric oxide pathway in the NANC neurotransmission process in these tissues. The ineffectiveness of L-NMMA in the BRP may suggest a species difference in the nitric oxide synthesizing enzyme from that in the rat and mouse anococcygeus. There is already evidence to suggest that the enzyme in the macrophage is different from that in the endothelial cell since the former is inhibited by L-NMMA and L-canavanine, but the latter is inhibited only by L-NMMA (Hibbs *et al.*, 1987; Iyengar *et al.*, 1987; Rees *et al.*, 1989).

15.2.12 **Other tissues**

Subsequent to the proposal that the L-arginine–nitric oxide system mediates NANC neurotransmission in the anococcygeus of the rat (Gillespie *et al.*, 1989; Li and Rand, 1989) and mouse (Gibson *et al.*, 1990), reports have been published suggesting the presence of a similar nerve in other tissues. The ability of haemoglobin or haemolysate to inhibit NANC vasodilation in cerebral arteries (Lee *et al.*, 1984; Toda, 1988), had previously suggested that the nerve was similar to that present in the anococcygeus and BRP. This suggestion was confirmed by the finding that L-NMMA inhibits NANC relaxation of dog cerebral artery in an L-arginine-reversible manner (Toda and Okamura, 1990). Although the major NANC relaxant nerve in the gut is an apamin-sensitive purinergic nerve (Burnstock, 1972; Banks *et al.*, 1979), the L-arginine–nitric oxide system may also be present. This is suggested by the finding that nerve stimulation of the canine ileocolonic junction induces release of a vasorelaxant indistinguishable from nitric oxide (Bult *et al.*, 1990). Part of the NANC relaxation of guinea-pig trachea is also blocked by L-NOARG (Tucker *et al.*, 1990). It is possible, therefore, that this NANC nerve may be more widespread than previously appreciated.

15.3. *Conclusions*

Experiments with L-NMMA and L-NOARG suggest that the L-arginine–nitric oxide system mediates NANC relaxant responses in the anococcygeus of the rat (Gillespie *et al.*, 1989; Li and Rand, 1989) and mouse (Gibson *et al.*, 1990), the BRP and penile artery, the trachea of the guinea-pig (Tucker *et al.*, 1990) and the cerebral artery (Toda and Okamura, 1990) and the ileocolonic junction of the dog (Bult *et al.*, 1990). The presence of this pathway in the CNS (Garthwaite *et al.*, 1988) suggests that here too, nitric oxide may act as a neurotransmitter. These findings clearly present a novel concept in neurotransmission, difficult to reconcile with the established view of preformed neurotransmitters in storge vesicles released in a quantal manner. Nitric oxide production from L-arginine occurs only when the nerve is activated, possibly following influx of calcium (Knowles *et al.*, 1989), and unless L-arginine is stored in vesicles, is unlikely to be quantal. Nevertheless, an enzyme capable of synthesizing nitric oxide is present in nervous tissue (Knowles *et al.*, 1989), inhibition of nitric oxide synthesis blocks NANC transmission (Gillespie *et al.*, 1989; Gibson *et al.*, 1990; Toda and Okamura, 1990), release of a nitric oxide-like substance can be detected following nerve stimulation (Bult *et al.*, 1990), nitric oxide mimics the action of the NANC neurotransmitter (Gillespie *et al.*, 1989), and drugs similarly inhibit the action of nitric oxide and the NANC neurotransmitter (Bowman *et al.*, 1982b; Martin *et al.*, 1986a; Gillespie and Sheng, 1988b). Thus, many of the criteria of Eccles (1964), which a neurotransmitter must satisfy, have been demonstrated for nitric oxide. It remains to be seen if all these criteria can be demonstrated in a single tissue and thereby conclusively establish nitric oxide as a neurotransmitter.

Acknowledgements

These studies were supported by the British Heart Foundation, the Nuffield Foundation and the Medical Research Funds of the University of Glasgow.

References

Ambache, N. and Killick, S.W. (1978). Species differences in post-ganglionic motor transmission to the retractor penis muscle. *British Journal of Pharmacology*, **63**, 25–34.

Ambache, N., Killick, S.W. and Zar, M.A. (1975). Extraction from ox retractor penis of an inhibitory substance which mimics its atropine-resistant neurogenic relaxation. *British Journal of Pharmacology*, **54**, 409–410.

Arnold, W.P., Mittal, C.K., Katsuki, S. and Murad, F. (1977). Nitric oxide activates guanylate cyclase and increases guanosine 3′,5′-cyclic monophosphate levels in various tissue preparations. *Proceedings of the National Academy of Sciences USA*, **74**, 3203–3207.

Banks, B.E.C., Brown, C., Burgess, G.M., Burnstock, G., Claret, M., Cocks, T.M. and Jenkinson, D.H. (1979). Apamin blocks certain neurotransmitter-induced increases in potassium permeability. Nature, **282**, 415–417.

Bargmann, W., Lindner, E. and Andres, K. (1967). Uber Synapsen an endokrinen Epithelzellen und die Definition sekretorischer Neurone. Untersuckungen am Zwischenlappen der Katzenhypophyse. *Zeitschrift Zellforschung Mikroskopische Anatomie,* **77**, 282–298.

Baumgarten, H.G., Hostein, A.F. and Owman, C. (1970). Auerbach's plexus of mammals and man; electron microscopic identification of three different types of neuronal processes in myenteric ganglia of the large intestinal from rhesus monkeys, guinea-pigs and man. *Zeitschrift Zellforschung Mikroskopische Anatomie*, **106**, 376–397.

Bell, C. and McLean, J.R. (1970). The distribution of cholinergic and adrenergic fibres in the retractor penis and vas deferens of the dog. *Zeitschrift Zellforschung Mikroskopische Anatomie*, **106**, 516–522.

Bowman, A. and Drummond, A.H. (1984). Cyclic GMP mediates neurogenic relaxation in the bovine retractor penis muscle. *British Journal of Pharmacology,* **81**, 651–674.

Bowman, A. and Gillespie, J.S. (1982). Block of some non-adrenergic inhibitory responses of smooth muscle by a substance from haemolysed erythrocytes. *Journal of Physiology*, **328**, 11–25.

Bowman, A. and Gillespie, J.S. (1983). Neurogenic vasodilatation in isolated bovine and canine penile arteries. *Journal of Physiology*, **341**, 603–616.

Bowman, A. and McGrath, J.C. (1985). The effect of hypoxia on neuroeffector transmission in the bovine retractor penis and rat anococcygeus muscles. *British Journal of Pharmacology,* **85**, 869–875.

Bowman, A., Gillespie, J.S. and Martin, W. (1979). The inhibitory material in extracts from the bovine retractor penis muscle is not an adenine nucleotide. *British Journal of Pharmacology*, **67**, 327–328.

Bowman, A., Gillespie, J.S. and Martin, W. (1981). Actions on the cardiovascular system of an inhibitory material extracted from the bovine retractor penis. *British Journal of Pharmacology*, **72**, 365–372.

Bowman, A., Gillespie, J.S. and Hunter, J.C. (1982a). VIP (vasoactive intestinal polypeptide) is not the inhibitory transmitter in the bovine and dog retractor penis muscles. *Journal of Physiology*, **329**, 42–43.

Bowman, A., Gillespie, J.S. and Pollock, D. (1982b). Oxyhaemoglobin blocks non-adrenergic inhibition in the bovine retractor penis muscle. *European Journal of Pharmacology*, **85**, 221–224.

Bowman, A., Gillespie, J.S. and Soares-De-Silva, P. (1986). A comparison of the actions of endothelium-derived relaxant factor and the inhibitory factor from the bovine retractor penis on rabbit aortic smooth muscle. *British Journal of Pharmacology*, **87**, 175–181.

Braughler, M.J., Mittal, C.K. and Murad, F. (1979). Effects of thiols, sugars and proteins on nitric oxide activation of guanylate cyclase. *Journal of Biological Chemistry*, **254**, 12450–12454.

Bult, H., Boeckxstaens, G.E., Pelckmans, P.A., Jordaens, F.H., Van Maercke,

Y.M. and Herman, A.G. (1990). Nitric oxide as an inhibitory non-adrenergic non-cholinergic neurotransmitter. *Nature*, **345**, 346–247.

Burnstock, G. (1972). Purinergic nerves. *Pharmacological Reviews*, **24**, 509–581.

Burnstock, G. (1979). Past and current evidence for the purinergic nerve hypothesis. In: *Physiological and Regulatory Functions of Adenosine and Adenine Nucleotides*, edited by H.P. Baer and G.I. Drummond. New York: Raven Press, pp. 66–74.

Burnstock, G., Cocks, T.M. and Crowe, R. (1978). Evidence for purinergic innervation of the anococcygeus muscle. *British Journal of Pharmacology*, **64**, 13–20.

Burnstock, G., Campbell, G., Bennett, M. and Holman, M.E. (1963). Inhibition of the smooth muscle of the taenia coli. *Nature*, **200**, 581–582.

Byrne, N.G. and Muir, T.C. (1984). Electrical and mechanical responses of the bovine retractor penis to nerve stimulation and to drugs. *Journal of Autonomic Pharmacology*, **4**, 261–271.

Carvajal, A., Gibson, A. and Yu, O. (1986). Evidence against VIP – involvement in neurogenic relaxations of the mouse anococcygeus muscle. *Journal of Pharmacy and Pharmacology*, **38**, 767–769.

Cocks, T.M., Angus, J.A., Campbell, J.H. and Campbell, G.R. (1985). Release and properties of endothelium-derived relaxing factor (EDRF) from endothelial cells in culture. *Journal of Physiology*, **123**, 310–320.

Craven, P.A. and De Rubertis, F.R. (1978). Restoration of the responsiveness of purified guanylate cyclase to nitrosoguanidine, nitric oxide and related activators by heme and hemeproteins. *Journal of Biological Chemistry*, **253**, 8433–8443.

Creed, K.E., and Gillespie, J.S. (1977). Some electrical properties of the rabbit anococcygeus muscle and a comparison of the effects of inhibitory nerve stimulation in rat and rabbit. *Journal of Physiology*, **273**, 137–153.

Creed, K.E., Gillespie, J.S. and Muir, T.C. (1975). The electrical basis of excitation and inhibition in the rat anococcygeus muscle. *Journal of Physiology*, **245**, 33–47.

Creed, K.E., Gillespie, J.S. and McCaffery, H. (1977). The rabbit anococcygeus muscle and its response to field stimulation and to some drugs. *Journal of Physiology*, **273**, 121–135.

Crossley, A.W.A. and Gillespie, J.S. (1983). The effect of an inhibitory factor from the bovine retractor penis on the gastro-intestinal tract and gall bladder of the guinea-pig. *British Journal of Pharmacology*, **78**, 213–220.

Dale, H.H. (1906). On some physiological actions of ergot. *Journal of Physiology*, **34**, 163–206.

Dale, H.H. and Gaddum, J.H. (1930). Reactions of denervated voluntary muscle and their bearing on the mode of action of parasympathetic and related nerves. *Journal of Physiology*, **70**, 109–144.

Dusting, G.J. Read, M.A. and Stewart, A.G. (1988). Endothelium-derived relaxing factor released from cultured cells: differentiation from nitric oxide. *Clinical and Experimental Pharmacology and Physiology*, **15**, 83–92.

Eccles, J.C. (1964) *The Physiology of Synapses*. Berlin: Springer.

Eränkö, O., Klinge, E. and Sjöstrand, N.O. (1976). Different types of synaptic vesicles in axons of the retractor penis muscle of the bull. *Experientia*, **32**, 1335–1337.

Falck, G. (1962). Observations on the possibilities of the cellular localization of monoamines by a fluorescence method. Acta *Physiologica Scandinavica*, **56**, (Suppl. 197), 1–25.

Förstermann, U., Trogisch, G. and Busse, R. (1985). Species-dependent differences in the nature of endothelium-derived vascular relaxing factor. *European Journal of Pharmacology*, **106**, 639–643.

Furchgott, R.F. (1988). Studies on the relaxation of rabbit aorta by sodium nitrite: the basis for the proposal that the acid-activatable inhibitory factor from bovine retractor penis is inorganic nitrite and the endothelium-derived relaxing factor is nitric oxide. In: *Mechanisms of Vasodilatation*, edited by P.M. Vanhoutte. New York: Raven Press, pp. 31–36.

Furchgott, R.F. and Zawadzki, J.V. (1980). The obligatory role of endothelial cells in the relaxation of arterial smooth muscle by acetylcholine. *Nature*, **288**, 373–376.

Garrett, J.R., Howard, E.R. and Lansdale, J.M. (1972). Myenteric nerves in the hind gut of the cat. *Journal of Physiology*, **226**, 103–104.

Garthwaite, J., Charles, S.L. and Chess-Williams, R. (1988). Endothelium-derived relaxing factor release on activation of NMDA receptors suggest role as intercellular messenger in the brain. *Nature*, **336**, 385–388.

Gibbins, I.L. (1982). Lack of correlation between ultrastructural and pharmacological types of non-adrenergic autonomic nerves. *Cell and Tissue Research*, **221**, 551–581.

Gibbins, I.L. and Haller, C.J. (1979). Ultrastructural identification of non-adrenergic, non-cholinergic nerves in the rat anococcygeus muscle. *Cell and Tissue Research*, **200**, 257–271.

Gibson, A. and Gillespie, J.S. (1973). Effect of immunosympathectomy and 6-hydroxydopamine on the response of the rat anococcygeus to nerve stimulation and to some drugs. *British Journal of Pharmacology*, **47**, 261–267.

Gibson, A. and Mirzazadeh, S. (1989). *N*-methylhydroxylamine inhibits and M & B 22,948 potentiates relaxations of the mouse anococcygeus to non-adrenergic, non-cholinergic field stimulation and to nitrovasodilator drugs. *British Journal of Pharmacology*, **96**, 637–644.

Gibson, A. and Tucker, J.F. (1982). The effects of vasoactive intestinal polypeptide and of adenosine 5′-triphosphate on the isolated anococcygeus of the mouse. *British Journal of Pharmacology*, **77**, 97–103.

Gibson, A., Mirzazadeh, S., Hobbs, A.J. and Moore, P.K. (1990). L-N^G-monomethyl arginine and L-N^G-nitro arginine inhibit non-adrenergic, non-cholinergic relaxation of the mouse anococcygeus muscle. *British Journal of Pharmacology*, **99**, 602–606.

Gillespie, J.S. (1972). The rat anococcygeus muscle and its response to nerve stimulation and to some drugs. *British Journal of Pharmacology*, **45**, 404–416.

Gillespie, J.S. and Hunter, J.C. (1982). Subcellular localisation of the smooth muscle inhibitory factor isolated from the bovine retractor penis muscle. *British Journal of Pharmacology*, **76**, 189P.

Gillespie, J.S. and Lüllmann-Rauch, R. (1974). On the ultrastructure of the rat anococcygeus muscle. *Cell and Tissue Research*, **149**, 91–104.

Gillespie, J.S. and McGrath, J.C. (1973). The spinal origin of the motor and inhibitory innervation of the rat anococcygeus muscles. *Journal of Physiology*, **230**, 656–672.

Gillespie, J.S. and McGrath, J.C. (1974). The response of the cat anococcygeus to nerve or drug stimulation and a comparison with the rat anococcygeus. *British Journal of Pharmacology*, **50**, 109–118.

Gillespie, J.S. and McKnight, A.T. (1978). The actions of some polypeptides and their antagonists on the anococcygeus muscle. *British Journal of Pharmacology*, **62**, 267–274.

Gillespie, J.S. and Martin, W. (1980). A smooth muscle inhibitory material from the bovine retractor penis and rat anococcygeus muscles. *Journal of Physiology*, **304**, 55–64.

Gillespie, J.S. and Sheng, H. (1988a). A comparison of haemoglobin and erythrocytes as inhibitors of smooth muscle relaxation by the NANC transmitter in the BRP and rat anococcygeus and by EDRF in the rabbit aortic strip. *British Journal of Pharmacology*, **98**, 445–450.

Gillespie, J.S and Sheng, H. (1988b). Influence of haemoglobin and erythrocytes on the effects of EDRF, a smooth muscle inhibitory factor, and nitric oxide on vascular and non-vascular smooth muscle. *British Journal of Pharmacology*, **95**, 1151–1156.

Gillespie, J.S. and Sheng, H. (1990). The effects of pyrogallol and hydroquinone on the response to NANC nerve stimulation in the rat anococcygeus and the bovine retractor penis muscles. *British Journal of Pharmacology*, **99**, 194–196.

Gillespie, J.S. and Xiaorong, L. (1989). The effect of arginine and L-*N*-monomethyl arginine on the response of the bovine retractor penis to stimulation of its NANC nerve. *British Journal of Pharmacology*, **97**, 453P.

Gillespie, J.S., Hunter, J.C. and Martin, W. (1981). Some physical and chemical properties of the smooth muscle inhibitory factor in extracts of bovine retractor penis muscle. *Journal of Physiology*, **315**, 111–125.

Gillespie, J.S., Hunter, J.C. and McKnight, A.T. (1982). The effect of ethanol on inhibitory and motor responses in the rat and rabbit anococcygeus and the bovine retractor penis muscles. *British Journal of Pharmacology*, **75**, 189–198.

Gillespie, J.S., Liu, X. and Martin, W. (1989). The effects of L-arginine and N^{G}-monomethyl L-arginine on the response of the rat anococcygeus to NANC nerve stimulation. *British Journal of Pharmacology*, **98**, 1080–1082.

Greeff, K., Kasperat, H. and Osswald, W. (1962). Paradoxe Wirkungen der elektrischen Vagusreizung am isolierten Magen- und Herzvorhofpräparat des Meerschweinchens sowie deren Beeinflussung durch Ganglien blocker, Sympathicolytica, Reserpin und Cocain. *Naunyn-Schmiedeberg's Archiv Pharmakologie Experimentelle Pathologi*, **243**, 528–545.

Griffith, T.M., Edwards, D.H., Lewis, M.J., Newby, A.C. and Henderson, A.H. (1984). The nature of endothelium-derived vascular relaxant factor. *Nature*, **308**, 645–647.

Gryglewski, R.J., Palmer, R.M.J. and Moncada, S. (1986). Superoxide anion is involved in the breakdown of endothelium-derived vascular relaxing factor. *Nature*, **320**, 454–456.

Hibbs, J.B., Jr, Vavrin, Z. and Taintor, R.R. (1987). L-Arginine is required for expression of the activated macrophage effector mechanism causing selective metabolic inhibition in target cells. *Journal of Immunology*, **138**, 550–565.

Hoyes, A.D. and Barber, P. (1976). Parameters of fixation of the putative pain afferents in the ureter: preservation of the dense cores of the large vesicles in the axon terminals. *Journal of Anatomy*, **122**, 113–120.

Hunter, J.C., Maggio, J.E. and Mantyk, P.W. (1984). Evidence for vasoactive intestinal polypeptide as a neurotransmitter in smooth muscle of the urogenital tract. *Brain Research*, **305**, 221–229.

Ignarro, L.J., Harbison, R.G., Wood, K.S. and Kadowitz, P.J. (1986). Activation of purified soluble guanylate cyclase by endothelium-derived relaxing factor from intrapulmonary artery and vein: stimulation by acetylcholine, bradykinin and arachidonic acid. *Journal of Pharmacology and Experimental Therapeutics*, **237**, 893–900.

Ignarro, L.J., Buga, G.M., Wood, K.S. and Byrnes, R.E. (1987). Endothelium-derived relaxing factor produced and released from artery and vein is nitric oxide. *Proceedings of the National Academy of Sciences USA*, **84**, 9265–9269.

Iijima, T. (1983). Quinacrine-induced degeneration of non-adrenergic, non-cholinergic autonomic nerves in the rat anococcygeus muscle. *Cell and Tissue Research*, **230**, 639–648.

Iyengar, R., Stuehr, D.J. and Marletta, M.A. (1987). Macrophage synthesis of nitrite, nitrate and *N*-nitrosamines: precursors and role of the respiratory burst. *Proceedings of the National Academy of Sciences USA*, **84**, 6369–6373.

Jang, C.S. (1940). The potentiation and paralysis of adrenergic effects by ergotoxine and other substances. *Journal of Pharmacology and Experimental Therapeutics*, **71**, 87–94.

Katsuki, S., Arnold, W., Mittal, C.K. and Murad, F. (1977). Stimulation of guanylate cyclase by sodium nitroprusside, nitroglycerin and nitric oxide in various tissue preparations and comparison to the effects of sodium azide and hydroxylamine. *Journal of Cyclic Nucleotide Research*, **3**, 23–25.

Kelm, M. and Schrader, J. (1988). Nitric oxide release from the isolated guinea pig heart. *European Journal of Pharmacology*, **155**, 317–321.

Klinge, E. and Sjöstrand, N.O. (1974). Contraction and relaxation of the retractor penis muscle and the penile artery of the bull. *Acta Physiologica Scandinavica*, (Suppl.), **420**, 1–88.

Klinge, E. Pohto, P. and Solatunturi, E. (1970). Adrenergic innervation and structure of bull retractor penis muscle. *Acta Physiologica Scandinavica*, **78**, 110–116.

Knowles, R.G., Palacios, M., Palmer, R.M.J. and Moncada, S. (1989). Formation of nitric oxide from L-arginine in the central nervous system: A transduction mechanism for the stimulation of soluble guanylate cyclase. *Proceedings of the National Academy of Sciences USA*, **86**, 5159–5162.

Langley, J.N. and Anderson, H.K. (1895). Innervation of the pelvic and adjoining viscera. Part III. *Journal of Physiology*, **19**, 85–121.

Langley, J.N. and Anderson, H.K. (1896). Innervation of the pelvic and adjoining viscera VI. Anatomical observations. *Journal of Physiology*, **20**, 372–406.

Lee, T.J.-F., McIlhany, M.P. and Sarwinski, S. (1984). Erythrocyte extracts enhance neurogenic vasoconstriction of dog cerebral arteries. *Journal of Cerebral Blood Flow and Metabolism*, **4**, 474–476.

Li, C.G. and Rand, M.J. (1989). Evidence for a role of nitric oxide in the neurotransmitter system mediating relaxation of the rat anococcygeus muscle. *Clinical and Experimental Pharmacology and Physiology*, **16**, 933–938.

Loewi, O. (1921). Über Humorale Übertagbarkeit der Herznervenwirkung. *Pflügers Archiv Gesamte Physiologie Menschen Tiere*, **189**, 239–242.

Long, C.J. and Berkowitz, B.A. (1989). What is the relationship between endothelium-derived relaxant factor and nitric oxide? *Life Sciences*, **45**, 1–14.

Luduena, F.P. and Grigas, E.O. (1966). Pharmacological study of antonomic innervation of dog retractor penis. *American Journal of Physiology*, **210**, 435–444.

Luduena, F.P. and Grigas, E.O. (1972). Effect of some biological substances on dog retractor penis *in vitro*. *Archives Internationales Pharmacodynamie Therapie*, **196**, 269–274.

Martin, W., Smith, J.A. and White, D.G. (1986a). The mechanism by which haemoglobin inhibits relaxation of rabbit aorta induced by nitrovasodilators, nitric oxide and bovine retractor penis inhibitory factor. *British Journal of Pharmacology*, **89**, 563–572.

Martin, W., Smith, J.A. Lewis, M.J. and Henderson, A.H. (1988). Evidence that inhibitory factor extracted from bovine retractor penis is nitrite, whose acid-activated derivative is stabilized nitric oxide. *British Journal of Pharmacology*, **93**, 579–586.

Martin, W., Villani, G.M., Jothianandan, D. and Furchgott, R.F. (1985). Selective blockade of endothelium-dependent and glyceryl trinitrate-induced relaxation by hemoglobin and by methylene blue in the rabbit aorta. *Journal of Pharmacology and Experimental Therapeutics*, **232**, 708–716.

Martin, W., Morgan, R.D., Smith, J.A. and White D.G. (1986b). Atriopeptin

II-induced relaxation of rabbit aorta is potentiated by M & B 22,948 but not blocked by haemoglobin. *British Journal of Pharmacology*, **89**, 557–561.
Moncada, S., Palmer, R.M.J. and Gryglewski, R.J. (1986). Mechanism of action of some inhibitors of endothelium-derived relaxing factor. *Proceedings of the National Academy of Sciences USA*, **83**, 9164–9168.
Mülsch, A., Bohme, E. and Busse, R. (1987). Stimulation of soluble guanylate cyclase by endothelium-derived relaxing factor from cultured endothelial cells. *European Journal of Pharmacology*, **135**, 247–250.
Murray, J.J., Fridovich, I., Makhoul, R.G. and Hagen, P.-O. (1986). Characterisation of endothelium-derived relaxing factor from cultured bovine aortic endothelial cells. *Biochemical and Biophysical Research Communications*, **144**, 689–696.
Myers, P.R., Guerra, R., Jr and Harrison, D.G. (1989). Release of NO and EDRF from cultured bovine aortic endothelial cells. *American Journal of Physiology*, **256**, H1030–H1037.
Myers, P.R., Minor, R.L., Jr, Guerra, R., Jr, Bates, J.N. and Harrison, D.G. (1990). Vasorelaxant properties of the endothelium-derived relaxing factor more closely resemble S-nitrosocyotein than nitric oxide. *Nature*, **343**, 161–163.
Olson, L. and Alund, M. (1979). Quinacrine-binding nerves: presence in the mouse anococcygeus muscle, disappearance after muscle transection. *Medical Biology*, **57**, 182–186.
Palmer, R.M.J., Ferrige, A.G. and Moncada, S. (1987). Nitric oxide release accounts for the biological activity of endothelium-derived relaxing factor. *Nature*, **327**, 524–526.
Palmer, R.M.J. Ashton, D.S. and Moncada, S. (1988). Vascular endothelial cells sythesize nitric oxide from L-arginine. *Nature*, **333**, 664–666.
Paton, W. and Vane, J.R. (1963). An analysis of the responses of the isolated stomach to electrical field stimulation and to drugs. *Journal of Physiology*, **165**, 10–46.
Rapoport, R.M. and Murad, F. (1983). Agonist-induced endothelium-dependent relaxation in rat thoracic aorta may be mediated through cGMP. *Circulation Research*, **52**, 352–357.
Rees, D.D., Palmer, R.M.J., Hodson, H.F. and Moncada, S. (1989). A specific inhibitor of nitric oxide formation from L-arginine attenuates endothelium-dependent relaxation. *British Journal of Pharmacology*, **96**, 418–424.
Rubanyi, G.M. and Vanhoutte, P.M. (1986). Superoxide anions and hyperoxia inactivate endothelium-derived relaxing factor. *American Journal of Physiology*, **250**, H822–H827.
Schmidt, H.H.H.W., Hau, H., Wittfoht, W., Gerlach, J., Prescher, K.-E., Klein, M.M., Niroomand, F. and Bohme, E. (1988). Arginine is a physiological precursor of endothelium-derived nitric oxide. *European Journal of Pharmacology*, **154**, 213–216.
Sisler, H.H. (1956). Nitrogen, phosphorus, arsenic, antimony and bismuth. In *Comprehensive Inorganic Chemistry. Vol 5*, edited by M.C. Sneed and R.C. Brasted. Princeton, New Jersey: Van Nostrand Inc., pp. 60–77.
Sjöstrand, N.O., Klinge, E. and Himberg, J.-J. (1981). Effects of VIP and other putative neurotransmitters on smooth muscle effectors of penile erection. *Acta Physiologica Scandinavica*, **113**, 403–405.
Sjöqvist, A., Delbro, D., Jodal, M. and Lundgren, O. (1980). The effect of apamin on non-adrenergic, non-cholinergic nervous vasodilations in the cat small intestines. *Experientia*, **36**, 4202.
Sneddon, P. and Burnstock, G. (1984). ATP as a co-transmitter in rat tail artery. *European Journal of Pharmacology*, **106**, 149–152.
Toda, N. (1988). Haemolysate inhibits cerebral artery relaxation. *Journal of Cerebral Blood Flow and Metabolism*, **8**, 46–53.

Toda, N. and Okamura, T. (1990). Modification by LN^G-monomethyl arginine (L-NMMA) of the response to nerve stimulation in isolated dog mesenteric and cerebral arteries. *Japanese Journal of Pharmacology*, **52**, 170–173.

Tucker, J.F., Brave, S.R., Charalambous, L., Hobbs, A.J. and Gibson, A. (1990). L-N^G-nitro arginine inhibits non-adrenergic, non-cholinergic relaxations, of guinea-pig isolated tracheal smooth muscle. *British Journal of Pharmacology*, **100**, 633–634.

Part V

5-Hydroxytryptamine (5-HT)

Chapter 16

Physiological and pharmacological aspects of 5-HT_3 receptor function

John A. Peters, Jeremy J. Lambert and Hilary M. Malone

16.1. *Introduction*

It is now nearly 40 years since the groups of Gaddum in Edinburgh and Rocha e. Silva in São Paulo analysed the contractile effect of 5-hydroxytryptamine (5-HT) upon the guinea-pig ileum, and attributed the response to the activation of a 'tryptamine' receptor distinct from other receptor types present in the gut (Gaddum, 1953; Rocha e. Silva *et al.*, 1953). From the outset of this research, the pharmacology of 'tryptamine' receptor-mediated contractile responses was noted to vary between different smooth muscle preparations, prompting Gaddum and Hameed (1954) to postulate the existence of two types of 'tryptamine' receptor. This theory was stated trenchantly in the seminal paper of Gaddum and Picarelli (1957), where the action of 5-HT upon the ileum was proposed to be due to the activation of two receptor subtypes; namely a 'D' receptor located upon muscular elements, and a pharmacologically distinct 'M' receptor situated upon intramural cholinergic neurones. The latter was suggested to mediate an indirect contractile response by stimulating the release of acetylcholine. The choice of nomenclature was perhaps unfortunate, since much of the criticism that this report attracted was directed at the use of morphine and dibenzyline (the drugs giving rise to the terminology M and D) as specific receptor antagonists. Although semantically flawed, the M and D receptor terminology was widely adopted by pharmacologists and continued to appear in the literature until recently. Alternative schemes of 5-HT receptor classification, which attempted to encompass a growing number of functional responses fitting into neither the M nor D categories, were received with little enthusiasm.

The identification of 5-HT recognition sites in the central nervous system (CNS) by the use of radioligand binding techniques further emphasized the heterogeneity of putative 5-HT receptors. In an influential paper, Peroutka and Snyder (1979) described the properties of two distinct 5-HT recognition sites, termed 5-HT_1 and 5-HT_2, which were selectively labelled by [^{3}H]-5-HT and [^{3}-H]-spiperone, respectively. Subsequent investigations have revealed far greater complexity, with at least five subtypes of 5-HT_1 recognition site, termed 5-HT_{1A}, 5-HT_{1B}, 5-HT_{1C}, 5-HT_{1D} and 5-HT_{1E}, being demonstrated to date (see Peroutka, 1988; Leonhardt *et al.*, 1989) along with possible heterogeneity, or multiple affinity states, within the 5-HT_2 category (Lyon *et al.*, 1987; McKenna and Peroutka, 1989). In an attempt to reconcile the differing terminologies introduced by Gaddum and Picarelli (1957) and Peroutka and Snyder (1979), Bradley *et al.* (1986) proposed a new classification and nomenclature for functional 5-HT receptors, based largely on data obtained from isolated peripheral tissues. A comparison of the pharmacological profiles of the 5-HT_2 recognition site and the 'D' receptor led to the conclusion that the two were essentially identical. The appellation 'D' receptor became redundant in favour of the more prevalent term 5-HT_2. The category '5-HT_1-like' was introduced to include functional receptors demonstrating pharmacological similarities to the heterogenous 5-HT_1 binding sites described in the CNS. The 'M' receptor was incorporated within a newly defined 5-HT_3 class, which is the subject of this chapter. The central binding site equivalent of the 5-HT_3 receptor (Kilpatrick *et al.*, 1987) emerged subsequent to the recommendations of Bradley *et al.* (1986) along with the discovery of further subtypes of 5-HT receptor e.g. 5-HT_{1P} (Mawe *et al.* 1986) and 5-HT_4 (Clarke *et al.*, 1989).

The scheme developed by Bradley *et al.* (1986) quite properly stressed the role of functional responses and the use of potent, selective and competitively acting receptor antagonists in the classification of 5-HT receptors. However, the nature of the linkage between the receptor activation and response was not considered, and the powerful contributions currently emanating from molecular biological studies could not have been envisaged. When these factors are taken into account, 5-HT receptors might be broadly divided into two families: receptors definitely (or most probably) coupled to G-proteins and exerting their effects via the phospholipase C cascade (5-HT_{1C}, 5-HT_2) or adenylate cyclase (5-HT_{1A}, 5-HT_{1B}, 5-HT_{1D} and 5-HT_4), and those in which an ion channel is likely to be integral to the receptor protein (5-HT_3; see reviews by Hoyer, 1989; Hartig, 1989; Frazer *et al.*, 1990). The properties of the latter, which are described in detail below, suggest similarities with the nicotinic/γ-aminobutyric acid $(GABA)_A$/glycine channel 'superfamily'.

16.2. *Functional responses mediated by 5-HT_3 receptors*

Bradley *et al.* (1986) clearly defined the criteria that must be satisfied before associating a functional response with the activation of the 5-HT_3 receptor subtype. Firstly, the action of 5-HT should be blocked by selective 5-HT_3 receptor antagonists, such as MDL-72222, ICS 205-930, ondansetron or granisetron, but be resistant to antagonism by compounds interacting with '5-HT_1-like' receptors (e.g. methiothepin) or 5-HT_2 receptors (e.g. methysergide, ketanserin). Secondly, 2-methyl-5-HT and other agonists selective for the 5-HT_3 receptor should mimic the effect of 5-HT. 5-HT receptors satisfying these criteria are present in both the central and peripheral nervous systems, and occur in several neuronal clonal cell lines.

16.2.1. **Peripheral nervous system**

5-HT_3 receptors are widely distributed in the periphery, but unlike other 5-HT receptor subtypes, they appear to be confined to nervous tissue. 5-HT_3 receptor activation most frequently elicits excitatory responses, the underlying mechanism probably being neuronal depolarization contingent upon an increase in membrane cation conductance (see Section 16.4). Within the sympathetic division of the autonomic nervous system, 5-HT_3 receptors have been documented to occur on the axons, and possibly terminals of preganglionic neurones and the somata and terminals of some, but not all, postganglionic neurones (reviewed by Wallis, 1989). At the terminals of stellate ganglion cells innervating the rabbit heart, 5-HT_3 receptor activation evokes the release of noradrenaline, resulting in a positive chronotropic and inotropic response (Fozard and Mobarok Ali, 1978b; Gothert and Duhrsen, 1979). The release of transmitter is calcium-dependent (Fozard and Mwaluko, 1976) and presumably due to a membrane depolarization, similar in character to that recorded directly from the somata of postganglionic sympathetic neurones. In contrast, 5-HT evoked release of noradrenaline from sympathetic terminals in vascular smooth muscle appears to be due to a 'tyramine-like' action, involving the uptake of 5-HT and stoichiometric displacement of noradrenaline from storage vesicles, rather than 5-HT_3 receptor activation (Humphrey *et al.*, 1983).

5-HT_3 receptor-mediated release of transmitter substances has been reported to occur from the terminals of postganglionic parasympathetic neurones located in the guinea-pig urinary bladder and rabbit heart (Fozard, 1984a; Saxena *et al.*, 1985). By analogy to the action of 5-HT at the somata of parasympathetic neurones in the ciliary and vesicle pelvic ganglia of the rabbit (Akasu *et al.*, 1987; Tatsumi and Katayama, 1987), membrane depolarization most likely underlies this effect. We are not aware of any report demonstrating the existence of 5-HT_3 receptors on preganglionic parasympathetic neurones.

Within the enteric nervous system, 5-HT_3 receptors have been found on neurones of the myenteric and submucous plexus of the ileum (e.g. Mawe *et al.*, 1986; Suprenant and Crist, 1988). Their activation results in a fast, phasic, membrane depolarization that is distinct in its pharmacology and electrogenesis from other electrical responses to 5-HT in these cells (see review by Gershon *et al.*, 1989). The relationship between the 5-HT_3

receptor-mediated depolarization, seen in both Type I (or S) and Type II (or AH) myenteric neurones, and that component of the contractile response of the ileum which can be blocked by 5-HT_3 receptor antagonists, is unclear. The orthodox view that contraction via 5-HT_3 receptor stimulation is solely the result of the release of acetylcholine from intramural cholinergic neurones is open to a number of objections. Space precludes their discussion here, but the interested reader is referred to the papers by Chahl (1983), Bucheit *et al.* (1985), Gunning and Humphrey (1987) and Gershon *et al.* (1989). 5-HT_3 receptors located on submucous neurones have recently been implicated in 5-HT-induced water and electrolyte secretion in the ileum (Baird and Cuthbert, 1987; Hendriks *et al.*, 1989). The available evidence suggests that a 5-HT_3 receptor-mediated depolarization of cholinergic secretomotor neurones contributes to this effect.

5-HT is a powerful excitant of many sensory nerve endings, an effect emphasized by the earliest investigations of the indoleamine's physiological actions. Cutaneous pain in humans, following the application of 5-HT to a blister base on the forearm, was first reported by Armstrong *et al.* (1953). Subsequent electrophysiological investigations directly demonstrated the excitatory effect of 5-HT upon nerve endings associated with cutaneous afferent fibres of groups II, III and IV (e.g. Fjallbrandt and Iggo, 1961; Beck and Handwerker, 1974). The presence of 5-HT_3 receptors on cutaneous sensory nerve endings appears likely in view of the fact that ICS 205–930 selectively blocks the pain experienced when 5-HT, or 2-methyl-5-HT, is applied to a blister base (Richardson *et al.*, 1985). Furthermore, subcutaneously administered 5-HT_3 receptor antagonists produce analgesia against acute and chronic inflammatory pain in rats (Eschalier *et al.*, 1989; Giordano and Rogers, 1989). Electrophysiological studies indicate that 5-HT_3 receptors mediating transient membrane depolarization also occur upon the somata of some somatosensory primary afferent neurones (Bevan and Robertson, 1987; Todorovic and Anderson, 1990). Additionally, 5-HT is thought to depolarize the central terminals of afferent neurones in the spinal cord (Shirasawa and Koketsu, 1977; Carstens *et al.*, 1981; Holz and Anderson, 1984), but the subtype(s) of 5-HT receptor involved is at present uncertain. 5-HT_3 recognition sites have been found in synaptosomal membranes prepared from the dorsal spinal cord (Hamon *et al.*, 1989). Quantitative autoradiography performed on spinal tissue slices indicates that many of these sites may be associated with afferents terminating in the superficial layers of the dorsal horn (Hamon *et al.*, 1989).

Even prior to the chemical synthesis and widespread availability of 5-HT itself, Dawes and Mott (1950) had documented the prominant reflex cardiovascular and respiratory responses occurring to an intravenous injection of phenylbiguanide, a compound latterly identified as a relatively selective 5-HT_3 receptor agonist (see Section 16.3). The presence of 5-HT_3 receptors on the terminals, perhaps even the entire surface, of certain primary visceral afferent neurones has subsequently been demonstrated by many workers.

The activation of 5-HT$_3$ receptors associated with cardiac sensory receptors innervated by unmyelinated vagal afferent fibres leads to a reflex bradycardia and hypotension, known as the Bezold–Jarisch effect of 5-HT (e.g. Fastier *et al.*, 1959; Paintal, 1973). This reflex provides a convenient measure of receptor stimulation *in vivo*, and has proved useful in the characterization of 5-HT$_3$ receptors and the development of ligands selective for them (Fozard, 1984c, 1989). 5-HT$_3$ receptor-mediated electrical responses recorded from the vagus nerve and the somata of primary visceral afferents in the nodose ganglion have been particularly well studied, and are described in detail in Sections 16.3 and 16.4. The existence of 5-HT$_3$ recognition sites on the central terminals of visceral afferent neurones is strongly suggested by the results of recent autoradiographic studies (Pratt and Bowery, 1989; Pratt *et al.*, 1990).

16.2.2. **Central nervous system**

The presence of 5-HT$_3$ receptors in the CNS was originally inferred from behavioural studies attributing anxiolytic and antipsychotic properties to highly selective 5-HT$_3$ receptor antagonists (for references and comprehensive review of the psychopharmacology of 5-HT$_3$ receptors see Costall *et al.*, 1990). Recognition sites, displaying the pharmacological profile of 5-HT$_3$ receptors, were subsequently detected in rat brain by the use of high affinity, tritium-labelled 5-HT$_3$ receptor antagonists of varied chemical structure (e.g. [^{3}H]-GR 65630 — Kilpatrick *et al.*, 1987; [^{3}H]-zacopride — Barnes *et al.*, 1988; [^{3}H]-quipazine — Peroutka and Hamik, 1988; [^{3}H]-quaternized ICS 205–930 — Watling *et al.*, 1988). In the rat forebrain, these recognition sites are differentially localized, occurring most prominently in the entorhinal cortex and other cortical areas, amygdala, hippocampus and nucleus accumbens (Kilpatrick *et al.*, 1987). In other species, such as the mouse, ferret and rabbit, a different distribution of forebrain 5-HT$_3$ binding sites may apply (Kilpatrick *et al.*, 1989). Regardless of species, the highest density of 5-HT$_3$ recognition sites in the mammalian CNS occurs in hindbrain regions; primarily within the subnucleus gelatinosus of the nucleus tractus solitarius, but also in association with the area postrema, the dorsal motor nucleus of the vagus nerve and the nucleus of the spinal tract of the trigemminal nerve (Pratt *et al.*, 1990). 5-HT$_3$ receptors in the area postrema and nucleus tractus solitarius, together with those present on the peripheral terminals of primary visceral afferents, are potential sites at which 5-HT$_3$ receptor antagonists may exert their well-established action against cytotoxic drug- and radiation-evoked emesis (reviewed by Andrews *et al.*, 1988).

In contrast to the substantial literature describing the behavioural effects of 5-HT$_3$ receptor antagonists (see Costall *et al.*, 1990), there have been relatively few reports of biochemical or electrophysiological responses that can be attributed to the activation of central 5-HT$_3$ receptors. In mouse hippocampal and striatal neurones in cell culture, 5-HT evokes a fast inward membrane current response similar to that mediated by 5-HT_3 receptors in voltage-clamped peripheral neurones and various neuronal clonal cell lines (Yakel and Jackson, 1988; see Section 16.4). In the hippocampal cells, this response is undoubtedly due to 5-HT_3 receptor activation (Yakel and Jackson, 1988), but pharmacological characterization of the striatal receptor is as yet incomplete (Yakel *et al.*, 1988). Recent microiontophoretic studies have demonstrated a suppressant action of 1-phenylbiguanide and 2-methyl-5-HT upon the firing rate of medial prefrontal cortical neurones *in vivo* (Ashby *et al.*, 1989, 1990; Wang *et al.*, 1990). The effect of 2-methyl-5-HT was blocked by the iontophoretic ejection of 5-HT_3 receptor antagonists, but not by antagonists acting at '5-HT_1-like', 5-HT_2 dopamine D_1 or dopamine D_2 receptors. Magnesium ions and a $GABA_A$ receptor antagonist were also ineffective, suggesting a direct action of 2-methyl-5-HT upon the unit under study, rather than an effect secondary to the activation of a GABA-ergic interneurone. The inhibitory response to 1-phenylbiguanide and 2-methyl-5-HT is surprising, because at all other sites examined to date, 5-HT_3 receptor activation generates a membrane depolarization and action potential discharge (see Sections 16.3 and 16.4). Moreover, it has been claimed that 5-HT_3 receptors in rat entorhinal and frontal cortices are coupled to a second messenger system, rather than the direct gating of a cation selective ion channel. Wang, Ashby and their colleagues (Ashby *et al.*, 1990; Edwards *et al.*, 1991) have reported a stimulation of phosphoinositide (PI) hydrolysis in cortical slices challenged with 2-methyl-5-HT and phenylbiguanide. The response displayed a pharmacological profile consistent with 5-HT_3 receptor mediation, being completely blocked by ondansetron, ICS 205–930, granisetron and zacopride (albeit at very high concentrations. 10 μM; Ashby *et al.*, 1990), but unaffected by methysergide or ritanserin. The lack of effect of the 5-HT_{1C} and 5-HT_2 receptor antagonist, ritanserin, is significant, because these 5-HT receptor subtypes are known to be coupled to PI hydrolysis, (e.g. Frazer *et al.*, 1990) and indeed contribute to the stimulation of PI turnover in cortical slices when 5-HT itself is employed as the agonist (Wang *et al.*, 1990). Although the effect of the 5-HT_3 receptor agonists was unaltered by tetrodotoxin, this should not be taken as conclusive evidence against stimulation of PI hydrolysis consequent to neurotransmitter release in the slice. Detailed and rigorous investigations of the conductance mechanisms subserving the inhibitory effect of 5-HT_3 receptor activation in the frontal cortex, and the purported intermediacy of PI turnover in this response, are now urgently required. Verification of these provocative claims would suggest not merely 5-HT_3 receptor subtypes, but two completely different molecular forms of the 5-HT_3 receptor.

Recent studies indicate that 5-HT_3 receptor activation modulates the release of several neurotransmitter substances in the CNS. Blandina *et al.* (1988, 1989) have demonstrated that 5-HT and 2-methyl-5-HT increase the release of endogenous dopamine from rat striatal slices in a concentration and Ca^{2+}-dependent manner. The effect of these agonists was antagonized by low concentrations of ICS 205–930, but was resistant to blockade by methiothepin or methysergide. 5-HT$_1$-like and 5-HT$_2$ receptor agonists failed to elicit an increase in the release of dopamine. Interestingly, transmitter release evoked by 5-HT or 2-methyl-5-HT was maintained throughout the period of agonist application (24 min). Similarly 5-HT$_3$ receptors seem to mediate the release of dopamine from the rat nucleus accumbens (Jiang *et al.*, 1990). In the presence of the 5-HT$_2$ and 5-HT$_{1C}$ receptor antagonist, ritanserin, 5-HT inhibits the release of acetylcholine from rat entorhinal cortex (Barnes *et al.*, 1989). Preliminary evidence suggests that 5-HT$_3$ receptors may also inhibit the release of noradrenaline from rat hypothalamus (Blandina *et al.*, 1990) and enhance the electrically-evoked release of 5-HT from guinea-pig cortex (Galzin *et al.*, 1990). Clearly these investigations are at an early stage, but further work in this area may give an insight into the physiological role of 5-HT$_3$ receptors in the CNS and allow an understanding of the neurochemistry underlying the purported behavioural effects of 5-HT$_3$ antagonists (Costall *et al.*, 1990).

16.3. *Electrophysiological studies of 5-HT$_3$ receptor pharmacology*

From the stance of an electrophysiologist, studies which aim to understand the details of agonist and antagonist interactions with the 5-HT$_3$ receptor should use the most powerful techniques available, namely the direct observation of membrane currents elicited by receptor activation. That this approach is at a very early stage and presents many practical difficulties becomes apparent below. Quantitative pharmacological data can often be obtained by less direct electrophysiological methods, such as the extracellular measurement of voltage changes in multicellular tissues in response to superfused agonists. Tissues which have proved suitable for this purpose include isolated sympathetic ganglia, ganglia of primary visceral afferent neurones and the vagus nerve, all of which possess 5-HT$_3$ receptors mediating membrane depolarization (e.g. Wallis and Woodward, 1975; Wallis *et al.*, 1982; Ireland and Tyers, 1987).

16.3.1 **Agonist pharmacology**

In the preparations mentioned above, 5-HT and certain related compounds evoke a concentration-dependent depolarization that is blocked by selective 5-HT$_3$ receptor antagonists (see Section 16.3.2.). Such responses demonstrate tachyphylaxis, presumably due to receptor desensitization, an effect which is pronounced in the rabbit nodose and superior cervical ganglia (e.g. Wallis and Woodward, 1975), but apparently less marked in the rat vagus nerve (e.g. Ireland and Tyers, 1987). The depolarizing action of 5-HT is mimicked by several compounds which are purported to be selective 5-HT$_3$ receptor agonists including 2-methyl-5-HT (Richardson *et al.*, 1985), 1-phenylbiguanide (Wallis and Nash, 1981) and *m*-chlorophenylbiguanide (*m*-CPBG) (Kilpatrick *et al.*, 1990a).

2-Methyl-5-HT was identified as a relatively selective agonist from a range of methylated derivatives of 5-HT synthesized in the rational development of novel 5-HT_3 receptor ligands (Richardson *et al.*, 1985). In the vagus nerve of rat, rabbit and guinea-pig, and preganglionic cervical sympathetic nerves of the rabbit, 2-methyl-5-HT appears to act as a partial agonist with a potency approximately equal to, or seven-fold lower than, that of 5-HT. The maximal effect of 2-methyl-5-HT in these tissues ranges between 60 to 85% of that evoked by 5-HT (Richardson *et al.*, 1985; Ireland and Tyers, 1987; Elliot and Wallis, 1988; Burridge *et al.*, 1989; Cramer *et al.*, 1990; Kilpatrick *et al.*, 1990b). The selectivity of 2-methyl-5-HT has been questioned on the basis of radioligand binding studies which have shown that the compound binds to 5-HT_{1A}, 5-HT_{1B}, 5-HT_{1C} and 5-HT_{1D} recognition sites with affinity values similar to, or higher than, those reported for the 5-HT_3 receptor (Hoyer, 1989; Cramer *et al.*, 1990; Van Wijngaarden *et al.*, 1990). Additionally, in voltage-clamped, guinea-pig submucous plexus neurones, 2-methyl-5-HT activates an inward current response which is insensitive to ICS 205–930, a potent 5-HT_3 receptor antagonist (Suprenant and Crist, 1988).

Data from functional studies and radioligand binding assays indicate 1-phenylbiguanide to be a relatively selective 5-HT_3 receptor agonist (see review by Fozard, 1990). In the rat superior cervical ganglion, the potency and maximal depolarizing action of 1-phenylbiguanide appears to be similar to that of 5-HT (Fortune *et al.*, 1983; Newberry and Gilbert, 1989). However, in vagus nerve excised from the same species, the potency of 1-phenylbiguanide is about two-fold lower than that of 5-HT and the compound displays the properties of a partial agonist (Ireland and Tyers, 1987; Kilpatrick *et al.*, 1990a). Interestingly, 1-phenylbiguanide is neither an agonist nor an antagonist at 5-HT_3 receptors in guinea-pig vagus nerve (Burridge *et al.*, 1989), and its potency in the rabbit superior cervical ganglion appears to be substantially lower than that reported for the corresponding structure in the rat (Wallis and Nash, 1981). Possible species differences in the characteristics of 5-HT_3 receptors will be considered in greater detail in this chapter. Although 1-phenylbiguanide possesses little affinity for 5-HT receptor subtypes other than those of the 5-HT_3 class, it is known to interact with α_2-adrenoceptors and central ‘tryptamine’ binding sites (Van Wijngaarden *et al.*, 1990). Furthermore, the compound induces carrier-mediated release of [^{3}H]-dopamine from rat striatum (Schmidt and Black, 1989). These drawbacks have prompted the development of other guanidine derivatives in an effort to achieve greater pharmacological selectivity and potency at the 5-HT_3 receptor, *m*CPBG (Kilpatrick *et al.*, 1990a) has recently been reported to act as a highly potent, but partial, agonist at 5-HT_3 receptors in rat vagus nerve. Data on the compound's selectivity derived from functional assays indicate minimal effects at 5-HT$_1$-like and 5-HT$_2$ receptors. Additionally, the concentration range over which *m*CPBG activates 5-HT$_3$ receptors lies well below that necessary for the release of [^{3}H]-dopamine (Kilpatrick *et al.*, 1990a). Radioligand binding and functional studies suggest that 3,4-dichlorophenylbiguanide may also prove useful as a selective 5-HT$_3$ receptor agonist, but quantitative electrophysiological data have not yet been published (Krijzer and Tulp, 1990).

16.3.2. **Antagonist pharmacology**

The pharmacology of 5-HT$_3$ receptor antagonists, their potential as therapeutic agents and the history of their development have recently been reviewed in detail (Fozard, 1989, 1990; Costall *et al.*, 1990), so only a brief account of a few salient points are presented here. Until quite recently, no satisfactory antagonists of the 5-HT$_3$ receptor were available. Early investigations demonstrated blockade of 5-HT$_3$ receptor-mediated responses by metoclopramide (Fozard and Mobarok Ali, 1978a), quipazine (Lansdown *et al.*, 1980) and (−)-nor-cocaine (Fozard, 1983), but also noted the deficiencies of these compounds as pharmacological tools due to their interactions with other receptor types and/or neurotransmitter uptake systems. The first potent and selective 5-HT$_3$ receptor antagonists, MDL-72222 and ICS 205–930, appeared in the mid 1980s (Fozard, 1984b; Richardson *et al.*, 1985). Since then, numerous other compounds have been synthesized. Those most thoroughly studied to date are listed in Table 16.1, which summarizes their antagonist potencies (as pA$_2$ values or apparent pA$_2$ values) in a variety of preparations from several species.

The mechanism of action of the compounds listed in Table 16.1 has been investigated in radioligand binding assays employing tritiated 5-HT$_3$ receptor antagonists and functional tests. With the exception of quipazine and (+)-tubocurarine, the compounds displace specifically bound radioligands from 5-HT$_3$ recognition sites in membranes from rat cortex (Kilpatrick *et al.*, 1987) and the clonal cell lines N1E–115 and NG 108–15 (Hoyer and Neijt, 1988; Neijt *et al.*, 1988b) in a manner consistent with competitive antagonism. However, functional assays using extracellular recording techniques, or measuring contractile responses, have given inconsistent results. For example, ICS 205–930 was originally reported to competitively block the action of 5-HT$_3$ receptor agonists in the rabbit vagus, heart and guinea-pig ileum preparations (Richardson *et al.*, 1985), but a later study conducted on rat vagus nerve concluded that antagonism was non-competitive in nature (Ireland and Tyers, 1987). In voltage-clamped N1E-115 cells, the maximum and slope of the concentration–response curve to 5-HT was reduced by ICS 205–930, superficially suggesting a non-competitive mode of action (Neijt *et al.*, 1988a). J.A. Peters, H.M. Malone and J.J. Lambert (unpublished

Table 16.1. Antagonist potencies of 5-HT_3 receptor antagonists in various preparations and species.

	Mouse	Rat		Rabbit				Guinea-pig		
Compound	SCG	SCG	VN	SCG	NG	VN	Heart	SCG	VN	Ileum
ICS 205–930	8·7[a]	9·4[a]	8·8[b] 11·0[c]	10·4[d]	10·2[d]	10·2[e,3]	10·6[e]	7·2[a]	7·6[b,f]	7·6[b] 7·9[e]
MDL-72222	—	—	7·9[c]	7·8[g]	7·7[g]	8·0[h]	9·3[i]	—	6·4[f]	6·2[j,1]
Ondansetron	—	8·1[k]	8·6[k,2]	—	—	9·4[k]	<10·5[k]	—	7·0[b,f]	7·1[b] 7·3[k,2]
Granisetron	—	—	—	—	—	10·1[l]	—	—	7·9[f]	8·1[m]
Zacopride	—	—	9·1[b]	—	—	10·1[h]	—	—	7·6[b,f]	7·6[b] 8·5[h]
Metoclopramide	—	6·3[n]	6·6[c,2]	7·2[g]	7·1[g]	7·4[l]	7·2[o]	—	5·4[f]	5·5[k,1]
Quipazine	—	—	8·5[c]	7·6[g]	7·5[g]	—	—	—	—	—
SDZ 206–830	—	—	—	—	—	13·1[e,3]	10·1[e]	—	—	9·1[e]
SDZ 206–792	—	—	—	—	—	8·9[e,3]	9·8[e]	—	—	7·7[e]
GR 67330	—	—	10·2[p]	—	—	—	—	—	8·2[f]	—
(+)-Tubocurarine	8·1[a]	7·1[a]	—	—	—	—	—	4·8[a]	—	—

pA_2 (or apparent pA_2) values for antagonists acting against the extracellularly recorded depolarization elicited by 5-HT (or 2-methyl-5-HT) in superior cervical ganglia (SCG), nodose ganglia (NG) and vagus nerve (VN). For the heart and ileum, agonist induced responses were quantified as positive chronotropic and contractile effects, respectively.

Sources: [a] N.R. Newberry, S.H. Cheshire and M.J. Gilbert, personal communication; [b] Lattimer *et al.*, 1989; [c] Ireland and Tyers, 1987; [d] Round and Wallis, 1986; [e] Richardson *et al.*, 1985; [f] Burridge *et al.*, 1989; [g] Round and Wallis, 1987; [h] Smith *et al.*, 1988; [i] Fozard, 1984b; [j] Donatsch *et al.*, 1984; [k] Butler *et al.*, 1988; [l] Elliot *et al.*, 1990; [m] Sanger and Nelson, 1989; [n] Ireland *et al.*, 1982; [o] Fozard and Mobarok Ali, 1978a; [p] Kilpatrick *et al.*, 1990c.

[1] pD_2 value; [2] pK_B value; [3] agonist-induced responses quantified from depression of 'C' fibre spike amplitude rather than membrane depolarization.

observations) have noted similar effects with ondansetron in voltage-clamped rabbit nodose ganglion neurones, whereas Butler *et al.* (1988) found this antagonist to act competitively in other functional assays including the rat vagus nerve. A plausible explanation for these discrepancies, forwarded by Neijt *et al.*, (1988a), assumes that the antagonists do act competitively, but apparent non-competitive antagonism may be observed in certain functional tests as a consequence of the rapid desensitization of 5-HT_3 receptor populations. A comparison of the time course of 5-HT_3 receptor-mediated electrical events recorded in single cell studies, and the rate constants of dissociation of high affinity antagonists such as ICS 205–930 and ondansetron, indicates that equilibrium between agonist and antagonist binding cannot be attained before the onset of desensitization truncates the response. If receptor desensitization underlies the apparently non-competitive action of some 5-HT_3 receptor antagonists at the level of the single cell, why does this not transfer through to all functional assays? A consideration of the agonist-evoked responses that are typically quantified may provide a part of the answer to this question. Substantial receptor reserve may exist when contractile responses to 5-HT_3 receptor activation are measured. A similar limitation applies when extra- or intracellularly recorded depolarizing responses are quantified. This is due to the agonist-evoked change in membrane potential having a maximal value that is set by the difference between cell resting potential and the reversal potential of the response. Thus, in the above situations, a fraction of the 5-HT_3 receptor population may be 'pseudo-irreversibly' occupied by antagonist without any decrement in the maximal response that can be elicited from the tissue or cell. Whether or not a slowly dissociating antagonist will demonstrate competitive or non-competitive behaviour is likely to be strongly influenced by the degree of receptor reserve in the system under study. When agonist-evoked membrane currents are recorded under voltage-clamp conditions, receptor reserve should not exist.

Richardson and Engel (1986) have proposed the existence of three subtypes of 5-HT_3 receptor, termed 5-HT_{3A}, 5-HT_{3B} and 5-HT_{3C}. The evidence for this subclassification stems from substancial differences in the affinities of certain antagonists (e.g. SDZ 206–830, SDZ 206–792 and MDL-72222) for the 5-HT_3 receptors present on: sympathetic ganglion cell somata and primary visceral afferents (3A subtype); the terminals of postganglionic sympathetic neurones in the rabbit heart (3B subtype); and enteric neurones of the guinea-pig ileum (3C subtype) (see Table 16.1). However, recent evidence suggests that species, rather than tissue differences, might at least in part contribute to the purported heterogeneity of 5-HT_3 receptors (Butler *et al.*, 1990). Burridge *et al.* (1989) and Lattimer *et al.* (1989) have demonstrated that several 5-HT_3 receptor antagonists display lower affinities in guinea-pig vagus nerve compared to rat vagus nerve. Furthermore, as shown in Table 16.1, antagonist affinities in guinea-pig vagus agree well with those determined in the ileum from the same species, suggesting a common receptor

Table 16.2. Antagonist potencies of 5-HT_3 receptor antagonists reported from single-cell studies.

	Mouse			Rabbit	Guinea-pig		
Compound	N1E-115 cells	NG 108–15 cells	Hippocampal neurones	Nodose ganglion cells	Nodose ganglion cells	Coeliac ganglion cells	Submucous plexus neurones
ICS 205–930	9·7[b]	-	—	10·3[a,d]	—	—	7·9[f]
MDL-72222	8·7[b]	—	—	9·4[a,e]	6·5[a,e]	5·8[g]	5·5[f]
Ondansetron	9·6[a,h]	—	—	10·1[a,d]	7·6[a,e]	—	7·0[f]
Metoclopramide	7·6[a,e]	6·7[a,c]	6·4[a,c]	7·9[a,d]	5·9[a,e]	—	—
Cocaine	5·1[a,e]	—	—	7·1[a,d]	5·7[a,e]	—	5·5[f]
(+)-Tubocurarine	9·1[a,i]	9·1[a,c]	8·8[a,c]	6·8[a,d]	5·0[a,e]	4·4[g]	4·7[f]

p1C_{50} values [i.e. $-\log_{10} IC_{50}$ (M)] determined for the antagonists acting against 5-HT-induced depolarizing responses, or 5-HT-evoked inward membrane currents ([a]) recorded under voltage-clamp conditions.

Sources: [b] Neijt *et al.*, 1988b; [c] Yakel and Jackson, 1988; [d] Peters *et al.*, 1990b,c; [e] J.A. Peters, H.M. Malone and J.J. Lambert, unpublished observations; [f] Vanner and Suprenant, 1990; [g] Wallis and Dun, 1988; [h] Lambert *et al.*, 1989; [i] Peters *et al.*, 1990a.

type in the two tissues. This point is reinforced by the results of current- and voltage-clamp recordings performed on single cells. Table 16.2 lists pIC_{50} values for a number of 5-HT$_3$ receptor antagonists acting against 5-HT-induced depolarizing, or inward current responses, in neuronal cell lines of murine origin (N1E-115 and NG 108–15), rabbit and guinea-pig nodose ganglion neurones and guinea-pig coeliac ganglion and submucous plexus neurones. These data, albeit limited, strongly suggest species differences in the characteristics of 5-HT$_3$ receptors and a reappraisal of the scheme forwarded by Richardson and Engel (1986) now appears to be warranted.

16.4. *Electrophysiological investigations of the 5-HT$_3$ receptor channel complex*

Much of our knowledge concerning the possible mechanisms underlying 5-HT$_3$ receptor mediated excitation stems from studies performed on peripheral neurones. Intracellular recordings from single neurones within sympathetic (Wallis and North, 1978; Wallis and Dun, 1987, 1988) and parasympathetic (Akasu *et al.*, 1987; Tatsumi and Katayama, 1987) autonomic ganglia *in vitro*, have demonstrated that 5-HT$_3$ receptor activation results in a phasic depolarization associated with an apparent increase in membrane conductance. Similar responses occur in sensory neurones, notably visceral primary afferent neurones, whose cell bodies lie in the nodose ganglion (Higashi, 1977; Higashi and Nishi, 1982; Stansfield and Wallis, 1985), and dorsal root ganglion cells (Bevan and Robertson, 1987; Todorovic and Anderson, 1990). Within the enteric nervous system, locally applied 5-HT elicits a complex depolarizing response from neurones of the myenteric and submucous plexus that is mediated in part via 5-HT$_3$ receptors (Mawe *et al.*, 1986; Suprenant and Crist, 1988; Vanner and Suprenant, 1990).

It should be emphasized that in several of the neuronal cell types mentioned above, 5-HT interacts with additional subtypes of 5-HT receptor (e.g. 5-HT$_{1P}$, 5-HT$_2$ or unidentified) to produce complex effects upon membrane potential and conductance, of which the rapid phasic depolarization attributable to 5-HT$_3$ receptor activation is but one component (see reviews by Gershon *et al.*, 1989; Wallis, 1989). Additionally, in primary visceral afferents and sympathetic neurones, the depolarization due to 5-HT$_3$ receptor stimulation is frequently succeeded by a prominent after-hyperpolarization (e.g. Wallis and Woodward, 1975; Higashi, 1977). In neurones of the rabbit nodose ganglion at least, the after-hyperpolarization appears to occur secondary to an influx of Ca^{2+} during the 5-HT-induced depolarization (see below) and the subsequent activation of a Ca^{2+}-sensitive K^+ conductance (Higashi and Nishi, 1982). This slow after-hyperpolarization may itself be subject to modulation by a 5-HT receptor subtype distinct from the 5-HT$_3$ class (Christian *et al.*, 1989).

Complementary to the work performed on peripheral neurones, a number of investigations have demonstrated the existence of 5-HT_3 receptors in clonal neuronal cell lines and central neurones maintained in culture (for a review, see Peters and Lambert, 1989). The characteristics of the 5-HT_3 receptor-mediated electrical response in these systems, which will be discussed in detail below, closely resemble those determined in the periphery.

16.4.1. Ion selectivity and permeation in the 5-HT_3 receptor channel complex

The ionic basis of the 5-HT_3 receptor-mediated electrical response was first examined using an extracellular recording (sucrose-gap) technique applied to superior cervical ganglia excised from rabbits (Wallis and Woodward, 1975). Ion substitution experiments suggested that the depolarization resulted from an increase in membrane conductance to Na^+ (and to a lesser extent Ca^{2+}), but with no involvement of Cl^-. Subsequent intracellular recordings from neurones of the superior cervical ganglion established the reversal potential of the 5-HT response ($E_{5\text{-HT}}$) to be −24 mV, a value incompatible with an increase in membrane Na^+ conductance alone, but consistent with a simultaneous increase in Na^+ and K^+ conductance (Wallis and North, 1978). Single-cell studies on other preparations have amply confirmed the involvement of Na^+-influx in the generation of 5-HT_3 receptor-mediated depolarizing responses. In coeliac ganglion cells (Wallis and Dun, 1987, 1988) and submucous plexus neurones of the guinea-pig (Suprenant and Crist, 1988), rabbit ciliary ganglion cells (Tatsumi and Katayama, 1987) and the clonal neuronal cell lines N1E-115 (Peters and Usherwood, 1983) and NG 108–15 (Reiser *et al.*, 1988), replacement of extracellular Na^+ by poorly permeant cations (e.g. $Tris^+$, see below) abolishes or greatly reduces depolarizing responses to 5-HT. However, in common with the superior cervical ganglion, ions other than Na^+ (K^+ presumably, see below) must also contribute to the response, since $E_{5\text{-HT}}$ is generally reported to be close to 0 mV or negative (see Table 16.3).

The identity of the ions permeating the 5-HT_3 receptor channel complex was first examined under voltage-clamp conditions in an elegant study of 5-HT-induced membrane currents in rabbit nodose ganglion neurones (Higashi and Nishi, 1982). Such currents were reduced in amplitude when the extracellular concentrations of either Na^+ ($[Na^+]_o$) or K^+ ($[K^+]_o$) were decreased, but were unaffected when the ganglion was superfused with a Cl^- deficient solution. From a quantitative analysis of the effects of $[Na^+]_o$, $[K^+]_o$, $[Cl^-]_o$ and also $[Ca^{2+}]_o$, upon $E_{5\text{-HT}}$, Higashi and Nishi (1982) concluded that the channel gated by 5-HT primarily conducts monovalent cations. Although an increase in membrane Ca^{2+} conductance could not be detected from reversal potential measurements, 5-HT-induced currents were slightly depressed in response to a reduction in the external concentration of

Table 16.3. A summary of electrophysiological characteristics of 5-HT_3 receptor-mediated responses reported from single-cell studies.

Preparation	Recording technique	$E_{5\text{-HT}}$ (mV)	P_K/P_{Na}	γ (pS)	Reference
N1E-115 neuroblastoma	WCR/FA	−2·1	1·09	0·31	Lambert *et al.*, 1989
N1E-115 neuroblastoma	WCR	+20·0	0·42	—	Neijt *et al.*, 1989
N18 neuroblastoma	WCR/FA	−1·6[a]	1·10	0·59	Yang, 1990
NG 108–15 hybrid cells	WCR/FA	+3·5	0·89	4·40	Yakel *et al.*, 1990b
NCB-20 hybrid cells	WCR	−2·0	1·09	—	Lambert *et al.*, 1989
Rabbit nodose ganglion neurones	VC	+7·0	0·43	—	Higashi and Nishi, 1982
Rabbit nodose ganglion neurones	WCR/SCR	−1·6	1·06	17·0	Peters *et al.*, 1990b,c and unpublished
Rabbit superior cervical ganglion cells	CC	−24·0	—	—	Wallis and North, 1978
Rabbit ciliary ganglion cells	CC	−12·0	—	—	Tatsumi and Katayama, 1987
Rat dorsal root ganglion cells	WCR/SCR	+6·9[a]	—	(Below limit of resolution on membrane patches)	B. Robertson and S. Bevan, personal communication
Guinea-pig submucous neurones	WCR/SCR	+3·3[a]	0·44	15·0/9·2	Derkach *et al.*, 1989
Guinea-pig coeliac ganglion cells	CC	−22·8	—	—	Wallis and Dun, 1988

$E_{5\text{-HT}}$, reversal potential of response; P_K/P_{Na}, potassium/sodium permeability ratio; γ, single-channel conductance; CC and VC, constant current and voltage-clamp recordings with intracellular electrodes; WCR, whole-cell voltage-clamp recording with internal dialysis; SCR, single-channel recording; FA, fluctuation analysis.

[a] Reversal potential measurement made with Cs^+, rather than K^+, as the predominant internal cation.

Ca^{2+}. The question of a significant Ca^{2+} permeability, first raised by the work of Wallis and Woodward (1975), was not resolved.

Further analysis of ion selectivity and permeation in the 5-HT_3 receptor channel complex has recently been attempted by several groups of workers employing the 'whole-cell' recording mode of the patch-clamp technique (Hamill *et al.*, 1981), or suction electrodes in conjunction with voltage-clamp circuitry. Apart from providing accurate control of membrane voltage when used judiciously, these techniques have the considerable advantage, for ion permeation studies, of introducing known concentrations of ions into the cell interior. Such studies, recording macroscopic currents from clonal N1E-115 (Lambert *et al.*, 1989) and N18 (Yang and Hille, 1990; Yang, 1990) neuroblastoma cells, and the neuroblastoma × glioma hybrid cell line NG 108–15 (Yakel and Jackson, 1988; Yakel *et al.*, 1990b), have confirmed that the 5-HT_3 receptor channel is permeable to monovalent cations, but largely excludes anions. The permeability of K^+ relative to Na^+ (P_K/P_{Na}) calculated according to the Goldman–Hodgkin–Katz equation (see Hille, 1984) from the known extra- and intracellular concentrations of Na^+ and K^+, and the empirically determined value of $E_{5\text{-HT}}$, has generally been determined to be close to unity (see Table 16.3). However, using N1E-115 cells, Neijt *et al.* (1989) found K^+ to be considerably less permeant than Na^+ ($P_K/P_{Na} = 0{\cdot}41$) a value similar to that reported for 5-HT_3 receptor channels in guinea-pig submucous plexus neurones (0·44; Derkach *et al.*, 1989) and that of 0·43 for rabbit nodose ganglion neurones (estimated by the authors using the data of Higashi and Nishi, 1982). In contrast to the latter value, J.A. Peters, H.M. Malone and J.J. Lambert (unpublished observations) have found a permeability ratio of 1·06 in voltage-clamped rabbit nodose ganglion neurones (in culture) dialysed with known concentrations of permeant ions (cf. Higashi and Nishi, 1982). The apparent disparity in P_K/P_{Na} ratios does not correlate with cell type and might instead be explained by relatively small errors in the determination of $E_{5\text{-HT}}$. Additionally, it should be pointed out that estimates of the permeability ratio have, with the exception of the studies of Yang and Hille (1990) and Yang (1990), assumed divalent cations and anions to be impermeant. This may be an oversimplification (see below).

The relationship between the amplitude of 5-HT-induced whole-cell currents and membrane potential, from which the value of $E_{5\text{-HT}}$ is commonly estimated by interpolation, is itself the subject of conflicting reports: Higashi and Nishi (1982) and Neijt *et al.* (1989), recording from nodose ganglion and N1E-115 cells, respectively, observed a linear current–voltage (*I–V*) relationship over a wide range of holding potentials. In contrast, the *I–V* relationship in mouse hippocampal neurones (Yakel and Jackson, 1988) and adult rat dorsal root ganglion neurones (Robertson and Bevan, 1991) in culture shows modest inward rectification. Several studies conducted on clonal N1E-115, NCB-20, NG 108–15 and N18 cells also indicate that the whole-cell current evoked by 5-HT is inwardly rectifying (Peters *et al.*, 1988; Yakel and Jackson, 1988; Lambert *et al.*, 1989; Yakel *et al.*, 1990b, Yang, 1990). Yakel *et al.* (1990b) have suggested that inward rectification is more pronounced when recording solutions giving rise to a high internal concentration (140–150 mM) of Cl^- are used, but other studies do not support this view (Lambert *et al.*, 1989; Yang, 1990). Inward rectification might arise in several ways. It may be intrinsic to the 5-HT ion channel (i.e. a voltage-dependence of single-channel conductance) or result from a voltage-dependence of agonist effectiveness (i.e. voltage-dependent gating). For example, it is known that the rate constants governing opening and closing of the nicotinic channel of the neuromuscular junction (which demonstrates striking parallels with the 5-HT$_3$ channel; see below) are differentially influenced by membrane potential (Lambert *et al.*, 1983). The conductance of single 5-HT$_3$ channels (see below) in guinea-pig submucous neurones (Derkach *et al.*, 1989) and rabbit nodose ganglion cells (J.A. Peters, H.M. Malone and J.J. Lambert, unpublished observations) shows no evidence of voltage-dependence, at least over a wide range of negative holding potentials. However, this basic information is lacking for those systems mentioned above where rectification of whole-cell currents seems most pronounced. Further work is clearly necessary to establish the origin of this phenomenon.

A detailed study of ion permeation in 5-HT$_3$ receptor-gated channels using a wide range of metalic and organic monovalent cations has recently been performed on N18 cells (Yang, 1990). In brief, the 5-HT$_3$ receptor channel was found to be essentially non-selective among alkali metal ions, all of which were highly permeant. Small organic cations such as ammonium and methylamine were more permeant than Na^+, and the permeabilities of other organic cations tested decreased as their molecular weight, or size, increased. Qualitatively similar results have been obtained by Yakel *et al.* (1990b) using NG 108–15 cells. However, a quantitative difference in the results from N18 and NG 108–15 cells arises in the case of the largest organic cation tested, *N*-methyl-D-glucamine (NMDG), which is reported to be virtually impermeant in the former cell line but appreciably permeant (as *N*-methyl glucamine; P_{NMG}/P_{Na} = 0·14) in the latter. Divalent cations such as Ca^{2+}, Mg^{2+} and Ba^{2+} permeate 5-HT$_3$ receptor channels in N18 cells but apparently do not do so in NG 108–15 (Yakel *et al.*, 1990b) or N1E-115 cells (Peters *et al.*, 1988). Clearly, the issue of divalent cation permeability is of considerable significance because of the pivotal role of Ca^{2+} in many intracellular processes. The data of Yang (1990) suggest that a small influx of Ca^{2+} through 5-HT$_3$ receptor-operated channels would occur under physiological conditions, and this may be of importance in several of the biochemical effects of 5-HT$_3$ receptor activation that have recently been documented (see below).

It is possible that the discrepant results obtained with NMDG and divalent cations indicate true differences in the ionic selectivity of 5-HT$_3$ receptor channels in the various neuronal cell lines examined. However, a more parsimonious explanation might be found by examining differences in experimental protocol. In the study of Yang (1990) permeability ratios for divalent cations were determined using an extracellular test solution containing only the chloride salt of the divalent cation under investigation, or a mixture of the divalent and the 'poorly' permeant monovalent NMDG. Other workers (e.g. Higashi and Nishi, 1982; Peters *et al.*, 1988; Yakel *et al.*, 1990b) have attempted to determine the relative permeabilities of Ca^{2+} or Mg^{2+} in the presence of highly permeant monovalent cations. The exclusion of Na^+ from the extracellular test solution might also explain why Yang (1990) detected a finite permeability to monovalent anions (e.g. Cl^-, NO_3 and F^-), whereas others have reported Cl^- to be impermeant (Higashi and Nishi, 1982; Lambert *et al.*, 1989; Yakel *et al.*, 1990b).

A consistent finding across several cell types and tissues is the pronounced modulatory effect of divalent cations upon 5-HT_3 receptor-mediated electrical responses. Early intracellular recordings performed on NG108–15 (Christian *et al.*, 1978) and N1E-115 cells (Peters and Usherwood, 1983) demonstrated that depolarizing responses to 5-HT were augmented by the omission of Ca^{2+} from the recording solution. A similar influence of divalent cations was reported by Wallis and Nash (1981) using the sucrose-gap technique to record 5-HT_3 receptor-mediated depolarizations in rabbit isolated superior cervical ganglion. More recent voltage-clamp studies on N1E-115, N18 and NG 108–15 cells (Peters *et al.*, 1988; Yang, 1990; Yakel *et al.*, 1990b) and adult rabbit nodose ganglion neurones (J.A. Peters, H.M. Malone and J.J. Lambert, unpublished observations), have collectively shown that Ca^{2+}, Mg^{2+} and other divalent cations modulate the amplitude and duration of 5-HT-induced currents. Exactly how a reduction in the extracellular concentrations of Ca^{2+} or Mg^{2+} facilitates the response remains unclear, but the effect occurs in the absence of any change in $E_{5\text{-HT}}$, excluding a gross alteration in the ion selectivity of the channel, and shows no obvious voltage-dependency (Peters *et al.*, 1988; Yang, 1990). Divalent cations could influence the affinity of 5-HT for its receptor, but radioligand binding studies examining this possibility have given inconsistent results. In membranes prepared from N1E-115 cells, varying the Ca^{2+} content of the incubation medium had no effect upon the binding of [^{3}H]-ICS 205–930 or the ability of 5-HT to displace such binding (Hoyer and Neijt, 1988). Conversely, at 5-HT_3 recognition sites in rat brain cortex labelled with [^{3}H]-Q ICS 205–930, the inclusion of Ca^{2+} and Mg^{2+} in the assay medium increased the affinity of antagonist binding and decreased the affinity of agonist binding (Stanton *et al.*, 1990).

16.4.2. **The 5-HT_3 receptor complex probably incorporates the ion channel**

Recent electrophysiological experiments lend considerable support to the prevalent notion that the 5-HT_3 receptor protein contains both the 5-HT recognition site and an integral transmembrane ion channel. The time course of the current produced by activation of the 5-HT_3 receptor of voltage-clamped neuroblastoma cells is extremely rapid (Yakel and Jackson, 1988; Yang, 1990). The local iontophoretic application of 5-HT from high resistance micropipettes to N18 cells produced a detectable current within 10 ms. Due to agonist diffusion such experiments must overestimate the time required for channel opening to occur as a consequence of receptor activation. Such fast kinetics would appear to preclude the essential involvement of second messengers and G-proteins in channel activation. Consistent with this suggestion, well-maintained 5-HT-induced currents can be recorded over a period of hours from whole cells and isolated membrane patches dialysed on their intracellular face with a nucleotide-free solution (Derkach *et al.*, 1989; Lambert *et al.*, 1989; Yakel *et al.*, 1988; Yang, 1990). Furthermore, 5-HT-induced whole-cell currents are not influenced by the internal application of G-protein activators and inactivators (Derkach *et al.*, 1989; Yang, 1990). Similarly, neither the binding of radiolabelled antagonists nor the ability of agonists to displace such binding is influenced by GTP or Gpp(NH)p (5′-guanylylimidodi-phosphate) (Hoyer and Neijt, 1988; Kilpatrick *et al.*, 1987).

Although second messengers are not an essential prerequisite for channel activation, the above observations do not exclude the possibility that some aspects of receptor channel function may be influenced by intracellular nucleotides. Indeed, we have observed that the time course of the inward current induced by locally applied 5-HT in N1E-115 cells becomes reduced during whole-cell recordings, perhaps due to the loss of some cytoplasmic factor(s) caused by the intracellular dialysis which accompanies this technique. Interestingly, under identical recording conditions the time course of the 5-HT-induced current of rabbit nodose ganglion neurones remained constant (J.A. Peters, H.M. Malone and J.J. Lambert, unpublished observations). A role for cAMP in the regulation of 5-HT_3 receptor function is suggested by the observation that agents that increase cAMP levels in NG 108–15 cells (forskolin, 3-isobutyl-1-methyl xanthine, dibutyryl cAMP, cholera toxin and prostaglandin E_1) enhance the rate at which the 5-HT-induced current desensitizes (Yakel and Jackson, 1988). However, the observation that these effects are mimicked by 1,9-dideoxyforskolin, an analogue of forskolin that does not activate adenylate cyclase, suggests that further experimentation is required before assigning a role for cAMP in the 5-HT_3 response. (Yakel *et al.*, 1990a)

16.4.3. The single-channel properties of 5-HT_3 receptors

The advent of the patch-clamp technique (Hamill *et al.*, 1981) allowed the direct determination of the characteristics of single agonist-gated ion channels. This approach has been used to great advantage in determining the kinetic and ion conducting properties of a number of ligand-gated ion channels including those of the nicotinic receptor, the excitatory amino acid receptors (Colquhoun *et al.*, 1987; Ascher and Nowak, 1988; Ascher *et al.*, 1988; Cull-Candy *et al.*, 1988) and the inhibitory amino acid receptors for glycine and GABA (Borman *et al.*, 1987). Furthermore, when employed in conjunction with molecular biology techniques, new insights into the influence of subunit composition and primary amino acid sequence on the physiological and pharmacological properties of the receptor channel complex have been revealed (Sakmann *et al.*, 1985; Imoto *et al.*, 1988; Schofield, 1989).

Comparatively few reports have investigated the single-channel properties of 5-HT_3 receptors and little is known of their protein structure and composition. On outside-out membrane patches of adult rabbit nodose ganglion neurones, 5-HT (1 μM) activated single-channel currents with a conductance of 17 pS (Malone *et al.*, 1990; Peters *et al.*, 1990b,c). The channel open probability was reduced by 5-HT_3 antagonists (Peters *et al.*, 1990c). 5-HT_3 receptor activation in guinea-pig submucous plexus neurones opens a comparable channel of 15–17 pS, and additionally activates a conductance of 9 pS (Derkach *et al.*, 1989; Suprenant, 1990). It is not yet clear whether this reflects subconductance states of the same receptor-channel or the activation of distinct molecular entities (See Table 16.3).

The conductance properties of 5-HT-activated ion channels of the murine neuroblastoma N1E-115, NCB-20 and N18 cells appear quite distinct from those described above. Fluctuation analysis of high gain a.c.-coupled records of the 5-HT-induced whole-cell current from N1E-115 cells suggest that this agonist activates single channels of an extremely low conductance of 0·3 pS (Lambert *et al.*, 1989; Peters and Lambert, 1989). Using a similar approach, a value of 0·6 pS (see Table 16.3) has recently been reported for the murine N18 neuroblastoma cell line (Yang, 1990). 5-HT can induce substantial currents in N1E-115 cells (Lambert *et al.*, 1989; Neijt *et al.*, 1989). If such currents are mediated by low conductance channels, then this necessitates a high density of receptor channel complexes within the cell membrane. However, the binding of [^{3}H]-ICS 205–930 to N1E-115 cell membrane fragments suggests a modest number of 5-HT_3 antagonist recognition sites in these cells (Hoyer and Neijt, 1988). Arguably, of more physiological relevance are the antagonist binding characteristics to whole cells. A recent study has investigated the binding of the 5-HT_3 antagonist [^{3}H]-GR 65630 to intact N1E-115 cells (Lummis *et al.*, 1990a). This investigation revealed a high density of 5-HT_3 recognition sites (200 000 per cell) sufficient to support a whole-cell current despite the small single-channel conductance.

Adding a further complexity, a recent investigation reports a larger single-channel conductance of 4 pS (Yakel *et al.*, 1990b) for the 5-HT_3 receptor of differentiated NG 108–15 cells (a murine neuroblastoma–rat glioma hybrid). Notwithstanding, the single-channel conductances reported for the mouse neuroblastoma cell lines are much smaller than those of guinea-pig submucous plexus neurones (Derkach *et al.*, 1989; Suprenant, 1990), guinea-pig nodose ganglion neurones (J.A. Peters, H.M. Malone and J.J. Lambert, unpublished observations) and rabbit nodose ganglion neurones (Malone *et al.*, 1990; Peters *et al.*, 1990b,c). Whether the small single-channel conductance is a characteristic of the transformed neuroblastoma cell or is species-dependent, remains to be determined. Future experiments utilizing untransformed cells, e.g. mouse hippocampal neurones (Yakel and Jackson, 1988), are urgently required to resolve this question.

As mentioned above, ion substitution experiments have established that, like the nicotinic receptor, the 5-HT$_3$ channel of the N18 neuroblastoma cell discriminates weakly amongst the alkali metal ions (Yang, 1990). An investigation of the ion conducting properties of this channel, using organic cations of increasing molecular size, advocates an ion channel with a minimum pore size of 7·6 Å. This value is similar to that deduced for the nicotinic ion channel (Adams *et al.*, 1980; Dwyer *et al.*, 1980; Hille, 1984) and the kainate ion channel, although it is somewhat larger than that proposed for the NMDA ion channel (Vyklicky, 1988).

The single-channel conductance estimates for the 5-HT$_3$ receptor of mouse neuroblastomas (0·3–4 pS) are comparable to those reported for the kainate-activated ion channel of 0·14–4 pS (Ascher and Nowak, 1988; Cull-Candy *et al.*, 1988), but clearly much smaller (40–60 pS) than those of the nicotinic receptor (Sakmann *et al.*, 1985; Colquhoun, *et al.*, 1987; Imoto *et al.*, 1988). Yet these three channels have a similar pore size. What dictates the ion conducting properties of a channel? Do the large differences in the conductance properties of the 5-HT$_3$ receptors of murine neuroblastomas and those of rabbit and guinea-pig neurones suggest a completely different structural composition of these receptors?

We are only beginning to understand the structural determinants of ionic conductance (Krueger, 1989; Miller, 1989; Montal, 1990) which include the size and shape of the channel entrances, the minimum open pore size, its length and the amino acid composition of the ionic pore (Dani, 1986; Imoto *et al.*, 1988). Of particular interest is a study which combined genetic and biophysical approaches to investigate the role of amino acids thought to form three rings of negative charge in the nicotinic channel entry ways (Imoto *et al.*, 1988). Patch-clamp recordings from nicotinic receptor subunits, modified by site-directed mutagenesis, demonstrated that the single-channel conductance decreases as the total number of negatively charged amino acids is reduced (Imoto *et al.*, 1988). Hence, the 5-HT$_3$ channel of the mouse neuroblastoma cells may differ from its counterparts in the rabbit and guinea-pig neurones by only a few critical amino acids, or by their relative position within the channel. Alternatively, it may not be coincidental that the recently cloned kainate channel — which, like the neuroblastoma 5-HT$_3$ channel, has a very low conductance — appears to share very little sequence homology with other ligand-gated ion channels (Hollman *et al.*, 1989). Until the 5-HT$_3$ receptor(s) structure has been determined we can only continue to speculate.

16.5. *The molecular properties of the 5-HT$_3$ receptor*

As mentioned above, electrophysiological experiments suggest that 5-HT$_3$ receptors are directly linked to their ion channel. In contrast to other ligand-gated ion channels, including those of the GABA$_A$, glycine and nicotinic receptor, relatively little is known of their molecular properties.

Recently the 5-HT$_3$ receptor present in rabbit small bowel and NCB-20 cells, has been successfully solubilized (Gordon *et al.*, 1990; McKernan, *et al.*, 1990a,b). Using sucrose density centrifugation the molecular weight of the NCB-20 receptor was estimated to be 249 kDa. This is similar to that reported for other ligand-gated ion channels (Strange, 1988). Using a 5-HT$_3$ antagonist affinity column the receptor has now been purified to homogeneity (McKernan *et al.*, 1990c). The purified protein when run on a polyacrylamide gel reveals two bands of molecular weight 38 kDa and 54 kDa, which presumably represent subunits of the 249 kDa receptor. Using the alternative technique of radiation inactivation, molecular weights of 35·4 kDa (Gozlan *et al.*, 1989) and 49·1 kDa (Lummis *et al.*, 1990b) have been reported for the rat brain receptor and 34·9 kDa (Miguel *et al.*, 1990) and 98·6 kDa (Lummis *et al.*, 1990b) for the neuroblastomas NG 108–15 and N1E-115, respectively. The relatively high value of 98·6 kDa may represent a subunit dimer (Lummis, *et al.*, 1990b).

Future work determining the subunit composition and molecular structure of the receptor is essential to allow a better understanding of the ion conducting and pharmacological properties of this ligand-gated ion channel.

Acknowledgements

The experimental work performed in the author's laboratory was supported by the Wellcome Trust (J.J.L.) and a Dundee University Research Initiative Grant (J.A.P.). We are grateful to the following individuals for preprints of papers in press, or permission to quote their unpublished observations: Professor D. Wallis; Drs M. Jackson, G. Kilpatrick, S. Lummis, I. Martin, R. McKernan, N. Newberry, B. Robertson, J. Yang and J. Yakel.

References

Adams, D.J., Dwyer, T.M. and Hille, B. (1980). The permeability of endplate channels to monovalent and divalent metal cations. *Journal of General Physiology*, **75**, 493–510.

Akasu, T., Hasuo, H. and Tokimasa, T. (1987). Activation of 5-HT$_3$ receptor subtypes causes rapid excitation of rabbit parasympathetic neurones. *British Journal of Pharmacology*, **91**, 453–455.

Andrews, P.L.R., Rapeport, W.G. and Sanger, G.J. (1988). Neuropharmacology of emesis induced by anti-cancer therapy. *Trends in Pharmacological Sciences*, **9**, 334–341.

Armstrong, D., Dry, R.M.L., Keele, C.A. and Markham, J.W. (1953). Observations on chemical excitants of cutaneous pain in man. *Journal of Physiology*, **120**, 326–351.

Ascher, P. and Nowak, L. (1988). Quisqualate- and kainate-activated channels in mouse central neurones in culture. *Journal of Physiology*, **399**, 227–245.

Ascher, P., Bregestovski, P. and Nowak, L. (1988). *N*-Methyl-D-aspartate-activated channels of mouse central neurones in magnesium-free solutions. *Journal of Physiology*, **399**, 207–226.

Ashby, C.R., Jr, Edwards, E., Harkins, K. and Wang, R.Y. (1989). Characterization of 5-hydroxytryptamine$_3$ receptors in the medial prefrontal cortex: a microiontophoretic study. *European Journal of Pharmacology*, **173**, 193–196.

Ashby, C.R., Jr, Edwards, E., Minabe, Y. and Wang, R.Y. (1990). Functional characterization of 5-HT$_3$-like receptors in the rat medial prefrontal cortex: biochemical and electrophysiological studies. *European Journal of Pharmacology*, **183**, 1958–1959.

Baird, A.W. and Cuthbert, A.W. (1987). Neuronal involvement in type 1 hypersensitivity reactions in gut epithelia. *British Journal of Pharmacology*, **92**, 647–655.

Barnes, J.M., Barnes, N.M., Costall, B., Naylor, R.J. and Tyers, M.B. (1989). 5-HT$_3$ receptors mediate inhibition of acetylcholine release in cortical tissue. Nature, **338**, 762–763.

Barnes, N.M., Costall, B. and Naylor, R.J. (1988). [^{3}H] Zacopride: a ligand for the identification of 5-HT$_3$ recognition sites. *Journal of Pharmacy and Pharmacology*, **40**, 548–551.

Beck, P.W. and Handwerker, H.O. (1974). Bradykinin and serotonin effects on various types of cutaneous nerve fibres. *Pflügers Archiv*, **347**, 209–222.

Bevan, S. and Robertson, B. (1987). 5-Hydroxytryptamine (5-HT) responses in adult rat dorsal root ganglion (DRG) neurones *in vitro*. *Journal of Physiology*, **390**, 256P.

Blandina, P., Goldfarb, J., Craddock-Royal, B. and Green, J.P. (1989). Release of endogenous dopamine by stimulation of 5-hydroxytryptamine$_3$ receptors in rat striatum. *Journal of Pharmacology and Experimental Therapeutics*, **251**, 803–809.

Blandina, P., Goldfarb, J. and Green, P.J. (1988). Activation of a 5-HT$_3$ receptor releases dopamine from rat striatal slice. *European Journal of Pharmacology*, **155**, 349–350.

Blandina, P., Goldfarb, J., Walcott, J. and Green, J.P. (1990). 5-HT$_3$ receptors inhibit release of endogenous noradrenaline from hypothalamus. In: *Serotonin: Molecular Biology, Receptors and Functional Aspects*, edited by P.R. Saxena and J.R. Fozzard. Basel: Birkhäuser (in press).

Borman, J., Hamill, O.P. and Sakmann, B. (1987). Mechanism of anion permeation through channels gated by glycine and γ-aminobutyric acid in mouse cultured spinal neurones. *Journal of Physiology*, **385**, 243–286.

Bradley, P.B., Engel, G., Feniuk, W., Fozard, J.R., Humphrey, P.P.A. Middlemiss, D.N., Mylecharane, E.J., Richardson, B.P. and Saxena, P.R. (1986). Proposals for the classfication and nomenclature of functional receptors for 5-hydroxytryptamine. *Neuropharmacology*, **25**, 563–576.

Bucheit, K.-H., Engel, G., Mutschler, E. and Richardson, B. (1985). Study of the contractile effect of 5-hydroxytryptamine (5-HT) in the isolated longitudinal muscle strip from guinea-pig ileum. Evidence for two, distinct release mechanisms. *Naunyn-Schmiedeberg's Archives of Pharmacology*, **329**, 36–41.

Burridge, J., Butler, A. and Kilpatrick, G.J. (1989). 5-HT$_3$ receptors mediate depolarization of the guinea-pig isolated nerve. *British Journal of Pharmacology*, **96**, 269P.

Butler, A., Hill, J.M., Ireland, S.J., Jordan, C.C. and Tyers, M.B. (1988). Pharma-

cological properties of GR38032F, a novel antagonist at 5-HT_3 receptors. *British Journal of Pharmacology*, **94**, 397–412.
Butler, A., Elswood, C.J., Burridge, J., Ireland, S.J., Bunce, K.T., Kilpatrick, G.J. and Tyres, M.B. (1990). The pharmacological characterization of 5-HT_3 receptors in three isolated preparations derived from guinea-pig tissues. *British Journal of Pharmacology*, **101**, 591–598.
Carstens, E., Klumpp, D., Randic, M. and Zimmermann, A. (1981). Effect of ionophoretically applied 5-hydroxytryptamine on the excitability of single primary afferent C- and A-fibres in cat spinal cord. *Brain Research*, **220**, 151–158.
Chahl, L.A. (1983). Substance P mediates atropine-sensitive response of guinea-pig ileum to serotonin. *European Journal of Pharmacology*, **87**, 485–489.
Christian, C.N., Nelson, P.G., Bullock, P., Mullinax, D. and Nirenberg, M. (1978). Pharmacologic responses of cells of a neuroblastoma × glioma hybrid clone and modulation of synapses between hybrid cells and mouse myotubes. *Brain Research*, **147**, 261–276.
Christian, E.P., Taylor, G.E. and Weinreich, D. (1989). Serotonin increases excitability of rabbit C-fibre neurons by two distinct mechanisms. *Journal of Applied Physiology*, **67** (2), 584–591.
Clarke, D.E., Craig, D.A. and Fozard, J.R. (1989). The 5-HT_4 receptor: naughty, but nice. *Trends in Pharmacological Sciences*, **10**, 385–386.
Colquhoun, D., Ogden, D.C. and Mathie, A. (1987). Nicotinic acetylcholine receptors of nerve and muscle: functional aspects. *Trends in Pharmacological Sciences*, **8**, 465–472.
Costall, B., Naylor, R.J. and Tyers, M.B. (1990). The psychopharmacology of 5-HT_3 receptors. *Pharmacology and Therapeutics*, **47**, 181–202.
Cramer, W., Van Drimmelen, M., Long, S. and Tulp, M. (1990). Bufotenin: actions on 5-HT_3 receptors. *European Journal of Pharmacology*, **183**, 2148–2149.
Cull-Candy, S.G., Howe, J.R. and Ogden, D.C. (1988). Noise and single channels activated by excitatory amino acids in rat cerebellar granule neurones. *Journal of Physiology*, **400**, 189–222.
Dani, J.A. (1986). Ion-channel entrances influence permeation. *Biophysical Journal*, **49**, 607–618.
Dawes, G.S. and Mott, J.C. (1950). Circulatory and respiratory reflexes caused by aromatic guanidines. *British Journal of Pharmacology*, **5**, 65–76.
Derkach, V., Suprenant, A. and North, R.A. (1989). 5-HT_3 receptors are membrane ion channels. *Nature*, **339**, 706–709.
Donatsch, P., Engel, G., Richardson, B.P. and Stadler, P. (1984). ICS 205–930: a highly selective and potent antagonist at peripheral neuronal 5-hydroxytryptamine (5-HT) receptors. *British Journal of Pharmacology*, **81**, 34P.
Dwyer, T.M., Adams, D.J. and Hille, B. (1980). The permeability of the endplate channel to organic cations in frog muscle. *Journal of General Physiology*, **75**, 469–492.
Edwards, E., Harkins, K.L., Ashby, C.R., Jr. and Wang, R.Y. (1991). The effects of 5-HT_3 receptor agonists on phosphoinositide hydrolysis in the rat frontocingulate and entorhinal cortices. *Journal of Pharmacology and Experimental Therapeutics*, **256**, 1025–1032.
Elliott, P. & Wallis, D.I. (1988). The depolarizing action of 5-hydroxytryptamine on rabbit isolated preganglionic cervical sympathetic nerves. *Naunyn-Schmiedeberg's Archives of Pharmacology*, **338**, 608–615.
Elliott, P., Seemungal, B.M. and Wallis, D.I. (1990). Antagonism of the effects of 5-hydroxytryptamine on the rabbit isolated vagus nerve by BRL 43694 and metoclopramide. *Naunyn-Schmiedeberg's Archives of Pharmacology*, **341**, 503–509.

Eschalier, A., Kayser, V. and Guilbaud, G. (1989). Influence of a specific 5-HT$_3$ antagonist on carrageenan-induced hyperalgesia in rats. *Pain*, **36**, 249–255.

Fastier, F.N., McDowall, M.A. and Waal, H. (1959). Pharmacological properties of phenylbiguanide and other amidine derivatives in relation to those of 5-hydroxytryptamine. *British Journal of Pharmacology and Chemotherapy*, **14**, 527–535.

Fjallbrant, N. and Iggo, A. (1961). The effect of histamine, 5-hydroxytryptamine and acetylcholine on cutaneous afferent fibres. *Journal of Physiology*, **156**, 578–590.

Fortune, D.H., Ireland, S.J. and Tyers, M.B. (1983). Phenylbiguanide mimics the effects of 5-hydroxytryptamine on the rat isolated vagus nerve and superior cervical ganglion. *British Journal of Pharmacology*, **79**, 298P.

Fozard, J.R. (1983). Differences between receptors for 5-hydroxytryptamine on autonomic neurones revealed by Nor (−) cocaine. *Journal of Autonomic Pharmacology*, **3**, 21–26.

Fozard, J.R. (1984a). Characteristics of the excitatory 5-HT receptor on the cholinergic nerves of the rabbit heart. *Proceedings of the IUPHAR 9th International Congress on Pharmacology*, 1189P.

Fozard, J.R. (1984b). MDL 72222: a potent and highly selective antagonist at neuronal 5-hydroxytryptamine receptors. *Naunyn-Schmiedeberg's Archives of Pharmacology*, **326**, 36–44.

Fozard, J.R. (1984c) Neuronal 5-HT receptors in the periphery. *Neuropharmacology*, **23**, 1473–1486.

Fozard, J.R. (1989). The development and early clinical evaluation of selective 5-HT$_3$ receptor antagonists. In: *The Peripheral Actions of 5-Hydroxytryptamine*, edited by J.R. Fozard. Oxford: Oxford University Press, pp. 354–376.

Fozard, J.R. (1990). Agonists and antagonists of 5-HT$_3$ receptors. In: *Cardiovascular Pharmacology of 5-Hydroxytryptamine: Prospective Therapeutic Applications*, edited by P.R. Saxena, D. Kluwer, D.I. Wallis, W. Wouters and P. Bevan. Dordrecht: Kluwer Academic Publishers, pp. 101–115.

Fozard, J.R. and Mobarok Ali, A.T.M. (1978a). Blockade of neuronal tryptamine receptors by metoclopramide. *European Journal of Pharmacology*, **49**, 109–112.

Fozard, J.R. and Mobarok Ali, A.T.M. (1978b). Receptors for 5-hydroxytryptamine on the sympathetic nerves of the rabbit heart. *Naunyn-Schmiedeberg's Archives of Pharmacology*, **301**, 223–235.

Fozard, J.R. and Mwaluko, G.M.P. (1976). Mechanism of the indirect sympathomimetic effect of 5-hydroxytryptamine on the isolated heart of the rabbit. *British Journal of Pharmacology*, **57**, 115–125.

Frazer, A., Maayani, S., and Wolfe, B.B. (1990). Subtypes of receptors for serotonin. *Annual Review of Pharmacology and Toxicology*, **30**, 307–348.

Gaddum, J.H. (1953). Tryptamine receptors. *Journal of Physiology*, **119**, 363–368.

Gaddum, J.H. and Hameed, K.A. (1954). Drugs which antagonise 5-hydroxytryptamine. *British Journal of Pharmacology*, **9**, 240–248.

Gaddum, J.H. and Picarelli, Z.P. (1957). Two kinds of tryptamine receptor. *British Journal of Pharmacology*, **12**, 323–328.

Galzin, A.M., Poncet, V. and Langer, S.Z. (1990). 5-HT$_3$ receptor agonists enhance the electrically-evoked release of [^{3}H]-5-HT in guinea-pig frontal cortex slices. *British Journal of Pharmacology*, **100**, 307P.

Gershon, M.D., Mawe, G.M. and Branchek, T.A. (1989). 5-Hydroxytryptamine and enteric neurones. In: *The Peripheral Actions of 5-Hydroxytryptamine*, edited by J.R. Fozard. Oxford: Oxford University Press, pp. 247–273.

Giordano, J. and Rogers, L.A. (1989). Peripherally administered serotonin 5-HT$_3$ receptor antagonists reduce inflammatory pain in rats. *European Journal of Pharmacology*, **170**, 83–86.

Gordon, J.C., Sarbin, N.S., Barefoot, D.S. and Pinkus, L.M. (1990). Solubilization of a 5-HT_3 binding site from rabbit small bowel muscularis membranes. *European Journal of Pharmacology*, **188**, 313–319.

Gothert, M. and Duhrsen, U. (1979). Effects of 5-hydroxytryptamine and related compounds on the sympathetic nerves of the rabbit heart. *Naunyn-Schmiedeberg's Archives of Pharmacology*, **308**, 9–18.

Gozlan, H., Schecter, L.E., Bolanos, F., Emerit, M.B., Miquel, M.C., Nielsen, M. and Hamon, M. (1989). Determination of the molecular size of the 5-HT_3 receptor binding site by radiation inactivation. *European Journal of Pharmacology (Molecular Pharmacology Section)*, **172**, 497–500.

Gunning, S.J. and Humphrey, P.P.A. (1987). Evidence for 5-HT_3-receptor mediated release of an inhibitory transmitter in guinea-pig isolated ileum. *British Journal of Pharmacology*, **91**, 359P.

Hamill, O.P., Marty, A., Neher, E., Sakmann, B. and Sigworth, F.J. (1981). Improved patch-clamp techniques for high resolution current recordings from cells and cell-free membrane patches. *Pflügers Archiv*, **391**, 85–100.

Hamon, M., Gallissot, M.C., Mernard, F., Gozlan, H., Bourgoin, S. and Verge, D. (1989). 5-HT_3 receptor binding sites are on capsaicin-sensitive fibres in the rat spinal cord. *European Journal of Pharmacology*, **164**, 315–322.

Hartig, P. (1989). Molecular biology of 5-HT receptors. *Trends in Pharmacological Sciences*, **10**, 64–69.

Hendriks, R., Bornstein, J.C. and Furness, J.B. (1989). Evidence for two types of 5-hydroxytryptamine receptor on secretomotor neurons of the guinea-pig ileum. *Naunyn-Schmiedeberg's Archives of Pharmacology*, **339**, 409–414.

Higashi, S. (1977). 5-hydroxytryptamine receptors on visceral primary afferent neurones in the nodose ganglion of the rabbit. *Nature*, **267**, 448–449.

Higashi, H. and Nishi, S. (1982). 5-Hydroxytryptamine receptors on visceral primary afferent neurones of rabbit nodose ganglia. *Journal of Physiology*, **323**, 543–567.

Hille, B. (1984). *Ionic Channels of Excitable Membranes*. Sunderland, MS: Sinaeur Associates.

Hollman, M., O'Shea-Greenfield, A., Rogers, S.W. and Heinemann, S. (1989). Cloning by functional expression of a member of the glutamate receptor family. *Nature*, **342**, 643–648.

Holz, G. and Anderson, E.G. (1984). The actions of serotonin on frog primary afferent terminals and cell bodies. *Comparative Biochemistry and Physiology*, **77C**, 13–21.

Hoyer, D. (1989). 5-Hydroxytryptamine receptors and effector coupling mechanisms in peripheral tissues. In: *The Peripheral Actions of 5-Hydroxytryptamine*, edited by J.R. Fozard. Oxford: Oxford University Press, pp. 72–99.

Hoyer, D. and Neijt, H.C. (1988). Identification of serotonin 5-HT_3 recognition sites in membranes of N1E-115 neuroblastoma cells by radioligand binding. *Molecular Pharmacology*, **33**, 303–309.

Humphrey, P.P.A., Feniuk, W. and Watts, A.D. (1983). Prejunctional effects of 5-hydroxytryptamine on noradrenergic nerves in the cardiovascular system. *Federation Proceedings*, **42**, 218–222.

Imoto, K., Busch, C., Sakmann, B., Mishina, M., Konno, T., Nakai, J., Bujo, H., Mori, Y., Fukuda, K. and Numa, S. (1988). Rings of negatively charged amino acids determine the acetylcholine receptor channel conductance. *Nature*, **335**, 645–648.

Ireland, S.J. and Tyers, M.B. (1987). Pharmacological characterization of 5-hydroxytryptamine-induced depolarizations of the rat isolated vagus nerve. *British Journal of Pharmacology*, **90**, 229–238

Ireland, S.J., Straughan, D.W. and Tyers, M.B. (1982). Antagonism by metoclopramide and quipazine of 5-hydroxytryptamine-induced depolarization of rat isolated vagus nerve. *British Journal of Pharmacology*, **75**, 16P.

Jiang, L.H., Ashby, C.R., Jr, Kasser, R.J. and Wang, R.Y. (1990). The effect of intraventricular administration of the 5-HT$_3$ receptor agonist 2-methylserotonin on the release of dopamine in the nucleus accumbens: an *in vivo* chronocoulometric study. *Brain Research*, **513**, 156–160.

Kilpatrick, G.J. Jones, B.J. and Tyers, M.B. (1987). Identification and distribution of 5-HT$_3$ receptors in rat brain using radioligand binding. *Nature*, **330**, 746–748.

Kilpatrick, G.J., Jones, B.J. and Tyers, M.B. (1989). Binding of the 5-HT$_3$ ligand, [^{3}H] GR65630, to rat area postrema, vagus nerve and the brains of several species. *European Journal of Pharmacology*, **159**, 157–164.

Kilpatrick, G.J., Butler, A., Burridge, J., Oxford, A.W. (1990a). 1-(*m*-Chloropheny)-biguanide, a potent high affinity 5-HT$_3$ receptor agonist. *European Journal of Pharmacology*, **182**, 193–197.

Kilpatrick, G.J., Butler, A., Hagan, R.M., Jones, B.J. and Tyers, M.B. (1990b). [^{3}H] GR67330, a very high affinity ligand for 5-HT$_3$ receptors. *Naunyn-Schmiedeberg's Archives of Pharmacology*, **342**, 22–30.

Krijzer, F.N.C. and Tulp, M.Th.M. (1990). Remarkable effects of 5-HT$_3$-antagonists on spontaneous and induced electrocortical activity in the rat. *European Journal of Pharmacology*, **183**, 1969.

Krueger, B.K. (1989). Toward an understanding of structure and function of ion channels. *FASEB Journal*, **3**, 1906–1914.

Lambert, J.J., Durant, N.N. and Henderson, E.G. (1983). Drug-induced modification of ionic conductance at the neuromuscular junction. *Annual Review of Pharmacology and Toxicology*, **23**, 505–539.

Lambert, J.J., Peters, J.A., Hales, T.G. and Dempster, J. (1989). The properties of 5-HT$_3$ receptors in clonal cell lines studied by patch-clamp techniques. *British Journal of Pharmacology*, **97**, 27–40.

Lansdown, M.J.R., Nash, H.L., Preston, P.R., Wallis, D.I. and Williams, R.G. (1980). Antagonism of 5-hydroxytryptamine receptors by quipazine. *British Journal of Pharmacology*, **68**, 525–532.

Lattimer, N., Rhodes, K.F. and Saville, V.L. (1989). Possible differences in 5-HT$_3$-like receptors in the rat and the guinea-pig. *British Journal of Pharmacology*, **96**, 270P.

Leonhardt, S., Herrick-Davis, K. and Titeler, M. (1989). Detection of a novel serotonin receptor subtype (5-HT$_{1E}$) in human brain: interaction with a GTP binding protein. *Journal of Neurochemistry*, **53**, 465–471.

Lummis, S.C.R., Kilpatrick, G.J. and Martin, I.L. (1990a). Characterization of 5-HT$_3$ receptors in intact N1E-115 neuroblastoma cells. *European Journal of Pharmacology*, (*Molecular Pharmacology Section*), **189**, 223–227.

Lummis, S.C.R., Nielsen, M., Kilpatrick, G.J. and Martin, I.L. (1990b). Target size of 5-HT$_3$ receptors in N1E-115 neuroblastoma cells and rat brain. *European Journal of Pharmacology*, (*Molecular Pharmacology Section*), **189**, 229–232.

Lyon, R.A., Davis, K.H. and Titeler, M. (1987). ^{3}H-DOB (4-Bromo-2,5-dimethoxyphenyliso-propylamine) labels a guanyl nucleotide-sensitive state of cortical 5-HT$_2$ receptors. *Molecular Pharmacology*, **31**, 194–199.

McKenna, D.J. and Peroutka, S.J. (1989). Differentiation of 5-hydroxytryptamine$_2$ receptor subtypes using ^{125}I-R-(−)2,5-dimethoxy-4-iodo-phenylisopropylamine and ^{3}H-ketanserin. *Journal of Neuroscience*, **9**, 3482–3490.

McKernan, R.M., Quirk, K., Jackson, R.G. and Ragan, I.C. (1990a). Solubilisation of the 5-hydroxytryptamine$_3$ receptor from pooled rat cortical and hippocampal membranes. *Journal of Neurochemistry*, **54**, 924–930.

McKernan, R.M., Biggs, C.S., Gillard, N., Quirk, K. and Ragan, I.C. (1990b).

Molecular size of the 5-HT_3 receptor solubilized from NCB-20 cells. *Biochemical Journal*, **269**, 623–628.
McKernan, R.M., Gillard, N.P., Quirk, K., Kneen, C.O., Stevenson, G.I., Swan, C.J. and Ragan, I. (1990c). Purification of the 5-hydroxytryptamine 5-HT_3 receptor from NCB-20 cells. *Journal of Biological Chemistry*, **265**, (23), 13572–13577.
Malone, H.M., Callachan, H., Lambert, J.J. and Peters, J.A. (1990). The effects of 5-hydroxytryptamine on adult rabbit nodose ganglion neurones in cell culture. *Neuroscience Letters*, **38**, S116.
Mawe, G.M., Branchek, T.A. and Gershon, M.D. (1986). Peripheral neural serotonin receptors: identification and characterization with specific agonists and antagonists. *Proceedings of the National Academy of Sciences USA*, **83**, 9799–9803.
Miller, C. (1989). Genetic manipulation of ion channels: a new approach to structure and mechanism. *Neuron*, **2**, 1195–1205.
Miguel, M.-C., Emerit, M.B., Bolanos, F.J., Schechter, L.E., Gozlan, H. and Hamon, M. (1990). Physicochemical properties of serotonin 5-HT_3 binding sites solubilized from membranes of NG 108–15 neuroblastoma-glioma cells. *Journal of Neurochemistry*, **55**, 1526–1536.
Montal, M. (1990). Molecular anatomy and molecular design of channel proteins. *FASEB Journal*, **4**, 2622–2635.
Neijt, H.C., Plomp, J.J. and Vijverberg, H.P.M. (1989). Kinetics of the membrane current mediated by serotonin 5-HT_3 receptors in cultured mouse neuroblastoma cells. *Journal of Physiology*, **411**, 257–269.
Neijt, H.C., Te Duits, I.J. and Vijverberg, H.P.M. (1988a). Pharmacological characterization of serotonin 5-HT_3 receptor-mediated electrical response in cultured mouse neuroblastoma cells. *Neuropharmacology*, **27**, 301–307.
Neijt, H.C., Karpf, A., Schoeffter, P., Engel, G. and Hoyer, D. (1988b). Characterization of 5-HT_3 recognition sites in membranes of NG 108–15 neuroblastoma-glioma cells with [^{3}H] ICS 205–930. *Naunyn-Schmiedeberg's Archives of Pharmacology*, **337**, 493–499.
Newberry, N.R. and Gilbert, M.J. (1989). 5-Hydroxytryptamine evokes three distinct responses in the rat superior cervical ganglion *in vitro*. *European Journal of Pharmacology*, **162**, 197–205.
Paintal, A.S. (1973). Sensory mechanisms involved in the Bezold-Jarisch effect. *Australian Journal of Biology and Medical Science*, **51**, 3–15.
Peroutka, S.J. (1988). 5-Hydroxytryptamine receptor subtypes: molecular, biochemical and physiological characterization. *Trends in Neurosciences*, **11**, 496–500.
Peroutka, S.J. and Hamik, A. (1988). [^{3}H] Quipazine labels 5-HT_3 recognition sites in rat cortical membranes. *European Journal of Pharmacology*, **148**, 297–299.
Peroutka, S.J. and Snyder, S.H. (1979). Multiple serotonin receptors: differential binding of [^{3}H] lysergic acid diethylamide and [^{3}H] spiperidol. *Molecular Pharmacology*, **16**, 687–699.
Peters, J.A. and Lambert, J.J. (1989). Electrophysiology of 5-HT_3 receptors in neuronal cell lines. *Trends in Pharmacological Sciences*, **10**, 172–175.
Peters, J.A. and Usherwood, P.N.R. (1983). 5-Hydroxytryptamine responses of murine neuroblastoma cells; ions and putative antagonists. *British Journal of Pharmacology*, **80**, 523P.
Peters, J.A., Hales, T.G. and Lambert, J.J. (1988). Divalent cations modulate 5-HT_3 receptor-induced currents in N1E-115 neuroblastoma cells. *European Journal of Pharmacology*, **151**, 491–495.
Peters, J.A., Malone, H.M. and Lambert, J.J. (1990a). Antagonism of 5-HT_3

receptor mediated currents in murine N1E-115 neuroblastoma cells by (+)-tubocurarine. *Neuroscience Letters*, **10**, 107–112.

Peters, J.A., Malone, H.M. and Lambert, J.J. (1990b). 5-Hydroxytryptamine$_3$ receptor mediated responses on adult rabbit nodose ganglion neurones in cell culture. *European Journal of Pharmacology*, **183**, 1112.

Peters, J.A., Malone, H.M. and Lambert, J.J. (1990c). Whole cell and single channel currents mediated by 5-HT$_3$ receptor activation in adult rabbit nodose ganglion neurones in culture. In: *Serotonin: Molecular Biology, Receptors and Functional Aspects*, edited by P.R. Saxena and J.R. Fozard. Basel: Birhäuser (in press).

Pratt, G.D. and Bowery, N.G. (1989). The 5-HT$_3$ receptor ligand, [^{3}H] BRL 43694, binds to presynaptic sites in the nucleus tractus solitarius of the rat. *Neuropharmacology*, **28**, 1367–1376.

Pratt, G.D., Bowery, N.G., Kilpatrick, G.J., Leslie, R.A., Barnes, N.M., Naylor, R.J., Jones, B.R., Nelson, D.R., Palacios, J.M., Slater, P. and Reynolds, D.J.M. (1990). Consensus meeting agrees distribution of 5-HT$_3$ receptors in mammalian hindbrain. *Trends in Pharmacological Sciences*, **11**, 135–137.

Reiser, G., Binmoller, F.-J. and Koch, R. (1988). Memantine (1-amino-3,5- dimethyl adamantane) blocks the serotonin-induced depolarization response in a neuronal cell line. *Brain Reseach*, **443**, 338–344.

Richardson, B.P. and Engel, G. (1986). The pharmacology and function of 5-HT$_3$ receptors. *Trends in Neurosciences*, **9**, 424–428.

Richardson, B.P., Engel, G., Donatsch, P. and Stadler, P.A. (1985). Identification of serotonin M-receptor subtypes and their specific blockade by a new class of drugs. *Nature*, **316**, 126–131.

Robertson, B. and Bevan, S. (1991). Properties of 5-hydroxytryptamine, 3-receptor-gated currents in adult rat dorsal root ganglion neurones. *British Journal of Pharmacology*, **102**, 272–276.

Rochae., Silva, M., Valle, J.R. and Picarelli, Z.P. (1953). A pharmacological analysis of the mode of action of serotonin (5-hydroxytryptamine) upon the guinea-pig ileum. *British Journal of Pharmacology*, **8**, 378–388.

Round, A.A. and Wallis, D.I. (1986). The depolarizing action of 5-hydroxytryptamine on rabbit vagal afferent and sympathetic neurones and its selective blockade by ICS 205–930. *British Journal of Pharmacology*, **88**, 485–494.

Round, A. and Wallis, D.I. (1987). Further studies on the blockade of 5-HT depolarizations of rabbit vagal afferent and sympathetic ganglion cells by MDL 72222 and other antagonists. *Neuropharmacology*, **26**, 39–48.

Sakmann, B., Methfessel, C. Mishina, M., Takahashi, T., Takai, T., Kurasaki, M., Fukuda, K. and Numa, S. (1985). Role of acetylcholine receptor subunits in gating of the channel. *Nature*, **318**, 538–543.

Sanger, G.J. and Nelson, D.R. (1989). Selective and functional 5-hydroxytryptamine$_3$ receptor antagonism by BRL 43694 (granisetron). *European Journal of Pharmacology*, **159**, 113–124.

Saxena, P.R., Heiligers, J., Mylecharane, E.J. and Tio, R. (1985). Excitatory 5-hydroxytryptamine receptors in the cat urinary bladder are of the M- and 5-HT$_2$ type. *Journal of Autonomic Pharmacology*, **5**, 101–107.

Schmidt, C.J. and Black, C.K. (1989). The putative 5-HT$_3$ agonist phenylbiguanide induces carrier mediated release of [^{3}H] dopamine. *European Journal of Pharmacology*, **167**, 309–310.

Schofield, P.R. (1989). The GABA$_A$ receptor: molecular biology reveals a complex picture. *Trends in Pharmacological Science*, **10**, 476–478.

Shirasawa, Y. and Koketsu, K. (1977). Action of 5-hydroxytryptamine on isolated spinal cord of bullfrogs. *Japanese Journal of Pharmacology*, **27**, 23–29.

Smith, W.W., Sancilio, L.F., Owera-Atepo, J.B., Naylor, R.J. and Lambert, L.L. (1988). Zacopride, a potent 5-HT_3 antagonist. *Journal of Pharmacy and Pharmacology*, **40**, 301–302.

Stansfeld, C.E. and Wallis, D.I. (1985). Properties of visceral primary afferent neurons in the nodose ganglion of the rabbit. *Journal of Neurophysiology*, **54**, 245–260.

Stanton, J.A., Watling, K.J. and Beer, M.S. (1990). The effect of Ca^{2+} and Mg^{2+} ions on the binding of [^{3}H]-QICS 205–930 to the 5-HT_3 recognition site in rat brain whole cortex. *British Journal of Pharmacology*, **100**, 395P.

Strange, P.G. (1988). The structure and mechanism of neurotransmitter receptors. *Biochemical Journal*, **249**, 309–318.

Suprenant, A. (1990). Whole cell and single channel currents produced by activation of 5-HT_3 receptors in enteric neurones. *Neuroscience Letters*, **38**, S115.

Suprenant, A. and Crist, J. (1988). Electrophysiological characterization of functionally distinct 5-hydroxytryptamine receptors on guinea-pig submucous plexus. *Neuroscience*, **24**, 283–295.

Tatsumi, H. and Katayama, Y. (1987). The actions of 5-hydroxytryptamine in the rabbit ciliary ganglion. *Journal of the Autonomic Nervous System*, **20**, 137–145.

Todorovic, S. and Anderson, E.G. (1990). 5-HT_2 and 5-HT_3 receptors mediate two distinct depolarizing responses in rat dorsal root ganglion neurons. *Brain Research*, **511**, 71–79.

Vanner, S. and Suprenant, A. (1990). Effects of 5-HT_3 receptor antagonists on 5-HT and nicotinic depolarizations in guinea-pig submucosal neurones. *British Journal of Pharmacology*, **99**, 840–844.

Van Wijngaarden, I., Tulp, M.Th.M. and Soudjin, W. (1990). The concept of selectivity of 5-HT receptor research. *European Journal of Pharmacology (Molecular Pharmacology Section)*, **188**, 301–312.

Vyklicky, L., Jr, Krusek, J. and Edwards, C. (1988). Differences in the pore sizes of the *N*-methyl-D-aspartate and kainate cation channels. *Neuroscience Letters*, **89**, 313–318.

Wallis, D.I. (1989). Interaction of 5-hydroxytryptamine with autonomic and sensory neurones. In: *The Peripheral Actions of 5-Hydroxytryptamine*, edited by J.R. Fozard. Oxford: Oxford University Press, pp. 220–246.

Wallis, D.I. and Dun, N.J. (1987). Fast and slow depolarizing responses of guinea-pig coeliac ganglion cells to 5-hydroxytryptamine. *Journal of the Autonomic Nervous System*, **21**, 185–194.

Wallis, D.I. and Dun, N.J. (1988). A comparison of fast and slow depolarizations evoked by 5-HT in guinea-pig coeliac ganglion cells *in vitro*. *British Journal of Pharmacology*, **93**, 110–120.

Wallis, D.I. and Nash, H. (1981). Relative activities of substances related to 5-hydroxytryptamine as depolarising agents of superior cervical ganglion cells. *European Journal of Pharmacology*, **70**, 381–392.

Wallis, D.I. and North, R.A. (1978). The action of 5-hydoxytryptamine on single neurones of the rabbit superior cervical ganglion. *Neuropharmacology*, **17**, 1023–1028.

Wallis, D.I. and Woodward, B. (1975). Membrane potential changes induced by 5-hydroxytryptamine in the superior cervical ganglion of the rabbit. *British Journal of Pharmacology*, **55**, 199–212.

Wallis, D.I., Stansfeld, C.E. and Nash, H.L. (1982). Depolarizing responses recorded from nodose ganglion cells of the rabbit evoked by 5-hydroxytryptamine and other substances. *Neuropharmacology*, **21**, 31–40.

Watling, K.J., Aspley, S., Swain, C.J. and Saunders, J. (1988). [^{3}H] Quaternised ICS 205–930 labels 5-HT_3 receptor binding sites in rat brain. *European Journal of Pharmacology*, **149**, 397–398.

Yakel, J.L. and Jackson, M.B. (1988). 5-HT_3 receptors mediate rapid responses in cultured hippocampus and a clonal cell line. *Neuron*, **1**, 615–621.

Yakel, J.L., Trussel, L.O. and Jackson, M.B. (1988). Three serotonin responses in cultured mouse hippocampal and striatal neurones. *Journal of Neuroscience*, **8**, 1273–1285.

Yakel, J.L., Shao, X.M. and Jackson, M.B. (1990a). Desensitisation and modulation of the 5-HT_3 receptor of NG108–15 cells. *Neuroscience Letters*, **38**, S118.

Yakel, J.L. Shao, X.M. and Jackson, M.B. (1990b). The selectivity of the channel coupled to the 5-HT_3 receptor. *Brain Research*, **533**, 46–52.

Yang, J. (1990). Ion permeation through 5-HT-gated channels in neuroblastoma N18 cells. *Journal of General Physiology*, **96**, 1177–1198.

Yang, J. and Hille, B. (1990). Cation permeability of 5-HT_3 receptor channels in cultured cells. *Biophysical Journal*, **57**, 127a.

Chapter 17

Presynaptic effects of 5-HT

Manfred Göthert

17.1. *General introductory remarks*

17.1.1. Mechanisms and sites of action and source of 5-HT involved in presynaptic effects

Neuronal function in the central and peripheral nervous system can be influenced by serotonin (5-hydroxytryptamine; 5-HT) not only via somadendritic 5-HT receptors but also by presynaptic mechanisms. The latter comprise receptor-independent 5-HT-induced noradrenaline release from postganglionic sympathetic nerve endings by a tyramine-like mechanism and, above all, receptor-mediated presynaptic effects on various neurones (Göthert, 1982; Moret, 1985; Starke *et al.*, 1989; Göthert, 1990b; Göthert *et al.*, 1990). Both presynaptic 5-HT *auto*receptors and presynaptic 5-HT *hetero*receptors can be discussed in this context.

Presynaptic 5-HT autoreceptors are located on the seretoninergic nerve terminals themselves and can be activated by 5-HT released from the neurone on which they are located. Presynaptic 5-HT heteroreceptors are located on nerve terminals which store and release other neurotransmitters. Such non-serotoninergic axon terminals may form axo-axonal synapses with serotoninergic terminals. As an alternative, 5-HT released from central neurones may, after diffusion within the tissue, also reach presynaptic 5-HT heteroreceptors on varicosities which do not form synapses with the serotoninergic ones. The functional state of these receptors can be modified by local changes of the concentration of 5-HT in the vicinity of the nerve terminal involved. Accordingly, such presynaptic receptors can play a role in the fine regulation of neurotransmitter release from varicosities of those axon branches at which the local change of 5-HT concentration occurs. In contrast, somadendritic 5-HT receptors modify the function of the whole neurone with all axon branches.

In the central nervous system (CNS), the 5-HT which activates presynaptic 5-HT receptors under physiological or pathological conditions may be assumed to be of neuronal origin. However, the source of endogenous 5-HT which might stimulate inhibitory or facilitatory presynaptic 5-HT heteroreceptors on peripheral noradrenergic neurones must primarily be non-neuronal in origin. As an exception only, serotoninergic neurones seem to innervate cerebral blood vessels, and they have been identified in the enteric nervous system, but as a rule they do not occur in the peripheral nervous system. Hence, platelets have to be considered as a potential source of 5-HT, which may come into play at these receptors under pathological rather than physiological conditions. Presynaptic 5-HT auto- and hetero-receptors may also be the target of exogenous 5-HT or other drugs, and hence may be involved in the main therapeutic and/or side-effects of such drugs.

In the present account, the tyramine-like, receptor-independent 5-HT-induced noradrenaline release from sympathetic nerves is briefly touched upon. Mainly, this chapter focuses on effects of serotonin mediated by presynaptic 5-HT autoreceptors, in the CNS, since they have been the most extensively investigated. A short synopsis is given of the presynaptic 5-HT heteroreceptors in the CNS and on peripheral noradrenergic neurones.

In the last decade, considerable progress has been made in the general classification of 5-HT receptors (for reviews see Bradley *et al.*, 1986; Leff and Martin, 1988; Peroutka, 1988; Frazer *et al.*, 1990; Göthert, 1990a), irrespective of their location in the synaptic cleft. As a framework for the more detailed discussion of receptor-mediated presynaptic effects of 5-HT, a brief outline of the current classification scheme of 5-HT receptors is given first, and some key drugs suitable for discriminating between the various 5-HT receptor classes and subclasses are mentioned in this context.

17.1.2. Main 5-HT receptor classes and subclasses, and some key drugs used for their identification

At least three main classes of 5-HT receptors, 5-HT_1, 5-HT_2 and 5-HT_3, have been identified by means of pharmacological and molecular biological techniques (for references, see above). Recently, a 5-HT receptor with pharmacological properties distinct from the receptor classes defined so far was identified in the rat CNS and was tentatively named 5-HT_4 (Dumuis *et al.*, 1988). The 5-HT_1 receptor ‘family’ is heterogeneous and has been subclassified into at least four subtypes, 1A, 1B, 1C and 1D (Göthert and Schlicker, 1990a; for further references, see above). The classification of a given receptor as belonging to one of the 5-HT receptor classes or subclasses is complicated by the fact that only a few drugs are available which selectively activate or block certain 5-HT receptors. This holds true for 5-HT_2 and 5-HT_3 receptors, for which more or less selective antagonists have been developed. Ketanserin has been the most widely used 5-HT_2 receptor antagonist, and several 5-HT_3 receptor antagonists have recently been synthesized, such as MDL-72222 (1αH,3αH-tropan-3-yl-3,5-diclorobenzoate), ICS 205–930 ((3α-tropanyl)-1-H-indole-3-carboxylic acid ester) and ondansetron.

However, selective drugs are missing for most of the 5-HT_1 receptor subtypes. Therefore, the subclassification of 5-HT_1 receptors by means of pharmacological techniques has to be based on experiments with several putative 5-HT receptor agonists and antagonists with an overlapping profile of affinities for the various 5-HT_1 receptor subtypes, in many cases, also for the other main classes of 5-HT receptors. Thus, the key antagonist at 5-HT_1 receptors metitepine (suggested International Nonproprietary Name; frequently termed methiothepine) also blocks 5-HT_2 receptors. The few antagonists which are suitable for discriminating between the 5-HT_1 subtypes, such as spiperone (5-HT_{1A}), propranolol (5-HT_{1A} and 5-HT_{1B}) and mesulergine (5-HT_{1C}), also, or even predominantly, block other 5-HT receptors or non-5-HT receptors. Subtype-selective 5-HT_1 receptor agonists are, as a rule, also not available; exceptions are, for example, 8-OH-DPAT (8-hydroxy-2-(di-*n*-propylamino-tetralin)), ipsapirone and urapidil, which preferentially activate 5-HT_{1A} receptors.

Problems arising from the lack of subtype-selective 5-HT_1 receptor agonists and antagonists had frequently to be overcome in attempts to classify presynaptic inhibitory 5-HT receptors in the central and peripheral nervous system, since in most cases they possess the characteristics of 5-HT_1 receptors (see below). Therefore, in many investigations, subclassification could only be based on the determination of the potencies of several 5-HT receptor agonists in inhibiting transmitter release and of some antagonists in blocking this effect. These potencies were then compared with the affinities of the drugs for the various 5-HT sites determined in radioligand binding studies.

17.2. *Presynaptic effects of 5-HT in the CNS*

Synaptosomes or slices prepared from certain brain regions and the spinal cord were used to identify and characterize presynaptic 5-HT auto- and heteroreceptors. The overflow of the relevant endogenous or tritiated neurotransmitter (previously taken up or synthesized from its ^3H-precursor) from the superfused preparations was stimulated either by electrical impulses or by high K^+ or, when a stimulatory effect of 5-HT itself was investigated, by introduction of 5-HT into the superfusion fluid. Under appropriate experimental conditions, the evoked overflow reflects transmitter release from the corresponding neurone (see Starke *et al.*, 1989; Göthert, 1990b).

17.2.1. **Inhibition of 5-HT release by presynaptic 5-HT autoreceptors**

The first report on the ability of a 5-HT receptor agonist to inhibit 5-HT release was published in 1971 by Farnebo and Hamberger: the electrically evoked [^3H]-5-HT release from rat brain cortex slices was found to be inhibited by lysergide (LSD), a non-selective 5-HT receptor agonist. Evidence for the assumption that this effect is receptor-mediated was provided by the additional findings that other 5-HT receptor agonists inhibit, and that metitepine facilitates, the evoked [^{3}H]-5-HT release (Farnebo and Hamberger, 1974; Hamon *et al.*, 1974). That 5-HT itself inhibits 5-HT release was shown in rat hypothalmic synaptosomes (Cerrito and Raiteri, 1979) and cortical slices (Göthert and Weinheimer, 1979). Since the inhibitory effect of 5-HT was competitively antagonized by metitepine, it could be concluded that both compounds compete for the same site, namely the inhibitory presynaptic 5-HT receptor (Göthert, 1980).

The results summarized in this brief historical account represent a basis for the scheme shown in Figure 17.1 (right panel). 5-HT released from the serotoninergic varicosites activates the presynaptic 5-HT autoreceptor, thus inhibiting further 5-HT release. Such an autoinhibitory feedback mechanism may play a role in fine regulation of 5-HT release. The facilitatory effect of metitepine and other 5-HT receptor antagonists on 5-HT release is due to blockade of the 5-HT autoreceptors, thus disinhibiting, i.e. increasing, 5-HT release. Part of the 5-HT released into the synaptic cleft is transported back into the nerve terminal by the specific 5-HT transporter in the cell membrane and, if not metabolized, is further transported by the vesicular uptake mechanism into the storage vesicles (Figure 17.1, right panel). It has been claimed that a functional link may exist between the 5-HT autoreceptor and the 5-HT transporter (Langer and Moret, 1982; Galzin *et al.*, 1985), but more recent results obtained in synaptosomes (Bonanno and Raiteri, 1987) and slices (Limberger and Späth, 1990) argue against this possibility.

The literature on presynaptic 5-HT autoreceptors has been reviewed extensively by several authors (e.g. Moret, 1985; Timmermans and Thoolen, 1987; Starke *et al.*, 1989; Göthert, 1990b), and should be consulted for more detailed information. In the present chapter, only a few important points are briefly touched upon and some emphasis is laid on future trends of research. Table 17.1 makes clear that presynaptic 5-HT autoreceptors have been identified in every region of the CNS of all mammalian species investigated for this purpose, including human cerebral cortex. Experimental attempts to classify these receptors revealed that in the rat and the mouse they belong to the 5-HT_{1B} subclass (for references, see review articles quoted above). However, radioligand binding studies revealed that 5-HT_{1B} recognition sites are not present in the brain of, for example, guinea-pig, pig, calf and human, but that in these species another subclass of 5-HT_1 receptors, namely the 5-HT_{1D} subtype, was found which seems to subserve the same function as 5-HT_{1B} receptors in the rat and the mouse brain. Accordingly, pig and guinea-pig (rather than rat and mouse brain preparations) appear to represent a model for the human brain with respect to its 5-HT autoreceptor. Therefore, it is of interest that in the guinea-pig (Hoyer and Middlemiss, 1989) and pig brain (Schlicker *et al.*, 1989), the presynaptic 5-HT autoreceptor has been classified as 5-HT_{1D}.

In the pig brain, the potency of 5-HT receptor agonists to inhibit 5-HT release was found to be correlated with the potency of these drugs to inhibit

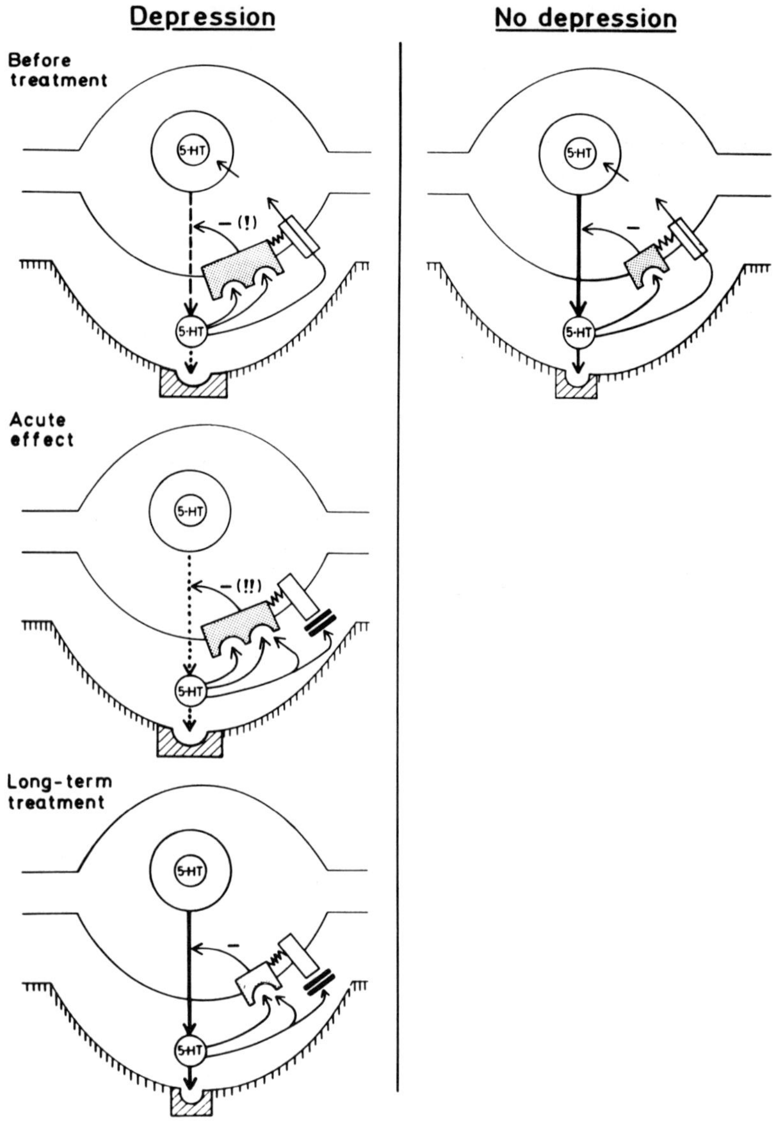

Figure 17.1. Function of presynaptic 5-HT autoreceptors in the brain under normal conditions (right panel), and hypothesized function in depressed patients before and after treatment with 5-HT uptake inhibitors (left panel). Stippled area in the membrane of the seretoninergic varicosity, 5-HT autoreceptor. Vertical arrows: solid, normal 5-HT release, resulting in normal 5-HT concentration at postsynaptic 5-HT receptors; broken, decreased release and decreased 5-HT concentration at postsynaptic 5-HT receptors. Thin solid arrows, binding of 5-HT to presynaptic autoreceptors and 5-HT uptake by the 5-HT transporter. Autoreceptor-mediated inhibition of 5-HT release: – , normal inhibition; –(!) and –(!!), reinforced inhibition. In untreated, depressed patients, autoreceptor function is assumed to be increased, symbolized by the increased stippled area, by the two recognition sites for 5-HT and by –(!). Blockade of the transporter by certain antidepressants first results in an increased concentration of 5-HT at the autoreceptor, leading immediately to further reinforcement of autoreceptor function, symbolized by –(!!). As a result of both effects (uptake blockade and increased autoreceptor function) the 5-HT concentration at postsynaptic receptors remains decreased. After long-term treatment with such antidepressants, a down-regulation of the autoreceptor occurs, resulting in normal serotoninergic synaptic transmission.

Table 17.1. Occurence of inhibitory presynaptic 5-HT autoreceptors in the CNS.

Species and area of the CNS investigated[a]	
Rat	Guinea-pig
Cerebral cortex	Cerebral cortex
Hippocampus	
Nucleus accumbens	Rabbit
Corpus striatum	Cerebral cortex
Hypothalamus	Hippocampus
Cerebellum	Hypothalamus
Medulla oblongata	Superior colliculus
Spinal cord	
	Pig
Mouse	Cerebral cortex
Cerebellum	
	Human
	Cerebral cortex

[a] For references, see text, Starke *et al.*, 1989 and Göthert, 1990b.

forskolin-stimulated cAMP formation (Schlicker *et al.*, 1989), suggesting that an inhibition of adenylate cyclase may be involved in autoinhibition of 5-HT release. Inhibition of Ca^{2+} influx also seems to play a role in signal transduction following autoreceptor activation (Göthert, 1980). Future investigations should focus on attempts to obtain more direct and more detailed information concerning the mechanism of action underlying the autoreceptor-mediated inhibition of 5-HT release, in particular the role of G-proteins in signal transduction and in changes in the ion conductance of the cell membrane.

Other open questions can be derived from information contained in Figure 17.2. The 5-HT nerve terminals are endowed not only with the 5-HT autoreceptor, but also with heteroreceptors for other endogenous compounds. Thus, presynaptic prostaglandin, γ-aminobutyric acid ($GABA_B$), histamine H_3 receptors and α_2-adrenoceptors have been identified, activation of which inhibits 5-HT release (for review see Göthert and Schlicker, 1990b). On the other hand, evidence has been presented that on noradrenergic neurones of the CNS, inhibitory presynaptic receptors interact with each other (Limberger *et al.*, 1988; Allgaier *et al.*, 1989). The question of whether such interactions also occur between the presynaptic 5-HT autoreceptors and the presynaptic heteroreceptors on the 5-HT neurones should be addressed in future studies.

The role of the 5-HT autoreceptor in depression also needs further clarification (see Göthert, 1986). It has been suggested that depression may be related to an increased activity and/or density of presynaptic 5-HT autoreceptor, leading to a decrease in 5-HT release and, as a consequence, in 5-HT concentration at the postsynaptic 5-HT receptors (Figure 17.1, left panel). The acute effect of 5-HT uptake inhibitors used as antidepressant drugs seems to consist of a transient increase in 5-HT concentration in the

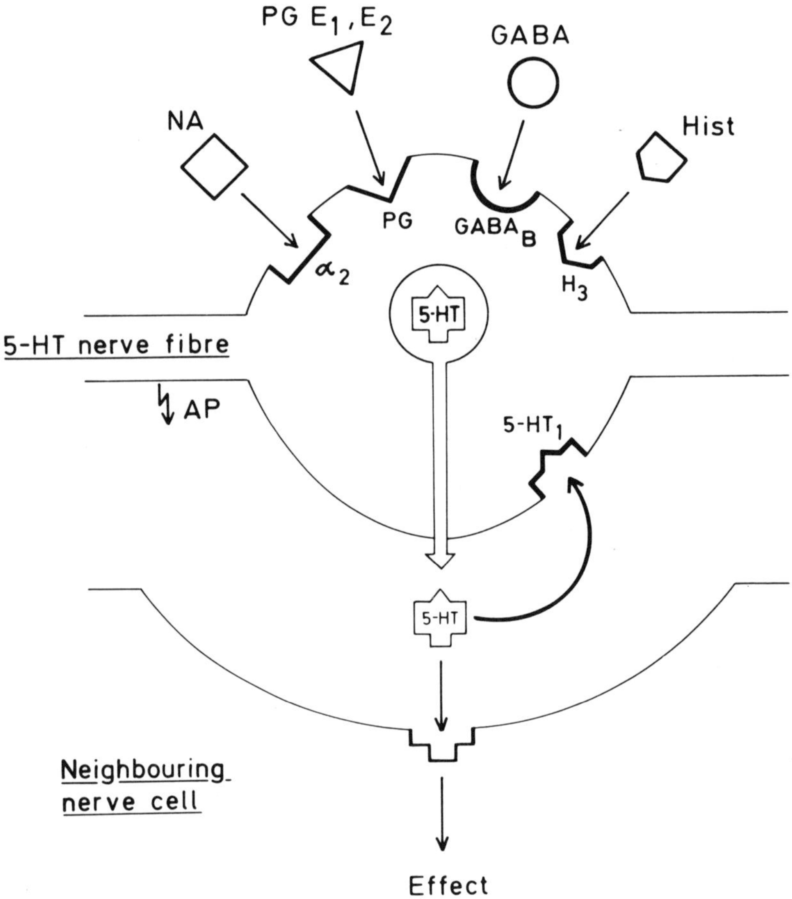

Figure 17.2. Presynaptic 5-HT_1 autoreceptor (5-HT_{1B} in rat and mouse; 5-HT_{1D} in pig and guinea-pig) and presynaptic heteroreceptors for other neurotransmitters or prostaglandins (upper part of the scheme) involved in inhibition of 5-HT release from serotoninergic varicosities in the CNS. AP, action potential; NA, noradrenaline; PG, prostaglandin; Hist, histamine; GABA, γ-aminobutyric acid.

biophase of the 5-HT autoreceptor, which immediately induces an even more pronounced activation of the 5-HT autoreceptor. In this phase, the 5-HT concentration at the postsynaptic 5-HT receptors is not yet increased. However, after long-term administration of such antidepressants, a down-regulation of presynaptic autoreceptors may occur. This in turn may restore autoreceptor function to normal. This model would explain the latency period characteristic for the therapeutic effect of uptake inhibitors. In support of this hypothesis, it was found (1) that acute *in vitro* application of such antidepressants does not increase ^3H overflow from slices preincubated with [^{3}H]-5-HT (Langer and Moret, 1982; Galzin *et al.*, 1985), or at best produces a very weak effect (Gross *et al.*, 1987), and (2) that long-term (but not acute) treatment of rats with antidepressants results in a decreased function of presynaptic 5-HT autoreceptors (Maura and Raiteri, 1984; Schoups and De Potter, 1988). In agreement with the above considerations (summarized in Figure 17.1, left panel), specific autoreceptor antagonists may be developed as a new class of antidepressants which may be assumed to exhibit the advantage of a relatively rapid onset of therapeutic effect.

17.2.2. Inhibition of transmitter release by presynaptic 5-HT heteroreceptors

Inhibitory presynaptic 5-HT heteroreceptors in the CNS have been investigated far less extensively than 5-HT autoreceptors. Much of the available information has recently been reviewed (Göthert, 1990a) and is summarized in Table 17.2.

Table 17.2. Occurrence, function and classification of presynaptic 5-HT heteroreceptors in the rat brain.[a]

Function	Neurone	Brain region	5-HT receptor class or subclass
Inhibition of release	DA	Striatum Nucleus accumbens	Unknown
	ACH	Striatum	5-HT_1
		Hippocampus	5-HT_{1B}
	GLU	Cerebellum	5-HT_1
Stimulation of release	DA	Striatum	5-HT_3

[a] For references, see text, and Göthert, 1990b.
DA, dopamine; ACH, acetylcholine; GLU, glutamate.

Inhibitory 5-HT heteroreceptors were identified on dopamine nerve terminals of the rat striatum and the nucleus accumbens (Ennis *et al.*, 1981; Westfall and Tittermary, 1982; Hetey and Drescher, 1986). 5-HT possesses only low affinity for these receptors which have not yet been classified in detail. Presynaptic 5-HT heteroreceptors also mediate inhibition of neurotransmitter release from cholinergic neurones of the rat striatum (Vizi *et al.*, 1981; Gillet *et al.*, 1985) and hippocampus (Maura and Raiteri, 1986) as well as from the glutamatergic neurones of the rat cerebellum (Raiteri *et al.*, 1986). The pharmacological properties of these receptors conform to the basic properties of the 5-HT_1 class, and the presynaptic 5-HT heteroreceptor on the cholinergic neurone of the hippocampus could be subclassified as 5-HT_{1B}.

The serotoninergic nerve terminals are endowed with inhibitory α_2-heteroreceptors (Figure 17.2: Göthert *et al.*, 1981); conversely, 5-HT did not inhibit the electrically evoked noradrenaline release in rat brain cortex slices (Taube *et al.*, 1977) suggesting that presynaptic 5-HT heteroreceptors are probably not present on noradrenergic nerve endings.

17.3.3. Stimulation or facilitation of transmitter release by presynaptic 5-HT heteroreceptors

The possibility that 5-HT induces receptor-mediated stimulation and facilitation of transmitter release has been examined in brain slices. The term facilitation of release describes the ability of 5-HT to enhance the release induced by other depolarizing stimuli, such as electrical impulses; in this case, 5-HT acts as a presynaptic modulator. A receptor-mediated stimulation of release occurs with 5-HT if it induces Ca^{2+}-dependent transmitter release by itself, i.e. without additional depolarizing stimulus. Such stimulatory presynaptic 5-HT heteroreceptors have been identified on the dopaminergic neurones of the rat striatum (Table 17.2). These receptors exhibit the pharmacological properties of the 5-HT_3 class (Blandina *et al.*, 1988, 1989). Data published very recently in abstract form suggest that presynaptic 5-HT_3 heteroreceptors are also involved in facilitation of transmitter release. This was observed in guinea-pig cortex slices, in which 5-HT_3 receptor agonists increased the electrically evoked [^{3}H]-5-HT release in a manner sensitive to blockade by the 5-HT receptor antagonist ICS 205–930 (Galzin *et al.*, 1990).

17.3. *Presynaptic effects of 5-HT on sympathetic nerves*

The effects of 5-HT on noradrenaline release were investigated in isolated preparations of sympathetically innervated tissues, which were superfused, perfused or incubated. Either end organ response (e.g. contraction, increase in heart rate) or the efflux of radioactively labelled or endogenous noradrenaline from the preparation under study was determined. Receptor-mediated inhibition of noradrenaline release was studied in tissues in which the sympathetic nerves were stimulated by electrical impulses.

17.3.1. Inhibition of noradrenaline release by presynaptic 5-HT heteroreceptors

The first account of the ability of 5-HT to inhibit noradrenaline release appeared in 1977: the electrically evoked [^{3}H]-noradrenaline release in the dog saphenous vein was found to be inhibited by 5-HT (McGrath, 1977). This observation was confirmed and extended by other groups of investigators (e.g. Feniuk *et al.*, 1979; Lorenz and Vanhoutte, 1985). Support for the suggestion that a 5-HT heteroreceptor is involved in this effect was derived from experiments in various blood vessels, in which the mixed 5-HT_1/5-HT_2 receptor antagonist metitepine was shown to block the 5-HT-induced inhibition of noradrenaline release (Cohen, 1985; Charlton *et al.*, 1986; Göthert *et al.*, 1986a,b). Table 17.3 contains a synopsis of the cardiovascular tissues and species in which such inhibitory presynaptic 5-HT receptors have been

Table 17.3. Occurence of inhibitory presynaptic 5-HT heteroreceptors on the sympathetic nerves of cardiovascular tissue.

Species and tissue investigated[a]	
Rat	Pig
Iliac artery	Coronary artery
Vena cava	
Renal vascular bed	Dog
Heart	Tibial artery
	Femoral arterial circulation
Guinea-pig	Saphenous vein
Atrium	Coronary artery
	Heart
	Human
	Saphenous vein

[a] For references, see text and Göthert *et al.*, 1990.

identified. The references on which this table is based are given in a more detailed review article on presynaptic effects of 5-HT in the cardiovascular system (Göthert *et al.*, 1990).

Attempts to classify the inhibitory 5-HT heteroreceptor on the sympathetic nerves were first made in the rat vena cava and renal vascular bed as well as in the human saphenous vein (Göthert *et al.*, 1986a,b; Charlton *et al.*, 1986). In these blood vessels, only metitepine (see above), but not the preferential 5-HT_2 receptor antagonist ketanserin, blocked the 5-HT-induced inhibition of noradrenaline release, suggesting that the receptor involved belongs to the 5-HT_1 'family'. On the basis of a more detailed pharmacological analysis, the inhibitory 5-HT receptor on the sympathetic nerves could be subclassified as 5-HT_{1B} in the rat vena cava and as 5-HT_{1D} in the human saphenous vein; in the pig coronary artery, it represents a novel, so far unknown, class of 5-HT receptors (Göthert *et al.*, 1991).

The possibility that presynaptic 5-HT receptors may interact with other presynaptic receptor systems on the same neurone has already been discussed above. Evidence has been presented that this occurs in the rat vena cava between the inhibitory 5-HT heteroreceptor and the α_2-autoreceptor on the sympathetic nerve terminals: activation of the former receptor decreases the ability of α_2-adrenoceptor agonists to inhibit, and of α_2-antagonists to facilitate, noradrenaline release (Molderings and Göthert, 1990).

17.3.2. Stimulation of noradrenaline release by presynaptic 5-HT heteroreceptors

Stimulatory 5-HT receptors are also located on the sympathetic nerve terminals. The characteristics of such a receptor-mediated indirect sympathomimetic effect are summarized in Table 17.4. The experiments on which this table is based were carried out in the isolated rabbit heart perfused according to the Langendorff technique; either the positive chronotropic response to 5-HT (and other indolethyamines; Fozard and Mwaluko, 1976; Fozard and Mobarok Ali, 1978) or the overflow of endogenous noradrenaline into the perfusion fluid was determined (Göthert and Dührsen, 1979). Criteria nos 1–5 of Table 17.4 are suitable for discriminating between receptor-mediated and tyramine-like sympathomimetic effects (cf. table 17.5), whereas criterion no. 6 does not. Unequivocal proof for the involvement of a receptor in the indirect sympathomimetic effect characterized in Table 17.4 could be derived from the development of specific competitive antagonists, such as MDL-72222 (Fozard, 1984) and ICS 205–930 (Richardson *et al.*, 1985). These are highly selective in blocking 5-HT_3 receptors. Accordingly, the stimulatory presynaptic 5-HT heteroreceptors can be classified as 5-HT_3. Further details and a more comprehensive survey of the literature are given in a recent review article (Göthert *et al.*, 1990).

17.3.3. Receptor-independent stimulation of noradrenaline release

High concentrations or doses of 5-HT are necessary to induce noradrenaline release by a tyramine-like mechanism (e.g. see McGrath, 1977; Freeman *et al.*, 1981), the criteria of which are listed in Table 17.5. Among these criteria, the abolition of end organ response by neuronal noradrenaline uptake inhibitors (e.g. cocaine), and the resistance of this type of 5-HT-induced noradrenaline release to 5-HT receptor antagonists or omission of Ca^{2+}, are the most characteristic and discriminative features of the receptor-independent sympathomimetic effect of 5-HT (for further details see Humphrey *et al.*, 1983; Göthert *et al.*, 1990).

17.4. *Concluding remarks*

As summarized in the previous sections, 5-HT can induce presynaptic effects by stimulation of various presynaptic receptors and by a receptor-independent, tyramine-like mechanism. The latter is of more academic interest, since it comes into play only at very high concentrations of 5-HT, which under extreme conditions may occur *in vivo*. However, the receptor-mediated responses, in particular in the CNS, may play a role under physiological and/or pathological conditions. All presynaptic 5-HT receptors have to be considered as potential targets of drugs and may be involved in their therapeutic or side-effects. Concerning the classification of presynaptic 5-HT receptors it may be stated that, as a rule, those mediating an inhibition of transmitter release belong to the 5-HT_1 ‘family’, whereas the stimulatory and facilatory receptors conform to the characteristics of the 5-HT_3 class.

Table 17.4. Characteristics of receptor-mediated indirect sympathomimetic effects of 5-HT in the rabbit heart.[a]

(1)	Rapid onset of noradrenaline release and of end organ response
(2)	Ca^{2+}-dependence
(3)	Blockade by colchicine, an inhibitor of exocytosis
(4)	Rapid desensitization to 5-HT and related drugs (but not to tyramine)
(5)	Failure of desipramine to inhibit the effect of 5-HT
(6)	Responses to 5-HT abolished by:
	β-adrenoceptor antagonists[b]
	pretreatment with reserpine[b]
	chemical sympathectomy (6-hydroxydopamine)[b]

[a] For references, see Fozard and Mwaluko, 1976; Fozard and Mobarok Ali, 1978; Göthert and Dührsen, 1979.
[b] Pharmacological manipulations not suitable for differentiating between receptor-mediated and tyramine-like mechanisms.

Table 17.5. Criteria for 5-HT-induced noradrenaline release by a tyramine-like mechanism.[a]

Slowly developing responses (noradrenaline release or end organ effects)	
End organ responses abolished by:	
(1)	α- (blood vessels) or β-adrenoceptor antagonists (heart)
(2)	neuronal uptake inhibitors
(3)	depletion of noradrenaline storage sites
(4)	surgical or chemical sympathectomy
Stimulation of noradrenaline release resistant to:	
(1)	omission of Ca^{2+} ions
(2)	drugs assumed to inhibit exocytosis
(3)	$5\text{-}HT_3$ receptor antagonists

[a] For references, see text.

Acknowledgement

The author's own work in this field was supported by the Deutsche Forschungsgemeinschaft. The expert secretarial assistance of Mrs R. Korneli is gratefully acknowledged.

References

Allgaier, C., Jäger, T. and Hertting, G. (1989). Endogenous noradrenaline impairs the prostaglandin-induced inhibition of noradrenaline release. *Naunyn-Schmiedeberg's Archives of Pharmacology*, **340**, 472–474.

Blandina, P., Goldfarb, J. and Green, J.P. (1988). Activation of a $5\text{-}HT_3$ receptor releases dopamine from rat striatal slice. *European Journal of Pharmacology*, **54**, 285–350.

Blandina, P., Goldfarb, J., Craddock-Royal, B. and Green, J.P. (1989). Release of endogenous dopamine by stimulation of 5-hydroxytryptamine$_3$ receptors in rat striatum. *Journal of Pharmacology and Experimental Therapeutics*, **251**, 803–809.

Bonanno, G. and Raiteri, M. (1987). Interaction between 5-HT uptake inhibition and activation of 5-HT autoreceptors by exogenous agonists in rat cerebral cortex slices and synaptosomes. *Naunyn-Schmiedeberg's Archives of Pharmacology*, **336**, 219–225.

Bradley, P.B., Engel, G., Feniuk, W., Fozard, J.R., Humphrey, P.P.A., Middlemiss, D.N., Mylecharane, E.J., Richardson, B.P. and Saxena, P.R. (1986). Proposals for the classification and nomenclature of functional receptors for 5-hydroxytryptamine. *Neuropharmacology*, **25**, 563–576.

Cerrito, F. and Raiteri, M. (1979). Serotonin release is modulated by presynaptic autoreceptors. *European Journal of Pharmacology*, **57**, 427–430.

Charlton, K.G., Bon, R.A. and Clarke, D.E. (1986). An inhibitory prejunctional 5-HT_1-like receptor in the isolated perfused rat kidney. Apparent distinction from the 5-HT_{1A}, 5-HT_{1B} and 5-HT_{1C} subtypes. *Naunyn-Schmiedeberg's Archives of Pharmacology*, **332**, 8–15.

Cohen, R.A. (1985). Serotonergic prejunctional inhibition of canine coronary adrenergic nerves. *Journal of Pharmacology and Experimental Therapeutics*, **235**, 76–80.

Dumuis, A., Bouhelal, R., Sebben, M., Cory, R. and Bockaert, J. (1988). A non-classical 5-hydroxytryptamine receptor positively coupled with adenylate cyclase in the central nervous system. *Molecular Pharmacology*, **34**, 880–887.

Ennis, C., Kemp, J.D. and Cox, B. (1981). Characterisation of inhibitory 5-hydroxytryptamine receptors that modulate dopamine release in the striatum. *Journal of Neurochemistry*, **36**, 1515–1520.

Farnebo, L.-O. and Hamberger, B. (1971). Drug-induced changes in the release of ^{3}H-monoamines from field stimulated rat brain slices. *Acta Physiologica Scandinavica*, **371**, 35–44.

Farnebo, L.-O. and Hamberger, B. (1974). Regulation of [^{3}H]-hydroxytryptamine release from rat brain slices. *Journal of Pharmacy and Pharmacology*, **26**, 642–644.

Feniuk, W., Humphrey, P.P.A. and Watts, A.D. (1979). Presynaptic inhibitory action of 5-hydroxytryptamine in dog isolated saphenous vein. *British Journal of Pharmacology*, **67**, 247–254.

Fozard, J.R. (1984). MDL 72222: a potent and highly selective antagonist at neuronal 5-hydroxytryptamine receptors. *Naunyn-Schmiedeberg's Archives of Pharmacology*, **326**, 36–44.

Fozard, J.R. and Mobarok Ali, A.T.M. (1978). Receptors for 5-hydroxytryptamine on the sympathetic nerves of the rabbit heart. *Naunyn-Schmiedeberg's Archives of Pharmacology*, **301**, 223–235.

Fozard, J.R. and Mwaluko, G.M.P. (1976). Mechanism of the indirect sympathomimetic effect of 5-hydroxytryptamine on the isolated heart of the rabbit. *British Journal of Pharmacology*, **57**, 115–125.

Frazer, A., Maayani, S. and Wolfe, B.B. (1990). Subtypes of receptors for serotonin. *Annual Review of Pharmacology and Toxicology*, **30**, 307–348.

Freeman, W.K., Rorie, D.K. and Tyce, G.M. (1981). Effects of 5-hydroxytryptamine on neuroeffector junction in human pulmonary artery. *Journal of Applied Physiology*, **51**, 693–698.

Galzin, A.M. Poncet, V. and Langer, S.Z. (1990). 5-HT_3 receptor agonists enhance the electrically-evoked release of [^{3}H]-5-HT in guinea-pig frontal cortex slices. *British Journal of Pharmacology*, **100**, 307P.

Galzin, A.M., Moret, C., Verzier, B. and Langer, S.Z. (1985). Interaction between tricyclic and nontricyclic 5-hydroxytryptamine uptake inhibitors and the presynaptic 5-hydroxytryptamine inhibitory autoreceptors in the rat hypothalamus. *Journal of Pharmacology and Experimental Therapeutics*, **235**, 200–211.

Gillet, G., Ammor, S. and Fillion, G. (1985). Serotonin inhibits acetylcholine release from rat striatum slices: evidence for a presynaptic receptor-mediated effect. *Journal of Neurochemistry*, **45**, 1687–1691.

Göthert, M. (1980). Serotonin-receptor-mediated modulation of Ca^{2+}-dependent 5-hydroxytryptamine release from neurones of the rat brain cortex. *Naunyn-Schmiedeberg's Archives of Pharmacology*, **314**, 223–230.

Göthert, M. (1982). Modulation of serotonin release in the brain via presynaptic receptors. *Trends in Pharmacological Sciences*, **3**, 437–440.

Göthert, M. (1986). Presynaptic 5-HT autoreceptors and the modulation of the release of 5-HT. *Clinical Neuropharmacology*, **9**, 308–310.

Göthert, M. (1990a). Pharmacological, biochemical and molecular classification schemes of serotonin (5-HT) receptors with special reference to the 5-HT_2 class. In: *Serotonin and 5-HT_2 Receptor Blockade in the Cardiovascular System*, edited by M. Göthert. Stuttgart, New York: Fischer: pp. 3–15.

Göthert, M. (1990b). Presynaptic serotonin receptors in the CNS. *Annals of the New York Academy of Sciences*, **604**, 102–112.

Göthert, M. and Dührsen, U. (1979). Effects of 5-hydroxytryptamine and related compounds on the sympathetic nerves of the rabbit heart. *Naunyn-Schmiedeberg's Archives of Pharmacology*, **308**, 9–18.

Göthert, M. and Schlicker, E. (1990a). Identification and classification of 5-HT_1 receptor subtypes. *Journal of Cardiovascular Pharmacology*, **15**, 1–7.

Göthert, M. and Schlicker, E. (1990b). Regulation of serotonin release in the central nervous system by presynaptic heteroreceptors. In: *Presynaptic Regulation of Neurotransmitter Release: A Handbook*, edited by J. Feigenbaum. Tel Aviv: Freund Publishing House, in press.

Göthert, M. and Weinheimer, G. (1979). Extracellular 5-hydroxytryptamine inhibits 5-hydroxytryptamine release from rat brain cortex slices. *Naunyn-Schmiedeberg's Archives of Pharmacology*, **310**, 93–96.

Göthert, M. Huth, H. and Schlicker, E. (1981). Characterization of the receptor subtype involved in alpha-adrenoceptor-mediated modulation of serotonin release from rat brain cortex slices. *Naunyn-Schmiedeberg's Archives of Pharmacology*, **317**, 199–203.

Göthert, M. , Schlicker, E. and Kollecker, P. (1986a). Receptor-mediated effects of serotonin and 5-methoxytryptamine on noradrenaline release in the rat vena cava and in the heart of the pithed rat. *Naunyn-Schmiedeberg's Archives of Pharmacology*, **332**, 124–120.

Göthert, M., Fink, K., Molderings, G.J. and Schlicker, E. (1990). 5-Hydroxytryptamine and related drugs and transmitter release from autonomic nerves in the cardiovascular system. In: *Cardiovascular Pharmacology of 5-Hydroxytryptamine: Prospective Therapeutic Applications*, edited by P.R. Saxena, D.I. Wallis, W. Wouters and P. Bevan. Dordrecht: Kluwer, pp. 285–294.

Göthert, M., Molderings, G.J., Fink, K. and Schlicker, E. (1991). Heterogeneity of presynaptic serotonin receptors on sympathetic neurones in blood vessels. *Blood Vessels*, **28**, 11–18.

Göthert, M., Kollecker, P., Rohm, N. and Zerkowski, H.R. (1986b). Inhibitory presynaptic 5-hydroxytryptamine (5-HT) receptors on the sympathetic nerves of the human saphenous vein. *Naunyn-Schmiedeberg's Archives of Pharmacology*, **332**, 317–323.

Gross, G., Hante, K. and Göthert, M. (1987). Effect of antidepressant and neuroleptic drugs on the electrically evoked release of serotonin from rat cerebral cortex. *Psychopharmacology*, **91**, 175–181.

Hamon, M., Bourgoin, S., Jagger, J. and Glowinski, J. (1974). Effects of LSD on synthesis and release of 5-HT in rat brain slices. *Brain Research*, **69**, 265–280.

Hetey, L. and Drescher, K. (1986). Influence of antipsychotics on presynaptic receptors modulating the release of dopamine in synaptosomes of the nucleus accumbens of rats. *Neuropharmacology*, **25**, 1103–1109.

Hoyer, D. and Middlemiss, D.N. (1989). Species differences in the pharmacology of terminal 5-HT autoreceptors in mammalian brain. *Trends in Pharmacological Sciences,* **10**, 130–132.

Humphrey, P.P.A., Feniuk, W. and Watts, A.D. (1983). Prejunctional effects of 5-hydroxytryptamine on noradrenergic nerves in the cardiovascular system. *Federation Proceedings*, **42**, 218–222.

Langer, S.Z. and Moret, C. (1982). Citalopram antagonizes the stimulation by lysergic acid diethylamide of presynaptic inhibitory serotonin autoreceptors in the rat hypothalamus. *Journal of Pharmacology and Experimental Therapeutics*, **222**, 220–226.

Leff, P. and Martin, G.R. (1988). The classification of 5-hydroxytryptamine receptors. *Medicinal Research Reviews*, **8**, 187–202.

Limberger, N. and Späth, L. (1990). What is the 'functional link' between serotonin uptake sites and presynaptic serotonin autoreceptors? *Naunyn-Schmiedeberg's Archives of Pharmacology*, **341** (Suppl.), R 88.

Limberger, N., Späth, L. and Starke, K. (1988). Presynaptic α_2-adrenoceptor, opioid κ-receptor and adenosine A_1-receptor interactions on noradrenaline release in rabbit brain cortex. *Naunyn-Schmiedeberg's Archives of Pharmacology*, **338**, 53–61.

Lorenz, R.R. and Vanhoutte, P.M. (1985). Prejunctional adrenergic inhibition by aggregating platelets in canine blood vessels. *American Journal of Physiology*, **249**, H685–H689.

McGrath, M.A. (1977). 5-Hydroxytryptamine and neurotransmitter release in canine blood vessels. Inhibition by low and augmentation by high concentrations. *Circulation Research*, **41**, 428–435.

Maura, G. and Raiteri, M. (1984). Functional evidence that chronic drugs induce adaptive changes of central autoreceptors regulating serotonin release. *European Journal of Pharmacology*, **97**, 309–313.

Maura, G. and Raiteri, M. (1986). Cholinergic terminals in rat hippocampus possess 5-HT_{1B} receptors mediating inhibition of acetylcholine release. *European Journal of Pharmacology*, **129**, 333–337.

Molderings, G.J. and Göthert, M. (1990). Mutual interaction between presynaptic α_2-adrenoceptors and 5-HT_{1B} receptors on the sympathetic nerve terminals of the rat inferior vena cava. *Naunyn-Schmiedeberg's Archives of Pharmacology*, **341**, 391–397.

Moret, C. (1985). Pharmacology of the serotonin autoreceptor. In: *Neuropharmacology of Serotonin*, edited by A.R. Green. Oxford: Oxford University Press, pp. 21–49.

Peroutka, S.J. (1988). 5-Hydroxytryptamine receptor subtypes. *Annual Review of Neuroscience*, **11**, 496–500.

Raiteri, M., Maura, G., Bonanno, G. and Pittaluga, A. (1986). Differential pharmacology and function of two 5-HT_1 receptors modulating transmitter release in rat cerebellum. *Journal of Pharmacology and Experimental Therapeutics*, **237**, 644–648.

Richardson, B.P., Engel, G., Donatsch, P. and Stadler, P.A. (1985). Identification of serotonin M-receptor subtypes and their specific blockade by a new class of drugs. *Nature*, **316**, 126–131.

Schlicker, E., Fink, K., Göthert, M., Hoyer, D., Molderings, G., Roschke, I. and Schoeffter, P. (1989). The pharmacological properties of the presynaptic serotonin autoreceptor in the pig brain cortex conform to the 5-HT_{1D} receptor subtype. *Naunyn-Schmiedeberg's Archives of Pharmacology*, **340**, 45–51.

Schoups, A.A. and De Potter, W.P. (1988). Species dependence of adaptations at the pre- and postsynaptic serotonergic receptors following long-term anti-depressant drug treatment. *Biochemical Pharmacology*, **37**, 4451–4460.

Starke, K., Göthert, M. and Kilbinger, H. (1989). Modulation of neurotransmitter release by presynaptic autoreceptors. *Physiological Reviews*, **69**, 865–989.

Taube, H.D., Starke, K. and Borowski, E. (1977). Presynaptic receptor systems on the noradrenergic neurones of rat brain. *Naunyn-Schmiedeberg's Archives of Pharmacology*, **299**, 123–141.

Timmermans, P.B.M.W.M. and Thoolen, M.J.M.C. (1987). Autoreceptors in the central nervous system. *Medicinal Research Reviews*, **7**, 307–332.

Vizi, E.S., Hársing, G. and Zsilla, G. (1981). Evidence of the modulatory role of serotonin in acetylcholine release from striatal interneurons. *Brain Research*, **212**, 89–99.

Westfall, T.C. and Tittermary, V. (1982). Inhibition of the electrically induced release of [^{3}H]dopamine by serotonin from superfused rat striatal slices. *Neuroscience Letters*, **28**, 205–209.

Chapter 18

Electrophysiological effects of 5-HT on vertebrate motoneurones

Ole Kiehn

18.1. *Introduction*

Serotonin (5-hydroxytryptamine; 5-HT) was first discovered in the vertebrate brain by Twarog and Page (1953). Since then, and especially since the mapping of serotonergic neurones in the rat brain (Dahlström and Fuxe, 1964, 1965; Fuxe, 1965), it has become a major goal to understand the functional role of 5-HT in the central nervous system. It is now apparent that 5-HT influences several types of complex behaviour including sleeping, temperature regulation, memory and mental states. Simpler behaviours like motor function also appear to be regulated by serotonergic systems. Thus, very early it was shown that 5-HT precursors given intravenously (i.v.) could enhance reflex activity in spinal animals (Carlsson *et al.*, 1963; Andén *et al.*, 1964a,b; Lundberg, 1965) and more recent studies also show that injection of 5-HT agonists into intact rats cause a behavioural 'serotonin syndrome', consisting of a number of motor symptoms, including tremor, rigidity, Straub tail and hindlimb abduction (Jacobs, 1976). While those experiments clearly indicate that 5-HT affects motor behaviour, the site of serotonergic action is not so clear. Considering the extensive ramification of the serotonergic system in the vertebrate nervous system (Björklund and Skagerberg, 1982; Kuypers and Huisman, 1982; Holstege and Kuypers, 1987), the 5-HT effects can theoretically be mediated at many, and possibly all, levels of a motor network. The neuronal circuits underlying motor behaviour in most vertebrates are, however, only partly known or more commonly, unknown. This review therefore focuses on the modulatory effects of 5-HT on motoneurones, the final common pathway for motor behaviour.

This review is not intended to be encyclopaedic, but rather focuses on selected issues which may promote our understanding of 5-HT regulation of motoneurone output. More comprehensive reviews on 5-HT-induced changes in spinal reflex patterns, which may or may not be mediated by a direct effect on motoneurone properties, can be found (Lundberg, 1965, 1982; Baldissera *et al.*, 1981; Krnjevic, 1981; Commissiong, 1981; Anderson,

1983), as well as more detailed reviews on aspects of the effects of 5-HT on motoneurone firing (VanderMaelen, 1985; Aghajanian and VanderMaelen, 1986; Sigvardt, 1989). However, many of the results discussed here have not been reviewed before, especially those obtained with newly developed *in vitro* brain-stem or spinal cord preparations. Experiments with such preparations have allowed a detailed analysis of some of the postsynaptic changes induced by 5-HT. They have shown that 5-HT regulation of vertebrate motoneurone membrane properties is as intricate and diverse as in other brain areas in which *in vitro* preparations have been a prerequisite for studies of electrical membrane properties and transmitter regulation for many years (see Dingledine, 1984; Jahnsen, 1986; Llinás, 1988). Electrophysiological studies of neurones have shown that 5-HT can have both inhibitory and facilitatory (or excitatory) effects, even in the same cell (VanderMaelen, 1985; Aghajanian and VanderMaelen, 1986; Nicoll, 1988). This is also the case for the 5-HT-mediated effects on motoneurone excitability.

18.2. *5-HT enhances glutamate induced firing and produces a slow depolarization in motoneurones*

Extracellular studies of motoneurones have shown that iontophoretic application of 5-HT onto facial motoneurones in the anaesthetized rat (McCall and Aghajanian, 1979) and onto lumbar motoneurones in the anaesthetized rat and cat (White and Neuman 1980, 1983) facilitated glutamate-induced motoneurone firing, while 5-HT by itself seldom evoked spike activity. 5-HT also enhanced other excitatory inputs to the motoneurones (McCall and Aghajanian, 1979).

The membrane mechanisms responsible for the facilitatory 5-HT effect have been investigated in some detail by intracellular recording techniques *in vivo*. VanderMaelen and Aghajanian (1980, 1982a,b) found that iontophoretic application of 5-HT or i.v. injection of 5-HT agonists caused a slow depolarization in facial motoneurones (Figure 18.1A). The depolarization often remained below threshold for action potentials and the response was concentration-dependent (Figure 18.1A). The cell responded more vigorously to excitatory inputs after 5-HT than before (Figure 18.1C). In addition, the depolarization was accompanied by an apparent increase in neuronal input resistance (Figure 18.1B), which suggested that 5-HT mediated its effect through a conductance decrease. Thus, the effect of 5-HT on facial motoneurone membrane properties could be characterized as neuromodulatory (Kupfermann, 1979; Kaczmarek and Levitan, 1987; Harris-Warrick, 1988): the 5-HT-mediated depolarization is slow in onset, the change in membrane properties outlasts the presence of transmitter, and the transmitter action is often first seen when other synaptic inputs are simultaneously active.

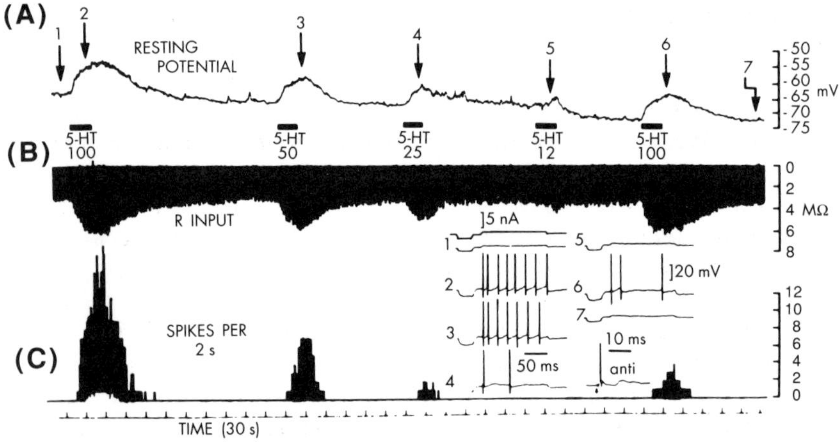

Figure 18.1. Response of a rat facial motoneurone to varying amounts of iontophoretically applied 5-HT, recorded intracellularly in an anaesthetized rat. (A), (B) and (C) are simultaneous chart recordings of resting membrane potential, neuronal input resistance and number of spikes, respectively. (A) Resting potential, with electrotonic displacements of membrane potential and spike potentials electronically removed. (B) Amplitude of voltage displacements in response to hyperpolarizing current pulses with the scale on the right adjusted by Ohm's law to give the input resistance in MΩ. (C) Output of a spike counter that was reset every 2 s. Most spikes that occurred were triggered by intracellular depolarizing current pulses. The bars below the intracellular trace in (A) indicate the duration and ejection currents (in nA) of iontophoretically applied 5-HT. 5-HT induced a slow membrane depolarization which was accompanied by an increase in excitability and an apparent increase in the input resistance. The inset shows individual oscilloscope traces taken at points indicated in (A). From VanderMaelen and Aghajanian, 1982b with permission.

Since the depolarization was not affected by intracellular chloride injection and it was reduced or abolished by hyperpolarizing the membrane potential to the vicinity of E_K, VanderMaelen and Aghajanian (1982a) suggested that 5-HT decreases the resting conductance to potassium ions. The inherent constraints in studying ionic membrane properties *in vivo*, did not allow a more rigourous examination of the 5-HT effect. However, this is now possible with the recent development of a thin slice preparation of the brain-stem containing viable facial motoneurones (Aghajanian and Rasmussen, 1989; Nishimura *et al.*, 1989; Larkman *et al.*, 1989). In this preparation bath application of 5-HT evokes a reversible depolarization associated with an apparent increase in input resistance measured in current-clamp (Aghajanian and Rasmussen, 1989; Larkman *et al.*, 1989) and an inward current and decrease in neuronal conductance measured in voltage-clamp (Aghajanian and Rasmussen, 1989). The 5-HT effect is probably direct since it persists in tetrodotoxin (TTX) (Larkman *et al.*, 1989). Ion-substitution or blockade of the 5-HT effect with potassium channel blockers was not attempted, and the 5-HT-regulated conductance or conductances on facial motoneurones still needs to be identified.

A 5-HT-evoked facilitation of motoneurones has also been observed in a variety of preparations using indirect measurements. 5-HT evokes depolarizing ventral root potentials in isolated hemisected neonatal rats (Komissarov and Abramets, 1980; Kitazawa *et al.*, 1985; Neuman, 1985; Connell and Wallis, 1987, 1988, 1989) and adult frog spinal cord (Tebecis and Phillis, 1967; Neuman, 1985; Holohean *et al.*, 1990). It also potentiates motoneurone field potentials in anaesthetized rats (Parry and Roberts, 1980; Roberts *et al.*, 1988) and 5-HT precursors given i.v. in spinal cats facilitate the monosynaptic reflex (Andén *et al.*, 1964a,b; Anderson and Shibuya, 1966; Banna and Anderson, 1968; Myslinski and Anderson, 1978). The depolarizing effect of 5-HT persists in TTX (Neuman, 1985; Connell and Wallis, 1987) or low Ca^{2+}/high Mg^{2+} Ringer (Komissarov and Abramets, 1980; Neuman, 1985), indicating that 5-HT mediates its excitatory effect via a direct action on motoneurone membrane properties (see, however, Holohean *et al.*, 1990). Whether these effects are caused by an ionic mechanism similar to the one described in facial motoneurones will have to await intracellular studies.

5-HT has also recently been shown to enhance motoneurone firing by induction of plateau properties in cat and turtle spinal motoneurones, to influence lamprey swimming by a decrease in the size of the spike afterhyperpolarization (AHP) and to enhance specific currents in neonatal rat motoneurones. These effects will be described separately in the next three sections.

18.3. *Serotonergic regulation of plateau properties in vertebrate motoneurones*

Plateau potentials are intrinsic properties of neurones (Hartline *et al.*, 1988; Llinás, 1988) and are expressed as prolonged endogenously maintained depolarized states. Transient depolarizations, e.g. a short barrage of excitatory postsynaptic potentials (EPSPs), can initiate the plateau potential which may remain for long periods before it either terminates spontaneously or is actively turned off by a brief inhibition. The plateau potential therefore allows the cell to possess two stable states of activity: one around rest and a second at a more depolarized level. This property of two levels of excitability is referred to as a *bistable behaviour*.

In an extensive series of experiments from our laboratory we have shown that plateau potential capabilities are spontaneously present in motoneurones of decerebrate unanaesthetized cats (Crone *et al.*, 1988; Hounsgaard *et al.*, 1984, 1986, 1988b; Kiehn, 1990). The bistable behaviour is illustrated in Figure 18.2. The motoneurone was shifted between two stable firing states by short-lasting synaptic excitation and inhibition (Figure

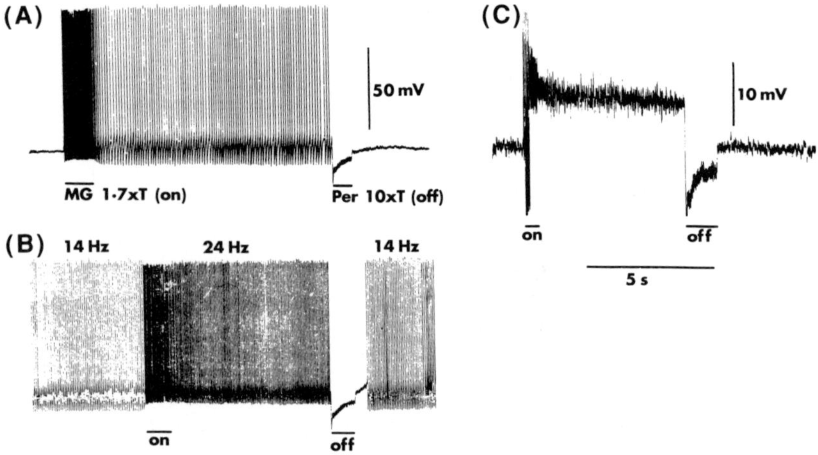

Figure 18.2. Bistable firing behaviour and plateau potentials in motoneurones. (A)–(C) Intracellular recordings from lateral gastrocnemius-soleus (LG-sol) motoneurones in unanaethetized decerebrate cats. (A) Brief synaptic excitation from the medial gastrocnemius (MG) nerve (indicated by the bar below the intracellular record; on, 1·7 × threshold, 300 Hz) initiates sustained firing in the LG-sol neurone, which is terminated by a brief synaptic inhibition from the peroneal nerve (off, 10 × threshold, 200 Hz). (B) When the cell is firing at a slow tonic rate identical inputs shift the motoneurone between two stable states of firing frequency. (C) In a different cell the spike initiating mechanism was inactivated by excessive prolonged depolarization. Brief synaptic excitation (on, MG 2 × threshold, 300 Hz) and inhibition (off, Per 10 × threshold, 200 Hz) now initiates and terminates a prolonged depolarizing plateau potential.
After Hounsgaard *et al.*, 1988b.

18.2A,B). The underlying plateau was revealed by inactivating the spike generating mechanism (Figure 18.2C). A bistable firing pattern could also be initiated and terminated by short-lasting depolarizing and hyperpolarizing current pulses injected into the motoneurones.

The ability to generate plateau potentials in motoneurones is a conditional rather than an endogenous property. We found that bistable behaviour in the decerebrate cat was dependent on activity in serotonergic and noradrenergic fibres (Hounsgaard *et al.*, 1986, 1988b; Conway *et al.*, 1988) descending from nuclei in the brain-stem (Björklund and Skagerberg, 1982; Kuypers and Huisman, 1982; Holstege and Kuypers, 1987). Motoneurones located below an acute spinal transection were not able to generate plateau potentials unless high doses of serotonergic (5-HTP) or noradrenergic (L-DOPA) precursors were given i.v. Studies in a newly developed *in vitro* preparation of the turtle spinal cord (Hounsgaard and Kiehn, 1985; Hounsgaard *et al.*, 1988a) confirmed these findings and showed that bath-applied 5-HT induced plateau properties in motoneurones (Figure 18.3A–E; Hounsgaard and Kiehn, 1985, 1989). The plateau activates slowly. This causes an accelerated firing rate during the current pulse (Figure 18.3B–E) which is opposite to the time-dependent adaptation so well known from previous

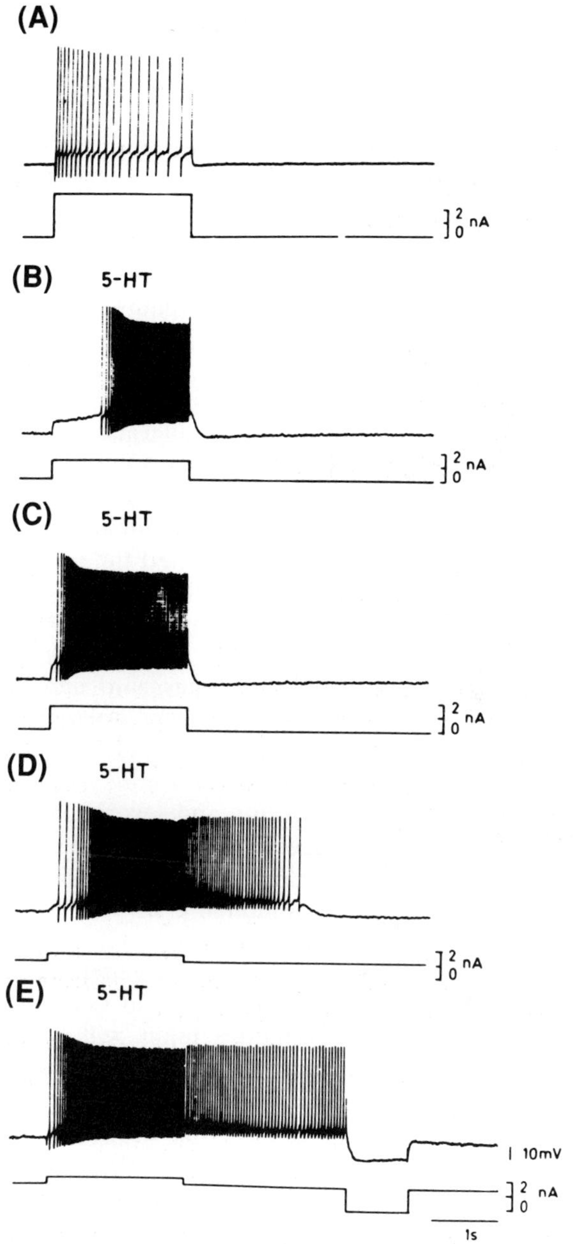

Figure 18.3. 5-HT-induced changes in response properties of turtle motoneurones *in vitro*. (A) Adaptation of rhythmic firing (upper trace) in normal medium in response to current injection (lower trace). (B),(C) Accelerated firing evoked from resting potential in 5-HT containing medium. Note low threshold and the late onset of firing in (B) and the shift in onset in (C) in response to a higher amplitude. (D) When the cell was depolarized by a steady holding current the current pulse also evoked an after-discharge following termination of the pulse. From a more depolarized level (E) a bistable firing was initiated and terminated by short-lasting depolarizing and hyperpolarizing current pulses, respectively. This firing behaviour reflects the activation of the underlying plateau potential.
From Hounsgaard and Kiehn, 1985, with permission from Springer-Verlag, Heidelberg©.

motoneurone studies (Figure 18.3A; Kernell, 1965; Kernell and Monster, 1982).

Plateau potentials have been studied in various cells from both vertebrates and invertebrates (Hartline *et al.*, 1988; Llinás, 1988). Generation of the plateau potential involves a negative slope region in the steady-state current–voltage (I–V) relationship, produced by a slowly- or non-inactivating inward current mechanism. If the plateau is conditional and not endogenous, induction of the plateau would require a change in the balance between outward and inward currents. Schwindt and Crill (1977) found that 40% of spinal motoneurones in the intact anaesthetized cat possess a region of negative slope and a net inward current in their I–V relation. However, a bistable behaviour was mainly seen after pharmacological reduction of outward currents and/or enhancement of inward currents (Schwindt and Crill 1977, 1980, 1984). Schwindt and Crill (1980) described a persistent inward current, I_i, as responsible for the plateau potential and suggested that I_i was mediated by Ca^{2+} ions. We have investigated the ionic basis for serotonin-dependent bistable behaviour in the turtle spinal cord and found that the plateau potentials are Ca^{2+}-dependent (Figure 18.4A,B), and most probably mediated at least in part by an L-like Ca^{2+} channel since the plateau capability is blocked by nifedipine (Hounsgaard and Kiehn, 1985, 1989). 5-HT reduces the size of the slow after-hyperpolarization (s-AHP; Figure 18.4C), which is mediated by a calcium-dependent potassium current. This current is blocked by apamin (Hounsgaard *et al.*, 1988a), and Hounsgaard and Mintz (1988) showed that apamin and several other potassium channel blockers can, like 5-HT, induce nifidepine-sensitive plateau potentials in turtle motoneurones. 5-HT might therefore induce bistable behaviour by removal of an outward current, although a direct simultaneous activation of the plateau current is also possible.

Since the size of the AHP is a major factor in determining spike frequency and adaptation (Kernell, 1965; Baldissera and Gustafsson, 1974; Madison and Nicoll, 1982), a given excitatory input will cause a stronger spike response after 5-HT than before, even if the stimulus is below the threshold for triggering a plateau potential. The input–output relation of the cell is altered by 5-HT, as seen by plotting the instantaneous frequency versus current (f–I) relation for the first three interspike intervals and steady state (after 2 s) before and after 5-HT (Figure 18.4D). The f–I slopes increase after 5-HT, i.e. the gain in the conversion from synaptic input to spike-coded output increases. A similar change in input–output gain was seen in spinal cat motoneurones after i.v. 5-HTP (Hounsgaard *et al.*, 1988b). The induction of plateau potentials in cat motoneurones may therefore be explained by a reduction in the size of the AHP, although it was not investigated systematically. In fact, White and Fung (1989) have found that 5-HT applied iontophoretically onto lumbar motoneurones in unanaesthetized decerebrate cats, reduced the size of the post-spike AHP. The authors do not mention however, whether 5-HT induced plateau properties

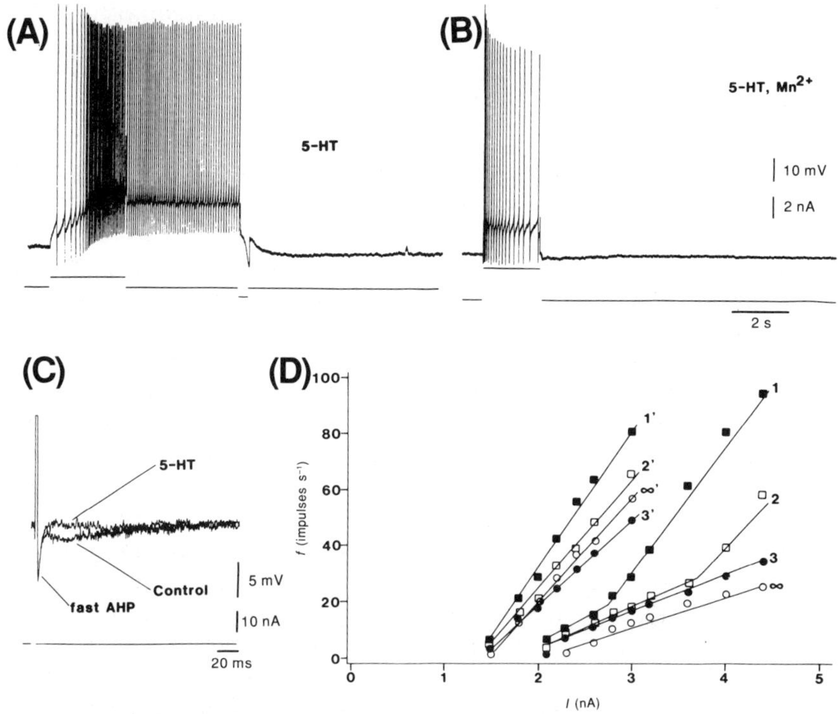

Figure 18.4. Ionic mechanism for the plateau properties in turtle motoneurones. (A),(B) 5-HT plateau properties (A) blocked after replacing the extracellular calcium with manganese (B; Mn^{2+}). (C) Superimposed sweeps of action potentials evoked by short (1 ms) intracellular current pulses showing that the s-AHP was reduced by 5-HT. (D) *f–I* relation in normal medium for the first three interspike intervals (1,2,3) and steady state (∞) and for the same intervals (1′,2′,3′ and ∞′) after 5-HT.
After Hounsgaard & Kiehn, 1989.

when iontophoretically applied under those circumstances. The mode of administration as well as the actual concentration of 5-HT could, however, be important for the ability of 5-HT to induce plateau properties. The fact that the postsynaptic effect of 5-HT can be concentration-dependent has been noted in other experiments (see below).

Normally, I_i is curtailed by outward currents, so self-sustained firing is rarely seen in normal motoneurones (Schwindt and Crill, 1984), explaining why plateau properties have been long overlooked. An additional explanation might be that bistable behaviour is depressed by babiturates (Hounsgaard *et al.*, 1986), which have been used extensively in *in vivo* studies of motoneurones.

These experiments demonstrate that 5-HT (and noradrenaline) can induce a very complex response pattern in motoneurones. The plateau properties give motoneurones a substantial computational power, and we suggest that motoneurones are not only acting as passive followers on the output side of the spinal cord, but can actively interpret their synaptic input in a non-linear way. It is likely that the plateau properties are behaviourally relevant and may account for the sharp discontinuities in motor neurone firing frequency seen in electromyographic recordings from intact rats during quiet standing (Eken and Kiehn, 1989). A plateau mechanism in the output stage will thus reduce the need for ongoing synaptic drive to the motoneurone pool, and the serotonergic and noradrenergic systems will play an import role in defining the final motor output. A more comprehensive discussion of the possible functional significance of plateau potentials in motor behaviour can be found in Kiehn (1991).

18.4. *5-HT modulates locomotor activity in the lamprey spinal cord by affecting a calcium-dependent potassium conductance*

The brain-stem and spinal cord of the lamprey, a fish-like vertebrate, can be isolated and maintained *in vitro* (see Rovanian, 1979; Grillner *et al.*, 1987). The *in vitro* preparation has allowed a detailed analysis of the neuronal circuitry underlying locomotor activity, and a network model for generating the basic locomotor rhythm has been proposed (Grillner *et al.*, 1987, 1988). Some of the properties of individual neurones and transmitters involved in the system have also been described. Even though the rhythmic motor pattern, corresponding to alternating swimming movements in the intact animal, is mimicked in the isolated spinal cord, the efferent motor pattern can be strongly modulated by several inputs. One of these modulatory inputs originates from central serotonergic terminals which are abundant in the lamprey spinal cord. In addition to a descending fibre system (Harris-Warrick *et al.*, 1985; Brodin *et al.*, 1986) contributing to the serotonergic innervation of the lateral and ventral spinal cord, there is an afferent system with cell bodies in the spinal ganglia. Unlike most other vertebrates there is also a well-developed intrinsic spinal 5-HT system composed of small interneurones located ventrally to the central canal (Harris-Warrick *et al.*, 1985; Van Dongen *et al.*, 1985b). The dendrites of these neurones form a very dense ventromedial plexus, within which identified motoneurones and premotor interneurones have their dendrites (Van Dongen *et al.*, 1985a).

When 5-HT is bath-applied during excitatory amino acid-induced fictive locomotion, the burst pattern is markedly influenced (Harris-Warrick and Cohen, 1985). The frequency of rhythmic ventral root discharge is reduced, the intersegmental phase lag is prolonged and both intensity and duration of burst discharges is increased (Figure 18.5A,B). Similar effects on the burst pattern have been seen after blocking the 5-HT uptake system (Christenson *et al.*, 1989) suggesting that 5-HT is released and acts on neurones in the neuronal network underlying locomotion.

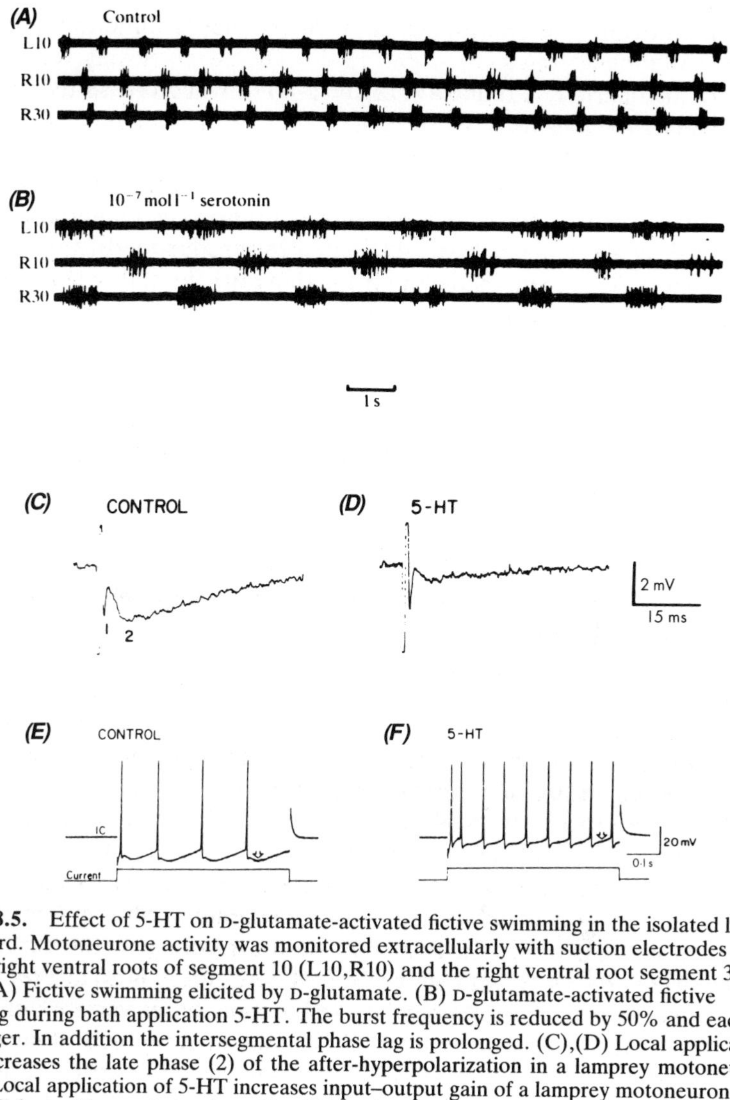

Figure 18.5. Effect of 5-HT on D-glutamate-activated fictive swimming in the isolated lamprey spinal cord. Motoneurone activity was monitored extracellularly with suction electrodes on the left and right ventral roots of segment 10 (L10,R10) and the right ventral root segment 30 (R30). (A) Fictive swimming elicited by D-glutamate. (B) D-glutamate-activated fictive swimming during bath application 5-HT. The burst frequency is reduced by 50% and each burst lasts longer. In addition the intersegmental phase lag is prolonged. (C),(D) Local application of 5-HT decreases the late phase (2) of the after-hyperpolarization in a lamprey motoneurone. (E),(F) Local application of 5-HT increases input–output gain of a lamprey motoneurone. (A),(B) Taken with permission from Harris-Warrick and Cohen, 1985, Company of Biologist LTD©. (C)–(F) Taken with permission from Wallén *et al.*, 1989a.

Some of the modulatory effects of 5-HT on the ongoing rhythmic activity can be attributed to its effect on a particular ionic conductance. 5-HT applied locally outside motoneurones depresses the duration and amplitude of the s-AHP following an action potential (Figure 18.5C,D; Van Dongen *et al.*, 1986; Wallén *et al.*, 1989a,b). Interestingly, 5-HT did not induce a bistable firing behaviour in lamprey motoneurones. Thus, although 5-HT regulates the same conductance in turtle and lamprey motoneurones, the cell's total sum of conductances may determine the functional outcome of the modulation.

As described earlier, a reduction of the s-AHP will increase the neuronal input–output gain (Figure 18.5E,F), so when 5-HT is added to the bath during excitatory amino acid-induced swimming, it will cause a more intense ventral root discharge and a higher discharge frequency of active motoneurones. However, the increased burst duration and decreased swim rate induced by 5-HT is not easily explained by a reduction of the s-AHP in motoneurones. A possible explanation for these effects is that the s-AHP of interneurones in the network controlling locomotion is also depressed by 5-HT (Wallén *et al.*, 1989a,b). In computer simulation experiments of the activity of the interneuronal network, a reduction of the s-AHP of interneurones led to slowing of the burst rate in a manner similar to that observed behaviourally during fictive swimming (Grillner *et al.*, 1988). This led Wallén *et al.* (1989a,b) to conclude that the action of 5-HT on the AHP accounts for the influence of 5-HT on locomotor activity. This conclusion may be premature for the following reasons: first, results from the model seem to be based on the assumption that 5-HT reduces the size of the AHP in excitatory interneurones while the experimental data only give evidence for an effect on inhibitory and unidentified interneurones (Wallén *et al.*, 1989a,b); secondly, the neuronal network underlying locomotion and the membrane properties of the individual neurones may be more complex than in the model; finally, results from other systems (Kaczmarek and Levitan, 1987; Harris-Warrick, 1988; Nicoll, 1988; Bobker and Williams, 1990) indicate that 5-HT has multiple effects on neurones and their connections. In fact, 5-HT has already been shown to depress the excitatory amino acid EPSPs evoked in lamprey motoneurones and certain premotor neurones from large reticulospinal neurones (Buchanan and Grillner, 1987).

Despite these comments, the work on 5-HT systems in the lamprey provides a good example of how we can start to understand regulatory changes of motor behaviour in vertebrates at the cellular level. It also demonstrates how modulatory systems can increase versatility in the spinal motor system and can create a basis for the changing requirements opposed from the exterior. Further experiments are needed to clarify the normal mode of activation and the interaction between the different 5-HT systems in the lamprey.

Locomotion has also been shown to be modulated by serotonin in other species. 5-HTP modulates efferent discharge in rabbits (Viala and Buser, 1969, 1971) and 5-HTP and 5-HT antagonists enhance locomotor pattern in chronic spinal cats by an increase in the step length and an augmentation in the electromyograph (EMG) amplitude (Barbeau and Rossignol, 1990). In an *in vitro* preparation of the spinal cord of the neonatal rat, 5-HT induces a slow rhythmic activity of left and right alternating ventral root bursts (Cazalets *et al.*, 1990). Characteristically, in these preparations 5-HT had a different effect on the locomotor pattern from that of noradrenaline, supporting a view that each system mediates its modulatory effect by specific neurochemical mechanisms and by acting on different subpopulations of cells.

18.5. *5-HT modulation of an inward rectifier and a low-voltage-activated calcium current in neonatal rat motoneurones*

The electrophysiology of motoneurones has recently been analysed in thin slices from the neonatal rat spinal cord (Takahashi, 1990a,b), using a newly developed technique which allows patch-clamp recordings from neurones in the mammalian brain (Edwards *et al.*, 1989). In addition to describing some of the basic properties of the ionic conductances present in those neurones, Takahashi and Berger (1990) found that 5-HT causes a marked depolarization when bath-applied (Figure 18.6A). The depolarization exceeded firing threshold and could last for minutes after wash-out of 5-HT. When measured in voltage-clamp, 5-HT caused an inward current, $I_{5\text{-HT}}$, which was accompanied by an increase in the conductance in the hyperpolarizing direction (Figure 18.6B). $I_{5\text{-HT}}$ was not blocked by various K^+-channel blockers or low extracellular Ca^{2+}. However, $I_{5\text{-HT}}$ was blocked by Cs^+ (Figure 18.6C, left) and displayed inward rectification. The current generated by 5-HT thus displayed characteristics similar to the intrinsic inward rectifying current in motoneurones (Figure 18.6D; Takahashi, 1990a). This current is a mixed K^+/Na^+-current activated by membrane hyperpolarization. The authors therefore conclude that the 5-HT excitation is mediated by activation of the intrinsic inward rectifier. This is interesting because the inward rectifier has been known to exist in motoneurones for a long time (Ito and Oshima, 1965; Nelson and Frank, 1967), but little has been known about its function. 5-HT augmentation of inward rectifying currents has also been found in guinea-pig thalamus neurones (Pape and McCormick, 1989), rat prepositus hypoglossi neurones (Bobker and Williams, 1989) and in identified motoneurones in *Aplysia* (Kirk *et al.*, 1988; Taussig *et al.*, 1989), and in the crab, *Cancer borealis* (O. Kiehn and R.M. Harris-Warrick, unpublished observations).

Enhancement of an inward rectifier is not the only effect of 5-HT on neonatal motoneurones. In normal calcium-containing medium, 5-HT, in addition to depolarizing the motoneurones (activation of the inward rectifying current), also enhances a transient low-voltage-activated (LVA; see Llinás, 1988) calcium current (Berger and Takahashi, 1990). Interestingly, the inward rectifying current is enhanced by submicromolar concentrations of 5-HT, while the LVA calcium current was only enhanced at concentrations above 10 μM, and it is suggested that different types of 5-HT receptors mediate these effects. The initial 5-HT-induced hyperpolarization seen in

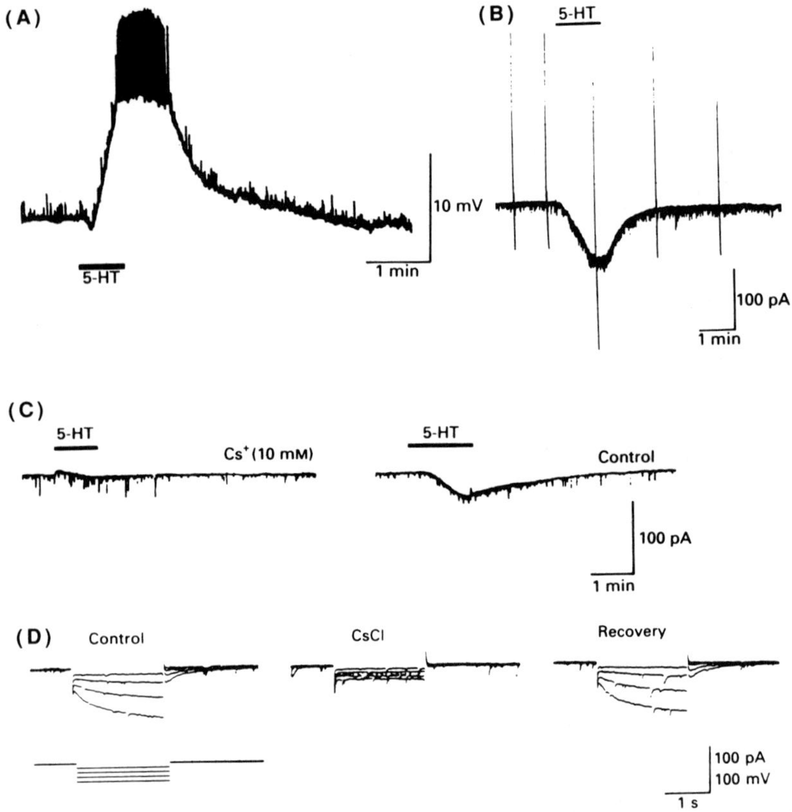

Figure 18.6. Effect of 5-HT applied to motoneurone in a slice preparation of the neonatal spinal cord. (A) The 5-HT response in current-clamp mode in Ca^{2+}-free-Mg^{2+} Krebs' solution. 5-HT was applied during the period indicated by the horizontal bar. Note the initial hyperpolarization. (B) In voltage-clamp mode 5-HT application caused an inward current, which was accompanied by an increase in input conductance as indicated by the size of the downward deflections of the voltage steps (tetrodotoxin added to the medium). (C) Responses of motoneurone to 5-HT in the presence of Cs^+ (left) and to a second application after 9 min wash-out of Cs^+ (right). (D) Time- and voltage-dependent inward rectification evoked in a neonatal spinal motoneurone by hyperpolarizing command pulses. All records show voltage-clamp data from the same cell. Upper traces illustrate superimposed current traces in control (left, standard Krebs' solution), when CsCl (2 mM) was added in substitution for $CaCl_2$ (middle) and recovery after wash-out of Cs^+ (right). The voltage steps are indicated below the control. (A)–(C) Taken with permission from Takahashi and Berger, 1990. (D) Taken with permission from Takahashi, 1990a.

Figure 18.6A is also indicative of multiple 5-HT receptors on neonatal motoneurones (see below).

While the functional outcome of enhancing the inward rectifier by 5-HT is obvious, the functional significance of enhancing the LVA Ca^{2+} current is not so clear. LVA calcium spikes have been attributed a role in generating low frequency oscillations in central neurones (Jahnsen and Llinás, 1984;

Llinás, 1988) and Berger and Takahashi (1990) suggest that 5-HT may physiologically facilitate such behaviour in neonatal motoneurones. In fact, L-DOPA and clonidine can induce low frequency oscillations in motoneurones in the acute spinal cat (Conway *et al.*, 1988). Although such oscillatory behaviour has been described in neonatal rat motoneurones *in vitro* (Walton and Llinás, 1986), its functional role is still obscure.

The studies of neonatal motoneurones emphasize the point made in the previous section that 5-HT can be expected to have multiple effects in the vertebrate motor system. This is already supported by results of experiments on invertebrate motoneurones where the facilitatory effect of 5-HT is caused by modulation of several different conductances in the same cell (Kirk *et al.*, 1988; Taussig *et al.*, 1989; Kiehn and Harris-Warrick, 1990).

18.6. *Inhibitory effects of 5-HT*

Despite the substantial evidence that 5-HT facilitates motoneurone excitability, several investigators have found inhibitory effects of 5-HT. 5-HT-mediated hyperpolarization and decreased excitability were described in an early intracellular *in vivo* study on cat spinal motoneurones (Phillis *et al.*, 1968). Similar effects have also been seen in more recent studies (Engberg *et al.*, 1976; Zhang and Krnjevic, 1986, 1989). There are, however, differences between the studies. The hyperpolarization found by Engberg *et al.* (1976) was short-lived and accompanied by an increase in input resistance. In contrast, Zhang and Krnjevic (1989), found that 5-HT induced a long-lasting hyperpolarization (up to 60 min) without a change in input resistance, and the authors suggested that the hyperpolarization was due to activation of an electrogenic Na–K pump.

Inhibition of motoneurone excitability by 5-HT has also been demonstrated in the isolated frog spinal cord (Caulford and Coceani, 1977; Holohean *et al.*, 1990) and rat spinal cord (Komissarov and Abramets, 1980). Interestingly, a low concentration of 5-HT causes hyperpolarization in the frog spinal cord while a high concentration of 5-HT causes depolarization (Holohean *et al.*, 1990). The exact reverse concentration profile was seen in rat spinal cord (Komissarov and Abramets, 1980). Other investigators have found that 5-HT only infrequently depresses motoneurone excitability and that the effect, when present, was transient and preceded a much more pronounced excitatory component (White and Neuman, 1980, 1983; VanderMaelen and Aghajanian, 1982b; White and Fung, 1989; Wallén *et al.*, 1989a; Rasmussen and Aghajanian, 1990; Takahashi and Berger, 1990).

Thus, 5-HT has multiple (inhibitory and facilitatory) effects on motoneurones which can be expressed at different transmitter concentrations. As we shall see in the next section, the inhibitory and facilitatory effects seem to be mediated through different 5-HT receptors.

18.7. *Receptor profile for the 5-HT effects*

The classification of Bradley *et al.* (1986) designated three major classes of 5-HT receptors called 5-HT_1-like, 5-HT_2 and 5-HT_3. These three major classes have been further subdivided, and it has now been possible to assign many (pre- and) postsynaptic 5-HT effects to specific 5-HT receptor subtypes (Peroutka, 1988; Schmidt and Peroutka, 1989; Bobker and Williams, 1990). Binding studies have indicated the presence of 5-HT_{1A}, 5-HT_{1B}, 5-HT_{1C} and 5-HT_2 sites in the mammalian spinal cord (Pazos and Palacios, 1985; Pazos *et al.*, 1985; Huang and Peroutka, 1987), and the diverse actions of 5-HT on spinal motoneurones could result from activation of various classes of 5-HT receptors.

Table 18.1 provides a summary of some of the 5-HT antagonists and agonists which have been used to either block or mimic 5-HT-mediated effects on vertebrate motoneurones. Many of the experiments were carried out before the 5-HT receptor classification was established and only in a few studies have the experimenters used an extensive battery of drugs to determine the receptor subtype for the 5-HT effect.

The results on facial motoneurones indicate a role for 5-HT_2 and/or 5-HT_{1C}, but not 5-HT_{1A} receptors in the serotonergic enhancement of excitability, since the effect of 5-HT was: (1) mimicked by the selective 5-HT_2/5-HT_{1C} agonist DOM; (2) mimicked by the broad spectrum 5-HT_1 agonist 5-CT, but not the selective 5-HT_{1A} agonist, 8-OH-DPAT; and (3) blocked by the 5-HT_2/5-HT_{1C} antagonists, ritanserin, ketanserin, metergoline, methysergide, cyproheptadine and cinanserin (for references see footnotes 15–20 in Table 8.1). Based on their study, Holohean *et al.* (1990) also concluded that the 5-HT-mediated depolarization in the frog spinal cord is mediated through a 5-HT_2/5-HT_{1C} receptor.

In contrast to these findings, Roberts *et al.* (1988) concluded that 5-HT depolarizes motoneurones in the intact rat by activation of a 5-HT_1-like receptor, different from the 5-HT_{1A} receptor since the effect of 5-HT was: (1) mimicked by 5-CT, but not by 8-OH-DPAT; and (2) blocked by methysergide, but not by ketanserin and unaffected by the specific 5-HT_3 receptor antagonist, MDL-72222. Connell and Wallis (1988, 1989) concluded that the 5-HT-induced depolarization seen in neonatal rat motoneurones could not be equated to an identified binding site, although they excluded the 5-HT_3 receptor site by use of specific 5-HT_3 receptor antagonists (MDL-72222, ICS 205–930) and agonists (2-Me-5-HT). It is noteworthy that, while Connell and Wallis (1989) found no effect of 8-OH-DPAT, Takahashi and Berger (1990) found that 8-OH-DPAT mimicked the 5-HT effect on the inward rectifier, also in neonatal motoneurones.

Whether the apparent differences in receptor profiles for the facilitatory effects reflect species differences, age differences (adult/neonatal) or differences in drug administration is still uncertain. Another possibility is that the discrepancies are because 5-HT-induced facilitation is mediated through

Table 18.1 Pharmacology of 5-HT effects on vertebrate motoneurones.

	Facilitatory		Inhibitory	
α-Me-5-HT	agonist	10,13[a]		
5-CT	agonist	2,10,20		
5-MeOT	agonist	10		
8-OH-DPAT	– agonist	2,10,11,13,20		
	agonist	22	agonist	7,11,13
Spiroxatrine	– antagonist	13	antagonist	13
Ipsapirone	– agonist	13	agonist	13
RU 24969	– agonist	10,11		
Cyanopindolol	– antagonist	2,11		
Spiperone	antagonist	11,22	antagonist	13
	– antagonist	13		
Methiothepin	– antagonist	10,17		
Mesulergine	antagonist	11		
Methysergide	antagonist	1,2,3,4,6,8,9,10,13, 15,16,18,17,19,21	– antagonist	6,13
	– antagonist	12,14		
Metergoline	antagonist	5,6,11,17	– antagonist	6
Mianserin	antagonist	13	– antagonist	13
DOM	agonist	19,20		
Ketanserin	antagonist	10,13,19	– antagonist	13
	– antagonist	2		
Ritanserin	antagonist	20		
	– antagonist	9,11		
Cinanserin	antagonist	1,3,4,17		
	– antagonist	14		
Cyproheptadine	antagonist	3,11,17		
2-Me-5-HT	– agonist	10,13		
MDL 72222	– antagonist	2,10,13	– antagonist	13
ICS 205–930	– antagonist	9,10		

[a] Numbers in table: (1) Barasi and Roberts, 1974; (2) Roberts *et al.*, 1988 (rat spinal-MN *in vivo*); (3) Banna and Anderson, 1968; (4) Myslinski and Anderson, 1978 (cat spinal-MN *in vivo*); (5),(6) White and Neuman, 1980, 1983; (7) Jackson and White, 1989 (rat and cat spinal-MN *in vivo*); (8) Crone *et al.*, 1988; (9) Hounsgaard and Kiehn, 1989 (cat spinal-MN *in vivo* and turtle spinal-MN *in vitro*); (10),(11) Connell and Wallis, 1988, 1989 (neonatal rat spinal-MN *in vitro*) (12) Tebecis and Phillis, 1967; (13) Holohean *et al.*, 1990 (adult frog spinal-MN *in vitro*) (14) Wallén *et al.*, 1989 (lamprey spinal-MN *in vitro*); (15) VanderMaelen and Aghajanian, 1980; (16),(17) McCall and Aghajanian, 1979, 1980; (18) VanderMaelen and Aghajanian, 1982; (19) Penington and Reiffenstein, 1986; (20) Rasmussen and Aghajanian, 1990 (rat facial-MN *in vivo* and *in vitro*): (21) Kommissarov and Abramets. 1980; (22) Takahashi and Berger, 1990 (neonatal rat spinal-MN *in vitro*).
MN, motoneurones;–, no agonist or antagonist effect.

several mechanisms (enhancement of inward rectifier, blockage of s-AHP, enhancement of calcium-current, etc.) each coupled to a separate receptor.

The receptor profile for the inhibitory effect is clearer, at least in the frog where it has been assigned to a receptor (5-HT_{1A}) different from the receptor(s) mediating the facilitatory effect (see Table 18.1).

In conclusion: vertebrate motoneurones contain distinct 5-HT receptors which mediate the various facilitatory and inhibitory effects of 5-HT. As more details of the electrophysiological 5-HT effects on motoneurones are revealed, it is likely that 5-HT facilitation will be coupled to distinct multiple subtypes of the 5-HT receptor.

18.8. *Second messenger systems*

In a variety of neurones the effects of 5-HT are mediated by intracellular messengers (Kaczmarek and Levitan, 1987; Nicoll, 1988; Bobker and Williams, 1990; Frazer *et al.*, 1990). The prolonged effects of 5-HT, and their slow onset in motoneurones, suggest intracellular messenger systems are involved. So far only a few studies have addressed this issue.

Wallén *et al.* (1989a) found no evidence for an involvement of cAMP, cGMP, diacylglycerol, arachidonic acid or a pertussis toxin-sensitive G-protein in the 5-HT-induced reduction of s-AHP in lamprey neurones. Similarly we found no evidence that the bistability in turtle motoneurones was mediated by cAMP, cGMP or protein kinase C (O. Kiehn and J. Hounsgaard, unpublished). In contrast to these negative findings, cAMP, cGMP and protein kinase C *increase* the size of the AHP in motoneurones in anaesthetized cats (Krnjevic and Van Meter, 1976; Zhang and Krnjevic, 1987a) while GTPγs mimics a carbachol-induced depolarization and depression of the AHP in those neurones (Zhang and Krnjevic, 1987b). The prolonged hyperpolarizing effect of 5-HT, which the same authors found in cat lumbar motoneurones, was mimicked by inositol triphosphate (IP_3) (Zhang and Krnjevic 1986, 1989).

Thus, at the moment the 5-HT facilitation has not been mimicked by a known second messenger system, while one study has demonstrated a hyperpolarizing effect of IP_3. Further studies are necessary to supplement the picture. It appears likely that the 5-HT-induced reduction of the s-AHP results from a direct action on the calcium-dependent potassium channel (similar to the 5-HT_3-mediated effect in enteric and cultured hippocampus neurones; Bobker and Williams, 1990), while other effects of 5-HT on vertebrate motoneurones may be mediated by specific, as yet undetermined, intracellular messenger systems. Some correlations between 5-HT receptor subtypes, electrophysiological effects, and use of intracellular messenger systems have been noted (Bobker and Williams, 1990; Frazer *et al.*, 1990). This information may be useful when searching for the second messengers signalling the 5-HT effect on motoneurones.

18.9. *Endogenous release of 5-HT from serotonergic neurones*

The 5-HT-mediated changes in motoneurone properties described so far were obtained after i.v. administration of 5-HT receptor activators or after direct iontophoresis or bath application of 5-HT. Although these methods of administration can give important information on changes in motoneuronal membrane properties, they are unlikely to mimic the spatial and temporal components of actual release. For example, local transmitter application by iontophoresis will mainly affect motoneurone somata and proximal dendrites, and not more distal dendrites which, like the former regions, are heavily innervated by serotonergic terminals (Kojima and Sano, 1983). Measurements of the time courses for induction and maintenance of the transmitter effects in relation to transmitter release for a given eletrophysiological change are also important for evaluating its possible behavioural relevance. In the case of the 5-HT-mediated effects on motoneurone membrane properties it will therefore be desirable to selectively activate the serotonergic neurones which project to motoneurones, and ultimately correlate their natural firing pattern in behaving animals with changes in motoneurone behaviour, like plateau properties, which are known to be 5-HT mediated.

Serotonergic projections to the medulla and spinal cord of higher vertebrates originate from discrete serotonergic cell groups located in the brain-stem. The ventral horn is innervated from nucleus raphe obscurus and nucleus raphe pallidus in the lower brain-stem, as originally described by Dahlström and Fuxe (1964, 1965) using a fluorescence technique, and confirmed in a substantial body of later studies using more modern anatomical techniques (for reviews see Björklund and Skagerberg, 1982; Kuypers and Huisman, 1982; Anderson, 1983; VanderMaelen, 1985; Holstege and Kuypers, 1987). Since the main innervation of motoneurones and premotoneurone interneurones in the ventral horn in higher vertebrates originates from the brain-stem, a selective activation of the serotonergic neurones in the raphe nuclei should mimic the direct effect imposed by the serotonergic system on the spinal motor system. So far surprisingly few studies have addressed that issue.

Anderson and co-workers (Clineschmidt and Anderson, 1970; Proudfit and Anderson, 1973, 1974) were the first to study the effect of raphe stimulation on motoneurone excitability in decerebrate cats. They found that stimulation of the raphe magnus caused a depression of spinal reflex activity, which was counteracted by serotonergic antagonists. In contrast, Barasi and Roberts (1974) found that raphe medianus stimulation in anaesthetized intact rats caused an increase in the monosynaptic reflex. The interpretation of these results is difficult since neither raphe magnus nor raphe medianus have direct projections to motoneurones.

Two more recent studies in rats (Roberts *et al.*, 1988) and in cats (Fung and Barnes, 1989) have, however, described raphe-produced excitation of motoneurones after stimulation of nucleus raphe obscurus or nucleus raphe pallidus. In the rat, long-lasting low frequency trains of stimuli given in nucleus raphe obscurus increased motoneurone excitability by a slowly, developing depolarization (Roberts *et al.*, 1988). This effect was blocked by methysergide, indicating that it was mediated through serotonergic receptors. A somewhat different effect was found in cat motoneurones (Fung and

Barnes, 1989). Stimulation in nucleus raphe pallidus produced a short latency (7–11 ms) EPSP, which caused an overall increase of motoneurone excitability. Serotonergic blockers were not used in these experiments, and one has to be cautious in interpreting the results. From the rat it is known that 5-HT axons are unmyelinated and thin (Dahlström and Fuxe, 1964), probably with low conduction velocities in the range of 1–2 $m\,s^{-1}$. If this is the case in the cat, the short-latency EPSP cannot be a result of serotonergic raphe activity. This comment addresses the well-known problem in getting a selective activation of serotonergic neurones (or other anatomically well-defined groups of neurones) when using electrical stimulation. Due to current spread, nearby neurones (in this case non-serotonergic neurones) will be activated in addition to fibres, which are just passing the nuclei. Additionally, non-serotonergic neurones are scattered within the raphe nuclei themselves (cf. Anderson, 1983).

The fact that 5-HT coexists with TRH, substance P and possibly other peptides or classical transmitters in the raphe neurones (Hökfelt, 1987) further complicates stimulation experiments, but is also a reason to perform them. The co-transmitters are expected to be released with 5-HT and affect either pre- or postsynaptic elements when the serotonergic cells are activated. Thus the combined actions of multiple transmitters may be more complex than the 5-HT action alone, and obviously are more in line with reality. This point has been illustrated by experiments carried out in the stomatogastric ganglion (STG) of crustacea. A group of propioceptors, called gastropyloric receptor (GRP) cells, monitor muscle tension in the foregut of the crab, *Cancer borealis* (Katz and Harris-Warrick, 1989). These cells contain both acetylcholine and 5-HT. Stimulation of GPR cells evokes rapid nicotinic ESPSs and plateau properties in the dorsal gastric (DG) motoneurones. The plateau properties are induced by 5-HT (Kiehn and Harris-Warrick, 1990) and require a minimum depolarization, which is provided by acetylcholine, to be triggered. The two transmitters thus play complimentary roles to generate DG plateau potentials.

Extracellular recordings from neurones in nucleus raphe pallidus and nucleus raphe obscurus in awake cats, have shown that serotonergic cells fire tonically with a firing frequency between 0·9 spikes per s and 5·3 spikes per s dependent on the state of arousal (Trulson and Trulson, 1982; Jacobs *et al.*, 1984). From other systems it is known that multiple transmitters are not released in the same ratio and concentrations when presynaptic fibres are fired at different frequencies within the physiological firing range (Hökfelt, 1987). Since changes in raphe cell firing frequency reflect changes in overall behaviour, it will be important to determine whether a differential release is present and whether it causes measurable changes on the final motor output. The newly developed *in vitro* brain-stem–spinal cord preparations (see Smith and Feldman, 1987) may be especially advantageous to answer some of these questions, and to develop more selective ways (perhaps chemically) of activating the serotonergic neurones.

More information on the correlation between firing behaviour of the serotonergic cells and actual motor behaviour, as well as the anatomical (see Holstege and Kuypers, 1987) and physiological organization of the afferent inputs to those cells, would also be very useful for a better understanding of the serotonergic regulation of motor behaviour.

18.10. *Concluding remarks*

It is clear from extracellular and intracellular *in vivo* and *in vitro* studies in a range of different species that 5-HT has both facilitatory (or excitatory) and inhibitory effects on motoneurone excitability. The postsynaptic membrane changes responsible for these effects have just started to be revealed. So far a calcium-dependent potassium conductance, an inward rectifier and a low-voltage-activated calcium conductance are known targets for 5-HT in motoneurones. The diversity of the 5-HT effects, which should be apparent from the review, may therefore reflect 5-HT regulation of multiple motoneuronal ionic conductances. Thus, the facilitatory effects of 5-HT can theoretically be obtained by regulation of different ionic conductances, dependent on the species, types of motoneurones (slow/fast; flexor/externsor; spinal-brain-stem), age (adult-neonatal) or preparation (anaesthetized/unanaesthetized). The route of drug administration (global/local) may also be important since ionic conductances are probably unevenly distributed throughout the motoneurone membrane. Future research, is expected to shed more light on these topics, especially by use of voltage-clamp and patch-clamp techniques in the growing numbers of spinal cord and brain-stem slice preparations and motoneurone cultures (O'Brien and Fischbach, 1986; Fruns *et al.*, 1987). These preparations will also allow detailed analyses of the receptor profiles for the 5-HT-induced effects as well as studies of the intracellular messengers mediating the effects.

From the experiments cited in this review, it is clear that 5-HT acts more like a slow modulator of the intrinsic membrane properties of motoneurones than a classical transmitter mediating rapid EPSPs or inhibitory postsynaptic potentials (IPSPs), i.e. 5-HT has a permissive effect on motoneurone properties. Thus, when 5-HT induces a prolonged depolarization or reduces the spike AHP, the motoneurone input–output function is changed and the cell responds more vigorously to synaptic excitation than when the transmitter is absent. Similarly, when 5-HT induces plateau properties, short-lasting synaptic excitation can be transformed into maintained motor output. In all cases the serotonergic system opposes a strong modulatory effect on the final motor output; an effect which is not exclusive for the serotonergic system, since other modulatory systems, like the noradrenergic system, are present.

The serotonergic (and noradrenergic systems) have long been regarded as 'global transmitter systems'. The small number of neurones in the brain-stem and the extensive ramification and divergent innervation pattern have led to this notion. Several authors (Kuypers and Huisman, 1982; Anderson, 1983) have, therefore, advanced the idea that the descending serotonergic (and noradrenergic) systems should work in concert facilitating motor output and depressing somatosensory, especially noxious, inputs. The combined effect should be a state of arousal or escape response.

Although this idea of an integrated functional role of the serotonergic system may seem attractive, a more selective action cannot been excluded. Anatomical studies suggest that motor nuclei innervating extensor muscles in the chicken are more densely surrounded by serotonergic fibres than are motor nuclei innervating flexor muscles (Kojima *et al.*, 1983; Homma *et al.*, 1988; Okado *et al.*, 1988). These findings may provide an anatomical basis for the physiological observation that extensor and flexor motoneurone activities are differently affected by serotonergic agonists (for references see Conway *et al.*, 1988). Taken together these data suggest that the descending serotonergic system can direct its effect more preferentially and modulate specific behavioural functions. Hopefully, future research will give us more knowledge about these aspects, and also about the functional significance of the 5-HT-induced changes of intrinsic motoneurone response properties and the circumstances under which they take place in the behaving animal.

Acknowledgements

The experiments on the plateau properties have been performed together with Hans Hultborn and Jørn Hounsgaard. I am grateful to them for many discussions and the development of ideas. Several other colleagues have contributed to the experiments, including B.A. Conway, C. Crone, T. Eken, B. Jespersen, L. Mazieres, I. Mintz and H. Wigström. I am also grateful to D. Baro and F. Richardson for their comments on the English text.

References

Aghajanian, G.K. and Rasmussen, K. (1989). Intracellular studies in the facial nucleus illustrating a simple new method for obtaining viable motoneurons in adult rat brain slices. *Synapse*, **3**, 331–338.

Aghajanian, G.K. and VanderMaelen, C.P. (1986). Specific systems of the reticular core: serotonin. In: *Handbook of Physiology*, *Vol. 4, Intrinsic Regulatory Systems of the Brain*, edited by F.E. Bloom. Bethesda: MD, American Physiological Society, pp. 237–256.

Anderson, E.G. (1983). The serotonin system of the spinal cord. In: *Handbook of the Spinal Cord*, Vol. 1, edited by R.A. Davidoff. New York: Marcel Dekker, pp. 241–274.

Anderson, E.G. and Shibuya, T. (1966). The effects of 5-hydroxytryptophan and l-tryptophan on spinal synaptic activity. *Journal of Pharmacology and Experimental Therapy*, **153**, 352–360.

Andén, N.-E., Jukes, M.G.M. and Lundberg, A. (1964a). Spinal reflexes and monoamine liberation. *Nature*, **202**, 1222–1223.

Andén, N.-E., Jukes, M.G.M., Lundberg, A. and Vyklicky, L. (1964b). A new spinal flexor reflex. *Nature*, **202**, 1344–1345.

Baldissera, F. and Gustafsson, B. (1974). Afterhyperpolarization conductance time course in lumbar motoneurones of the cat. *Acta Physiologica Scandinavica*, **91**, 512–527.

Baldissera, F., Hultborn, H. and Illert, M. (1981) Integration in spinal neuronal systems. In: *Handbook of Physiology, Vol. 2, Motor Control*, edited by V.B. Brooks. Bethesda, MD: American Physiological Society, pp. 509–595.

Banna, N.B. and Anderson, E.G. (1968). The effects of 5-hydroxytryptamine antagonists on spinal neuronal activity. *Journal of Pharmacology and Experimental Therapy*, **162**, 319–325.

Barasi, S. and Roberts, M.H.T. (1974). The modification of lumbar motoneurone excitability by stimulation of a putative 5-hydroxytryptamine pathway. *British Journal of Pharmacology*, **52**, 339–348.

Barbeau, H. and Rossignol, S. (1990). The effects of serotonergic drugs on the locomotor pattern and on cutaneous reflexes of the adult chronic spinal cat. *Brain Research*, **514**, 55–67.

Berger, A.J. and Takahashi, T. (1990). Serotonin enhances a low-voltage-activated calcium current in rat spinal motoneurons. *Journal of Neuroscience*, **10**, 1922–1928.

Björklund, A. and Skagerberg, G. (1982). Descending monoaminergic projections to the spinal cord. In: *Brain Stem Control of Spinal Mechanisms*, edited by B. Sjölund and A. Björklund. Amsterdam: Elsevier Biomedical Press, pp. 55–88.

Bobker, D.H. and Williams, J.T. (1989). Serotonin augments the cationic current I_h in central neurons. *Neuron*, **2**, 1535–1540.

Bobker, D.H. and Williams, J.T. (1990). Ion conductances affected by 5-HT receptor subtypes in mammalian neurons. *Trends in Neuroscience*, **13**, 169–173.

Bradley, P.B., Engel, G., Feniuk, W., Fozard, J.R., Humphrey, P.P.A., Middlemiss, D.N., Mylecharane, E.J., Richardson, B.P. and Saxena, P.R. (1986). Proposals for the classification and nomenclature of functional receptors for 5-hydroxytryptamine. *Neuropharmacology*, **25**, 563–576.

Brodin, L., Buchanan, J.T., Hökfelt, T., Grillner, S. and Verhofstad, A.A.J. (1986). A spinal projection of 5-hydroxytryptamine neurons in the lamprey brainstem; evidence from combined retrograde tracing and immunohistochemistry. *Neuroscience Letters*, **67**, 53–57.

Buchanan, J.T. and Grillner, S. (1987). 5-hydroxytryptamine depresses reticulospinal excitatory postsynaptic potentials in motoneurons of the lamprey. *Society of Neuroscience, Abstracts*, **13**, 1272.

Carlsson, A., Magnusson, T. and Rosengren, E. (1963). 5-Hydroxytryptamine of the spinal cord normally and after transection. *Experientia*, **15**, 358.

Caulford, P.G. and Coceani, F. (1977). Microiontophoresis of 5-hydroxytryptamine, epinephrine, and prostaglandin E_1 on spinal neurons in the frog. *Canadian Journal of Physiology and Pharmacology*, **55**, 293–300.

Cazalets, J.R., Grillner, P., Menard, I., Cremieux, J. and Clarac, F. (1990). Two types of motor rhythm induced by NMDA and amines in an *in vitro* spinal cord preparation of neonatal rat. *Neuroscience Letters*, **111** 116–121.

Christenson, J., Franck, J. and Grillner, S. (1989). Increase in endogenous 5-hydroxytryptamine levels modulates the central network underlying locomotion in the lamprey spinal cord. *Neuroscience Letters*, **100**, 188–192.

Clineschmidt, B.V. and Anderson, E.G. (1970). The blockade of bulbospinal inhibi-

tion by 5-hydroxytryptamine antagonists. *Experimental Brain Research*, **11**, 175–186.
Commissiong, J.W. (1981). Spinal monoaminergic systems: an aspect of somatic motor function. *Federation Proceedings*, **40**, 2771–2777.
Connell, L.A. and Wallis, D.I. (1987). Effects of 5-hydroxytryptamine (5-HT) in the isolated, hemisected spinal cord of the neonate rat. *Journal of Physiology*, **390**, 44P.
Connell, L.A. and Wallis, D.I. (1988). Responses to 5-hydroxytryptamine evoked in the hemisected spinal cord of the neonate rat. *British Journal of Pharmacology*, **94**, 1101–1114.
Connell, L.A. and Wallis, D.I. (1989). 5-Hydroxytryptamine depolarizes neonatal rat motoneurones through a receptor unrelated to an identified binding site. *Neuropharmacology*, **28**, 625–634.
Conway, B.A., Hultborn, H., Kiehn, O. and Mintz, I. (1988). Plateau potentials in α-motoneurones induced by intravenous injection of L-DOPA and clonidine in the spinal cat. *Journal of Physiology*, **405**, 369–384.
Crone, C., Hultborn, H., Kiehn, O., Mazieres, L. and Wigström, H. (1988). Maintained changes in motoneuronal excitability by short-lasting inputs in the decerebrate cat. *Journal of Physiology*, **405**, 321–343.
Dahlström, A. and Fuxe, K. (1964). Evidence for the existence of monoamine-containing neurons in the central nervous system. I. Demonstration of monoamines in the cell bodies of brain stem neurons. *Acta Physiologica Scandinavica*, **62** (Suppl., 232).
Dahlström, A. and Fuxe, K. (1965). Evidence for the existence of monoamine neurons in the central nervous system. II. Experimentally induced changes in the intraneuronal amine levels of bulbospinal neuron systems. *Acta Physiologica Scandinavica*, **64** (Suppl. 247), 5–37.
Dingledine, R. (1984) *Brain Slices*. New York: Plenum Press.
Edwards, F.A., Konnerth, A., Sakmann, B. and Takahashi, T. (1989). A thin slice preparation for patch clamp recordings from neurones of the mammalian central nervous system. *Pflügers Archiv*, **414**, 600–612.
Eken, T. and Kiehn, O. (1989). Bistable firing properties of soleus motor units in unrestrained rats. *Acta Physiologica Scandinavica*, **136**, 383–394.
Engberg, I., Flatman, J.A. and Kadzielawa, K. (1976). Lack of specificity of motoneurone responses to microiontophoretically applied phenolic amines. *Acta Physiologica Scandinavica*, **96**, 137–139.
Frazer, A., Maayani, S. and Wolfe, B.B. (1990). Subtypes of receptors for serotonin. *Annual Review of Pharmacology and Toxicology*, **30**, 307–348.
Fruns, M., Krieger, C. and Sears, T.A. (1987). Identification and electrophysiological investigations of embryonic mammalian motoneurones in culture. *Neuroscience Letters*, **83**, 82–88.
Fung, S.J. and Barnes, C.D. (1989). Raphé-produced excitation of spinal cord motoneurons in the cat. *Neuroscience Letters*, **103**, 185–190.
Fuxe, K. (1965). Evidence for the existence of monoamine neurons in the central nervous system. IV. Distribution of monoamine terminals in the central nervous system. *Acta Physiologica Scandinavica,* **64** (Suppl. 247), 37–85.
Grillner, S., Buchanan, J.T. and Lansner, A. (1988). Simulation of the segmental burst generating network for locomotion in lamprey. *Neuroscience Letters*, **89**, 31–35.
Grillner, S., Wallén, P., Dale, N., Brodin, L., Buchanan, J. and Hill, R. (1987). Transmitters, membrane properties and network circuitry in the control of locomotion in lamprey. *Trends in Neuroscience*, **10**, 34–41.
Harris-Warrick, R.M. (1988). Chemical modulation of central pattern generators.

In: *Neural Control of Rhythmic Movements in Vertebrates*, edited by A. Cohen, S. Rossignol and S. Grillner. New York: Wiley, pp. 285–331.

Harris-Warrick, R.M. and Cohen, A.V. (1985). Serotonin modulates the central pattern generator for locomotion in the isolated lamprey spinal cord. *Journal of Experimental Biology*, **116**, 27–46.

Harris-Warrick, R.M., McPhee, J.C. and Filler, J.A. (1985). Distribution of serotonergic neurons and processes in the lamprey spinal cord. *Neuroscience*, **14**, 1127–1140.

Hartline, D.K., Russel, D.F., Raper, J.A. and Graubard, K. (1988). Special cellular and synaptic mechanisms in motor pattern generation. *Comparative Biochemistry and Physiology*, **91C**, 115–131.

Holohean, A.M., Hackman, J.C. and Davidoff, R.A. (1990). Changes in membrane potential of frog motoneurons induced by activation serotonin receptor subtypes. *Neuroscience*, **34**, 555–564.

Hökfelt, T. (1987). Neuronal communication through multiple coexisting messengers. In: *Synaptic Function*, edited by G.M. Edelman, W.E. Gall and W.M. Cowan. New York: Wiley, pp. 179–212.

Holstege, J.C. and Kuypers, H.G.J.M. (1987). Brainstem projections to spinal motoneurons: an update. *Neuroscience*, **23**, 809–821.

Homma, S., Sako, H., Kohno, K. and Okado, N. (1988). The pattern of distribution of serotoninergic fibers in the anterior horn of the chick spinal cord. *Anatomy and Embryology*, **179**, 25–31.

Hounsgaard, J. and Kiehn, O. (1985). Ca^{++} dependent bistability induced by serotonin in spinal motoneurons. *Experimental Brain Research*, **57**, 422–425.

Hounsgaard, J. and Kiehn, O. (1989). Serotonin-induced bistability of turtle motoneurones caused by a nifedipine-sensitive calcium plateau potential. *Journal of Physiology*, **414**, 265–282.

Hounsgaard J. and Mintz, I. (1988). Calcium conductance and firing properties of spinal motoneurones in the turtle. *Journal of Physiology*, **398**, 591–603.

Hounsgaard, J., Hultborn, H. and Kiehn, O. (1986). Transmitter-controled properties of α-motoneurones causing long-lasting motor discharge to brief excitatory inputs. In *Progress in Brain Research*, Vol. 64, edited by H.J. Freund, U. Büttner, B. Cohen and J. Noth. Amsterdam: Elsevier, pp. 39–49.

Hounsgaard, J., Kiehn, O. and Mintz, I. (1988a). Response properties of motoneurones in a thin slice preparation of the turtle spinal cord. *Journal of Physiology*, **398**, 575–589.

Hounsgaard, J., Hultborn, H., Jespersen, B. and Kiehn, O. (1984). Intrinsic membrane properties causing a bistable behaviour of α-motoneurones. *Experimental Brain Research*, **55**, 391–394.

Hounsgaard, J., Hultborn, H. Jespersen, B. and Kiehn, O. (1988b). Bistability of α-motoneurones in the decerebrate cat and in the acute spinal cat after intravenous 5-hydroxytryptophan. *Journal of Physiology*, **405**, 345–367.

Huang, J.C. and Peroutka, S.J. (1987). Identification of 5-hydroxytryptamine$_1$, binding site subtypes in rat spinal cord. *Brain Research*, **436**, 173–176.

Ito, M. and Oshima, T. (1965). Electrical behaviour of the motoneurone membrane during intracellular applied current steps. *Journal of Physiology*, **180**, 607–635.

Jackson, D.A. and White, S.R. (1989). Opposite effects of intravenous and iontophoretic administration of the 5-HT_{1A} agonist, 8-OHDPAT, on spinal motoneuron excitability. *Society of Neuroscience, Abstracts*, **15**, 225.

Jacobs, B.L. (1976). An animal behavioral model for studying central serotonergic synapses. *Life Sciences*, **19**, 777–785.

Jacobs, B.L., Heym, J. and Steinfels, G.F. (1984). Physiological and behavioral analysis of raphe unit activity. In: *Handbook of Psychopharmacology*, vol. 18, edited by L.L. Iversen, S.D. Iversen and S.H. Snyder. New York: Plenum, pp. 343–395.

Jahnsen, H. (1986). Responses of neurons in isolated preparations of the mammalian central nervous system. *Progress in Neurobiology*, **27**, 351–372.

Jahnsen, H. and Llinás, R. (1984). Ionic basis for the electroresponsiveness and oscillatory properties of guinea-pig thalamic neurones *in vitro*. *Journal of Physiology*, **349**, 227–247.

Kaczmarek, L.K. and Levitan, I.B. (1987). *Neuromodulation: The Biochemical Control of Neuronal Excitability*. Oxford: Oxford University Press.

Katz, P.S. and Harris-Warrick, R.M. (1989). Serotonergic/cholinergic muscle receptor cells in the crab stomatogastric nervous system. II. Rapid nicotinic and prolonged modulatory effects on neurons in the stomatogastric ganglion. *Journal of Neurophysiology*, **62**, 571–581.

Kernell, D. (1965). The limits of firing frequency in cat lumbosacral motoneurones possessing different time course of afterhyperpolarization. *Acta Physiologica Scandinavica*, **65**, 87–100.

Kernell, D. and Monster, A.W. (1982). Time course and properties of late adaptation in spinal motoneurones of the cat. *Experimental Brain Research*, **46**, 191–196.

Kiehn, O. (1990). Monoaminergic regulation of plateau potentials in vertebrate motoneurones — Basic mechanism and possible functional role. Thesis. University of Copenhagen.

Kiehn, O. (1991). Plateau potentials and active integration in the 'final common pathway' for motor behaviour. *Trends in Neuroscience*, **14**, 68–74.

Kiehn, O. and Harris-Warrick, R.M. (1990). Serotonin induces plateau properties in a stomatogastric motoneurone by a mixed conductance decrease and increase mechanism. *Society of Neuroscience, Abstracts*, **16**, 633.

Kirk, M.D., Taussig, R. and Scheller, R.H. (1988). Egg-laying hormone, serotonin, and cyclic nucleotide modulation of ionic currents in the identified motoneuron B16 of *Aplysia*. *Journal of Neuroscience*, **8**, 1181–1193.

Kitazawa, T., Saito, K. and Ohga, A. (1985). Effects of catecholamines on spinal motoneurones and spinal reflex discharges in the isolated spinal cord of the newborn rat. *Developmental Brain Research*, **19**, 31–36.

Kojima, M. and Sano, Y. (1983). The organization of serotonin fibers in the anterior column of the mammalian spinal cord. An immunohistochemical study. *Anatomy and Embryology*, **167**, 1–11.

Kojima, M., Takeuchi, Y., Kawat, M. and Sano, Y. (1983). Motoneurones innervating the cremaster muscle of the rat are characteristically densely innervated by serotonergic fibers as revealed by combined immunohistochemistry and retrograde fluorescence DAPI-labelling. *Anatomy and Embryology*, **168**, 41–49.

Komissarov, I.V. and Abramets, I.I. (1980). Effect of monoamines on motoneurons of the isolated rat spinal cord. *Neurophysiology*, **12**, 258–262 (translation).

Krnjevic, K. (1981). Transmitters in motor systems. In: *Handbook of Physiology, Vol. 2, Motor Control*, edited by V.B. Brooks. Bethesda, MD: American Physiological Society, pp. 107–154.

Krnjevic, K. and Van Meter, W.G. (1976). Cyclic nucleotides in spinal cells. *Canadian Journal of Physiological Pharmacology*, **54**, 416–421.

Kupfermann, I. (1979). Modulatory actions of neurotransmitters. *Annual Review of Neuroscience*, **2**, 447–465.

Kuypers, H.G.J.M. and Huisman, A.M. (1982). The new anatomy of the descending brain pathways. In: *Brain Stem Control of Spinal Mechanisms*, edited by B. Sjölund and A. Björklund. Amsterdam: Elsevier Biomedical Press, pp. 29–54.

Larkman, P.M., Penington, N.J. and Kelly, J.S. (1989). Electrophysiology of adult rat facial motoneurones: the effects of serotonin (5-HT) in a novel *in vitro* brainstem slice. *Journal of Neuroscience Methods*, **28**, 133–146.

Llinás, R. (1988). The intrinsic electrophysiological properties of mammalian neurons: insights into central nervous system function. *Science*, **242**, 1654–1664.

Lundberg, A. (1965). Monoamines and spinal reflexes. In: *Studies in Physiology*. Berlin: Springer, pp. 186–190.

Lundberg, A. (1982). Inhibitory control from the brain stem of transmission from primary afferents to motoneurons, primary afferent terminals and ascending pathways. In: *Brain Stem Control of Spinal Mechanisms*, edited by B. Sjölund and A. Björklund. Amsterdam: Elsevier Biomedical Press, pp. 179–224.

McCall, R.B. and Aghajanian, G.K. (1979). Serotonergic facilitation of facial motoneuron excitation. *Brain Research*, **169**, 11–27.

McCall, R.B. and Aghajanian, G.K. (1980). Pharmacological characterization of serotonin receptors in the facial motor nucleus: a microiontophoretic study. *European Journal of Pharmacology*, **65**, 175–183.

Madison, D.V. and Nicoll, R.A. (1982). Noradrenaline blocks accomodation of pyramidal cell discharge in the hippocampus. *Nature*, **299**, 636–638.

Myslinski, N.R. and Anderson, E.G. (1978). The effect of serotonin precursors on α- and γ-motoneuron activity. *Journal of Pharmacology and Experimental Therapy*, **204**, 19–26.

Nelson, P.G. and Frank, K. (1967). Anomalous rectification in cat spinal motoneurones and effect of polarizing currents on excitatory postsynaptic potential *Journal of Neurophysiology*, **30**, 1097–1113.

Neuman, R.S. (1985). Action of serotonin and norepinephrine on spinal motoneurones following blockade of synaptic transmission. *Canadian Journal of Physiological Pharmacology*, **63**, 735–738.

Nicoll, R.A. (1988). The coupling of neurotransmitter receptors to ion channels in the brain. *Science*, **241**, 545–551.

Nishimura, Y., Schwindt, P.C. and Crill, W.E. (1989). Electrical properties of facial motoneurones in brainstem slices from guinea pig. *Brain Research*, **502**, 127–142.

O'Brien, R.J. and Fischbach, G.D. (1986). Isolation of embryonic chick motoneurones and their survival *in vitro*. *Journal of Neuroscience*, **6**, 3265–3274.

Okado, N., Homma, S., Ishihara, R., Sako, H. and Kohno, K. (1988). Differential innervation of specific motor neuron pools by serotoninergic fibers in the chick spinal cord. *Neuroscience Letters*, **94**, 29–32.

Pape, H.-C. and McCormick, D.A. (1989). Noradrenaline and serotonin selectively modulate thalamic burst firing by enhancing a hyperpolarization-activated cation current. *Nature*, **340**, 715–718.

Parry, O. and Roberts, M.H.T. (1980). The responses of motoneurones to 5-hydroxytryptamine. *Neuropharmacology*, **19**, 515–518.

Pazos, A. and Palacios, J.M. (1985). Quantitative autoradiographic mapping of serotonin receptors in the rat brain. I. Serotonin-1 receptors. *Brain Research*, **346**, 205–230.

Pazos, A., Cortés, R. and Palacios, J.M. (1985). Quantitative autoradiographic mapping of serotonin receptors in the rat brain. II. Serotonin-2 receptors. *Brain Research*, **346**, 231–249.

Penington, N.J. and Reiffenstein, R.J. (1986). Possible involvement of serotonin receptors in the facilitatory effect of a hallucinogenic phenethylamine on single facial motoneurons. *Canadian Journal of Physiological Pharmacology*, **64**, 1302–1309.

Peroutka, S.J. (1988). 5-hydroxytryptamine receptor subtypes. *Annual Review of Neuroscience*, **11**, 45–60.

Phillis, J.W., Tebecis, A.K. and York, D.H. (1968). Depression of spinal motoneurones by noradrenaline, 5-hydroxytryptamine and histamine. *European Journal of Pharmacology*, **4**, 471–475.

Proudfit, H.K. and Anderson, E.G. (1973). Influence of serotonin antagonists on bulbospinal systems. *Brain Research*, **61**, 331–341.

Proudfit, H.K. and Anderson, E.G. (1974). New long-latency bulbospinal evoked potentials blocked by serotonin antagonists. *Brain Research*, **65**, 542–546.

Rasmussen, K. and Aghajanian, G.K. (1990). Serotonin excitation of facial motoneurons: receptor subtype characterization. *Synapse*, **5**, 324–332.

Roberts, M.H.T., Davis, M., Girdlestone, D. and Foster, G.A. (1988). Effects of 5-hydroxytryptamine agonists and antogonists on the responses of rat spinal motoneurones to raphe obscurus stimulation. *British Journal of Pharmacology*, **95**, 437–448.

Rovainen, C.M. (1979). Neurobiology of lampreys. *Physiology Review*, **59**, 1007–1077.

Schmidt, A.W. and Peroutka, S.J. (1989). 5-Hydroxytryptamine receptor 'families'. *FASEB Journal*, **3**, 2242–2249.

Schwindt, P.C. and Crill W.E. (1977). A persistent negative resistance in cat lumbar motoneurons. *Brain Research*, **120**, 173–178.

Schwindt, P.C. and Crill, W.E. (1980). Role of a persistent inward current in motoneuron bursting during spinal seizures. *Journal of Neurophysiology*, **43**, 1296–1318.

Schwindt, P.C. and Crill, W.E. (1984). Membrane properties of cat spinal motoneurons. In: *Handbook of the Spinal Cord*, Vols 2 and 3, edited by R.A. Davidoff. New York: Marcel Dekker, pp. 199–242.

Sigvardt, K.A. (1989). Modulation of properties of neurons underlying rhythmic movements in vertebrates. *Seminars in Neuroscience*, **1**, 55–65.

Smith, J.C. and Feldman, J.L. (1987). *In vitro* brainstem spinal cord preparation for study of motor system for mammalian respiration and locomotion. *Journal of Neuroscience Methods*, **21**, 321–333.

Takahashi, T. (1990a). Inward rectification in neonatal rat spinal motoneurones. *Journal of Physiology*, **423**, 47–62.

Takahashi, T. (1990b). Membrane currents in visually identified motoneurones of neonatal rat spinal cord. *Journal of Physiology*, **423**, 27–46.

Takahashi, T. and Berger, A.J. (1990). Direct excitation of rat spinal motoneurones by serotonin. *Journal of Physiology*, **423**, 63–76.

Taussig, R., Sweet-Cordero, A. and Scheller, R.H. (1989). Modulation of ionic currents in *Aplysia* motor neuron B15 by serotonin, neuropeptides, and second messengers. *Journal of Neuroscience*, **9**, 3218–3229.

Tebecis, A.K. and Phillis, J.W. (1967). The effects of topically applied biogenic monoamines on the isolated toad spinal cord. *Comparative Biochemistry and Physiology*, **23**, 553–563.

Trulson, M.E. and Trulson, V.M. (1982). Activity of nucleus raphe pallidus neurons across the sleep–waking cycle in freely moving cats. *Brain Research*, **237**, 232–237.

Twarog, B.M. and Page, I.H. (1953). Serotonin content of some mammalian tissues and urine and a method for its determination. *American Journal of Physiology*, **175**, 157–161.

VanderMaelen, C.P. (1985). Serotonin. In: *Neurotransmitter Actions in the Vertebrate Nervous System*, edited by M.A. Rogawski and J.L. Barker. New York: Plenum Press, pp. 201–240.

VanderMaelen, C.P. and Aghajanian, G.K. (1980). Intracellular studies showing modulation of facial motoneurone excitability by serotonin. *Nature*, **287**, 346–347.

VanderMaelen, C.P. and Aghajanian, G.K. (1982a). Intracellular studies on the effects of systemic administration of serotonin agonists on rat facial motoneurons. *European Journal of Pharmacology*, **78**, 233–236.

VanderMaelen, C.P. and Aghajanian, G.K. (1982b). Serotonin-induced depolarization of rat facial motoneurons *in vivo*: comparison with amino acid transmitters. *Brain Research*, **239**, 139–152.

Van Dongen, P.A.M., Grillner, S. and Hökfelt, T. (1986). 5-Hydroxytryptamine (serotonin) causes a reduction in the afterhyperpolarization following the action potential in lamprey motoneurones and premotor interneurons. *Brain Research*, **366**, 320–325.

Van Dongen, P.A.M., Hökfelt, T., Grillner, S., Verhofstad, A.A.J. and Steinbusch, H.W.M. (1985a). Possible target neurons of 5-hydroxytryptamine fibers in the lamprey spinal cord: immunohistochemistry combined with intracellular staining with lucifer yellow. *Journal of Comparative Neurology*, **234**, 523–535.

Van Dongen, P.A.M., Hökfelt, T., Grillner, S., Verhofstad, A.A.J., Steinbusch, H.W.M., Cuello, A.C. and Terenius, L. (1985b). Immunohistochemical demonstration of some putative neurotransmitters in the lamprey spinal cord and spinal ganglia: 5-hydroxytryptamine-, tachykinin- and neuropeptide-Y-immunoreactive neurons and fibers. *Journal of Comparative Neurology*, **234**, 501–522.

Viala, D. and Buser, P. (1969). The effects of DOPA and 5-HTP on rhythmic efferent discharges in hind limb nerves in the rabbit. *Brain Research*, **12**, 437–443.

Viala, D. and Buser, P. (1971). Modalités d'obtention de rythmes locomoteurs chez le lapin spinal par traitements pharmacologiques (DOPA, 5-HTP, D-amphétamine). *Brain Research*, 35, 151–165.

Wallén, P., Buchanan, J.T., Grillner, S., Hill, R.H., Christenson, J. and Hökfelt, T. (1989a). Effects of 5-hydroxytryptamine on the afterhyperpolarization, spike frequency regulation and oscillatory membrane properties in lamprey spinal cord neurons. *Journal of Neurophysiology*, **61**, 759–768.

Wallén, P., Christenson, J., Brodin, L., Hill, R., Lansner, A. and Grillner, S. (1989b). Mechanisms underlying the serotonergic modulation of the spinal circuitry for locomotion in lamprey. In *Progress in Brain Research*, Vol. 80, edited by J.H.J. Allum and M. Hulliger. Amsterdam: Elsevier Biomedical Press, pp. 321–327.

Walton, K. and Llinás, R. (1986). Calcium-dependent low threshold rebound potentials and oscillatory potentials in neonatal rat spinal motoneurons *in vitro*. *Society of Neuroscience, Abstracts,* **12**, 386.

White, S.R. and Fung, S.J. (1989). Serotonin depolarizes cat spinal motoneurons *in situ* and decreases motoneuron afterhyperpolarizing potentials. *Brain Research*, **502**, 205–213.

White, S.R. and Neuman, R.S. (1980). Facilitation of spinal motoneurone excitability by 5-hydroxytryptamine and noradrenaline. *Brain Research*, **188**, 119–127.

White, S.R. and Neuman, R.S. (1983). Pharmacological antagonism of facilitatory but not inhibitory effects of serotonin and norepinephrine on excitability of spinal motoneurons.. *Neuropharmacology*, **22**, 489–494.

Zhang, L. and Krnjevic, K. (1986). Inositol 1,4,5-triphosphate mimics the hyperpolarization induced by 5-HT in cat spinal motoneurons *in vivo*. *Society of Neuroscience*, *Abstracts*, **12**, 1648.

Zhang, L. and Krnjevic, K. (1987a). Effects of intracellular injections of phorbolester and protein kinase C on cat spinal motoneurons *in vivo*. *Neuroscience Letters*, **77**, 287–292.

Zhang, L. and Krnjevic, K. (1987b). GTPγs mimics effects of carbachol on cat spinal motoneurons. *Society of Neuroscience*, *Abstracts*, **13**, 280.

Zhang, L. and Krnjevic, K. (1989). A Ca^{2+}-dependent, long-lasting hyperpolarization induced by inositol triphosphate (IP_3) in cat spinal motoneurons. *Society of Neuroscience*, *Abstracts*, **15**, 1308.

Chapter 19

Vascular 5-HT receptors

A.H. Bom and P.R. Saxena

19.1. *Introduction*

The action of 5-hydroxytryptamine (5-HT, serotonin) on the cardiovascular system cannot be defined in a simple way. Both bradycardia and tachycardia, hypotension and hypertension, vasoconstriction and vasodilatation can be observed, depending on species, dose employed and experimental conditions (see, for example, Saxena, 1989). Recent advances in the classification of 5-HT receptors suggests that the heterogeneity of vascular responses, even within the same vascular bed, can be best explained by the presence of different types of 5-HT receptors in various parts of the vascular system.

19.2. *5-HT receptors*

In 1957 a first classification of 5-HT receptors was proposed by Gaddum and Picarelli, based on the study of 5-HT-induced contractions of isolated segments of guinea-pig eilum. These contractions could be partially blocked by morphine (M) or dibenzyline (D), but were completely antagonized by the combined use of both compounds. In the dibenzyline-pretreated ileum segments, atropine and cocaine were also able to antagonize the effect of 5-HT, whereas in the morphine-pretreated ileum segments, lysergic acid diethylamide (LSD), 2-bromo-LSD and dihydroergotamine were effective. It was concluded that 5-HT must act by two different mechanisms and receptors: an M-receptor located on enteric nerve fibres, mediating the release of acetylcholine, and a D-receptor, located on enteric smooth muscle. Later, several other compounds such as cyproheptadine, methysergide, methiothepin, metergoline and mianserin, became known as D-receptor antagonists. However, none of these drugs are selective in their antagonism of 5-HT receptor subtypes, so little further progress was made until Bennett and Aghajanian (1974) reported the first successful radioligand binding study of cerebral 5-HT receptors, using d-[^{3}H]-LSD. [^{3}H]-5-HT also showed a high affinity, but because of discrepancies between the binding of [^{3}H]-LSD and [^{3}H]-5-

a 5-HT_1 recognition site, which is labelled with [^{3}H]-5-HT, and a 5-HT_2 Snyder, 1976; Fillion *et al.*, 1978). However, further studies revealed that at least two distinct 5-HT recognition sites are present on cerebral membranes: a 5-HT_1 recognition site, which is labelled with [^{3}H]-5-HT, and a 5-HT_2 recognition site, which can be labelled with [^{3}H]-spiperone (Peroutka and Snyder, 1979). More recently, 5-HT_1 recognition sites have been shown to be heterogeneous: 5-HT_{1A}, 5-HT_{1B}, 5-HT_{1C}, and 5-HT_{1D} subtypes have been described (Pedigo *et al.*, 1981; Schnellman *et al.*, 1984; Asarch *et al.*, 1985; Hoyer *et al.*, 1985; Heuring and Peroutka, 1987).

The development of ketanserin, a compound with a high affinity for the 5-HT_2 recognition sites (Leysen *et al.*, 1981), made it possible to correlate 5-HT_2 recognition sites with functional D-receptors, which were renamed as 5-HT_2 receptors. The effects mediated by the neuronal M-receptor can be blocked by selective antagonists, e.g. MDL-72222 (Fozard, 1984) and ICS 205–930 (Donatsch *et al.*, 1984; Richardson *et al.*, 1985), but not by methiothepin or ketanserin; these receptors were called 5-HT_3 receptors. More recently, 5-HT_3 recognition sites have been demonstrated in the brain (Kilpatrick *et al.*, 1987) and in mouse neuroblastoma cells (Neijt *et al.*, 1988). Since 5-HT has a high affinity for 5-HT_1 recognition sites and some effects of 5-HT cannot be blocked by 5-HT_2 or 5-HT_3 receptor antagonists, an international committee proposed the presence of '5-HT_1-like' receptors (Bradley *et al.*, 1986). According to their criteria 5-HT_1-like receptors are not blocked by the 5-HT_2 receptor antagonists ketanserin and cyproheptadine or by the 5-HT_3 receptor antagonists MDL-72222 and ICS 205–930, but can be stimulated by 5-carboxamidotryptamine. Furthermore, methiothepin, a compound with affinity for both 5-HT_1 and 5-HT_2 recognition sites, must block the effects of 5-HT and 5-carboxamidotryptamine. Unfortunately, no selective 5-HT_1 receptor antagonist is available yet. Bradley *et al.* (1986) already indicated that further research would lead to the discovery of 5-HT receptors that cannot be classified as 5-HT_1-like, 5-HT_2 or 5-HT_3 receptors, and indeed, a 5-HT_4 receptor on mouse embryo colliculi (Dumuis *et al.*, 1989) and adult guinea-pig hippocampal (Bockaert *et al.*, 1989) neurones, positively coupled to adenyl cyclase, has been demonstrated. In functional studies, this receptor seems to correspond to the one mediating tachycardia in the pig (Bom *et al.*, 1988b; Villalón *et al.*, 1990), increase in contractile force of the human atrium (Kaumann *et al*, 1989) and enhancement of the cholinergically mediated submaximal twitch response in guinea-pig longitudinal muscle myenteric plexus (Craig and Clarke, 1990).

The present classification of functional 5-HT receptors is summarized in Table 19.1 (see Saxena and Villalón, 1990). It has to be emphasized that the classification of 5-HT receptors is still in development and it is envisaged that some rearrangement will take place in future. For example, pharmacologically the 5-HT_{1C} receptor resembles more the 5-HT_2 receptor and these may become known as 5-HT_{2A} and 5-HT_{2B}.

Table 19.1. Classification of and some functional responses mediated by 5-HT receptors.

Receptor subtype	'Selective' agonists	'Selective' antagonists	Binding site	Second messenger	Some functional responses
5-HT_1-like					
5-HT_{1A}	5-CT, 8-OH-DPAT, RU 24969, $5\text{-CH}_3\text{O-T}$, Sumatriptan	Cyanopindolol, methysergide, methiothepin, spiperone	5-HT_{1A}	Negative or positive coupling to adenylate cyclase, K^+ channel	Behavioral changes, centrally evoked hypotensive response, some endocrinological effects
5-HT_{1B}	RU 24969, 5-CT, $5\text{-CH}_3\text{O-T}$, Sumatriptan	Cyanopindolol, methiothepin,	5-HT_{1B}	Negative coupling to adenylate cyclase	Autoreceptor in the rat brain, inhibition of acetylcholine and noradrenaline release in rats
5-HT_{1C}[a]		Mesulergine, methiothepin, methysergide	5-HT_{1C}	Phosphoinositide specific phospho-lipase-C, Ca^{2+} channel	Not yet convincingly demonstrated due to unselective drugs
5-HT_{1D}	5-CT, RU-24969, Sumatriptan	Methiothepin	5-HT_{1D}	Negative coupling to adenylate cyclase	Not yet convincingly demonstrated due to unselective drugs
5-HT_{1x}[b]	5-CT, AH25086[c], Sumatriptan, 8-OH-DPAT, RU 24969	Methiothepin, methysergide[d]	Not yet found[e]	Ca^{2+} channel, Negative coupling to adenylate cyclase	Contraction of cephalic arteries (basilar, pial) and arteriovenous anastomoses in the carotid region, decrease of neuronal noradrenaline release

5-HT_{1y}[b]	5-CT	Methiothepin, methysergide	Not yet found[e]	Negative coupling to Adenylate cyclase	Vascular smooth muscle relaxation, hypotension, tachycardia in the cat
5-HT_2	α-CH_3-5-HT	Ketanserin, cyproheptadine, methysergide, methiothepin	5-HT_2	Phosphoinositide specific phospho-lipase-C, Ca^{2+} channel	Contraction of various vascular, gastrointestinal and bronchial smooth muscles, platelet aggregation, head twitch and convulsion
5-HT_3	5-HT, 2-CH_3-5-HT	MDL-72222, ICS 205-930, granisetron, ondansetron	5-HT_3	Fast cation channels	Membrane depolarization, dermal pain and flare response
5-HT_4	5-HT, Renzapride, 5-CH_3-O-T α-CH_3-5-HT	ICS 205–930	Not yet found	Positive coupling to adenylate cyclase	Gastrokinetic action, cholinergically mediated guinea-pig ileum contraction, myocardial stimulation in the pig

[a] Shows little difference from the 5-HT_2 receptor; [b] the receptor subtype is as yet unnamed and this name has been put for convenience in this manuscript to distinguish between the two unnamed 5-HT_1-like receptors; [c] ligand binding profile is not yet reported; [d] Partial agonist; [e] does not correlate with 5-HT_{1A}, 5-HT_{1B}, 5-HT_{1C} or 5-HT_{1D} binding sites. AH25086, 3-aminoethyl-*N*-methyl-1H-indole-5-methane carboxamide; 5-CH_3O-T, 5-methoxytryptamine; 5-CT, 5-carboxamidotryptamine; α-CH_3-5-HT, α-methyl-5-HT; 8-OH-DPAT, 8-hydroxy-2-(di-*N*,*N*-*n*-propylamino)tetralin; RU 24969, 5-methoxy-3-(1,2,3,6-tetrahydro-4-pyridinyl)-1H-indole.

19.3. *Mechanism of action of 5-HT*

19.3.1. **Vasoconstriction**

Stimulation of both 5-HT_1-like and 5-HT_2 receptors located on smooth muscle cells can result in contraction of blood vessels. However, in certain blood vessels, such as the rabbit ear artery and external carotid artery, 5-HT can act directly on α-receptors (Apperley *et al.*, 1976; Black *et al.*, 1981; Van Nueten, 1983). 5-HT can also cause vasoconstriction by indirect mechanisms, such as the 5-HT_2 receptor-mediated release of catecholamines from the adrenals (Feniuk *et al.*, 1981) or, in high doses, by a tyramine-like action (McGrath, 1977).

a. *5-HT_1-like receptor-mediated contractions*

This type of contraction has been demonstrated *in vitro* in the dog saphenous vein, dog auricular artery and basilar arteries of guinea-pigs, rabbits, dogs, pigs, sheep, monkeys and humans (Table 19.2). However, in dogs, sheep and humans 5-HT_2 receptors are also involved. Since the dog saphenous vein has been studied extensively, this vessel is discussed in more detail here.

5-HT causes a biphasic contraction curve in the dog saphenous vein. The first phase (low 5-HT concentrations) is caused by stimulation of specific 5-HT receptors, whereas the second phase (higher 5-HT concentrations) is related to the tyramine-like action of 5-HT, displacing noradrenaline from neuronal stores (Humphrey, 1978). Furthermore, at low 5-HT concentrations, the release of neuronal noradrenaline is inhibited, and this presynaptic action of 5-HT can be antagonized by methiothepin and methysergide, but not by yohimbine, (−)-pindolol or ketanserin. 5-Carboxamidotryptamine mimics this effect of 5-HT (Engel *et al.*, 1983), indicating that this response is mediated by a 5-HT_1-like receptor. Both 5-HT and 8-OH-DPAT cause contraction of the smooth muscle of the vein. However, the concentration–response curve for 8-OH-DPAT can be shifted to the right by methiothepin or yohimbine, but not by ketanserin (Paiva *et al.*, 1988), cyanopindolol (Humphrey *et al.*, 1988) or spiperone (Perren *et al.*, 1989). The 5-HT-induced contractions can be antagonized by methiothepin, yohimbine, ketanserin (Van Nueten *et al.*, 1981; Tuncer *et al.*, 1985) and methysergide, suggestive of the presence of both 5-HT_1-like and 5-HT_2 receptors (Paiva *et al.*, 1988), whereas phentolamine is also able to antagonize the contractile response to 5-HT (Curro *et al.*, 1978). In contrast, both ketanserin and spiperone showed no antagonism of the 5-HT-induced contraction of the dog saphenous vein in the study of Feniuk *et al.* (1985). Furthermore, Apperley *et al.* (1980) showed that methysergide was only a weak antagonist of 5-HT, and, in the lower dose range, even behaved as an agonist. 5-Carboxamidotryptamine, 5-*N*,*N*-dimethyl-carboxamidotryptamine and 5-*N*-ethyl-carboxamidotryptamine are potent agonists, although all

Table 19.2. 5-HT_1-like receptor-mediated blood vessel contractions.

Species	Blood vessel	References
Dog	Saphenous vein	Humphrey, 1978; Apperley *et al.*, 1980[a]
Dog	Auricular artery	Apperley *et al.*, 1980
Guinea-pig	Basilar artery	Chang and Owman, 1989
Rabbit	Basilar artery	Parsons and Whalley, 1989; Cain and Nicholson, 1989
Dog	Basilar artery	Connor *et al.*, 1989; Taylor *et al.*, 1986; Peroutka *et al.*, 1986
Pig	Basilar artery	Van Charldorp and Wouters, 1990
Sheep	Basilar artery	Gaw *et al.*, 1990
Monkey	Basilar artery	Connor *et al.*, 1989
Human	Basilar artery	Parsons *et al.*, 1989
Pig	Arteriovenous anastomoses	Saxena and Verdouw, 1982, 1984, 1985; Saxena *et al.*, 1986; Bom *et al.*, 1988b, 1989

[a] For further references, see text.

three compounds produce lower maximum responses than 5-HT (Feniuk *et al.*, 1985). Sumatriptan acts as a selective agonist for the 5-HT_1-like receptors in the dog saphenous vein. Sumatriptan induces both contraction of the smooth muscle cells and presynaptic inhibition of neuronally mediated contractions (Humphrey *et al.*, 1988). The contractile effect of sumatriptan cannot be antagonized by ketanserin, MDL-72222, cyanopindolol, mesulergine or metergoline, but methiothepin causes a shift to the right of the concentration–response curve. 5-HT, 5-carboxamidotryptamine and sumatriptan cause a concentration-dependent inhibition of prostaglandin E_2-stimulated cyclic AMP, suggesting that stimulation of a 5-HT_1-like receptor on smooth muscle cells induces inhibition of adenylate cyclase in this vessel. The response to sumatriptan was attenuated by methiothepin, but not by metergoline, spiperone or ondansetron (Summer and Humphrey, 1990).

5-HT_1-like receptor-mediated constriction has also been studied *in vivo*. Stimulation of 5-HT_1-like receptors in the carotid vascular bed of the pig results in a reduction of arteriovenous anastomotic blood flow, possibly by a constriction of arteriovenous anastomoses (Saxena and Verdouw, 1982, 1984, 1985; Saxena *et al.*, 1986; Bom *et al.*, 1988a, 1989; Den Boer *et al.*, 1990).

b. *5-HT_2 receptor-mediated contractions*

In the majority of large blood vessels this receptor type mediates the contractile response (Table 19.3). In many studies this receptor has been characterized using the 5-HT_2 receptor antagonist ketanserin, but it must be remembered that this compound also possesses α_1-adrenoceptor blocking activity. Fortunately, more selective 5-HT_2 receptors antagonists, e.g. ritanserin, have been identified.

Table 19.3. 5-HT_2 receptor-mediated blood vessel contraction.

Species	Blood vessel	References
Rat	Jugular vein	Cohen *et al.*, 1981; Leff and Martin, 1986
Rat	Portal vein	Lemberger *et al.*, 1984
Rat	Aorta	Cohen *et al.*, 1981; Bradley *et al.*, 1983; Forster and Whalley, 1982
Rat	Caudal artery	Leysen *et al.*, 1984
Rabbit	Aorta	Kohli, 1968; Apperly *et al.*, 1976[a]
Rabbit	Carotid artery	Black *et al.*, 1981
Rabbit	Femoral artery	Black *et al.*, 1981; Van Nueten, 1983
Cat	Saphenous vein	Feniuk *et al.*, 1983
Dog	Basilar artery	Van Nueten, *et al.*, 1981, 1984; Müller-Schweinitzer and Engel, 1983; Frenken, 1989
Dog	Carotid artery	Apperley *et al.*, 1980
Dog	Coronary artery	Van Nueten, 1983; M.L. Cohen *et al.*, 1983
Dog	Femoral artery	Apperley *et al.*, 1980
Sheep	Basilar artery	Gaw *et al.*, 1990
Calf	Coronary artery	Frenken and Kaumann, 1984
Calf	Pulmonary artery	Frenken and Kaumann, 1984
Human	Basilar artery	Blackburn *et al.*, 1988; Forster and Whalley, 1982
Human	Umbilical artery	McGrath *et al.*, 1985
Human	Femoral artery	Glusa and Markwardt, 1984

[a] For further references, see text.

A typical example of 5-HT_2 receptor-mediated blood vessel constriction is the rabbit aorta. 5-HT induces contraction of the rabbit aorta (Kohli, 1968; Maling, 1971) and the effect can be blocked by dibenamine (Furchgott, 1954), methysergide, cyproheptadine, pizotifen (Apperley *et al.*, 1976; Bradley *et al.*, 1983), trazodone (Leff and Martin, 1986), 2-bromo-LSD (Kohli, 1968; Stollack and Furchgott, 1984; Purdy *et al.*, 1981, 1987), 5-methylgramine, 5-methoxygramine (Stollack and Furchgott, 1984), spiperone (Maayani *et al.*, 1984; Clancy and Maayani, 1985), ICI 169,369 (Blackburn *et al.*, 1988) and ketanserin (Feniuk *et al.*, 1985). 5-Carboxamidotryptamine (Feniuk *et al.*, 1985) and sumatriptan (Humphrey *et al.*, 1988) are only weak agonists. Furthermore, α-methyl-5-HT mimics 5-HT and can be antagonized competitively by trazodone (Leff and Martin, 1986). However, at higher concentrations ($>10^{-5}$ M) 5-HT can also act on postsynaptic α-adrenoceptors (Purdy *et al.*, 1987).

19.3.2. **Vasodilatation**

5-HT-induced vasodilation is mainly mediated by 5-HT_1-like receptors, either by a direct action on vascular smooth muscle cells or by indirect mechanisms such as presynaptic inhibition of postganglionic sympathetic nerve fibre neurotransmitter release (McGrath, 1977) or endothelial-dependent relaxation (Cocks and Angus, 1983). In some blood vessels 5-HT induces vasodilation by the production of prostacyclin, which may be mediated by 5-HT_2 receptors (Kokkas and Boeymaens, 1988).

Table 19.4. 5-HT_1-like receptor-mediated blood vessel relaxation.

Species	Blood vessel	References
Cat	Saphenous vein	Feniuk *et al.*, 1983; Feniuk *et al.*, 1984 Humphrey *et al.*, 1988
Rabbit	Jugular vein	Martin *et al.*, 1987
Pig	Vena cava	Trevethick *et al.*, 1984; 1986
Pig	Carotid arterioles	Saxena and Verdouw, 1982; Verdouw *et al.*, 1985 Saxena *et al.*, 1986

a. *Direct vascular relaxation mediated by 5-HT_1 like receptors*

This phenomenon has been shown *in vitro* in precontracted cat saphenous vein, rabbit jugular vein and pig vena cava (Table 19.4). In the U46619-precontracted rabbit jugular vein, low 5-HT concentrations cause relaxation, which is endothelium-dependent, whereas higher 5-HT concentrations cause relaxation by an action directly on the vascular smooth muscle cells. Both responses are resistant to blockade by ketanserin or MDL-72222, but are susceptible to antagonism by methysergide. In endothelium-intact jugular veins 5-HT is more potent than 5-carboxamidotryptamine or α-methyl-5-HT, whereas in endothelium-denuded jugular veins 5-carboxamido-tryptamine is more potent than 5-HT, and α-methyl-5-HT is inactive (Martin *et al.*, 1987). In the cat saphenous vein, sumatriptan fails to elicit vasodilatation (Humphrey *et al.*, 1988).

In vivo, 5-HT and 5-carboxamidotryptamine elicit a potent 5-HT_1-like receptor-mediated vasodilatation in the pig, especially in the skin, which turns bright pink (Saxena and Verdouw, 1982, 1985; Saxena *et al.*, 1986). It should, however, be noted that 8-OH-DPAT (Bom *et al.*, 1988a), RU-24969 (Bom *et al.*, 1989) and sumatriptan (Den Boer *et al.*, 1990) do not increase arteriolar blood flow in the pig.

b. *Presynaptic inhibition mediated by 5-HT_1-like receptors*

5-HT-induced presynaptic inhibition has been described in dog saphenous vein and tibial artery, rat kidney and vena cava. This phenomenon is discussed in more detail in Chapter 17 of this book.

c. *Endothelium-dependent relaxation mediated by 5-HT_1-like receptors*

5-HT relaxes, isolated canine and porcine coronary arteries, chick jugular vein and rat aorta (Table 19.5) and this effect is mainly the result of release of endothelium-dependent relaxing factor (EDRF). Dysfunction or denudation of the endothelium in various pathological states might therefore enhance the vasoconstrictor effect of 5-HT.

The endothelial 5-HT receptor has been studied in detail in the canine coronary artery by Houston and Vanhoutte (1988). Neither ketanserin nor

Table 19.5. 5-HT_1-like receptor-mediated endothelial-dependent blood vessel relaxation.

Species	Blood vessel	References
Dog	Coronary artery	Cocks and Angus, 1983; R.A. Cohen *et al.*, 1983 Houston *et al.*, 1985; Houston and Vanhoutte, 1988
Pig	Coronary artery	Cocks and Angus, 1983; Shimokawa *et al.*, 1987
Rabbit	Coronary artery	Garland, 1985
Chicken	Jugular vein	Imaizumi *et al.*, 1984
Rat	Aorta	Lüscher and Vanhoutte, 1986
Rabbit	Jugular vein	Martin *et al.*, 1987

MDL-72222 is able to antagonize the endothelium-dependent relaxing action of 5-HT, whereas methiothepin and metergoline can block it, indicating that 5-HT_1-like receptors are involved. Since cyanopindolol and propranolol do not inhibit the action of 5-HT, and the 5-HT_{1A} agonist 8-OH-DPAT is inactive, a mediation by putative 5-HT_{1A} or 5-HT_{1B} receptors is unlikely.

19.4. *The nature of vascular smooth muscle 5-HT_1-like receptors*

As described above the 5-HT_1-like receptor present on vascular smooth muscle cells can cause either vasoconstriction or vasodilatation. In view of the heterogeneity of the 5-HT_1-like receptors, one has to consider whether vasodilatation and vasoconstriction in the different vessels are mediated by the same or different 5-HT_1-like receptor, and to which specific subtypes these receptors belong.

Concerning the first question, it is clear that the two 5-HT_1-like receptors are pharmacologically different. The main reason for this is that, while both vasodilatation and vasoconstriction are observed with 5-HT or 5-carboxamidotryptamine (see Saxena *et al.*, 1989), 8-OH-DPAT (5-HT_{1A} agonist; Middlemiss and Fozard, 1983), RU-24969 (5-HT_{1A} and 5-HT_{1B} agonist; Hoyer *et al.*, 1985), sumatriptan (5-HT_{1A}, 5-HT_{1B} and 5-HT_{1D}; Peroutka and McCarthy, 1989; Sumner and Humphrey, 1989) have only vasoconstrictor action (Bom *et al.*, 1988a, 1989; Humphrey *et al.*, 1988, 1990; Den Boer *et al.*, 1990). Since the vasoconstrictor effect of these drugs is not antagonized by spiperone (5-HT_{1A} antagonist; Hoyer *et al.*, 1985), cyanopindolol, pindolol, propranolol (all 5-HT_{1A} and 5-HT_{1B} antagonists; Hoyer *et al.*, 1985), mesulergine (5-HT_{1C} antagonist; Hoyer *et al.*, 1985) or metergoline (5-HT_{1A}, 5-HT_{1B}, 5-HT_{1C} and 5-HT_{1D} antagonist; Hoyer *et al.*, 1985) (see Feniuk *et al.*, 1985; Bom *et al.*, 1988a, 1989; Humphrey *et al.*, 1988, 1990), the 5-HT_1-like receptor mediating vascular constriction does not appear to be related to any of the 5-HT_{1A}, 5-HT_{1B}, 5-HT_{1C} or 5-HT_{1D} subtypes. Even the vasodilatory 5-HT_1-like receptor may not resemble these subtypes because of the inactivity of sumatriptan as an agonist in the cat saphenous vein (Humphrey *et al.*, 1988) and the poor activity of metergoline and mianserin as antagonists against depressor responses in the cat (see Saxena, 1988).

19.5. *Concluding remarks*

The effects of 5-HT in the cardiovascular system are complex and consist of bradycardia or tachycardia, hypotension or hypertension and vasodilatation or vasoconstriction. These cardiovascular effects are mediated by four different kinds of receptors called 5-HT_1-like, 5-HT_2, 5-HT_3 and 5-HT_4. The 5-HT-induced vasoconstriction in the majority of vessels occurs via the 5-HT_2 receptor, but the vasoconstrictor response in the dog saphenous vein and cephalic vessels (arteries and arteriovenous anastomoses) of several species is mediated exclusively, or in addition, by a 5-HT_1-like receptor. The peripheral vasodilator response also involves 5-HT_1-like receptors located at three different sites: sympathetic nerve terminals (reduction of transmitter release), vascular smooth muscle and vascular endothelium (release of EDRF). Arteriolar dilatation, together with the constriction of arteriovenous anastomoses, leads to an increase in nutrient (tissue; capillary) blood flow. The 5-HT_1-like receptors are heterogeneous in nature and the 5-HT_1-like receptors causing vasoconstriction and vasodilatation are different and do not seem to correlate to any of the 5-HT_1 binding subtypes (5-HT_{1A}, 5-HT_{1B}, 5-HT_{1C} or 5-HT_{1D}) recognized so far. Selective agonists and antagonists at the vascular 5-HT receptors are, or can be, used to develop drugs for hypertension, migraine and peripheral vascular diseases.

References

Apperley, E., Humphrey, P.P.A. and Levy, G.P. (1976). Receptors for 5-hydroxytryptamine and noradrenaline in rabbit isolated ear artery and aorta. *British Journal of Pharmacology*, **58**, 211–221.

Apperley, E., Feniuk, W., Humphrey, P.P.A. and Levy, G.P. (1980). Evidence for two types of excitatory receptor for 5-hydroxytryptamine in dog isolated vasculature. *British Journal of Pharmacology*, **68**, 215–224.

Asarch, K.B., Ransom, R.W. and Shih, J.C. (1985). 5-HT_{1A} and 5-HT_{1B} selectivity of two phenylpiperazine derivatives: evidence for 5-HT_{1B} heterogeneity. *Life Sciences*, **36**, 1265–1273.

Bennett, J.P. and Aghajanian, G.K. (1974). *d*-LSD binding to brain homogenates: possible relationship to serotonin receptors. *Life Sciences*, **15**, 1935–1944.

Bennett, J.P. and Snyder, S.H. (1976). Serotonin and lysergic acid diethylamide binding in rat brain membranes: relationship to postsynaptic serotonin receptors. *Molecular Pharmacology*, **12**, 373–389.

Black, J.L., French, R.J. and Mylecharane, E.J. (1981). Receptor mechanisms for 5-hydroxytryptamine in rabbit arteries. *British Journal of Pharmacology*, **74**, 619–626.

Blackburn, T.P., Thornber, C.W., Pearce, R.J. and Cox, B. (1988). *In vitro* studies with ICI 169,369, a chemical novel 5-HT antagonist. *European Journal of Pharmacology*, **150**, 247–256.

Bockaert, J., Sebben, M. and Dumuis, A. (1990). Pharmacological characterization of 5-hydroxytryptamine$_4$ (5-HT$_4$) receptors positively coupled to adenyl cyclase in adult guinea pig hippocampal membranes: effect of substituted benzamide derivatives. *Molecular Pharmacology*, **37**, 408–411.

Bom, A.H., Verdouw, P.D. and Saxena, P.R. (1988a). Carotid haemodynamics in pigs during infusions of 8-OH-DPAT: reduction in arteriovenous shunting is mediated by 5-HT$_1$-like receptors. *British Journal of Pharmacology*, **96**, 125–132.

Bom, A.H., Duncker, D.J., Saxena, P.R. and Verdouw, P.D. (1988b). 5-Hydroxytryptamine-induced tachycardia in the pig: possible involvement of a new type of 5-hydroxytryptamine receptor. *British Journal of Pharmacology*, **93**, 663–671.

Bom, A.H., Villalón, C.M., Verdouw, P.D. and Saxena, P.R. (1989). The 5-HT$_1$-like receptor mediating reduction in porcine carotid arteriovenous shunting by RU 24969 is unrelated to either 5-HT$_{1A}$ or 5-HT$_{1B}$ subtype. *European Journal of Pharmacology*, **171**, 87–96.

Bradley, P.B., Humphrey, P.P.A. and Williams. (1983). Are vascular 'D' and '5-HT$_2$' receptors for 5-hydroxytryptamine the same? *British Journal of Pharmacology*, **79**, 295P.

Bradley, P.B., Engel, G., Feniuk, W., Fozard, J.R., Humphrey, P.P.A., Middlemiss, D.N., Mylecharane, E.J., Richardson, B.P. and Saxena, P.R. (1986). Proposals for the classification and nomenclature of functional receptors for 5-hydroxytryptamine. *Neuropharmacology*, **25**, 563–576.

Cain, C.R. and Nicholson, C.D. (1989). Comparison of the effects of cromakalin, a potassium conductance enhancer, and nimodipine, a calcium antagonist, on 5-hydroxytryptamine responses in a variety of vascular smooth muscle preparations. *Naunyn-Schmiedeberg's Archives of Pharmacology*, **340**, 293–299.

Chang, J.-Y and Owman, Ch. (1989). Cerebrovascular serotonergic receptors mediating vasoconstriction: further evidence for the existence of 5-HT$_2$ receptors in rat and 5-HT$_1$-like receptors in guinea pig basilar arteries. *Acta Physiologica Scandinavica*, **136**, 59–67.

Clancy, B.M. and Maayani, S. (1985). 5-Hydroxytryptamine receptor in isolated rabbit aorta: characterization with tryptamine analogs. *Journal of Pharmacology and Experimental Therapy*, **233**, 761–769.

Cocks, T.M. and Angus, J.A. (1983). Endothelium-dependent relaxation of coronary arteries by noradrenaline and serotonin. *Nature*, **305**, 627–630.

Cohen, M.L., Fuller, R.W. and Wiley, K.S. (1981). Evidence for 5-HT$_2$ receptors mediating contraction in vascular smooth muscle. *Journal of Pharmacology and Experimental Therapy*, **218**, 421–425.

Cohen, M.L., Mason, N., Wiley, K.S. and Fuller, R.W. (1983). Further evidence that vascular serotonin receptors are of the 5-HT$_2$ type. *Biochemical Pharmacology*, **32**, 567–570.

Cohen, R.A., Shepherd, J.T. and Vanhoutte, P.M. (1983). 5-Hydroxytryptamine can mediate endothelium-dependent relaxation of coronary arteries. *American Journal of Physiology*, **245**, H1077–H1080.

Connor, H.E., Feniuk, W. and Humphrey, P.P.A. (1989). Characterization of 5-HT receptors mediating contraction of canine and primate basilar artery by use of GR43175, a selective 5-HT$_1$-like receptor agonist. *British Journal of Pharmacology*, **96**, 379–387.

Craig, D.A. and Clarke, D.E. (1990). Pharmacological characterization of a neuronal receptor for 5-hydroxytryptamine in guinea pig ileum with properties similar to the 5-hydroxytryptamine$_4$ receptor. *Journal of Pharmacology and Experimental Therapy*, **252**, 1378–1386.

Curro, F.A., Greenberg, S., Verbeuren, T.J. and Vanhoutte, P.M. (1978). Interaction between alpha adrenergic and serotonergic activation of canine saphenous vein. *Journal of Pharmacology and Experimental Therapy*, **207**, 936–949.

Den Boer, M.O., Villalón, C.M., Heiligers, J.P.C., Saxena, P.R. and Humphrey, P.P.A. (1990). The craniovascular effects of sumatriptan. *British Journal of Pharmacology*, **99**, 37P.

Donatsch, P., Engel, G., Richardson, B.P. and Stadler, P.A. (1984). ICS 205–930: a highly selective and potent antagonist at peripheral neuronal 5-hydroxytryptamine (5HT) receptors. *British Journal of Pharmacology*, **81**, 34P.

Dumuis, A., Sebben, M. and Bockaert, J. (1989). The gastrointestinal prokinetic benzamide derivatives are agonists at the non-classical 5-HT receptor (5-HT$_4$) positively coupled to adenylate cyclase in neurons. *Naunyn-Schmiedeberg's Archives of Pharmacology*, **340**, 403–410.

Engel, G., Göthert, M., Müller-Schweinitzer, E., Schlicker, E., Sistonen, L. and Stadler, P.A. (1983). Evidence for common pharmacological properties of [^{3}H]5-hydroxytryptamine binding sites, presynaptic 5-hydroxytryptamine autoreceptors in CNS and inhibitory presynaptic 5-hydroxytryptamine receptors on sympathetic nerves. *Naunyn-Schmiedeberg's Archives of Pharmacology*, **324**, 116–124.

Feniuk, W., Hare, J. and Humphrey, P.P.A. (1981). Analysis of the mechanism of 5-hydroxytryptamine-induced vasopressor responses in ganglion-blocked anaesthetized dogs. *Journal of Pharmacy and Pharmacology*, **33**, 155–160.

Feniuk, W., Humphrey, P.P.A. and Watts, A.D. (1983). 5-Hydroxytryptamine-induced relaxation of isolated mammalian smooth muscle. *European Journal of Pharmacology*, **96**, 71–78.

Feniuk, W., Humphrey, P.P.A. and Watts, A.D. (1984). 5-Carboxamidotryptamine — a potent agonist at 5-hydroxytryptamine receptors mediating relaxation. *British Journal of Pharmacology*, **82**, 209P.

Feniuk, W., Humphrey, P.P.A. Perren, M.J. and Watts, A.D. (1985). A comparison of 5-hydroxytryptamine receptors mediating contraction in rabbit aorta and dog saphenous vein: evidence for different receptor types obtained by use of selective agonists and antagonists. *British Journal of Pharmacology*, **86**, 697–704.

Fillion, G.M.B., Rouselle, J.-C., Fillion, M.-P., Beaudoin, D.M., Goiny, M.R., Deniau, J.-M. and Jacob, J.J. (1978). High affinity binding of [^{3}H]5-hydroxytryptamine to brain synaptosomal membranes: comparison with [^{3}H]lysergic acid diethylamide binding. *Molecular Pharmacology*, **14**, 50–59.

Forster, C. and Whalley, E.T. (1982). Analysis of the 5-hydroxytryptamine induced contractions of the human basilar arterial strip compared with the rat aortic strip *in vitro*. *Naunyn-Schmiedeberg's Archives of Pharmacology*, **319**, 12–17.

Fozard, J.R. (1984). MDL-72222, a potent and highly selective antagonist at neuronal 5-hydroxytryptamine receptors. *Naunyn-Schmiedeberg's Archives of Pharmacology*, **326**, 36–44.

Frenken, M. (1989). Evidence for two populations of 5-hydroxytryptamine receptors in dog basilar artery. *Journal of Pharmacology and Experimental Therapy*, **250**, 379–387.

Frenken, M. and Kaumann, A.J. (1984). Interaction of ketanserin and its metabolite ketanserinol with 5-HT$_2$ receptors in pulmonary and coronary arteries of calf. *Naunyn-Schmiedeberg's Archives of Pharmacology*, **326**, 334–339.

Furchgott, R.F. (1954). Dibenamine blockade in strips of rabbit aorta and its use in differentiating receptors. *Journal of Pharmacology and Experimental Therapy*, **111**, 265–284.

Gaddum, J.H. and Picarelli, Z.P. (1957). Two kinds of tryptamine receptors. *British Journal of Pharmacology*, **2**, 239–249.

Garland, C.J. (1985). Endothelial cells and the electrical and mechanical responses of the rabbit coronary artery to 5-hydroxytryptamine. *Journal of Pharmacology and Experimental Therapy*, **233**, 158–162.

Gaw, A.J., Wadsworth, R.M. and Humphrey, P.P.A. (1990). Pharmacological characterization of postjunctional 5-HT receptors in cerebral arteries from the sheep. *European Journal of Pharmacology*, **179**, 35–44.

Glusa, E. and Markwardt, F. (1984). Studies on 5-hydroxytryptamine receptors on isolated human femoral veins and arteries and the influence of dihydroergotamine. *Pharmacology*, **29**, 336–342.

Heuring, R.E. and Peroutka, S.J. (1987). Characterization of a novel ^{3}H-5-hydroxytryptamine binding site subtype in bovine brain membranes. *Journal of Neuroscience*, **7**, 894–903.

Houston, D.S. and Vanhoutte, P.M. (1988). Comparison of serotonergic receptor subtypes on the smooth muscle and endothelium of the canine coronary artery. *Journal of Pharmacology and Experimental Therapy*, **244**, 1–10.

Houston, D.S., Shepherd, J.T. and Vanhoutte, P.M. (1985). Adenine nucleotides, serotonin, and endothelium-dependent relaxations to platelets. *American Journal of Physiology*, **248**, H389–H395.

Hoyer, D., Engel, G. and Kalkman, H.O. (1985). Molecular pharmacology of 5-HT_1 and 5-HT_2 recognition sites in rat and pig membranes: radioligand binding studies with [^{3}H]5-HT, [^{3}H]8-OH-DPAT, (−)[^{125}I]iodocyanopindolol, [^{3}H]-mesulergine and [^{3}H]ketanserin. *European Journal of Pharmacology*, **118**, 13–23.

Humphrey, P.P.A. (1978). The effect of α-adrenoceptor antagonists on contractile responses to 5-hydroxytryptamine in dog saphenous vein. *British Journal of Pharmacology*, **63**, 671–675.

Humphrey, P.P.A., Apperley, E., Feniuk, W. and Perren, M.J. (1990). A rational approach to identifying a fundamentally new drug for the treatment of migraine. In: *Cardiovascular Pharmacology of 5-Hydroxytryptamine: Prospective Therapeutic Applications*, edited by P.R. Saxena, D.I. Wallis, W. Wouters and P. Bevan. Dordrecht: Kluwer, pp. 417–431.

Humphrey, P.P.A., Feniuk, W., Perren, M.J., Connor, H.E., Oxford, A.W., Coates, I.H. and Butina, D. (1988). GR43175, a selective agonist for the 5-HT_1-like receptor in dog isolated saphenous vein. *British Journal of Pharmacology*, **94**, 1123–1132.

Imaizumi, Y., Baba, M., Imaizumi, Y. and Watanabe, M. (1984). Involvement of endothelium in the relaxation of isolated chick jugular vein by 5-hydroxytryptamine. *European Journal of Pharmacology*, **97**, 335–336.

Kaumann, A.J., Murray, K.J., Brown, A.M., Sanders, L. and Brown, M.J. (1989). A receptor for 5-HT in human atrium. *British Journal of Parmacology*, **98**, 664P.

Kilpatrick, G.J., Jones, B.J. and Tyers, M.B. (1987). Identification of 5-HT_3 receptors in rat brain using radioligand binding. *Nature*, **330**, 746–748.

Kohli, J.D. (1968). Receptors for sympathomimetic amines in the rabbit aorta: differentiation by specific antagonists. *British Journal of Pharmacology*, **32**, 273–279.

Kokkas, B. and Boeymaens, J.-M. (1988). Release of prostacyclin from the dog saphenous vein by 5-hydroxytryptamine. *European Journal of Pharmacology*, **147**, 473–476.

Leff, P. and Martin, G.R. (1986). Peripheral 5-HT_2-like receptors. Can they be classified with the available antagonists? *British Journal of Pharmacology*, **88** 585–593.

Lemberger, H.F., Mason, N. and Cohen, M.L. (1984). 5-HT_2 receptors in the rat portal vein: desensitization following cumulative serotonin addition. *Life Sciences*, **35**, 71–77.

Leysen, J.E., Awouters, F., Kennis, L., Laduron, P.M., Vandenberk, J. and Janssen, P.A.J. (1981). Receptor binding profile of R 41468, a novel antagonist at 5-HT_2 receptors. *Life Sciences*, **28**, 1015–1022.

Leysen, J.E., De Chaffoy de Courcelles, D., De Clerck, F., Niemegeers, C.J.E. and Van Nueten, J.M. (1984). Serotonin-S_2 receptor binding sites and functional correlates. *Neuropharmacology*, **23**, 1493–1501.

Lüscher, T.F. and Vanhoutte, P.M. (1986). Endothelium-dependent responses to platelets and serotonin in spontaneously hypertensive rats. *Hypertension*, **88**, 55–60.

Maayani, S., Wilkinson, C.W. and Stollack, J.S. (1984). 5-Hydroxytryptamine receptor in rabbit aorta: characterization by butyrophenone analogs. *Journal of Pharmacology and Experimental Therapy*, **229**, 346–350.

McGrath, M.A. (1977). 5-Hydroxytryptamine and neurotransmitter release in canine blood vessels, inhibition by low and augmentation by high concentrations. *Circulation Research*, **41**, 428–435.

McGrath, J.C., MacLennan, S.J. and Stuart-Smith, K. (1985). Characterization of the receptor mediating contraction of human umbilical artery by 5-hydroxytryptamine. *British Journal of Pharmacology*, **84**, 199–202.

Maling, H.M., Fleisch, J.H. and Saul, W.F. (1971). Species differences in aortic response to vasoactive amines: the effects of compound 48/80, cocaine, reserpine and 6-hydroxydopamine. *Journal of Pharmacology and Experimental Therapy*, **176**, 672–683.

Martin, G.R., Leff, P., Cambridge, D. and Barrett, V.J. (1987). Comparative analysis of two types of 5-hydroxytryptamine receptor mediating vasorelaxation: differential classification using tryptamines. *Naunyn-Schmiedeberg's Archives of Pharmacology*, **336**, 365–373.

Middlemiss, D.N. and Fozard, J.R. (1983). 8-Hydroxy-2-(di-*n*-propylamino)-tetralin discriminates between subtypes of the 5-HT_1 recognition site. *European Journal of Pharmacology*, **90**, 151–157.

Müller-Schweinitzer, E. and Engel, G. (1983). Evidence for the mediation by 5-HT_2 receptors of 5-hydroxytryptamine-induced contractions of canine basilar artery. *Naunyn-Schmiedeberg's Archives of Pharmacology*, **324**, 287–292.

Neijt, H.C., Karpf, A., Schoeffer, P., Engel., G. and Hoyer, D. (1988). Characterization of 5-HT_3 recognition sites in membranes of NG 108–15 neuroblastoma-glioma cells with [^{3}H]ICS 205–930. *Naunyn-Schmiedeberg's Archives of Pharmacology*, **337**, 493–499.

Paiva, M.Q., Caramona, M.M. and Osswald, W. (1988). The actions of 5-hydroxytryptamine agonists and antagonists at pre- and postjunctional level on the canine saphenous vein. *Naunyn-Schmiedeberg's Archives of Pharmacology*, **338**, 616–622.

Parsons, A.A. and Whalley, E.T. (1989). Evidence for the presence of 5-HT_1-like receptors in rabbit isolated basilar arteries. *European Journal of Pharmacology*, **174**, 189–196.

Parsons, A.A., Whalley, E.T., Feniuk, W., Connor, H.E. and Humphrey, P.P.A. (1989). 5-HT_1-like receptors mediate 5-hydroxytryptamine-induced contraction of human isolated basilar artery. *British Journal of Pharmacology*, **96**, 434–440.

Pedigo, N.W., Yamamura, H.I. and Nelson, D.D. (1981). Discrimination of multiple [^{3}H]5-hydroxytryptamine binding sites by the neuroleptic spiperone in rat brain. *Journal of Neurochemistry*, **36**, 220–226.

Perren, M.J., Feniuk, W., Humphrey, P.P.A. (1989). Vascular actions of 8-OH-

DPAT mediated via activation of non-5-HT_{1A} receptors. *British Journal of Pharmacology*, **98**, 797P.
Peroutka, S.J. and Snyder, S.H. (1979). Multiple serotonin receptors: differential binding of [^{3}H]5-hydroxytryptamine, [^{3}H]lysergic acid diethylamide and [^{3}H]spiroperidol. *Molecular Pharmacology*, **16**, 687–699.
Peroutka, S.J., Huang, S. and Allen, G.S. (1986). Canine basilar artery contractions mediated by 5-$hydroxytryptamine_{1A}$ receptors. *Journal of Pharmacology and Experimental Therapy*, **237**, 901–906.
Peroutka, S.J. and McCarthy, B.G. (1989). Sumatriptan (GR43175) interacts selectively with 5-HT_{1B} and 5-HT_{1D} binding sites. *European Journal of Pharmacology*, **163**, 133–136.
Purdy, R.E., Hurlbut, D.E. and Rains, L.A. (1981). Receptors for 5-hydroxytryptamine in rabbit isolated ear artery and aorta. *Blood Vessels*, **18**, 16–27.
Purdy, R.E., Murray, D.L. and Stupecky, G.L. (1987). Receptors for 5-hydroxytryptamine in rabbit blood vessels: activation of alpha adrenoceptors in rabbit thoracic aorta. *Journal of Pharmacology and Experimental Therapy*, **240**, 535–541.
Richardson, B.P., Engel, G., Donatsch, P. and Stadler, P.A. (1985). Identification of serotonin M-receptor subtypes and their specific blockade by a new class of drugs. *Nature*, **316**, 126–131.
Saxena, P.R. (1988). Further characterization of 5-$hydroxytryptamine_1$-like receptors mediating tachycardia in the cat: no apparent relationship to known subtypes of the 5-$hydroxytryptamine_1$ binding site. *Development and Research*, **13**, 245–258.
Saxena, P.R. (1989). Cardiovascular effects from stimulation of 5-hydroxytryptamine receptors. *Fundamental and Clinical Pharmacology*, **3**, 245–265.
Saxena, P.R. and Verdouw, P.D. (1982). Redistribution by 5-hydroxytryptamine of carotid arterial blood flow at the expense of arteriovenous blood flow. *Journal of Physiology (London)*, **332**, 501–520.
Saxena, P.R. and Verdouw, P.D. (1984). Effects of methysergide and 5-hydroxytryptamine on carotid blood flow distribution in pigs: further evidence for the presence of atypical 5-HT receptors. *British Journal of Pharmacology*, **82**, 817–826.
Saxena, P.R. and Verdouw, P.D. (1985). 5-Carboxamidotryptamine, a compound with high affinity for 5-HT_1 binding sites, dilates arterioles and constricts arteriovenous anastomoses. *British Journal of Pharmacology*, **84**, 533–544.
Saxena, P.R. and Villalón, C.M. (1990). Cardiovascular effects of serotonin agonists and antagonists. *Journal of Cardiovascular Pharmacology*, **15** (Suppl. 7), S17–S34.
Saxena, P.R., Bom, A.H. and Verdouw, P.D. (1989). Characterization of 5-hydroxytryptamine receptors in the cranial vasculature. *Cephalagia*, **9**, (Suppl. 9), 15–22.
Saxena, P.R., Duncker, D.J., Bom, A.H., Heiligers, J. and Verdouw, P.D. (1986). Effects of MDL-72222 and methiothepin on carotid vascular responses to 5-hydroxytryptamine in the pig: evidence for the presence of '5-$hydroxytryptamine_1$-like' receptors. *Naunyn-Schmiedeberg's Archives of Pharmacology*, **333**, 198–204.
Schnellman, R.G., Waters, S.J. and Nelson, D.L. (1984). [^{3}H]5-hydroxytryptamine binding sites: species and tissue variation. *Journal of Neurochemistry*, **42**, 65–70.
Shimokawa, H., Aarhus, L.L. and Vanhoutte, P.M. (1987). Porcine coronary arteries with regenerated endothelium have a reduced endothelium-dependent responsiveness to aggregating platelets and serotonin. *Circulation Research*, **61**, 256–270.
Stollack, J.S. and Furchgott, R.F. (1984). Use of selective antagonists for determining the types of receptors mediating the actions of 5-hydroxytryptamine and tryptamine in the isolated rabbit aorta. *Journal of Pharmacology and Experimental Therapy*, **224**, 215–221.

Sumner, M.J. and Humphrey, P.P.A. (1989). 5-HT_{1D} binding sites can be subdivided by GR43175. *British Journal of Pharmacology*, **98**, 29–31.

Sumner, M.J. and Humphrey, P.P.A. (1990). Sumatriptan (GR43175) inhibits cyclic-AMP accumulation in dog isolated saphenous vein. *British Journal of Pharmacology*, **99**, 219–220.

Taylor, E.W., Duckles, S.P. and Nelson, D.L. (1986). Dissociation constants of serotonin agonists in the canine basilar artery correlate to K_1 values at the 5-HT_{1A} binding site. *Journal of Pharmacology and Experimental Therapy*, **236**, 118–125.

Trevethic, M.A., Feniuk, W. and Humphrey, P.P.A. (1984). 5-Hydroxytryptamine-induced relaxation of neonatal porcine vena cava *in vitro*. *Life Sciences*, **35**, 477–486.

Travethick, M.A., Feniuk, W. and Humphrey, P.P.A. (1986). 5-Carboxamidotryptamine: a potent agonist mediating relaxation and elevation of cyclic AMP in the isolated neonatal procine vena cava. *Life Sciences*, **38**, 1512–1528.

Tuncer, M., Dogan, N., Ilhan, M. and Kayaalp, S.O. (1985). Serotonin-induced contraction of canine saphenous vein: mediation by 5-HT_1 receptors. *Archives Internationalés de Pharmacodynamie et de Thérapie*, **274**, 305–312.

Van Charldorp, K.J. and Wouters, W. (1990). Close similarity between contraction mediating 5-HT_1-like receptors in porcine basilar arteries and canine saphenous vein. *Naunyn Schmiedeberg's Archives of Pharmacology*, **341** (Suppl.), Abstract 353, R89.

Van Nueten, J.M. (1983). 5-hydroxytryptamine and precapillary vessels. *Federation Proceedings*, **42**, 223–227.

Van Nueten, J.M., Leysen, J.E., De Clerck, F. and Vanhoutte, P.M. (1984). Serotonergic receptor subtypes and vascular reactivity. *Journal of Cardiovascular Pharmacology*, **6**, S564–S574.

Van Nueten, J.M., Janssen, P.A.J., Van Beek, J., Xhonneux, R., Verbeuren, T.J. and Vanhoutte, P.M. (1981). Vascular effects of ketanserin (R 41 468), a novel antagonist of 5-HT_2 serotonergic receptors. *Journal of Pharmacology and Experimental Therapy*, **218**, 217–230.

Verdouw, P.D., Jennewein, H.M., Mierau, J. and Saxena, P.R. (1985). *N*-(3-Acetylaminophenil) piperazine hydrochloride (BEA 1654), a putative 5-HT_1 agonist, causes constriction of arteriovenous anastomoses and dilatation of arterioles. *European Journal of Pharmacology*, **107**, 337–346.

Villalón, C.M. den Boer, M.O. Heiligers, J.P.C. and Saxena, P.R. (1990). Mediation of 5-hydroxytryptamine-induced tachycardia in the pig by the putative 5-HT_4 receptor. *British Journal of Pharmacology*, **100**, 665–667.

Chapter 20

CNS effects of stimulating 5-HT receptor subtypes

Rosario Samanin

20.1. *Introduction*

Since the discovery of serotonin (5-HT) in the brain (Twarog and Page, 1953) research has been greatly facilitated by the mapping of 5-HT containing neurones with histofluorescence methods (Dahlström and Fuxe, 1965) and by the availability of substances that altered central serotonergic transmission with a certain degree of selectivity (Garattini and Samanin, 1978) e.g. *p*-chlorophenylalanine, an inhibitor of tryptophan hydroxylase, 5,6,- or 5,7-dihdydroxytryptamine, selective serotonergic neurotoxins in appropriate conditions, and several 5-HT receptor blockers (Garattini and Samanin, 1978). Recent studies, however, suggest that some 5-HT uptake blockers such as fluoxetine, have a less specific effect on 5-HT transmission than initially suggested (Samanin and Garattini, 1990).

The discovery that *d*-lysergic acid diethylamide (LSD-25), a 5-HT receptor antagonist in the periphery, mimicked the inhibitory action of 5-HT on serotonergic neurones in the raphe nuclei and that other hallucinogenic substances such as dimethyltryptamine, bufotenine and psilocybin had the same effects (Aghajanian and Haigler, 1975), was the first apparently well-documented description of a central effect related to activation of 5-HT receptors. 5-HT receptors are still considered to be involved in the perceptual effects of LSD-25 and the other substances, but the location and the nature of these receptors are not clear, nor is it known whether their action on 5-HT receptors is sufficient for the hallucinogenic effects (Glennon *et al.*, 1986).

20.2. *5-HT receptors*

20.2.1. **The discovery of subtypes**

By examining specific binding to frontal cortex of the rat, Peroutka and Synder (1979) suggested that [^{3}H]-5-HT and [^{3}H]-spiroperidol labelled two distinct classes of binding sites, named 5-HT_1 and 5-HT_2 respectively. [^{3}H]-LSD apparently labelled both receptors with the same affinity. The spiroperidol displacement of [^{3}H]-5-HT binding was not monophasic, and Pedigo *et al.* (1981) suggested that this indicated the existence of two populations of 5-HT receptors: they corresponded to the sites for which spiperone showed high or low affinity and were named 5-HT_{1A} and 5-HT_{1B} subtype, respectively. A third 5-HT receptor subtype, named 5-HT_{1C}, was discovered by Pazos *et al.* (1984) in the choroid plexus in autoradiographic studies with [^{3}H]-5-HT. Finally, in bovine brain, where there appear to be no 5-HT_{1B} sites, Heuring and Peroutka (1987) identified a fourth 5-HT_1 receptor, named 5-HT_{1D}, whose pharmacological characteristics did not correspond to any of the other 5-HT_1 receptor subtypes previously described.

Kilpatrick *et al.* (1987) provided evidence for 5-HT_3 receptors in the rat brain by studying the high-affinity binding of [^{3}H]-GR 65630, a selective antagonist of peripheral 5-HT_3 receptors. The 5-HT_3 receptor is pharmacologically indistinguishable from the M-receptors originally described in the guinea-pig ileum, whereas the 5-HT_2 type closely resembles the D-receptor (Frazer *et al.*, 1990).

Although the existence of other subtypes for 5-HT_1, 5-HT_2 and 5-HT_3 receptors and of a 5-HT_4 type has been suggested (see Frazer *et al.*, 1990), the 5-HT_{1A}–5-HT_{1D} subtypes and the 5-HT_2 and 5-HT_3 types are those best characterized so far and this review is essentially limited to examining the distribution, effects and suggested functions of these receptors in the mammalian central nervous system (CNS).

The existence of multiple 5-HT receptors in the CNS has been confirmed by biochemical, physiological and behavioural studies (see Conn and Sanders-Bush, 1987; Peroutka, 1988; Frazer *et al.*, 1990), although the lack of highly selective agonists and antagonists for most 5-HT receptor subtypes seriously limits progress (Glennon, 1990; Van Wijngaarden *et al.*, 1990).

The primary structure of some 5-HT receptor subtypes — 5-HT_{1C}, 5-HT_2, 5-HT_{1A} — has been recently described (see Hartig, 1989), confirming that they are distinct proteins mediating specific functions. Furthermore, it has been suggested (Hartig, 1989; Schmidt and Peroutka, 1989) that 5-HT receptors belong to three main families. One comprises the 5-HT_{1A}, 5-HT_{1B} and 5-HT_{1D} receptors: they are coupled to G-proteins and linked to adenylate cyclase as second messenger. The second family of 5-HT receptors is marked by structural homology between 5-HT_{1C} and 5-HT_2 receptors, their utilization of the phosphoinositide second messenger pathway through coupling to G-protein and their close pharmacological similarities. Finally, there is a family of ligands directly coupled to ion channels to which the 5-HT_3 receptors belong.

20.2.2. $5\text{-}HT_{1A}$ receptors

a. *Characteristics and distribution of binding sites*

A very useful agent for studying these receptors in the CNS is 8-hydroxy-2-(di-*n*-propyl-amino-tetraline; 8-OH-DPAT). This compound shows high affinity (lower than 10 nM) and selectivity for the $5\text{-}HT_{1A}$ binding sites (Hoyer, 1988), and the labelled compound has been used for mapping receptor distribution in the presence of different compounds (Pazos *et al.*, 1988).

Very high densities of $5\text{-}HT_{1A}$ binding sites labelled with [^{3}H]-8-OH-DPAT or [^{3}H]-5-HT are found in the hippocampus, raphe nuclei and some layers of the cerebral cortex in the human brain. A similar pattern is found in the rat although in the human the density of $5\text{-}HT_{1A}$ sites is highest over the CA1 field while in rat the dentate gyrus is the richest region. External layers of human frontal and striate cortex are particularly rich in $5\text{-}HT_{1A}$ sites while the internal layers of the rat cortex contain the highest density. Substantial amounts are also found in the nucleus centralis of the amygdala, the nucleus paramedianus of the thalamus and the locus coeruleus of human brain and in the lateral septal nucleus of the rat (Pazos *et al.*, 1987, 1988).

Except for raphe nuclei, these binding sites seem to be postsynaptic to 5-HT-containing neurones since autoreceptors in nerve terminals have been classified as the $5\text{-}HT_{1B}$ or $5\text{-}HT_{1D}$ type, depending on the animal species (Hoyer and Middlemiss, 1989). The binding of [^{3}H]-8-OH-DPAT in the striatum was reduced in animals with selective destruction of 5-HT neurones, but this was probably due to the affinity of 8-OH-DPAT for the sodium-dependent 5-HT uptake carrier in this region.

b. *Pharmacological agents*

Ipsapirone, gepirone and flesinoxan, like 8-OH-DPAT, behave as specific $5\text{-}HT_{1A}$ receptor agonists or partial agonists depending on the brain region examined whereas buspirone, a non-benzodiazepine anxiolytic agent, shows similar affinity for $5\text{-}HT_{1A}$ and D_2 binding sites (Van Wijngaarden *et al.*, 1990). β-Adrenergic receptor antagonists such as cyanopindolol, (−)-pindolol and (−)-propranolol are commonly used as they act as antagonists at $5\text{-}HT_{1A}$ and $5\text{-}HT_{1B}$ receptors (Hoyer, 1988). Non-selective antagonists such as spiperone, methysergide, metergoline and others are also occasionally used.

c. *Neurophysiological responses*

$5\text{-}HT_{1A}$ receptor agonists were found to suppress the spontaneous firing of serotonergic neurones in the dorsal raphe (DR) when administered microiontophoretically. The effect of 8-OH-DPAT was blocked by (−)-propranolol but the effect of 5-HT itself was not (Sprouse and Aghajanian,

Table 20.1. Characteristics of $5\text{-}HT_{1A}$ receptors.

Main ligands	[^{3}H]-5-HT (in the presence of compounds having affinity for other 5-HT binding sites), [^{3}H]-8-OH-DPAT, [^{3}H]-ipsapirone, [^{3}H]-PAPP
Highest densities in the brain	Hippocampus, raphe nuclei, some cerebral cortical layers
Pharmacological agents	8-OH-DPAT, gepirone, ipsapirone, buspirone flesinoxan, (−)-pindolol, cyanopindolol, (−)-propranolol, spiperone
Neurophysiological responses	Hyperpolarization of membrane potential of raphe and hippocampal cells through a cAMP-independent increase in potassium conductance
Biochemical effects	Stimulation or inhibition of adenylase cyclase. Reduction of 5-HT release from nerve terminals through activation of autoreceptors in the raphe area
Physiological and behavioural effects	Anxiolytic and antidepressive effects, increased appetite, hypotension, anticataleptic effect, complex influence on sexual behavior and pain responses

1986). This suggests that the firing rate of DR neurones is under inhibitory control of somatodendritic autoreceptors, some of which are of the $5\text{-}HT_{1A}$ type.

Intravenously administered 8-OH-DPAT also potently suppresses the firing rate of DR cells ($ED_{50} = 0{\cdot}4\,\mu g\ Kg^{-1}$) while a higher dose was required to inhibit neurones in the median raphe nucleus (MR, $ED_{50} = 11\,\mu g\,kg^{-1}$) (Sinton and Fallon, 1988). This difference may be of functional significance since these two nuclei seem to mediate different behavioural effects of $5\text{-}HT_{1A}$ agonists (Carli and Samanin, 1988; Cervo *et al.*, 1988a). The inhibition of 5-HT neurones in the DR is presumably mediated by a G-protein since it was blocked by pertussis toxin. Using intracellular recordings in brain slices it was seen that activation of $5\text{-}HT_{1A}$ receptors in the DR induced hyperpolarization through a cAMP-independent increase in potassium conductance (Innis *et al.*, 1988).

Microelectrophoresis and intracellular recording studies have found similar effects with $5\text{-}HT_{1A}$ receptor agonists on hippocampal CA1 pyramidal cells, although here they behave as partial agonists. In conditions in which the synaptic availability of 5-HT is elevated (for instance in some stressful situations), partial agonists may reduce the postsynaptic effects of 5-HT while at the same time activating inhibitory autoreceptors. The net result is complete blockade of 5-HT transmission. A preferential presynaptic effect of partial $5\text{-}HT_{1A}$ agonists appears to be facilitated by the purported existence of a large receptor reserve in the raphe nuclei autoreceptors. Ligands to $5\text{-}HT_{1B}$ receptors produce little or no effect on DR or hippocampal neurones (Sprouse and Aghajanian, 1988).

After 14 days treatment with the $5\text{-}HT_{1A}$ agonist gepirone, the reduction by iontophoretic 5-HT agonists in firing activity of DR 5-HT neurones was attenuated; the effect on hippocampal pyramidal cells was unchanged (Blier and de Montigny, 1987). These findings suggest that somatodendritic 5-HT_{1A} receptors are desensitized after chronic treatment with 5-HT_{1A} agonists.

5-HT_{1A} agonists also cause neuronal inhibition in the cerebral cortex, the ventromedial hypothalamus, the lateral septum and the locus coeruleus (Bobker and Williams, 1989).

d. *Biochemical effects*

The hypothesis that 5-HT_{1A} binding sites might mediate physiological responses to 5-HT was strongly corroborated by the finding that these sites are linked to adenylate cyclase in some brain regions (Shenker *et al.*, 1987; Bockaert *et al.*, 1990).

In agreement with the finding that 5-HT_{1A} agonists activate somatodendritic 5-HT receptors, 8-OH-DPAT at subcutaneous doses ranging from 30 to 300 $\mu g\,kg^{-1}$ reduced 5-HT synthesis in the rat brain. This effect was attributed to an action on cell bodies against terminal 5-HT autoreceptors since they depended on the impulse flow of serotonergic neurones (Hjorth and Magnusson, 1988). In support of the electrophysiological findings, 8-OH-DPAT reduces 5-HT metabolism in the DR more than the MR, and reduces 5-HT synthesis preferentially in their respective projection areas (striatum and cortex from DR, hypothalamus and hippocampus from MR) (Scatton *et al.*, 1989; Invernizzi *et al.*, 1990). These differences are important for interpreting the effects of systemically administered 5-HT_{1A} agonists, as various behavioural responses have been attributed to an action on somatodendritic autoreceptors in the raphe area (Bendotti and Samanin, 1986; Carli and Samanin, 1988; Cervo *et al.*, 1988a; Carli *et al.*, 1989; Invernizzi *et al.*, 1988).

In apparent contrast with electrophysiological and behavioural data (Blier and de Montigny, 1987; Kennett *et al.*, 1987b), no attenuation of the effect of 8-OH-DPAT or setraline (a 5-HT uptake blocker) on 5-HT turnover was found after chronic treatment (Larsson *et al.*, 1990; R. Invernizzi and R. Samanin, unpublished results). It appears that desensitization of 5-HT_{1A} autoreceptors does not easily develop after repeated treatment with agents which directly or indirectly activate them: continuous release of the drug (see Blier and de Montigny, 1987) might be necessary.

e. *Physiological and behavioural effects*

The bulk of data suggests that specific activation of presynaptic 5-HT_{1A} receptors causes anxiolytic-like effects not very different from those seen with benzodiazepines and barbiturates. Buspirone, a clinically-used non-benzodiazepine anxiolytic drug, shows affinity for 5-HT_{1A} binding sites (Peroutka, 1988), and 5-HT_{1A} receptors in the raphe area may be involved in the anxiolytic effect (Carli *et al.*, 1989). However buspirone has a similar affinity for D_2 receptors and its metabolite, 1-(2-pyrimidinyl)-piperazine (1-PP), acts as an antagonist at α_2-adrenoceptors. Dopamine receptors may also be involved (Merlo Pich and Samanin, 1986).

5-HT_{1A} agonists may possess antidepressant properties as 8-OH-DPAT is active in the forced swimming (Cervo and Samanin, 1987) and helplessness (Giral *et al.*, 1988) models. In the forced swimming test the effect of peripherally administered 8-OH-DPAT was found to depend on intact serotonergic neurones and could be produced by directly injecting 8-OH-DPAT in the DR (Cervo *et al.*, 1988a). The latter procedure was still effective after chronic treatment, suggesting that no desensitization of 5-HT_{1A} autoreceptors had occurred (Cervo and Samanin, 1991). Interestingly, buspirone was active in this test only when administered directly in the DR, probably because the α_2-adrenergic blocking effect of its metabolite, 1-PP, interfered with the antidepressant-like effect (Cervo *et al.*, 1988b).

It is not clear whether pre- or postsynaptic 5-HT_{1A} sites are involved in the effect of 5-HT_{1A} agonists in the helpless behaviour of rats. It was suggested that postsynaptic receptors were involved in the ability of 5-HT_{1A} agonists to block the behaviour of restrained rats in an open field, a suggested model of animal depression (Kennett *et al.*, 1987a).

A robust effect of 5-HT_{1A} agonists is to increase feeding in rats (Dourish *et al.*, 1985), a behaviour widely assumed to be under the inhibitory control of the central 5-HT system. 8-OH-DPAT usually enhances feeding in satiated rats, whereas in starved rats food intake is reduced, probably because of motor effects which are particularly evident in food-deprived rats (Bendotti and Samanin, 1987). The increase in eating with 8-OH-DPAT was prevented by intracerebroventricular injection of a 5-HT neurotoxin (Bendotti and Samanin, 1986) suggesting that 5-HT neurones were involved. Moreover, 8-OH-DPAT injection in the raphe nuclei significantly increased eating by free-feeding rats (Bendotti and Samanin, 1986). This effect was attributed to 8-OH-DPAT's ability to stimulate somatodendritic autoreceptors and confirmed that a reduction in central 5-HT transmission may facilitate feeding.

It has been argued that 8-OH-DPAT causes animals to eat solid foods by inducing gnawing since glucose consumption was reduced, not raised, by $60\text{–}120\,\mu g\,kg^{-1}$ in non-deprived rats. However, studies have shown that 8-OH-DPAT also increases consumption of palatable wet mash and liquid diets (Dourish *et al.*, 1988) and 8-OH-DPAT injected in the raphe nuclei elicited no gnawing response (Bendotti and Samanin, 1986). Other 5-HT_{1A} agonists such as buspirone and ipsapirone, which do not cause gnawing, enhance food intake in non-fasted rats (Dourish *et al.*, 1986; Wong and Reid, 1987).

8-OH-DPAT facilitates some aspects of sexual behaviour in male rats, but inhibits lordosis in female rats and has little effect on sexual behaviour in mice. The effects in male rats are probably not mediated by 5-HT_{1A} receptors as they are not blocked by appropriate 5-HT antagonists — effects on sensorimotor and motivational levels may be responsible (see Bevan, 1989). Studies with 5-HT_{1A} agonists on pain responses are also complex, as both hyperalgesia and analgesia have been reported. The type of stimulus may influence the response (see Hamon *et al.*, 1990).

Preliminary findings suggest that 5-HT_{1A} agonists impair passive avoidance and spatial learning, but further studies are needed to assess the role of 5-HT_{1A} receptors in the control of cognitive behaviour. Of particular interest is the fact that 5-HT_{1A} agonists such as 8-OH-DPAT and fesinoxan cause hypotension and bradycardia by acting on various central nuclei including the DR (Fozard *et al.*, 1987; Connor and Higgins, 1990). Thus, 5-HT_{1A} agonists may be helpful in the treatment of hypertension.

For more details on the behavioural effects of 5-HT_{1A} agonists, including those not mentioned here, the reader is referred to recent literature (Osborne and Hamon, 1988; Paoletti *et al.*, 1990; Semanin and Garattini, 1990).

20.2.3. **5-HT_{1B} receptors**

a. *Characteristics and distribution of binding sites*

The 5-HT_{1B} binding site was initially characterized by the low-affinity spiperone-competition curve for [^{3}H]-5-HT binding to rat brain cortex (Pedigo *et al.*, 1981), but most information on their distribution derives from studies on specific binding of [^{3}H]-5-HT in the presence of drugs blocking other 5-HT_1 receptor subtypes (8-OH-DPAT for 5-HT_{1A} and mesulergine for 5-HT_{1C}). Competition curves with ($\pm$)-SDZ 21-009, a compound with very high affinity for 5-HT_{1B} sites, have also been used to identify these sites (Waeber *et al.*, 1989b).

In the mouse and rat brain, the highest densities of 5-HT_{1B} binding sites are found in the globus pallidus and substantia nigra pars reticulata. The dorsal subiculum and central grey also have high densities. Although the density is moderate in the caudate-putamen of rat brain, most binding sites in this region are of the 5-HT_{1B} type. Substantial amounts of 5-HT_{1B} binding sites are found in the dentate gyrus and in the superficial layers of the cerebral cortex (Pazos *et al.*, 1988).

Interestingly, only mice and rats appear to have 5-HT_{1B} binding sites; brain regions that in the rat have the highest density of 5-HT_{1B} sites contain in higher mammals a 5-HT_1 subtype, named 5-HT_{1D}, whose pharmacological characteristics differ from those of 5-HT_{1B} sites (Waeber *et al.*, 1989a,b).

b. *Pharmacological agents*

As mentioned above, no specific agonist exists for the 5-HT_{1B} receptor, with the possible exception of two agents, CGS-1266B and CP-93,129. RU-24 969, which has agonist high affinity for 5-HT_{1A} and 5-HT_{1B} sites has been

Table 20.2. Characteristics of 5-HT_{1B} receptors.

Main ligands	[^{3}H]-5-HT (in the presence of compounds having affinity for other 5-HT binding sites), [^{125}I]-cyanopindolol
Highest densities in the brain	Globus pallidus, substantia nigra pars reticulata, dorsal subiculum in mouse and rat brain. Absent in higher mammals
Pharmacological agents	CGS-1266B, CP-93,129, RU-24 969, mCPP, TFMPP, (−)-pindolol, (−)-propranolol
Neurophysiological responses	Inhibition of neuronal activity in the locus coeruleus
Biochemical effects	Inhibition of adenylate cyclase Inhibitory effect on the release of 5-HT and other transmitters from nerve terminals
Behavioural effects	Decreased appetite, increased anxiety, depression, inhibitory influence on nociceptive responses

used to study 5-HT_{1B} receptors (Carli *et al.*, 1988; Hoyer, 1988). Antagonism of its effects by (−)-pindolol, an antagonist at 5-HT_{1A} and 5-HT_{1B} sites, and a lack of effect of spiperone, an agent blocking 5-HT_{1A} but not 5-HT_{1B} receptors, suggests 5-HT_{1B} involvement. Differences between 8-OH-DPAT and RU-24 969 may serve to clarify 5-HT_{1B} functions. Phenylpiperazines such as *m*-chlorophenylpiperazine (*m*CPP) and 1-(3-trifluoromethylphenyl) piperazine (TFMPP) have been used as 5-HT_{1B} agonists (Kennett *et al.*, 1987a, 1988), but they act on several 5-HT receptors, with a high affinity for the 5-HT_{1C} subtype.

c. *Neurophysiological responses*

To our knowledge the only region where responses to 5-HT have been classified as 5-HT_{1B} is the locus coeruleus (LC). 5-Carboxamidotryptamine (5-CT), which has high agonist affinity for 5-HT_{1A} and 5-HT_{1B} sites, inhibited γ-aminobutyric acid (GABA) and glutamate-mediated synaptic potentials in this area (Bobker and Williams, 1989).

d. *Biochemical effects*

High affinity agonists at 5-HT sites inhibited the forskolin-stimulated adenylate cyclase in membranes from rat substantia nigra with an order of potency correlating with their affinity for 5-HT_{1B} sites. Ergolines such as metergoline and methysergide behave as agonists at these receptors (Schoeffter and Hoyer, 1989).

Using the release of [^{3}H]-5-HT, a correlation was found between the drugs' potency in reducing release and affinity for the 5-HT_{1B} site. In synaptosomes from rat brain, 5-HT autoreceptors are of the 5-HT_{1B} type (Raiteri *et al.*, 1986). Postsynaptic 5-HT_{1B} receptors may also act as inhibitory heteroreceptors on nerve terminals containing acetylcholine and dopamine.

e. *Behavioural studies*

RU-24969 has been reported to reduce food intake dose-dependently in rats. At higher doses it caused hyperlocomotion and hyper-reactivity but this did not interfere with eating since metergoline, a non-selective 5-HT antagonist, reduced the anorectic effect but not the motor stimulation; the reverse applied to haloperidol (Bendotti and Samanin, 1987).

Quipazine and mCPP also reduced rats' food intake by a metergoline-sensitive mechanism (Samanin *et al.*, 1979), but 5-HT_2 receptors are involved in quipazine's effect. Both *m*CPP and TFMPP apparently use 5-HT_{1B} and 5-HT_{1C} sites to cause anorexia (Kennet and Curzon, 1988). Recently CP-93,129, a specific 5-HT_{1B} receptor agonist, was found to reduce food intake when administered into the paraventricular nucleus of the hypothalamus.

RU-24969 appears to have 'anxiogenic' effects in a test of conditioned suppression of drinking (Carli *et al.*, 1988). Moreover, studies with TFMPP administered into the ventral tegmentum suggest that 5-HT_{1B} receptors here act by opposing antidepressant-like effects in the forced swimming test (Cervo *et al.*, 1989). TFMPP, mCPP and quipazine were reported to reduce nociceptive responses in conditions in which 8-OH-DPAT increased rats' sensitivity to noxious stimuli (see Hamon *et al.*, 1990).

20.2.4. **5-HT_{1C} receptors**

a. *Characteristics and distribution of binding sites*

These sites were first detected in choroid plexus epithelial cells (Pazos *et al.*, 1985). Using mRNA isolated from choroid plexus and injected into frog oocytes, a 5-HT-stimulated chloride current was produced which showed a profile typical of a 5-HT_{1C} site (Julius *et al.*, 1988). *In situ* hybridization was then used to map the distribution of the 5-HT_{1C} mRNA in mouse and rat brain (Molineaux *et al.*, 1989; Mengod *et al.*, 1990). Besides the choroid plexus other regions, such as hippocampus, sriatum, substantia nigra and brain-stem nuclie, contained high levels. The general distribution of 5-HT_{1C} binding sites in rat and human brain are reported to be similar.

b. *Pharmacological agents*

Mesulergine, commonly used as a 5-HT_{1C} antagonist has high affinity for 5-HT_2 sites and D2 receptors. TFMPP and *m*CPP behave as agonists at 5-HT_{1C} sites and have been used to study the behavioural output of 5-HT_{1C} sites. Even when used with appropriate antagonists, however, their selectivity is poor (Hoyer, 1988; Van Wijngaarden *et al.*, 1990).

Table 20.3. Characteristics of 5-HT_{1C} receptors.

Main ligands	[^{3}H]-5-HT (in the presence of compounds having affinity for other 5-HT_1 binding sites), [^{3}H]-mesulergine
Highest densities in the brain	Choroid plexus, limbic system, ventral striatum, substantia nigra, some nuclei in the lower brain-stem
Pharmacological agents	TFMPP, *m*CPP, mesulergine
Biochemical effects	Stimulation of phosphoinositide hydrolysis in the choroid plexus
Behavioural effects	Hypophagia, anxiety, penil erection, migraine, hallucinogenesis

c. *Biochemical effects*

5-HT_{1C} receptors are positively linked to phosphatidylinositol turnover in the choroid plexus, but it is not known whether this is true in other brain regions or whether the hyperpolarization and increased chloride current seen in oocytes is a characteristic of 5-HT_{1C} receptors in the CNS of mammals.

d. *Behavioural effects*

It has been suggested that part of the hypophagic effect of *m*CPP and TFMPP is mediated by 5-HT_{1C} receptors (Kennett and Curzon, 1988) since drugs with high affinity for 5-HT_{1C} sites partially reduced their effects. However, cyproheptadine did not modify the effects of *m*CPP, and the effect of mesulergine depends on the time of day. Ritanserin, with affinity at 5-HT_{1C} sites at least equal to mesulergine, did not modify feeding or the effect of *m*CPP (Dourish *et al.*, 1989).

The proposal that *m*CPP causes anxiety, penile erection and migraine via activation of 5-HT_{1C} receptors needs confirmation with more selective ligands. Hallucinogens such as 1-(2,5-dimethoxy-4-methylphenyl)-2-aminopropane (DOM) and 1-(2,5-dimethoxy-4-iodophenyl)-2-aminopropane (DOI) behave as high affinity agonists at 5-HT_{1C} and 5-HT_2 sites (Van Wijngaarden *et al.*, 1990), but the importance of these receptors in human hallucinogenesis remains to be established.

20.2.5. **5-HT_{1D} receptors**

a. *Characteristics and distribution of binding sites*

Binding sites were identified in bovine brain using [^{3}H]-5-HT in the presence of 5-HT_{1A} and 5-HT_{1C} ligands (Heuring and Peroutka, 1987). Although

Table 20.4. Characteristics of 5-HT_{1D} receptors.

Main ligands	$[^3H]$-5-HT (in the presence of compounds having affinity for other 5-HT_1 binding sites)
Highest densities in the brain	Basal ganglia, dorsal subiculum, central grey, superior colliculus
Pharmacological agents	Several tryptamines, 5-CT, ergolines
Biochemical effects	Inhibition of adenylate cyclase in calf substantia nigra Inhibition of 5-HT release from nerve terminals (autoreceptors) in guinea-pig, pig and human cerebral cortex
Physiological effects	Alleviation of migraine attacks

present in rat brain, 5-HT_{1D} sites are also found in those brain regions of higher mammals, including humans, which correspond to those possessing 5-HT_{1B} sites in the rat. In the basal ganglia of cat, guinea-pig and human, most $[^3H]$5-HT binding sites are of the 5-HT_{1D} type: the dorsal subiculum, central grey and superior colliculus are rich in these sites.

A human cDNA clone transfected into mouse fibroblast cells led to the expression of a 5-HT_{1D}-like receptor. In view of the low homology with other 5-HT receptors, it was suggested that this may represent a novel 5-HT receptor family.

b. *Pharmacological agents*

Several tryptamines, 5-CT and ergolines show high affinity for 5-HT_{1D} binding sites although they also act at other 5-HT sites (Hoyer, 1988). Certain drugs behaving as antagonists at 5-HT_{1B} receptors act as agonists at 5-HT_{1D} sites (Schoeffter and Hoyer, 1989), including β-adrenoceptor antagonists (e.g. (−)-propranolol) and α-adrenoceptor antagonists (e.g. yohimbine). These findings further indicate that 5-HT_{1B} and 5-HT_{1D} receptors have different pahrmacology.

c. *Biochemical effects*

Since both 5-HT and 5-CT inhibit forskolin-stimulated adenylate cyclase in the presence of 5-HT antagonists, 5-HT_{1D} receptors may be negatively linked to the cyclase in calf substantia nigra. In human prefrontal cortex and striatum 5-HT_{1D} receptors are coupled to a G-protein, but the second messenger or ion channel is not known. There is evidence that autoreceptors on 5-HT nerve terminals of human, pig and guinea-pig cerebral cortex are of the 5-HT_{1D} type.

Table 20.5. Characteristics of 5-HT_2 receptors.

Main ligands	[^{3}H]-LSD, [^{3}H]-spiperone, [^{3}H]-ketanserin, [^{H}]-DOB, [^{3}H]-DOI
Highest densities in the brain	Cerebral cortex, claustrum, olfactory system
Pharmacological agents	Ketanserin, ritanserin, DOB, DOI, quipazine
Neurophysiological effects	Neuronal facilitation, tonic inhibition of other 5-HT receptors
Biochemical effects	Stimulation of inositol hydrolisis in cerebral cortex but not in subcortical regions Activation of phospholipase A_2 in hippocampal and cortical neurones
Physiological and behavioural effects	Hallucinogenesis, modulation of pain perception, influence on motor, feeding, sexual, affective and cognitive behaviour

d. *Physiological and behavioural effects*

It has been proposed that sumatriptan reduces migraine attacks by activating 5-HT_{1D} receptors, but this agent displays high affinity for other 5-HT sites. Considering that autoreceptors on 5-HT terminals are of the 5-HT_{1D} variety, and the analogies between 5-HT_{1B} receptors in rat and 5-HT_{1D} sites in human, the latter are likely to be involved in the control of many brain functions, including feeding and emotional responses.

20.2.6. **5-HT_2 receptors**

a. *Characteristics and distribution of binding sites*

It has been suggested that two affinity states of the 5-HT_2 receptor exist: one with high affinity for agonists and sensitive to guanyl nucleotides, the other with low agonist affinity and unaffected by GTP (Lyon *et al.*, 1987). Since the high affinity site was not identified in bovine frontal cortex it was suggested that it indicated a receptor subtype named 5-HT_{2A} distinct from the low affinity 5-HT_{2B}. However species and experimental conditions are now thought to be responsible for these differences. Recently the hallucinogenic phenylisopropylamines [^{3}H]-DOB (4-bromo-2,5-dimethoxyphenyl isopropylamine) and [^{125}I]-DOI have been used to label the high affinity agonist state of the 5-HT_2 receptor.

On the basis that the pharmacology of 5-HT_2 and 5-HT_{1C} sites is similar and both are coupled to phospholipase C, it has been suggested that 5-HT_{1C} sites belong to the 5-HT_2 receptor family. This has been supported by the isolation of a clone encoding the 5-HT_2 receptor which showed 49% identity with 5-HT_{1C} receptor and 80% within the transmembrane domains (Pritchett *et al.*, 1988; Julius *et al.*, 1990). This close similarity raises the question of whether, in brain regions rich in 5-HT_{1C} receptors, labelling of the high affinity 5-HT_2 site may coincide with the 5-HT_{1C} site.

The most complete studies on the distribution of 5-HT_2 binding sites in rat and human brain have been performed with [^{3}H]-ketanserin (Pazos *et al.*, 1987). High concentrations were found in cerebral cortex, claustrum and the olfactory system, with intermediate levels in striatum, nucleus accumbens and dentate gyrus.

b. *Pharmacological agents*

Ketanserin and ritanserin are frequently used as 5-HT_2 receptor antagonists, but their specificity is limited as the former displays high affinity for α-adrenoceptors and the latter for 5-HT_{1C} binding sites. Similar problems arise with DOI which has high affinity for 5-HT_{1C} receptors (Van Wijngaarden *et al.*, 1990). Potentially useful agents are *m*CPP and TFMPP since they act as antagonists at 5-HT_2 receptors and agonists at 5-HT_{1C} receptors (Conn and Sanders-Bush, 1987).

c. *Neurophysiological effects*

Neuronal facilitation or excitation by activation of presumed 5-HT_2 receptors has been described in facial motoneurones nucleus accumbens, neocortex, claustrum and olfactory system (see Bobker and Wiliams, 1990). The effect seem to be mediated by a decrease in K^+ conductance.

d. *Biochemical effects*

At micromolar concentrations 5-HT stimulates inositol phosphoinositide hydrolysis in rat cerebral cortex slices, and the effect is blocked by various 5-HT receptor antagonists with a rank order of potency indicating a 5-HT_2 receptor (Conn and Sanders-Bush, 1984; Kendall and Nahorski, 1985). The recently described translocation of protein kinase C caused by 5-HT and DOI in rat cortical slices, and its blockade by ketanserin, indirectly confirms that cortical 5-HT_2 receptors are coupled to phospholipase C, although there are alternative explanations.

Studies in hippocampal neurones co-cultured with glia cells have shown that 5-HT stimulated the release of arachidonic acid by an extracellular calcium-dependent mechanism (Felder *et al.*, 1990). A similar effect was found in cortical neurones, but not elsewhere. Pharmacological characterization suggested that this effect was mediated by 5-HT_2 receptors. The finding that 5-HT can activate phospholipase A2 in hippocampus and cerebral cortex is particularly interesting in view of recent evidence that arachidonic acid and its eicosanoid metabolites are involved in several central physiological and pathological processes.

5-HT receptors may act as inhibitory heteroreceptors on striatal dopaminergic, hippocampal cholinergic and cerebellar glutamatergic neurones in the rat.

e. *Regulation of other 5-HT receptor types*

An interesting characteristic of 5-HT_2 receptors is that their blockade facilitates the expression of other 5-HT receptor activity. This has been shown behaviourally (see Backus *et al.*, 1990) and electrophysiologically in the prefrontal cortex and lateral geniculate (but not DR) where blockade of 5-HT_2 receptors facilitated the neuronal inhibitory effect of activating 5-HT_1 receptors (Lakoski and Aghajanian, 1985). In the prefrontal cortex 8-OH-DPAT mimicked the effect of 5-HT. This is interesting since chronic treatment with tricycylic antidepressant agents reduced the density of 5-HT_2 receptors (Peroutka and Snyder, 1980), but enhanced the physiological effects of stimulating 5-HT_{1A} receptors (Welner *et al.*, 1989). Thus, enhanced transmission at 5-HT_1 receptors rather than decreased 5-HT_2 receptor activity may be involved in antidepressant activity. There is, however, no evidence that 5-HT_2 receptor antagonists exert antidepressant-like effects or facilitate the effect of 5-HT_{1A} receptor agonists in validated models of animal depression.

A tonic inhibitory influence of 5-HT_2 receptors on 5-HT_3 receptors governing the release of acetylcholine in rat entorhinal cortex is suggested by the fact that the inhibitory effect of 5-HT and 2-methyl-5-HT on acetylcholine release was seen only in the presence of ketanserin and was blocked by 5-HT_3 antagonists.

f. *Physiological and behavioural effects*

All the effects attributed to 5-HT_2 receptors should be considered provisional in view of the close similarities between 5-HT_2 and 5-HT_{1C} receptor pharmacology. Typical motor effects caused by activation of 5-HT_2 receptors are the head shakes (or twitches) observed in mice and, to a lesser extent, in rats. Preliminary reports suggest that activation of 5-HT_2 receptors reduces slow wave sleep and enhances rapid eye movement (REM) sleep (Idzikowski *et al.*, 1986; Pastel, 1988).

Correlative studies on human hallucinogenic properties, discriminative stimulus effects and affinity for 5-HT_2 binding sites suggest that indolealkylamine (tryptamines and LSD) and phenalkylamine (DOM, DOI) derivatives are hallucinogenic through agonist action at 5-HT_2 receptors (Glennon, 1990). However, the fact that some drugs to which the DOM-stimulus generalizes (fenfluramine, lisuride) are not hallucinogenic in humans suggests that 5-HT_2 receptor agonism may not be sufficient for hallucinogenesis (Glennon *et al.*, 1986). Moreover, most 5-HT_2 receptor agonists can act as agonists at 5-HT_{1C} receptors. Associational disturbances are probably in-

Table 20.6. Characteristics of 5-HT_3 receptors.

Main ligands	[^{3}H]-GR 65630 A, [^{3}H]-ICS 205-933, (S)-isomer of [^{3}H]-zacopride, [^{3}H]-quipazine, [^{3}H]-BRL 43694.
Highest densities in the brain	Nucleus of the tractus solitarius, area postrema, entorhinal, pyriform and temporal cortex, olfactory lobe and olfactory tubercle, some limbic regions
Pharmacological agents	2-Methyl-5-HT, 1-(*m*-chloropheynyl)-biguanide, GR 65630 A, ondansetron, ICS 205-993, BRL 43694 (granisetron)
Neurophysiological effects	Neuronal depolarization
Biochemical effects	Positively coupled to phospholipase C in rat entorhinal and frontal cortices. Facilitation of dopamine release in rat striatum (?) and inhibition of acetylcholine release in rat entorhinal cortex
Behavioural effects	5-HT_3 receptor antagonists may be useful in the treatment of emesis, anxiety, psychosis and memory disturbances

volved in the 5-HT_2 receptor-mediated hypophagia found with quipazine and DOI in rats (Hewson *et al.*, 1988; Schechter and Simansky, 1988). Several studies have found that 5-HT_2 receptor antagonists did not affect rat feeding (Dourish *et al.*, 1989; Samanin *et al.*, 1989).

Preliminary studies suggest that ritanserin may help alleviate some aspects of anxiety and depression in humans, but it has proved difficult to find clear-cut effects of ritanserin in established animal models of anxiety and depression (see Glennon, 1990). Using a new protocol for the elevated X-maze in rats, effects of ritanserin compatible with an anxiolytic activity were recently described. Antidepressant-like effects of ketanserin and ritanserin were found in one model presumed to measure impulse control (Marek *et al.*, 1989). Various antidepressant agents and 5-HT_2 receptor antagonists enhance rats' ability to wait for a food reward.

Various 5-HT_2 receptor antagonists have recently been found to improve the performance of hypoxic squirrel monkeys in a delayed match-to-sample task, suggesting that learning and/or memory processes are under the control of central 5-HT_2 receptors (DeNoble *et al.*, 1990).

20.2.7. **5-HT_3 receptors**

A detailed discussion of 5-HT_3 receptors can be found in Chapter 16 by Peters *et al.* (this volume).

a. *Characteristics and distribution of binding sites*

5-HT_3 binding sites have been identified in rat and human brain. Although in the periphery three 5-HT_3 receptor subtypes have been hypothesized

(Fozard, 1984), all the ligands used to date apparently label a single receptor site in the CNS. The highest levels of specific 5-HT_3 binding are found in discrete nuclei of the lower brain-stem, particularly the nucleus of the tractus solitarius and the area postrema (Pratt *et al.*, 1990).

b. *Pharmacological agents*

2-Methyl-5-HT, a 5-HT_3 receptor agonist, shows affinity for 5-HT_1 receptor subtypes similar to that for 5-HT_3 receptors (Van Wijngaarden *et al.*, 1990). Recently, 1-(*m*-chlorophenyl)-biguanide was found to be a potent 5-HT_3 receptor agonist with no significant effect on other 5-HT receptors (Kilpatrick *et al.*, 1990). A quaternized analogue of 5-HT (*N*,*N*,*N*-trimethyl-5-HT) also showed high affinity for 5-HT_3 receptors labelled by [^{3}H]-LY 278584 (Glennon *et al.*, 1990).

c. *Neurophysiology*

Activation of 5-HT_3 receptors causes depolarization and transmitter release in peripheral neurones. Voltage-clamp studies have shown that activating 5-HT_3 receptors causes an inward current by opening a cationic, non-selective, ligand-gated channel, permeable to Na, K and probably Ca ions. The rapid activation of the cationic channel, prompt desensitization and blockade by curare, have led to the suggestion that the 5-HT_3 receptor closely resembles the nicotinic receptor and probably belongs to the nicotine–$GABA_A$–glycine family of receptors directly coupled to ion channels (see Bobker and Williams, 1990).

Although GTP or ATP are not necessary for ion channel opening mediated by 5-HT_3 receptors, and studies using the radiation inactivation technique suggest that the 5-HT_3 receptor is not coupled to G-proteins in rat cortex, preliminary findings suggest that 5-HT_3 receptors, like 5-HT_2 ones, may be positively coupled to phospholipase C in rat entorhinal and frontal cortices (Wang *et al.*, 1990).

d. *Biochemical effects*

It has been reported that 5-HT and 2-methyl-5-HT increased spontaneous and K^+-evoked release of endogenous dopamine in superfused rat striatal slices and the effect was blocked by ICS 205-930. 5-HT and 2-methyl-5-HT appear to inhibit K^+-evoked release of acetylcholine in rat entorhinal cortex by a 5-HT_3-mediated mechanism only in the presence of ketanserin, a 5-HT_2 receptor antagonist (Barnes *et al.*, 1989a,b). Preliminary findings suggest that activation of 5-HT_3 receptors inhibits the release of noradrenaline in rat hypothalamus slices (Blandina *et al.*, 1990) and facilitates the electrically-evoked release of [^{3}H]-5-HT in guinea-pig frontal cortex (Galzin *et al.*, 1990).

e. *Behavioural effects*

One well-documented effect of 5-HT_3 receptor antagonists is their ability to suppress cytotoxic-induced vomiting in the ferret and dog (Costall *et al.*, 1986; Fozard, 1987). The exact site and mechanism of this action is not known, but these drugs might block the 5-HT_3 receptor-mediated excitatory effects of 5-HT on vagal afferent terminals in the nucleus tractus solitarius and area postrema.

Great interest was aroused by the finding that GR-38032F, a potent 5-HT_3 receptor antagonist, inhibited hyperlocomotion caused by drug-induced activation of the mesolimbic dopaminergic system in the rat and marmoset, as hyperactivity of this system has long been considered to be involved in psychosis (Costall *et al.*, 1987). An apparent indirect confirmation was provided by the finding that ICS 205-930, another potent 5-HT_3 receptor antagonist, blocked the place preference induced by morphine, an effect in which the mosolimbic dopaminergic system has been involved (Carboni *et al.*, 1988). These findings, if confirmed, might suggest that 5-HT_3 receptor antagonists may be of some help in the treatment of narcotic abuse (Tricklebank, 1989).

Anxiolytic-like effects of 5-HT_3 receptor antagonists have been described using animal models (Jones *et al.*, 1988), and Barnes *et al.* (1990) recently reported that ondansetron improved basal performance and scopolamine-induced deficit in some rodent and primate tests of cognition.

20.3. *Conclusions*

This review was written in mid 1990 to provide a brief outline of the functional effects of stimulating 5-HT receptors in the mammalian CNS. Progress in this area has been spectacular in the last 10 years, but we need more selective agonists and antagonists at the various 5-HT receptors to clarify the functional role of each receptor type and subtype. 5-HT in the CNS is involved in many physiological, and probably pathological, processes. Drugs acting on specific 5-HT receptors, therefore, will certainly find an important place in the treatment of CNS disorders. Changes induced by 5-HT_{1A} receptor agonists on the cardiovascular system, feeding and affective behaviour or favourable effects of 5-HT_3 receptor antagonists on drug-induced emesis, anxiety and cognitive disturbances, are a few suggested uses of 5-HT receptor agonists and antagonists.

References

Aghajanian, G.K. and Haigler, H.J. (1975). Hallucinogenic indoleamines: preferential action upon presynaptic serotonin receptors. *Psychopharmacology Communications*, **1**, 619–629.

Backus L.I., Sharp, T. and Grahame-Smith, D.G. (1990). Behavioural evidence for a functional interaction between central 5-HT_2 and 5-HT_{1A} receptors. *British Journal of Pharmacology*, **100**, 793–799.

Barnes, J.M., Barnes, N.M., Costall, B. and Naylor, R.J. (1989a). 5-Carboxamidotryptamine modulation of potassium-stimulated [^{3}H]-dopamine release in the rat nucleus accumbens. *British Journal of Pharmacology*, **97**, 378P.

Barnes, J.M., Barnes, N.M., Costall, B., Naylor, R.J. and Tyers, M.B. (1989b). 5-HT_3 receptors mediated inhibition of acetylcholine release in cortical tissue. *Nature*, **338**, 762–763.

Barnes, J.M., Costall, B., Coughlan, J., Domeney, A.M., Gerrard, P.A., Kelly, M.E., Naylor, R.J., Onaivi, E.S., Tomkins, D.M. and Tyers, M.B. (1990). The effects of ondansetron, a 5-HT_3 receptor antagonist, on cognition in rodents and primates. *Pharmacology, Biochemistry and Behaviour*, **35**, 955–962.

Bendotti, C. and Samanin, R. (1986). 8-Hydroxy-2-(di-*n*-propylamino)tetralin (8-OH-DPAT) elicits eating in free-feeding rats by acting on central serotonin neurons. *European Journal of Pharmacology*, **121**, 147–150.

Bendotti, C. and Samanin, R. (1987). The role of putative 5-HT_{1A} and 5-HT_{1B} receptors in the control of feeding in rats. *Life Sciences*, **41**, 635–642.

Bevan, P. (1989). 5-HT and sexual behaviour. In: *Behavioural Pharmacology of 5-HT*, edited by P. Bevan, A.R. Cools and T. Archer. Hillsdale, NJ: Lawrence Erlbaum, pp. 33–34.

Blandina, P., Goldfarb, J., Walcott, J. and Green, J.P. (1990). 5-HT_3 receptors inhibit release of endogenous noradrenaline from hypothalamus. In: *The Second IUPHAR Satellite Meeting on Serotonin*, Basel, Switzerland, 11–13 July. Final Programme and Abstracts. Abstr. no. 73, 71.

Blier, P. and de Montigny, C. (1987). Modification of 5-HT neuron properties by sustained administration of the 5-HT_{1A} agonist gepirone: electrophysiological studies in the rat brain. *Synapse*, **1**, 470–480.

Bobker, D.H. and Williams, J.T. (1989). Serotonin agonists inhibit synaptic potentials in the rat locus coeruleus *in vitro* via 5-$hydroxytryptamine_{1A}$ and 5-$hydroxytryptamine_{1B}$ receptors. *Journal of Pharmacology and Experimental Therapy*, **250**, 37–43.

Bobker, D.H. and Williams, J.T. (1990). Ion conductances affected by 5-HT receptor subtypes in mammalian neurons. *Trends in Neuroscience*, **13**, 169–173.

Bockaert, J., Sebben, M. and Dumuis, A. (1990). Pharmacological characterization of 5-$hydroxytryptamine_4$ (5-HT_4) receptors positively coupled to adenylate cyclase in adult guinea pig hippocampal membranes: effect of substituted benzamide derivatives. *Molecular Pharmacology*, **37**, 408–411.

Carboni, E., Acquas, E., Leone, P., Perezzani, L. and Di Chiara, G. (1988). 5-HT_3 receptor antagonists block morphine- and nicotine-induced place-preference conditioning. *European Journal of Pharmacology*, **151**, 159–160.

Carli, M. and Samanin, R. (1988). Potential anxiolytic properties of 8-hydroxy-2-(di-*N*-propylamino) tetralin, a selective $serotonin_{1A}$ receptor agonist. *Psychopharmacology*, **94**, 84–91.

Carli, M., Prontera, C. and Samanin, R. (1989). Evidence that central 5-hydroxytryptaminergic neurones are involved in the anxiolytic activity of buspirone. *British Journal of Pharmacology*, **96**, 829–836.

Carli, M., Invernizzi, R., Cervo, L. and Samanin, R. (1988). Neurochemical and behavioural studies with RU-24969 in the rat. *Psychopharmacology*, **945**, 359–364.

Cervo, L. and Samanin, R. (1987). Potential antidepressant properties of 8-hydroxy-2-(di-*n*-propylamino)tetralin, a selective $serotonin_{1A}$ receptor agonist. *European Journal of Pharmacology*, **144**, 223–229.

Cervo, L. and Samanin, R. (1991). The effect of chronic treatment with 8-OH-DPAT in the forced swimming test requires the integrity of presynaptic serotonergic mechanisms. *Psychopharmacology*, **103**, 524–528.

Cervo, L., Grignaschi, G. and Samanin, R. (1988a). 8-Hydroxy-2-(di-*n*-propylamino)tetralin, a selective serotonin$_{1A}$ receptor agonist, reduces the immobility of rats in the forced swimming test by acting on the nucleus raphe dorsalis. *European Journal of Pharmacology*, **158**, 53–59.

Cervo, L., Grignaschi, G. and Samanin, R. (1988b). Different effects of intracerebral and systemic administration of buspirone in the forced swimming test: involvement of a metabolite. *Life Sciences*, **43**, 2095–2102.

Cervo, L., Grignaschi, G., Nowakowska, E. and Samanin, R. (1989). 1-(3-Trifluoromethylphenyl)piperazine (TFMPP) in the ventral tegmental area reduces the effect of desipramine in the forced swimming test in rats: possible role of serotonin receptors. *European Journal of Pharmacology*, **171**, 119–125.

Conn, P. and Sanders-Bush, E. (1984). Selective 5-HT-2 antagonists inhibit serotonin stimulated phosphatidylinositol metabolism in cerebral cortex. *Neuropharmacology*, **8**, 993–994.

Conn, P.J. and Sanders-Bush, E. (1987). Relative efficacies of piperazines at the phosphoinositide hydrolysis-linked serotonergic (5-HT-2 and 5-HT-1c) receptors. *Journal of Pharmacology and Experimental Therapy*, **242**, 552–557.

Connor, H.E. and Higgins, G.A. (1990). Cardiovascular effects of 5-HT$_{1A}$ receptor agonists injected into the dorsal raphe nucleus of conscious rats. *European Journal of Pharmacology*, **182**, 63–72.

Costall, B., Domeney, A.M., Naylor, R.J. and Tattersall, F.D. (1986). 5-Hydroxytryptamine M-receptor antagonism to prevent cisplatin-induced emesis. *Neuropharmacology*, **25**, 959–961.

Costall, B., Domeney, A.M., Naylor, R.J. and Tyers, M.B. (1987). Effects of the 5-HT$_3$ receptor antagonist, GR38032F, on raised dopaminergic activity in the mesolimbic system of the rat and marmoset brain. *British Journal of Pharmacology*, **92**, 881–894.

Dahlström, A. and Fuxe, K. (1965). Evidence for the existence of monoamine-containing neurons in the central nervous system. I. Demonstration of monoamines in the cell bodies of brain stem neurons. *Acta Physiologica Scandinavica*, Suppl. 232, 1–55.

DeNoble, V.J. Schrack, L.M., Reigel, A.L. and Strek, K.F. (1990). Serotonin antagonists improve performance in two models of a delayed match to sample task in squirrel monkeys. *Psychopharmacology*, **101** (Suppl.), S14.

Dourish, C.T., Hutson, P.H. and Curzon, G. (1985). Low doses of the putative serotonin agonist 8-hydroxy-2-(di-*n*-propylamino)tetraline (8-OH-DPAT) elicit feeding in the rat. *Psychopharmacology*, **86**, 197–203.

Dourish, C.T., Clark, M.L. and Iversen, S.D. (1988). 8-OH-DPAT elicits feeding and not chewing: evidence from liquid diet studies and a diet choice test. *Psychopharmacology*, **95**, 185–188.

Dourish, C.T., Clark, M.L., Fletcher, A. and Iversen, S.D. (1989). Evidence that blockade of postsynaptic 5-HT$_1$ receptors elicits feeding in satiated rats. *Psychopharmacology*, **97**, 54–58.

Dourish, C.T., Hutson, P.H., Kennett, G.A. and Curzon, G. (1986). 8-OH-DPAT-induced hyperphagia: its neural basis and possible therapeutic relevance. *Appetite*, **7** (Suppl.), 127–140.

Felder, C.C., Kenterman, R.Y., Ma, A.L. and Axelrod, J. (1990). Serotonin stimulates phospholipase A2 and the release of arachidonic acid in hippocampal neurons by a type 2 serotonin receptor that is independent of inositolphospholipid hydrolysis. *Proceedings of the National Academy of Sciences USA*, **87**, 2187–2191.

Fozard, J.R. (1984). MDL 72222: a potent and highly selective antagonist at neuronal 5-hydroxytryptamine receptors. *Naunyn-Schmiedebergs' Archives of Pharmacology*, **326**, 36–44.

Fozard, J.R. (1987). 5-HT_3 receptors and cytotoxic drug-induced vomiting. *Trends in Pharmacological Sciences*, **8**, 44–45.

Frazer, A., Maayani, S. and Wolfe, B.B. (1990). Subtypes of receptor for serotonin. *Annual Review of Pharmacology and Toxicology*, **30**, 307–348.

Galzin, A.M., Poncet, V. and Langer, S.Z. (1990). Facilitation by 5-HT_3 receptor agonists of the electrically-evoked release of [^{3}H]-5-HT in guinea pig frontal cortex slices. In: *The Second IUPHAR Satellite Meeting on Serotonin*, Basel, Switzerland, 11–13 July. Final Programme and Abstracts. Abstr. no. 134, 103.

Garattini, S. and Samanin, R. (1978) Drugs affecting serotonin: a survey. In: *Serotonin in Health and Disease, Vol. 2: Physiological Action*, edited by W.B. Essman. New York: Spectrum, pp. 247–293.

Giral, P., Martin, P., Soubri, P. and Simon, P. (1988). Reversal of helpless behavior in rats by putative 5-HT_{1A} agonists. *Biological Psychiatry*, **23**, 237–242.

Glennon, R.A. (1990). Serotonin receptors: clinical implications. *Neuroscience and Biobehavioural Review*, **14**, 35–47.

Glennon, R.A., Titeler, M. and Young, R. (1986). Structure–activity relationships and mechanism of action of hallucinogenic agents based on drug discrimination and radioligand binding studies. *Psychopharmacology Bulletin*, **22**, 953–958.

Glennon, R.A., Peroutka, S.J. and Dukat, M. (1990). Binding characteristics of a quaternary salt of serotonin: 5-HTQ. In: *The Second IUPHAR Satellite Meeting on Serotonin*, Basel, Switzerland, 11–13 July. Final Programme and Abstracts. Abstr. no. 16, 42.

Hamon, M., Collin, E., Chantrel, D., Daval, G., Verge, D., Bourgoin S. and Cesselin, F. (1990). Serotonin receptors and the modulation of pain. In: *Serotonin and Pain*, edited by J.-M. Besson. Amsterdam: Elsevier, pp. 53–65.

Hartig, P.R. (1989). Molecular biology of 5-HT receptors. *Trends in Pharmacological Sciences*, **10**, 64–69.

Heuring, R.E. and Peroutka, S.J. (1987). Characterization of a novel ^{3}H-5-hydroxytryptamine binding site subtype in bovine brain membrane. *Journal of Neuroscience*, **7**, 894–903.

Hewson, G., Leighton, G.E., Hill, R.G. and Hughes, J. (1988). Quipazine reduces food intake in the rat by activation of 5-HT_2-receptors. *British Journal of Pharmacology*, **95**, 598–604.

Hjorth, S. and Magnusson, T. (1988). The 5-HT_{1A} receptor agonist, 8-OH-DPAT, preferentially activates cell body 5-HT autoreceptors in rat brain *in vivo*. *Naunyn-Schmiedeberg's Archives of Pharmacology*, **338**, 463–471.

Hoyer, D. (1988) Functional correlates of serotonin 5-HT_1 recognition sites. *Journal of Receptor Research*, **8**, 58–81.

Hoyer, D. and Middlemiss, D.N. (1989). Species differences in the pharmacology of terminal 5-HT autoreceptors in mammalian brain. *Trends in Pharmacological Sciences*, **10**, 130–132.

Idzikowski, C., Mills, F.J. and Glennard, R. (1986). 5-Hydroxytryptamine-2 antagonist increases human slow wave. *Brain Research*, **378**, 164–168.

Innis, R.B., Nestler, E.J. and Aghajanian, G.K. (1988). Evidence for G protein mediation of serotonin- and $GABA_B$-induced hyperpolarization of rat dorsal raphe neurones. *Brain Research*, **459**, 27–36.

Invernizzi, R., Cervo, L. and Samanin, R. (1988). 8-Hydroxy-2-(di-*n*-propylamino)-tetralin, a selective serotonin$_{1A}$ receptor agonist, blocks haloperidol-induced catalepsy by an action on raphe nuclei medianus and dorsalis. *Neuropharmacology*, **27**, 515–518.

Invernizzi, R., Carli, M., Di Clemente, A. and Samanin, R. (1990). Administration of 8-hydroxy-2-(di-*n*-propylamino)tetralin in raphe nuclei dorsalis and medianus reduces serotonin synthesis in the rat brain: differences in potency and regional sensitivity. *Journal of Neurochemistry*, **36**, 243–247.

Jones, B.J., Costall, B., Domeney, A.M., Kelly, M.E., Naylor, R., Oakley, N.R. and Tyers, M.B. (1988). The potential anxiolytic activity of GR38032F, a 5-HT_3-receptor antagonist. *British Journal of Pharmacology*, **93**, 985–993.

Julius, D., MacDermott, A.B., Axel, R. and Jessell, T.M. (1988). Molecular characterization of a functional cDNA encoding the $serotonin_{1C}$ receptor. *Science*, **241**, 558–564.

Julius, D., Huang, K.N., Livelli, T.J., Axel, R. and Jessell, T.M. (1990). The 5-HT_2 receptor defines a family of structurally distinct but functionally conserved serotonin receptors. *Proceedings of the National Academy of Sciences USA*, **87**, 928–932.

Kendall, D.A. and Nahorski, S.R. (1985). 5-Hydroxytryptamine-stimulated inositol phospholipid hydrolysis in rat cerebral cortex slices: pharmacological characterization and effects of antidepressants. *Journal of Pharmacology and Experimental Therapy*, **233**, 473–479.

Kennett, G.A. and Curzon, G. (1988). Evidence that hypophagia induced by mCPP and TFMPP requires 5-HT_{1C} and 5-HT_{1B} receptors; hypophagia induced by RU 24969 only requires 5-HT_{1B} receptors. *Psychopharmacology*, **96**, 93–100.

Kennett, G.A., Dourish, C.T. and Curzon, G. (1987a). Antidepressant-like action of 5-HT_{1A} agonists and conventional antidepressants in an animal model of depression. *European Journal of Pharmacology*, **134**, 265–274.

Kennett, G.A., Marcou, M., Dourish, C.T. and Curzon, G. (1987b). Single administration of 5-HT_{1A} agonists decreases 5-HT_{1A} presynaptic, but not postsynaptic, receptor-mediated responses: relations to antidepressant-like action. *European Journal of Pharmacology*, **138**, 53–60.

Kilpatrick, G.J., Jones, B.J. and Tyers, M.B. (1987). Identification and distribution of 5-HT_3 receptors in rat brain using radioligand binding. *Nature*, **330**, 746–748.

Kilpatrick, G.J., Butler, A., Burridge, J. and Oxford, A.W. (1990). 1-(*m*-Chlorophenyl)-biguanide, a potent high affinity 5-HT_3 receptor agonist. *European Journal of Pharmacology*, **182**, 193–197.

Lakoski, J.M. and Aghajanian, G.K. (1985). Effects of ketanserin on neuronal responses to serotonin in the prefrontal cortex, lateral geniculate and dorsal raphe nucleus. *Neuropharmacology*, **24**, 265–273.

Larsson, L.-G., Renyi, L., Ross, S.B., Svensson, B. and Ängeby-Möller, K. (1990). Different effects on the responses of functional pre- and postsynaptic 5-HT_{1A} receptors by repeated treatment of rats with the 5-HT_{1A} receptor agonist 8-OH-DPAT. *Neuropharmacology*, **29**, 85–91.

Lyon, R.A., Davis, K.H. and Titeler, M. (1987). ^{3}H-DOB (4-Bromo-2,5- dimethoxyphenylisopropylamine) labels a guanyl nucleotide-sensitive state of cortical 5-HT_2 receptors. *Molecular Pharmacology*, **31**, 194–199.

Marek, G.J., Li, A.A. and Seiden, L.S. (1989). Selective $5\text{-hydroxytryptamine}_2$ antagonists have antidepressant-like effects on differential-reinforcement-of-low-rate 72-second schedule. *Journal of Pharmacology and Experimental Therapy*, **250**, 52–59.

Mengod, G., Nguyen, H., Waeber, C., Lbbert, H. and Palacios, J.M. (1990). The distribution and cellular localization of the $serotonin_{1C}$ receptor mRNA in the rodent brain examined by *in situ* hybridization histochemistry. Comparison with receptor binding distribution. *Neuroscience*, **35**, 577–591.

Merlo Pich, E. and Samanin, R. (1986). Disinhibitory effects of buspirone and low doses of sulpiride and haloperidol in two experimental anxiety models in rats: possible role of dopamine. *Psychopharmacology*, **89**, 125–130.

Molineaux, S.M., Jessell, T.M., Axel, R. and Julius, D. (1989). 5-HT_{1C} receptor is a prominent serotonin receptor subtype in the central nervous system. *Proceedings of the National Academy of Sciences USA*, **86**, 6793–6797.

Osborne, N.N. and Hamon, M. (Eds) (1988). *Neuronal Serotonin*. Chichester: Wiley.

Paoletti, R., Vanhoutte, P.M., Brunello, N. and Maggi, F.M. (Eds) (1990). *Serotonin. From Cell Biology to Pharmacology and Therapeutics*. Dordrecht: Kluwer.

Pastel, R.H. (1988). Effects of DOI, a selective serotonin-2 agonist, on sleep in the rat. Presented at *9th European Congress of Sleep Research*, September, Jerusalem, Israel.

Pazos, A., Cortes, R. and Palacios, M. (1985). Quantitative autoradiographgic mapping of serotonin receptors in the rat brain. II. Serotonin-2 receptors. *Brain Research*, **346**, 231–249.

Pazos, A., Hoyer, D. and Palacios, J.M. (1984). The binding of serotonergic ligands to the porcine choroid plexus: characterization of a new type of serotonin recognition site. *European Journal of Pharmacology*, **106**, 539–546.

Pazos, A., Probst, A. and Palacios, J.M. (1987). Serotonin receptors in the human brain. III. Autoradiographic mapping of serotonin-1 receptors. *Neuroscience*, **21**, 97–102.

Pazos, A., Hoyer, D., Dietl, M.M. and Palacios, J.M. (1988). Autoradiography of serotonin receptors. In: *Neuronal Serotonin*, edited by N.N. Osborne and M. Hamon. Chichester: Wiley, pp. 507–543.

Pedigo, N.W., Yamamura, H.I. and Nelson, D.L. (1981). Discrimination of multiple [^{3}H]5-hydroxytryptamine binding sites by the neuroleptic spiperone in rat brain. *Journal of Neurochemistry*, **36**, 220–226.

Peroutka, S.J. (1988). 5-Hydroxytryptamine receptor subtypes. *Annual Review of Neuroscience*, **11**, 45–60.

Peroutka, S.J. and Snyder, S.H. (1979). Multiple serotonin receptors: differential binding of [^{3}H]5-hydroxytryptamine, [^{3}H]-lysergic acid diethylamide and [^{3}H]-spiroperidol. *Molecular Pharmacology*, **16**, 687–699.

Peroutka, S.J. and Snyder, S.H. (1980). Long-term antidepressant treatment decreases spiroperidol-labelled serotonin receptor binding. *Science*, **210**, 88–90.

Pratt, G.D., Bowery, N.G., Kilpatrick, G.J., Leslie, R.A., Barnes, N.M., Naylor, R.J., Jones, B.J., Nelson, D.R., Palacios, J.M., Slater, P. and Reynolds, J.M. (1990). Consensus meeting agrees distribution of 5-HT$_3$ receptors in mammalian hindbrain. *Trends in Pharmacological Sciences*, **11**, 135–136.

Pritchett, D.R., Bach, A.W., Wozny, M., Taleb, O., Dal Toso, R., Shih, J.C. and Seeburg, P.H. (1988). Structure and functional expression of cloned rat serotonin 5HT$_2$ receptor. *EMBO Journal*, **7**, 4135–4140.

Raiteri, M., Maura, G., Bonanno, G. and Pittaluga, A. (1986). Differential pharmacology and function of two 5-HT$_1$ receptors modulating transmitter release in rat cerebellum. *Journal of Pharmacology and Experimental Therapy*, **237**, 644–648.

Samanin, R. and Garattini, S. (1990). The pharmacology of serotonergic drugs affecting appetite. In: *Nutrition and the Brain*, Vol. 8, edited by R.J. Wurtman and J.J. Wurtman. New York: Raven Press, pp. 163–192.

Samanin, R., Mennini, T., Ferraris, A., Bendotti, C., Brosini, F. and Garattini, S. (1979). *m*-Chlorophenylpiperazine: a central serotonin agonist causing powerful anorexia in rats. *Naunyn-Schmiedeberg's Archives of Pharmacology*, **308**, 159–163.

Samanin, R., Mennini, T., Bendotti, C. Barone, D., Caccia, S. and Garattini, S. (1989). Evidence that central 5-HT$_2$ receptors do not play an important role in the anorectic activity of *d*-fenfluramine in the rat. *Neuropharmacology*, **28**, 465–569.

Scatton, B., Blier, P. and Serrano, A. (1989). Differential functional properties of dorsal and median raphe serotonin systems in the rat. In: *International Symposium on Serotonin from Cell Biology to Pharmacology and Therapeutics*, Florence, 29 March–1 April. Abstract book, p. 84.

Schechter, L.E. and Simansky, K.J. (1988). 1-(2,5-Dimethoxy-4-iodophenyl)-2-aminopropane (DOI) exerts an anorectic action that is blocked by 5-HT_2 antagonists in rats. *Psychopharmacology*, **94**, 342–346.

Schmidt, A.W. and Peroutka, S.J. (1989). 5-Hydroxytryptamine receptor 'families'. *FASEB Journal*, **3**, 2242–2249.

Schoeffter, P. and Hoyer, D. (1989). 5-Hydroxytryptamine 5-HT_{1B} and 5-HT_{1D} receptors mediating inhibition of adenylate cyclase activity. Pharmacological comparison with special reference to the effects of yohimbine, rauwolscine and some β-adrenoceptor antagonists. *Naunyn-Schmiedeberg's Archives of Pharmacology*, **340**, 285–292.

Shenker, A., Maayani, S., Weinstein, H. and Green, J.P. (1987). Pharmacological characterization of two 5-hydroxytryptamine receptors coupled to adenylcyclase in guinea pig hippocampal membranes. *Molecular Pharmacology*, **31**, 357–367.

Sinton, C.M. and Fallon, S.L. (1988). Electrophysiological evidence for a functional differentiation between subtypes of the 5-HT_1 receptor. *European Journal of Pharmacology*, **157**, 173–181.

Sprouse, J.S. and Aghajanian, G.K. (1986). (−)-Propranolol blocks the inhibition of serotonergic dorsal raphe cell firing by 5-HT_{1A} selective agonists. *European Journal Pharmacology*, **128**, 295–298.

Sprouse, J.S. and Aghajanian, G.K. (1988). Responses of hippocampal pyramidal cells to putative serotonin 5-HT_{1A} and 5-HT_{1B} agonists: a comparative study with dorsal raphe neurons. *Neuropharmacology*, **27**, 707–715.

Tricklebank, M.D. (1989). Interactions between dopamine and 5-HT_3 receptors suggest new treatments for psychosis and drug addiction. *Trends in Pharmacological Science*, **10**, 127–129.

Twarog, B.M. and Page, I.H. (1953). Serotonin content of some mammalian tissues and urine and a method for its determination. *American Journal of Physiology*, **175**, 157–161.

Van Wijngaarden, I., Tulp, M.Th.M. and Soudijn, W. (1990). The concept of selectivity in 5-HT receptor research. *European Journal of Pharmacology*, **188**, 301–312.

Waeber, C., Hoyer, D. and Palacios, J.M. (1989a). 5-$Hydroxytryptamine_3$ receptors in the human brain: autoradiographic visualization using [^{3}H]ICS 205–930. *Neuroscience*, **31**, 393–400.

Waeber, C., Dietl, M.M., Hoyer, D. and Palacios, J.M. (1989b). 5-HT_1 receptors in the vertebrate brain. Regional distribution examined by autoradiography. *Naunyn-Schmiedebergs Archives of Pharmacology*, **340**, 486–494.

Wang, R.Y., Ashby, C.R., Jr. and Edwards, E. (1990). 5-HT_3-like receptors in the rat brain. In: *The Second IUPHAR Satellite Meeting on Serotonin*, Basel, Switzerland, 11–13 July. Final Programme and Abstracts. Abstr. no. 15, 41.

Wong, D.T. and Reid, L.R. (1987). Fenfluramine antagonizes the stimulation of food intake by the putative 5-$hydroxytryptamine_{1A}$ agonist, isapirone, in non-fasted rats. *Journal of Pharmaceutical Pharmacology*, **39**, 570–571.

Current research

Post-tetanic potentiation in autonomic nerves

The post-tetanic potentiation in vascular sympathetic nerve has many features in common with the post-tetanic potentiation in somatomotor and central neurones (1, 2). Both are prejunctional, calcium-dependent processes with a similar time course. However, they differ in frequency requirements, reflecting the difference in average discharge frequency between the systems.

Potentiation may be an important mechanism that can be utilized by the autonomic nervous system to further accentuate the effector responses at increasing discharge rates. An increased firing rate will enhance the effector response not only by temporal summation at the level of the effector, but also by increasing transmitter output per impulse. (Nina Sjoblom-Widfeldt, Department of Physiology, University of Goteborg, Gothenburg, Sweden).

(1) Rosenthal, J. (1969). *Journal of Physiology*, **203**, 121–133.
(2) Sjoblom-Widfeldt, N. (1990). *Acta Physiologica Scandinavica*, **138** (Suppl. 587), 1–52.

The Effects of (−)-Vesamicol on the Mobilization of Acetylcholine for Release from Rat Motor Nerve Terminals

(−)-Vesamicol blocks acetylcholine transport into synaptic vesicles (1). It produces rundown in endplate current (EPC) amplitudes in high frequency (50 Hz for 1 s) trains (2). (+)-Tubocurarine, by action on putative presynaptic nicotinic receptors, also produces EPC rundown (3).

We have compared the effects of (−)-vesamicol on train rundown with those of (+)-vesamicol and (+)-tubocurarine. (+)-Vesamicol has no effect on EPC rundown, showing that train rundown, and inhibition of vesicular filling, have the same stereoselectivity. The maximal rundown produced by (−)-vesamicol is less than that produced by (+)-tubocurarine, indicating separate sites of action. The effects of (−)-vesamicol and (+)-tubocurarine on train rundown are non-additive, suggesting that (+)-vesamicol acts at a site downstream from prejunctional nicotinic receptors. (−)-Vesamicol may produce rundown by inhibition of vesicular filling, or by action on an as yet undetermined site unrelated to vesicle filling. (C. Prior, T. Searl, K. Pemberton, W.C. Bowman and I.G. Marshall, Department of Physiology and Pharmacology, University of Strathclyde, Glasgow).

(1) Marshall, I.G. and Parsons, S.M. (1987). *Trends in Neurosciences*,
(2) Prior, C., Searl, T. & Marshall, I.G. (1989). *British Journal of Pharmacology*, **98**, 826P.
(3) Gibb, A.J. and Marshall, I.G. (1984). *Journal of Physiology*, **351**, 275–297.

Differing role for neuropeptide Y in sympathetic vasomotor activity in large and small arteries

Recent studies have supported the involvement of non-adrenergic chemical transmitters in sympathetic vascular control. One of these likely transmitters, neuropeptide Y (NPY), is present together with noradrenaline (NA) in certain perivascular nerves. Reported actions of NPY include vasoconstriction unrelated to α-adrenoceptor stimulation (1), inhibition of NA release via a prejunctional action (2), and enhancement of NA-induced vasoconstriction via a postjunctional action (2). In general, *in vitro* studies indicate that with a decrease in arterial diameter the ability of NPY *per se* to cause a vasoconstriction increases, while the ability to potentiate NA-induced contraction decreases (3, 4). The implication is that NPY has a differing role in sympathetic vasomotor activity in large and small arteries. (Mary P. Owen, Department of Pharmacology and Toxicology, Philadelphia College of Pharmacy and Science, USA)

(1) Lundberg, J.M. and Tatemoto, K. (1982). *Acta Physiologica Scandinavica*, **116**, 393–402.
(2) Lundberg, J.M., Pernow, J., Dahlof, C. and Tatemoto, K. (1985). *Acta Physiologica Scandinavica*, **123**, 511–513.
(3) Owen, M.P. and Taphorn, M.C. (1988). *Proceedings of the 2nd International Symposium on Resistance Arteries*, edited by W. Halpern *et al.* New York: Perinatology Press, pp. 74–79.
(4) Owen, M.P. and Taphorn, M.C. (1990). *Federation Proceedings*, **49**, A334.

Airway endocrine cells

The epithelium of the lower respiratory tract contains numerous cells with the properties of peptide hormone producing endocrine cells. In small bronchi and in the lungs they are arranged in clusters, so-called neuroepithelial bodies (NEBs). The NEBs are known to contain serotonin in some species and also regulatory peptides such as gastrin releasing peptide, leu-enkephalin, calcitonin and calcitonin gene-related peptide (1, 2, 3). In addition, the NEBs were recently found to store immunoreactive helodermin and pituitary adenylate cyclase activating peptide, both of which are newly identified vasoactive intestinal-like peptides (unpublished). In the endocrine cells serotonin seems to coexist with a variety of peptides such as calcitonin gene-related peptide (3), gastrin releasing peptide (4), somatostatin (4) and calcitonin.

The functional role of the NEBs is poorly understood. They have been shown to respond to hypoxia with reduced serotonin content and ultrastructural signs of exocytosis, suggesting their involvement in the adjustment to variations in the oxygen supply. The rich occurrence of such cells in the airways during the neonatal period and in connection with respiratory disorders (5) may also speak in favour of such a role. (Anders Lus, Rolf Uddman and Frank Sundler, Departments of Medical Cell Research and Otolaryngology, Malmo General Hospital, University of Lund, Sweden).

(1) Lauweryns, J.M., Cokelaere, M. and Theunynck, P. (1972). *Z. Zellforsch*, **135**, 569–592.
(2) Gosney, J.R. and Sissons, M.C.J. (1985). *Thorax*, **40**, 194–198.
(3) Keith, I.M. and Ekman, R. (1988) *Regulatory Peptides*, **22**, 315–325.
(4) Dayer, A.M., DeMey, J. and Will, S.A. (1985). *Cell and Tissue Research*, **239**, 621–625.
(5) Gosney, J., Heath, D., Smith, P., Harris, P. and Yacoub, M. (1989) *Archives of Pathology and Laboratory Medicine*, **113**, 337–341.

NANC-Innervation of the teleost swimbladder

An important function of the teleost swimbladder is to maintain neutral buoyancy in the water. Previous studies have shown that the swimbladder is innervated by the autonomic nervous system, probably via nerve fibres running in the vagus nerve. The secretion of gas from the gas gland is stimulated by cholinergic nerves and the resorption of gas by adrenergic nerves that increase the resorbing area and reduce the blood flow through the gas gland (1, 2). Later studies (3, 4) have demonstrated by immunohistochemistry that the mucosa of the teleost swimbladder also contains several other putative neurotransmitters, e.g. vasoactive intestinal polypeptide (VIP)-like and substance P (SP)-like immunoreactivity (IR) in nerve fibres. VIP-like IR could also be seen in nerve fibres in the gas gland of the cod and the goldsinny wrasse.

The physiological role of VIP, SP and 5-hydroxytryptamine (5-HT) has been studied *in vitro* using isolated strip preparations from the smooth muscles of the muscularis mucosae of the swimbladder from cod and eel. These were mounted in organ baths, and the different drugs were added. It was found that VIP was relaxatory and the SP and 5-HT were constrictory on the smooth muscles. New results in this field have been obtained by using an X-ray method, where it is possible to measure the area of the swimbladder *in vivo* for calculation of the volume. Drugs were injected through a catheter into a gill artery, and the swimbladder gas removed with syringe through the body wall, thus stimulating the fish to secrete new gas. The rate of secretion is inhibited partly by atropin and completely by vagotomy. The blockade obtained by atropine could be reversed back to control values by injections of VIP or SP, but vagotomized fish could not be induced to secrete gas either with VIP, SP, or with the cholinergic agonist carbachol. (K. Lundin, Comparative Neuroscience Unit, Department of Zoophysiology, University of Goteborg, Gothenburg, Sweden).

(1) Fange, R. (1953). *Acta Physiologica Scandinavica*, **30** (Suppl. 110), 1–133.
(2) Nilsson, S. (1971). *Comp. Gen. Pharmacology*, **3**, 371–375.
(3) Lundin, K. and Homgren, S. (1989). *Journal of Comparative Physiology*, **154B**, 627–623.
(4) Lundin, K. and Homgren, S. (1989). *Cell and Tissue Research*, **257**, 641–647.

Pharmacological modulation of non-cholinergic neurotransmission in guinea-pig bronchi

The guinea-pig bronchial smooth muscles are innervated by two types of excitatory nerves, cholinergic and non-cholinergic nerves, in contrast to the trachea where excitatory cholinergic and inhibitory non-adrenergic nerves were predominant. We have investigated the modulating effects of various drugs on electrically-induced neurogenic responses of the guinea-pig airways. Adenosine, ATP, dopamine, morphine dynorphin and β-endorphin selectively inhibited non-cholinergically mediated contraction of the guinea-pig isolated bronchi, while noradrenaline, adrenaline and prostaglandin E_2 inhibited both cholinergically and non-cholinergically mediated contractions. Since submaximal contractions of bronchial muscle evoked by exogenous acetylcholine or substance P were poorly inhibited by these drugs, the inhibitory actions on neurogenic contractions seem to be preferentially mediated by a prejunctional reduction of the transmitter release and partly by a post-junctional depression of the response.

These findings indicate that neuromodulating effects of the transmitter substances or auacoids are different between proximal and peripheral airways, or between cholinergic and non-cholinergic nerves. (Yuichiro Kamikawa and Yasuo Shimo, Department of Pharmacology, Dokkyo University School of Medicine, Mibu, Tochigi, Japan).

Influence of calcium antagonists on hippocampal LTP

A transient increase (10 min) in extracellular calcium concentrations (4 mM) causes a long-lasting enhancement of population spike responses evoked by radiatum fibres to CA1 pyramidal neurones in rat hippocampal slices (1). This phenomenon is similar to tetanic long-term potenitation (LTP). The influence of various drugs has been investigated on calcium-induced LTP. The *N*-methyl-D-aspartate (NMDA) antagonist, 2-amino-5-phosphonopentanoic acid (AP5, 100 μM), cadmium ions and aminoglycoside antibiotics neomycin and streptomycin, were able to prevent the calcium-induced LTP, while atropine sulphate (10 μM), propranolol hydrochloride (10 μM) and verapamil hydrochloride (100 μM) were ineffective. These results suggest an involvement of the NMDA receptor, and of N-type calcium channel in the development of calcium-induced LTP. (C. Frank, S. Sagratella and A. Scotti de Carolis, Dipartimento di Medicina Sperimetale Universita Tor Vergata, Roma et Laboratorio di Farmacolgia Instituto Superiore di Sanita, Roma).

(1) Turner, R.W. *et al.* (1982). *Neuroscience*, **7**, 1411–1416.

Adenosine and ATP

Both adenosine and ATP have been recognized as modulators of synaptic transmission for many years, but recent work has shown a selective ability of adenosine to inhibit postjunctional muscarinic sensitivity in hippocampal neurones while amino acid responses are unchanged (1). The inhibitory effects of adenosine on presynaptic terminals is dependent on magnesium ions however (2), and work in progress indicates that this can lead to interactions with other magnesium-sensitive receptors. These effects may be related to our observations that some dihydropyridine calcium antagonists can modify adenosine responses in the hippocampus (3). In neocortex, chronic treatment with methylxanthines has been found to reduce sensitivity to adenosine, even though binding studies have reported an increase of receptor density. The generality of this finding is under investigation. (J.T. Bartrup and T.W. Stone, Department of Pharmacology, University of Glasgow).

(1) Brookes, P.A. and Stone, T.W. (1988). *Brain Research*, **458**, 106–114.
(2) Bartrup, J.T. and Stone, T.W. (1988). *Brain Research*, **463**, 374–379.
(3) Bartrup, J.T. and Stone, T.W. (1990). *British Journal of Pharmacology*, in press.

5-HT

Our previous studies have shown that serotonergic agents tested (8-OH-DPAT, 5-Me-ODMT, LSD, methysergide and 5-HTP) decrease the spinal monosynaptic reflex and increase the polysynaptic reflex in acutely spinalized rats, and it has been difficult to discuss the functional significance of serotonergic receptors located on the spinal reflex pathway. Our recent study using DOI and ritanserin, a selective agonist and an antagonist to the 5-HT_2 receptor, respectively, showed that 5-HT_2 receptors located on the motoneurone somata or dendrites increased the monsynaptic reflex. Excitability texts suggested that the inhibitory effects of 5-Me-ODMT on the MSR were due to its action on the presynaptic terminals. (Hideki Ono, June Yamazaki and Taku Nagao, Department of Toxicology and Pharmacology, University of Tokyo, Japan).

$GABA_B$ receptors in synaptic plasticity

The function of $GABA_B$ receptors in the central nervous system (CNS) has remained elusive (1). Work in the hippocampus (2,3) and the cerebellum (4) indicates a role in synaptic plasticity. In both areas there are $GABA_B$ receptors on the terminals of inhibitory interneurones and on the postsynaptic cells. The autoreceptors seem to be responsible for shutting off inhibition during repeated stimulation and thus allow induction of plastic changes. The recent development of improved antagonists (5) is likely to assist in greater understanding of $GABA_B$-mediated functions at central synapses. (Andrew Batchelor and John Garthwaite, Department of Physiology, University of Liverpool).

(1) Bowery, N. (1989). *Trends in Pharmacological Science*, **10**, 401–407.
(2) Dutar, P. and Nicoll, R.A. (1988). *Neuron*, **1**, 585–591.
(3) Davies, C.H., Davies, C.N. and Collingridge, G.L. (1990). *Journal of Physiology*, **242**, 513–531.
(4) Batchelor, A.M. and Garthwaite, J., in preparation.
(5) Kerr, D.I.B. *et al.* (1989). *Neuroscience Letters*, **107**, 239–244.

Modulating the excitatory amino acid neurotransmitter changes in ischaemia

Experiments *in vivo* have shown inconsistent protective effects of L-glutamate antagonists against cerebral ischaemia (1, 2), partly due to different experimental paradigms, partly to the complex involvement of amines, free radicals and leukocytes. The development of undesirable side-effects to *N*-methyl-D-aspartate (NMDA) antagonists *in vivo*, e.g. neurodegeneration and behavioural abnormalities (3), mean that safer drugs (EAAs) have to be developed.

An alternative approach might be to enhance the apparent desensitization to EAAs seen with repeated or prolonged application to central nervous system (CNS) structures (4, 5). Such a desensitizing mechanism appears to be complex and may differ between the selective EAA agonists: channel block of the NMDA receptor complex is reduced by glycine whereas the faster desensitization with quisqualate is not (6). It will be interesting to determine whether such a desensitizing mechanism can protect neurones against the endogenous EAAs that are released during ischemia. (Jonas Addae, Faculty of Medical Science, The University of the West Indies, St Augustine, Trinidad and Tobago).

(1) Buchan A. and Pulsinelli, W.A. (1990). *Journal of Neuroscience*, **10**, 311–316.
(2) Jensen, M.L. and Auer, R.N. (1988). *British Journal of Anaesthesia*, **61**, 206–210.
(3) Olney, J.W., Labruyere, J. and Price, M.T. (1989). *Science*, **244**, 1360–1362.
(4) Fagni, L., Baudri, M. and Lynch, G. (1983). *Brain Research*, **261**, 167–171.
(5) Addae, J.I. and Stone, T.W. (1986). *European Journal of Pharmacology*, **121**, 337–343.
(6) Mayer, M.L., Vyklicky, L. and Clements, J. (1989). *Nature*, **338**, 425–427.

Habituation in a crayfish leg reflex

In recent years studies of habituation and other simple forms of learning in molluscs have provided important insights into our understanding of synaptic plasticity (1,2). We are extending the study of the cellular basis of habituation to an arthropod 'simple' nervous system. In decerebrate crayfish, the reflex leg levation that follows stimulation of force-sensitive afferents in the terminal segment of leg habituates with repetition of the stimulus. Neuronal correlates of habituation are being studied in an *in vitro* preparation (3) consisting of the isolated central nervous system and the distal portion of a walking leg. In this preparation, the decline in the number of impulses evoked in the levator nerve with repetition of the stimulus is correlated with excitatory postsynaptic potential amplitude rather than any change in motoneurone resting potential. By recording from interneurones during habituation of the reflex, we are attempting to localize the synapses at which it is taking place. (W.J.P. Barnes and A.R. Marchand, Department of Zoology, University of Glasgow and LNF2-CNRS, Marseille, France).

(1) Farley, J. and Alkon, D.L. (1987). In: *Invertebrate Models: Cell Receptors and Cell Communication*, edited by A.H. Greenberg. Basel and New York: Karger, pp. 220–226.
(2) Hawkins, R.D., Clark, G.A. and Kandel, E.R. (1987). In: *Handbook of Physiology*, edited by V.B. Mountcastle and F. Plum. Bethesda, MD: American Physiological Society, pp. 25–83.
(3) Chrachri, A. and Clarac, F. (1989). *Journal of Neurophysiology*, **62**, 1237–1250.

Galanin

Numerous immunohistochemical studies have revealed a widespread distribution of immunoreactive (ir)-galanin in the central and peripheral nervous systems. There is, however, much less information on the functional significance of these observations. Release of galanin from intrapancreatic nerves may regulate pancreatic hormone secretion; in the hypothalamus, galanin may modulate the release of pituitary hormones. In the spinal cord, ir-galanin release has been detected in the substantia gelatinosa and pia mater, exogenous galanin has biphasic effects on nociceptive flexor reflexes, and axotomy stimulates galanin synthesis. The underlying mechanisms have yet to be elucidated, but it seems likely that this neuropeptide plays some role(s) in sensory processing. (W.D. Hutchison and C.R. Morton, Division of Neurosciences, John Curtin School of Medical Research, Australian National University, Canberra, Australia).

Function of galanin in the regulation of insulin secretion

We have shown that: (1) in the dog, the intrapancreatic nerves and the nerve cell bodies in the coeliac ganlion that are immunoreactive for galanin are also immunoreactive for tyrosine hydroxylase, a marker for adrenergic nerves; (2) pretreatment with galanin antiserum in mice abolishes the swimming stress-induced inhibition of glucose-stimulated insulin secretion; and (3) galanin inhibits insulin secretion from isolated rat islets by increasing the membraneous permeability to potassium ions followed by decreased permeability to calcium ions as studied by efflux of $^{86}Rb^{+}$ and $^{45}Ca^{2+}$. Galanin might be a sympathetic mediator in the pancreas regulating islet hormone secretion. (S. Lindskog, S. Karlsson, B.E. Dunning, F. Sundler and B. Ahrén, Lund University, Lund, Sweden).